Themed Issue in Honor of Carlos Gutiérrez Merino: Forty Years of Research Excellence in the Field of Membrane Proteins and Bioenergetics

Themed Issue in Honor of Carlos Gutiérrez Merino: Forty Years of Research Excellence in the Field of Membrane Proteins and Bioenergetics

Guest Editors

Alejandro Samhan-Arias
Manuel Aureliano
Carmen Lopez-Sanchez

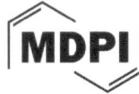

Basel • Beijing • Wuhan • Barcelona • Belgrade • Novi Sad • Cluj • Manchester

Guest Editors

Alejandro Samhan-Arias
Department of Biochemistry
Autonomous University
of Madrid
Madrid
Spain

Manuel Aureliano
Algarve Centre for Marine
Sciences (CCMar)
University of Algarve
Faro
Portugal

Carmen Lopez-Sanchez
Department of Human
Anatomy and Embryology
University of Extremadura
Badajoz
Spain

Editorial Office
MDPI AG
Grosspeteranlage 5
4052 Basel, Switzerland

This is a reprint of the Special Issue, published open access by the journal *Molecules* (ISSN 1420-3049), freely accessible at: www.mdpi.com/journal/molecules/special_issues/14L7T288TM.

For citation purposes, cite each article independently as indicated on the article page online and using the guide below:

Lastname, A.A.; Lastname, B.B. Article Title. *Journal Name* **Year**, *Volume Number*, Page Range.

ISBN 978-3-7258-3958-2 (Hbk)
ISBN 978-3-7258-3957-5 (PDF)
https://doi.org/10.3390/books978-3-7258-3957-5

© 2025 by the authors. Articles in this book are Open Access and distributed under the Creative Commons Attribution (CC BY) license. The book as a whole is distributed by MDPI under the terms and conditions of the Creative Commons Attribution-NonCommercial-NoDerivs (CC BY-NC-ND) license (https://creativecommons.org/licenses/by-nc-nd/4.0/).

Contents

About the Editors vii

Alejandro K. Samhan-Arias, Carmen López-Sánchez and Manuel Aureliano
Editorial on the Themed Issue in Honor of Carlos Gutiérrez Merino: Forty Years of Research Excellence in the Field of Membrane Proteins and Bioenergetics
Reprinted from: *Molecules* 2025, *30*, 1710, https://doi.org/10.3390/molecules30081710 1

Silvia S. Antollini and Francisco J. Barrantes
Carlos Gutiérrez-Merino: Synergy of Theory and Experimentation in Biological Membrane Research
Reprinted from: *Molecules* 2024, *29*, 820, https://doi.org/10.3390/molecules29040820 6

Adrián Povo-Retana, Rodrigo Landauro-Vera, Carlota Alvarez-Lucena, Marta Cascante and Lisardo Boscá
Trabectedin and Lurbinectedin Modulate the Interplay between Cells in the Tumour Microenvironment—Progresses in Their Use in Combined Cancer Therapy
Reprinted from: *Molecules* 2024, *29*, 331, https://doi.org/10.3390/molecules29020331 22

Luisa B. Maia, Biplab K. Maiti, Isabel Moura and José J. G. Moura
Selenium—More than Just a Fortuitous Sulfur Substitute in Redox Biology
Reprinted from: *Molecules* 2024, *29*, 120, https://doi.org/10.3390/molecules29010120 43

Natividad Chaves, Laura Nogales, Ismael Montero-Fernández, José Blanco-Salas and Juan Carlos Alías
Mediterranean Shrub Species as a Source of Biomolecules against Neurodegenerative Diseases
Reprinted from: *Molecules* 2023, *28*, 8133, https://doi.org/10.3390/molecules28248133 80

Alejandro K. Samhan-Arias, Joana Poejo, Dorinda Marques-da-Silva, Oscar H. Martínez-Costa and Carlos Gutierrez-Merino
Are There Lipid Membrane-Domain Subtypes in Neurons with Different Roles in Calcium Signaling?
Reprinted from: *Molecules* 2023, *28*, 7909, https://doi.org/10.3390/molecules28237909 115

Dorinda Marques-da-Silva and Ricardo Lagoa
Rafting on the Evidence for Lipid Raft-like Domains as Hubs Triggering Environmental Toxicants' Cellular Effects
Reprinted from: *Molecules* 2023, *28*, 6598, https://doi.org/10.3390/molecules28186598 149

Cándido Ortiz-Placín, Alba Castillejo-Rufo, Matías Estarás and Antonio González
Membrane Lipid Derivatives: Roles of Arachidonic Acid and Its Metabolites in Pancreatic Physiology and Pathophysiology
Reprinted from: *Molecules* 2023, *28*, 4316, https://doi.org/10.3390/molecules28114316 172

João Lopes, Dorinda Marques-da-Silva, Paula A. Videira, Alejandro K. Samhan-Arias and Ricardo Lagoa
Cardiolipin Membranes Promote Cytochrome *c* Transformation of Polycyclic Aromatic Hydrocarbons and Their In Vivo Metabolites
Reprinted from: *Molecules* 2024, *29*, 1129, https://doi.org/10.3390/molecules29051129 194

Jairo Salazar, Alejandro K. Samhan-Arias and Carlos Gutierrez-Merino
Hexa-Histidine, a Peptide with Versatile Applications in the Study of Amyloid-β(1–42) Molecular Mechanisms of Action
Reprinted from: *Molecules* 2023, *28*, 7138, https://doi.org/10.3390/molecules28207138 211

Joana Poejo, María Berrocal, Lucía Saez, Carlos Gutierrez-Merino and Ana M. Mata
Store-Operated Calcium Entry Inhibition and Plasma Membrane Calcium Pump Upregulation Contribute to the Maintenance of Resting Cytosolic Calcium Concentration in A1-like Astrocytes
Reprinted from: *Molecules* **2023**, *28*, 5363, https://doi.org/10.3390/molecules28145363 . . . . . . **231**

Seung Jun Jung, Kunn Hadinoto and Jin-Won Park
Mechanical Properties of 3-Hydroxybutyric Acid-Induced Vesicles
Reprinted from: *Molecules* **2023**, *28*, 2742, https://doi.org/10.3390/molecules28062742 . . . . . . **247**

Pilar Eraso, María J. Mazón, Victoria Jiménez, Patricia Pizarro-García, Eva P. Cuevas, Jara Majuelos-Melguizo, et al.
New Functions of Intracellular LOXL2: Modulation of RNA-Binding Proteins
Reprinted from: *Molecules* **2023**, *28*, 4433, https://doi.org/10.3390/molecules28114433 . . . . . . **252**

Beatriz Vieira-da-Silva and Miguel A. R. B. Castanho
Resazurin Reduction-Based Assays Revisited: Guidelines for Accurate Reporting of Relative Differences on Metabolic Status
Reprinted from: *Molecules* **2023**, *28*, 2283, https://doi.org/10.3390/molecules28052283 . . . . . . **268**

About the Editors

Alejandro Samhan-Arias

Alejandro K. Samhan-Arias is an associate professor and a coordinator of the Master's course in Biotechnology, Biochemistry Department, School of Medicine at the Universidad Autónoma de Madrid (UAM) and the Instituto de Investigaciones Biomédicas 'Sols-Morreale' (CSIC). He is dedicated to comprehending both the beneficial and harmful properties of free radicals and reactive oxygen and nitrogen species, with a particular focus on reactions occurring in biological membranes. His primary interests also encompass the physical biochemistry and structural biology of electron-transfer proteins, particularly metalloproteins, whose function might be altered by specific microenvironments, such as those provided by specific lipid membrane domains. He has expertise in a multitude of biophysical and spectroscopic techniques.

Manuel Aureliano

Manuel Aureliano is a full professor of Biochemistry (Aggregation in Inorganic Biochemistry) at the Faculty of Sciences and Technology, University of Algarve, Faro, Portugal. He was a director of the Biochemistry degree at the University of Algarve for about two decades, from 1998 to 2013 and from 2021 to 2025. His main research interests include the biological and biomedical applications of decavanadate (V10). At the Algarve Centre for Marine Sciences (CCMAR-Algarve), he explored the environmental and medicinal applications of V10 and others polyoxometalates (POMs). He was selected as a "Outstanding Reviewer" (Top 10 reviewers) for the journal *Metallomics* for three consecutive years (2017, 2018, and 2019). In the years 2021, 2022, 2023, and 2024, he was also included in the "World's Top 2% Scientists list". Recently, in 2024, he was the winner of the third edition of the "UAlg Researcher Award", awarded by the University of Algarve.

Carmen Lopez-Sanchez

Carmen López-Sánchez is a professor of Human Anatomy and Embryology at the Faculty of Medicine and Health Sciences and the Institute of Molecular Pathology Biomarkers of the University of Extremadura, Badajoz, Spain, where she teaches Human Anatomy and Embryology and develops her research lines. She has expertise in a multitude of research methods, including anatomical, histological, microscopy and molecular biology techniques. Her main research interests include the study of natural antioxidants in the field of neurodegenerative experimental diseases induced in adult rat models. Additionally, she also conducts experimental studies in avian models, thereby analyzing the cellular and molecular factors involved in cardiac development during the earliest embryological stages.

Editorial

Editorial on the Themed Issue in Honor of Carlos Gutiérrez Merino: Forty Years of Research Excellence in the Field of Membrane Proteins and Bioenergetics

Alejandro K. Samhan-Arias [1,2,*], Carmen López-Sánchez [3] and Manuel Aureliano [4,5,*]

1. Departamento de Bioquímica, Universidad Autónoma de Madrid (UAM), C/Arturo Duperier 4, 28029 Madrid, Spain
2. Instituto de Investigaciones Biomédicas Sols-Morreale, Consejo Superior de Investigaciones Científicas-Universidad Autónoma de Madrid (CSIC-UAM), 28029 Madrid, Spain
3. Department of Human Anatomy and Embryology, Faculty of Medicine and Health Sciences, Institute of Molecular Pathology Biomarkers, University of Extremadura, 06006 Badajoz, Spain; clopez@unex.es
4. Faculdade de Ciências e Tecnologia (FCT), Universidade do Algarve, 8005-139 Faro, Portugal
5. Centro de Ciências do Mar (CCMar), Universidade do Algarve, 8005-139 Faro, Portugal
* Correspondence: alejandro.samhan@uam.es (A.K.S.-A.); maalves@ualg.pt (M.A.)

Prof. Carlos Gutiérrez-Merino (Figure 1) has led over 30 research projects funded by national and international agencies and, under his guidance, numerous researchers have developed their doctoral theses, contributing to the growth of biomedical research in Extremadura. His career has been dedicated to the investigation of several topics, including calcium homeostasis in muscle and neuronal cells, oxidative stress, and cellular bioenergetics with a focus on proteins and biomolecules such as P-type ATPases and muscle proteins [1–4]; the neuronal plasma membrane L-type calcium channels [5,6], and its role in neurodegeneration, including Alzheimer's disease [7–10]; microsomal reductases function in oxidative stress [11–14]; the role of natural antioxidants [15–18]; and the toxicology of vanadium [19,20].

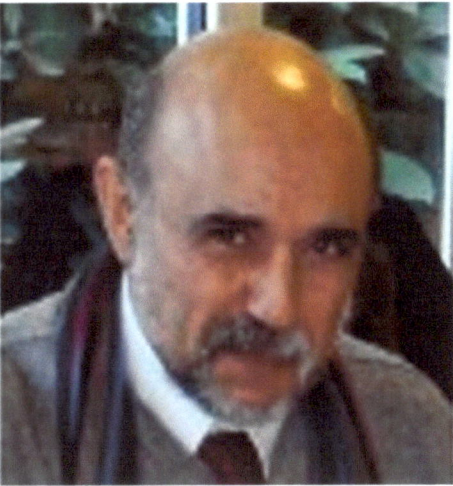

Figure 1. Prof. Carlos Gutiérrez-Merino (kindly provided by Carlos Gutiérrez-Merino).

The impact of his scientific work is reflected in more than 130 impact publications, and his participation in books and international conferences. His research has been widely cited, and has inspired new lines of study in biochemistry and neuroscience. His work has been instrumental in establishing the University of Extremadura as a reference center for biomedical research, and in positioning Extremadura on the national and international scientific map. Prof. Gutiérrez-Merino remains active in research, and maintains collaborations on projects with colleagues and friends that we want to dedicate this editorial letter to: Prof. Manuel Aureliano (University of Algarve, Portugal), Prof. Carmen López-Sánchez (University of Extremadura, Spain), and Prof. Alejandro K. Samhan-Arias (Autonomous University of Madrid, Spain).

In this Special Issue, "Themed Issue in Honor of Prof. Carlos Gutiérrez-Merino: Forty Years of Research Excellence in the Field of Membrane Proteins and Bioenergetics", a wide range of topics are addressed, including research directly related to his work, studies derived from his research conducted by his disciples, and contributions from collaborators and friends who wished to dedicate their work to him in this Special Issue. These areas include: Fluorescence Resonance Energy Transfer (FRET) to high-resolution cell imaging [21]; molecular mechanisms of trabectedin and lurbinectedin, alkaloid compounds originally isolated from *Ecteinascidia turbinata*, to induce cell death in tumoral cells [22]; selenocysteine-containing proteins [23]; extracts or isolated compounds for therapy against neurodegenerative diseases [24]; proteins that play major roles in calcium signaling [25]; plasma membrane raft-like domains operate as hubs for toxicants' cellular actions [26]; and membrane lipid derivative arachidonic acid and its metabolites in the development of pancreatitis and diabetes [27].

Moreover, six regular papers from different research areas were published at this Special Issue, highlighting: (1) the discovery of new routes for polycyclic aromatic hydrocarbons (PAHs') toxicity to mitochondria, highlight the importance of mitochondrial membranes and cytochrome *c* in bioenergetics and environmental detoxification [28]; (2) the description of the His_6-tag as a molecular target for neurotoxic Aβ peptides, suggesting its use to direct the action of these peptides toward selected cellular targets [29]; (3) the description of the role of store-operated calcium entry inhibition and the plasma membrane calcium pump in the maintenance of resting cytosolic calcium levels, leading to an increased production of amyloid precursor protein (APP) and Aβ peptides in A1-like astrocytes [30]; (4) a study of the vesicle mechanical behavior upon its exposure to 3-hydroxybutyric acid, using an atomic force microscope (AFM) [31]; (5) a description of the interaction of Lysyl oxidase-like 2 with numerous RNA-binding proteins, emphasizing the complexity of protein interactions in cellular signaling and cancer biology [32]; and (6) guidelines for resazurin reduction-based assays, opening new avenues to integrate chemistry, biology, toxicology, and pharmaceutical science into standardized and comparable applications for the resazurin assay [33]. So far (19 March 2025), these six papers and seven reviews have garnered a total of 85 citations and 41193 views, indicating an average of 7 citations and 3168 views per publication.

At the time at which he celebrated almost 50 years of active research since he started his PhD thesis, we wanted to celebrate his academic and research achievements, but also his human and professional legacy. His example of perseverance, rigor, and passion for science has left an indelible mark on those who have had the privilege of working and following him. We want to extend our deepest recognition and gratitude to Prof. Carlos Gutiérrez-Merino. His career stands as a testament to how dedication and effort can transform research with limited resources such as Extremadura, and turn them into benchmarks of scientific excellence. As recent contributions from Prof. Carlos Gutiérrez-Merino also include the direction several doctoral theses, whose more relevant results have been published in this Special Issue and in Molecules (MDPI) [25,29,30]. The most recent discovery of several polyoxometalates (POMs) as inhibitors of SERCA/PMCA, as well as agonists of ionotropic and metabotropic receptors in neurons [34,35], reflects indeed his perseverance, rigor, and passion for science.

Putting it all together, Prof. Carlos Gutiérrez-Merino has been responsible for a new generation of scientists across Spain and Portugal for four decades. Prof. Gutiérrez-Merino trained started to go deep into the understanding of molecular interactions of biomolecules with enzymes during their PhD studies. Fluorescence Resonance Energy Transfer (FRET) was used to study lipid state transitions and proteins distribution in membranes. Prof. Gutiérrez-Merino brought his knowledge to Spain, being the mentor of many students in interdisciplinary fields of biochemistry and biophysics, shaping the future of a new generation of scientists and professors. Prof. Gutiérrez-Merino has also promoted several collaborations with Portugal, allowing many students and professors to be involved in his wonderful mentoring. Emergent topics arose in this time, such as protein targets for nitrosative and oxidative stress, cross-talk between Ca^{2+} homeostasis and redox pathways in neurological diseases, antioxidants for cell protection, and disease prevention and polyoxometalates as agonists of ionotropic and metabotropic receptors and inhibitors of SERCA and PMCA, among many others. Altogether, Prof. Carlos Gutiérrez-Merino, shaped the future of many researchers in Spain and Portugal, and made a major and unique contribution to the advance of the knowledge in several interdisciplinary fields of biochemical sciences.

Funding: M.A. thanks to Portuguese national funds from FCT—Foundation for Science and Technology through projects UIDB/04326/2020, UIDP/04326/2020 and LA/P/0101/2020.

Acknowledgments: The authors wish to express their hearty thanks to Carlos Gutiérrez-Merino for providing his photograph and giving us permission to use it, as shown in the Figure in this manuscript.

Conflicts of Interest: The authors declare no conflicts of interest.

References

1. Biltonen, R.L.; Gutierrez-Merino, C. Membrane Structural Fluctuations and Modulation of Ca^{2+}-ATPase Activity in Reconstituted Systems. In *Developments in Biochemistry*; Calcium Binding Proteins: Structure and Function; Elsevier: Amsterdam, The Netherlands, 1980; Volume 14, pp. 75–77.
2. Gutiérrez-Martín, Y.; Martín-Romero, F.J.; Henao, F.; Gutiérrez-Merino, C. Synaptosomal Plasma Membrane Ca^{2+} Pump Activity Inhibition by Repetitive Micromolar $ONOO^-$ Pulses. *Free Radic. Biol. Med.* **2002**, *32*, 46–55. [CrossRef] [PubMed]
3. Tiago, T.; Simão, S.; Aureliano, M.; Martín-Romero, F.J.; Gutiérrez-Merino, C. Inhibition of Skeletal Muscle S1-Myosin ATPase by Peroxynitrite. *Biochemistry* **2006**, *45*, 3794–3804. [CrossRef] [PubMed]
4. Tiago, T.; Ramos, S.; Aureliano, M.; Gutiérrez-Merino, C. Peroxynitrite Induces F-Actin Depolymerization and Blockade of Myosin ATPase Stimulation. *Biochem. Biophys. Res. Commun.* **2006**, *342*, 44–49. [CrossRef] [PubMed]
5. Marques-da-Silva, D.; Samhan-Arias, A.K.; Tiago, T.; Gutierrez-Merino, C. L-Type Calcium Channels and Cytochrome B5 Reductase Are Components of Protein Complexes Tightly Associated with Lipid Rafts Microdomains of the Neuronal Plasma Membrane. *J. Proteom.* **2010**, *73*, 1502–1510. [CrossRef]
6. Marques-da-Silva, D.; Gutierrez-Merino, C. L-Type Voltage-Operated Calcium Channels, N-Methyl-d-Aspartate Receptors and Neuronal Nitric-Oxide Synthase Form a Calcium/Redox Nano-Transducer within Lipid Rafts. *Biochem. Biophys. Res. Commun.* **2012**, *420*, 257–262. [CrossRef]
7. Gutierrez-Merino, C.; Marques-da-Silva, D.; Fortalezas, S.; Samhan-Arias, A.K. Cytosolic Calcium Homeostasis in Neurons—Control Systems, Modulation by Reactive Oxygen and Nitrogen Species, and Space and Time Fluctuations. In *Neurochemistry*; Heinbockel, T., Ed.; IntechOpen: Rijeka, Croatia, 2014; Chapter 3.
8. Salazar, J.; Poejo, J.; Mata, A.M.; Samhan-Arias, A.K.; Gutierrez-Merino, C. Design and Experimental Evaluation of a Peptide Antagonist against Amyloid β(1-42) Interactions with Calmodulin and Calbindin-D28k. *Int. J. Mol. Sci.* **2022**, *23*, 2289. [CrossRef]
9. Poejo, J.; Salazar, J.; Mata, A.M.; Gutierrez-Merino, C. The Relevance of Amyloid β-Calmodulin Complexation in Neurons and Brain Degeneration in Alzheimer's Disease. *Int. J. Mol. Sci.* **2021**, *22*, 4976. [CrossRef]
10. Corbacho, I.; Berrocal, M.; Török, K.; Mata, A.M.; Gutierrez-Merino, C. High Affinity Binding of Amyloid β-Peptide to Calmodulin: Structural and Functional Implications. *Biochem. Biophys. Res. Commun.* **2017**, *486*, 992–997. [CrossRef]

11. Martín-Romero, F.J.; Gutiérrez-Martín, Y.; Henao, F.; Gutiérrez-Merino, C. The NADH Oxidase Activity of the Plasma Membrane of Synaptosomes Is a Major Source of Superoxide Anion and Is Inhibited by Peroxynitrite. *J. Neurochem.* **2002**, *82*, 604–614. [CrossRef]
12. Samhan-Arias, A.K.; Fortalezas, S.; Cordas, C.M.; Moura, I.; Moura, J.J.G.; Gutierrez-Merino, C. Cytochrome B5 Reductase Is the Component from Neuronal Synaptic Plasma Membrane Vesicles That Generates Superoxide Anion upon Stimulation by Cytochrome c. *Redox. Biol.* **2018**, *15*, 109–114. [CrossRef]
13. Samhan-Arias, A.K.; Marques-da-Silva, D.; Yanamala, N.; Gutierrez-Merino, C. Stimulation and Clustering of Cytochrome B5 Reductase in Caveolin-Rich Lipid Microdomains Is an Early Event in Oxidative Stress-Mediated Apoptosis of Cerebellar Granule Neurons. *J. Proteom.* **2012**, *75*, 2934–2949. [CrossRef] [PubMed]
14. Samhan-Arias, A.K.; Garcia-Bereguiain, M.A.; Martin-Romero, F.J.; Gutierrez-Merino, C. Clustering of Plasma Membrane-Bound Cytochrome B5 Reductase within 'Lipid Raft' Microdomains of the Neuronal Plasma Membrane. *Mol. Cell. Neurosci.* **2009**, *40*, 14–26. [CrossRef]
15. López-Sánchez, C.; Lagoa, R.; Poejo, J.; García-López, V.; García-Martínez, V.; Gutierrez-Merino, C. An Update of Kaempferol Protection against Brain Damage Induced by Ischemia-Reperfusion and by 3-Nitropropionic Acid. *Molecules* **2024**, *29*, 776. [CrossRef] [PubMed]
16. Lagoa, R.; Samhan-Arias, A.K.; Gutierrez-Merino, C. Correlation between the Potency of Flavonoids for Cytochrome c Reduction and Inhibition of Cardiolipin-Induced Peroxidase Activity. *Biofactors* **2017**, *43*, 451–468. [CrossRef]
17. Lagoa, R.; Graziani, I.; Lopez-Sanchez, C.; Garcia-Martinez, V.; Gutierrez-Merino, C. Complex I and Cytochrome c Are Molecular Targets of Flavonoids That Inhibit Hydrogen Peroxide Production by Mitochondria. *Biochim. Biophys. Acta.* **2011**, *1807*, 1562–1572. [CrossRef]
18. Lagoa, R.; Lopez-Sanchez, C.; Samhan-Arias, A.K.; Gañan, C.M.; Garcia-Martinez, V.; Gutierrez-Merino, C. Kaempferol Protects against Rat Striatal Degeneration Induced by 3-Nitropropionic Acid. *J. Neurochem.* **2009**, *111*, 473–487. [CrossRef] [PubMed]
19. Soares, S.S.; Gutiérrez-Merino, C.; Aureliano, M. Decavanadate Induces Mitochondrial Membrane Depolarization and Inhibits Oxygen Consumption. *J. Inorg. Biochem.* **2007**, *101*, 789–796. [CrossRef]
20. Tiago, T.; Aureliano, M.; Gutiérrez-Merino, C. Decavanadate Binding to a High Affinity Site near the Myosin Catalytic Centre Inhibits F-Actin-Stimulated Myosin ATPase Activity. *Biochemistry* **2004**, *43*, 5551–5561. [CrossRef]
21. Antollini, S.S.; Barrantes, F.J. Carlos Gutiérrez-Merino: Synergy of Theory and Experimentation in Biological Membrane Research. *Molecules* **2024**, *29*, 820. [CrossRef]
22. Povo-Retana, A.; Landauro-Vera, R.; Alvarez-Lucena, C.; Cascante, M.; Boscá, L. Trabectedin and Lurbinectedin Modulate the Interplay between Cells in the Tumour Microenvironment—Progresses in Their Use in Combined Cancer Therapy. *Molecules* **2024**, *29*, 331. [CrossRef]
23. Maia, L.B.; Maiti, B.K.; Moura, I.; Moura, J.J.G. Selenium—More than Just a Fortuitous Sulfur Substitute in Redox Biology. *Molecules* **2024**, *29*, 120. [CrossRef] [PubMed]
24. Chaves, N.; Nogales, L.; Montero-Fernández, I.; Blanco-Salas, J.; Alías, J.C. Mediterranean Shrub Species as a Source of Biomolecules against Neurodegenerative Diseases. *Molecules* **2023**, *28*, 8133. [CrossRef] [PubMed]
25. Samhan-Arias, A.K.; Poejo, J.; Marques-da-Silva, D.; Martínez-Costa, O.H.; Gutierrez-Merino, C. Are There Lipid Membrane-Domain Subtypes in Neurons with Different Roles in Calcium Signaling? *Molecules* **2023**, *28*, 7909. [CrossRef]
26. Marques-da-Silva, D.; Lagoa, R. Rafting on the Evidence for Lipid Raft-like Domains as Hubs Triggering Environmental Toxicants' Cellular Effects. *Molecules* **2023**, *28*, 6598. [CrossRef]
27. Ortiz-Placín, C.; Castillejo-Rufo, A.; Estarás, M.; González, A. Membrane Lipid Derivatives: Roles of Arachidonic Acid and Its Metabolites in Pancreatic Physiology and Pathophysiology. *Molecules* **2023**, *28*, 4316. [CrossRef] [PubMed]
28. Lopes, J.; Marques-da-Silva, D.; Videira, P.A.; Samhan-Arias, A.K.; Lagoa, R. Cardiolipin Membranes Promote Cytochrome c Transformation of Polycyclic Aromatic Hydrocarbons and Their In Vivo Metabolites. *Molecules* **2024**, *29*, 1129. [CrossRef]
29. Salazar, J.; Samhan-Arias, A.K.; Gutierrez-Merino, C. Hexa-Histidine, a Peptide with Versatile Applications in the Study of Amyloid-β(1–42) Molecular Mechanisms of Action. *Molecules* **2023**, *28*, 7138. [CrossRef]
30. Poejo, J.; Berrocal, M.; Saez, L.; Gutierrez-Merino, C.; Mata, A.M. Store-Operated Calcium Entry Inhibition and Plasma Membrane Calcium Pump Upregulation Contribute to the Maintenance of Resting Cytosolic Calcium Concentration in A1-like Astrocytes. *Molecules* **2023**, *28*, 5363. [CrossRef]
31. Jung, S.J.; Hadinoto, K.; Park, J.-W. Mechanical Properties of 3-Hydroxybutyric Acid-Induced Vesicles. *Molecules* **2023**, *28*, 2742. [CrossRef]
32. Eraso, P.; Mazón, M.J.; Jiménez, V.; Pizarro-García, P.; Cuevas, E.P.; Majuelos-Melguizo, J.; Morillo-Bernal, J.; Cano, A.; Portillo, F. New Functions of Intracellular LOXL2: Modulation of RNA-Binding Proteins. *Molecules* **2023**, *28*, 4433. [CrossRef]
33. Vieira-da-Silva, B.; Castanho, M.A.R.B. Resazurin Reduction-Based Assays Revisited: Guidelines for Accurate Reporting of Relative Differences on Metabolic Status. *Molecules* **2023**, *28*, 2283. [CrossRef] [PubMed]

34. Aureliano, M.; Fraqueza, G.; Berrocal, M.; Cordoba-Granados, J.J.; Gumerova, N.I.; Rompel, A.; Gutierrez-Merino, C.; Mata, A.M. Inhibition of SERCA and PMCA Ca^{2+}-ATPase Activities by Polyoxotungstates. *J. Inorg. Biochem.* **2022**, *236*, 111952. [CrossRef] [PubMed]
35. Poejo, J.; Gumerova, N.I.; Rompel, A.; Mata, A.M.; Aureliano, M.; Gutierrez-Merino, C. Unveiling the Agonistic Properties of Preyssler-Type Polyoxotungstates on Purinergic P2 Receptors. *J. Inorg. Biochem.* **2024**, *259*, 112640. [CrossRef] [PubMed]

Disclaimer/Publisher's Note: The statements, opinions and data contained in all publications are solely those of the individual author(s) and contributor(s) and not of MDPI and/or the editor(s). MDPI and/or the editor(s) disclaim responsibility for any injury to people or property resulting from any ideas, methods, instructions or products referred to in the content.

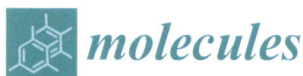 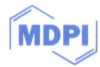

Review

Carlos Gutiérrez-Merino: Synergy of Theory and Experimentation in Biological Membrane Research

Silvia S. Antollini [1] and Francisco J. Barrantes [2,*]

[1] Departamento de Biología, Bioquímica y Farmacia, Universidad Nacional del Sur, Instituto de Investigaciones Bioquímicas de Bahía Blanca (CONICET-UNS), Bahía Blanca 8000, Argentina; silviant@criba.edu.ar
[2] Laboratory of Molecular Neurobiology, BIOMED UCA-CONICET, Buenos Aires C1107AAZ, Argentina
* Correspondence: francisco_barrantes@uca.edu.ar

Abstract: Professor Carlos Gutiérrez-Merino, a prominent scientist working in the complex realm of biological membranes, has made significant theoretical and experimental contributions to the field. Contemporaneous with the development of the fluid-mosaic model of Singer and Nicolson, the Förster resonance energy transfer (FRET) approach has become an invaluable tool for studying molecular interactions in membranes, providing structural insights on a scale of 1–10 nm and remaining important alongside evolving perspectives on membrane structures. In the last few decades, Gutiérrez-Merino's work has covered multiple facets in the field of FRET, with his contributions producing significant advances in quantitative membrane biology. His more recent experimental work expanded the ground concepts of FRET to high-resolution cell imaging. Commencing in the late 1980s, a series of collaborations between Gutiérrez-Merino and the authors involved research visits and joint investigations focused on the nicotinic acetylcholine receptor and its relation to membrane lipids, fostering a lasting friendship.

Keywords: Förster resonance energy transfer (FRET); membrane biophysics; membrane proteins; membrane lipids; lipid–protein interactions; nicotinic acetylcholine receptor

Citation: Antollini, S.S.; Barrantes, F.J. Carlos Gutiérrez-Merino: Synergy of Theory and Experimentation in Biological Membrane Research. *Molecules* **2024**, *29*, 820. https://doi.org/10.3390/molecules29040820

Academic Editors: Manuel Aureliano, Carmen Lopez-Sanchez and Alejandro Samhan-Arias

Received: 12 January 2024
Revised: 6 February 2024
Accepted: 7 February 2024
Published: 10 February 2024

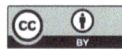

Copyright: © 2024 by the authors. Licensee MDPI, Basel, Switzerland. This article is an open access article distributed under the terms and conditions of the Creative Commons Attribution (CC BY) license (https://creativecommons.org/licenses/by/4.0/).

1. Introduction

Professor Carlos Gutiérrez-Merino belongs to a group of curious and restless scientists who have contributed with incisive theoretical approaches and solid experimental work to the advancement of our knowledge in the highly complex and competitive field of biological membranes. He first approached us in the late 1980s, leading to a fruitful scientific collaboration entailing several research visits to carry out experimental work at the Institute for Biochemical Research of the Universidad Nacional del Sur in Bahía Blanca, Argentina, and reciprocated by visits of F.J.B. to Prof. Gutiérrez-Merino's laboratory at the Department of Biochemistry and Molecular Biology of the University of Extremadura in Spain, catalyzed by the Cooperation Programme with Iberoamerica. These exchanges extended throughout two decades, resulted in the publication of eight research papers, and helped forge a strong friendship with Carlos, a cultivated and warm-hearted individual who generously devoted many hours to teaching and holding discussions with research students and members of staff in our laboratory.

Biological membranes are complex and dynamic and remain the subject of multiple controversies. Various theories and models were suggested before Singer and Nicolson proposed the fluid-mosaic model in 1972 [1]. The innovative depiction of a biological membrane of the Singer and Nicolson model gained wide acceptance, provoking ample discussions, triggering experiments, and ultimately shedding light on membrane structure and function. The model has withstood the test of time, with various modifications and extensions, despite the enormous amount of new information gained during the last decades, some of which openly challenged the fluid-mosaic depiction [2–5].

Currently, a biological membrane is conceptualized as an intricate, crowded structure with a diverse lipid and protein composition, featuring lateral and transverse asymmetry, variable patchiness, variable thickness, and high protein occupancy [2,5]. It is universally accepted that biological membranes act as barriers that separate two fluid media, preventing direct contact between the inner and outer compartments. However, constituting a physical barrier is not their sole function. Many essential biochemical reactions for cell life, involving metabolic and signaling processes with membrane-bound enzymes and transmembrane proteins such as G-protein coupled receptors (e.g., rhodopsin or muscarinic receptors) and ion channels (e.g., nicotinic, histaminergic, GABAergic, or glutamatergic receptors), take place in cell membranes. This makes membranes pivotal scenarios in nearly all cellular physiological and pathological processes. These essential reactions require molecular communication, involving both protein–protein and protein–lipid interactions, and the study of these processes posed formidable experimental challenges a few decades ago.

2. Gutiérrez-Merino's Development of Theoretical Approaches in Fluorescence Spectroscopy in Biological Membrane Research

At the time when the fluid-mosaic membrane model was being developed, Förster resonance energy transfer (FRET) emerged as a revolutionary and extremely useful technique for the study of molecular interactions in biological systems, as it allows the obtention of structural details in the 1–10 nm scale size [6–8]. FRET theoretical developments addressing the analysis of experimental data permitted biophysicists to extract quantitative information about a great variety of membrane properties [9–26].

One of Gutiérrez-Merino's contributions to the field of FRET took the form of two theoretical approaches that were presented almost simultaneously. One of these approaches was developed for model systems of binary lipid mixtures undergoing phase separation and involving four main conditions: (a) a triangular network of lipids in a gel phase [27]; (b) an insignificant relative population of small clusters; (c) donor and acceptor molecules oriented in the plane of the membrane (achieved at very low concentrations of labeled lipids, typically <5%); and (d) a substantial number of acceptor molecules for each donor molecule [17]. The acceptor molecules were assumed to be situated in concentric layers of lipid (discs) around a single donor molecule.

The rate of energy transfer (k_r) between a donor and an acceptor separated by a distance r was calculated using the value of $K_T(r)$ obtained with Förster's equation [28], and the relative number of phospholipid molecules in each disc with respect to the number of phospholipid molecules in the first disc around a given molecule (Equation (1)) was formulated as follows:

$$k_T(r) = \tau_o^{-1} (R_0/r)^{-6} \text{ with } k_r = [k_T(r)/k_T(r_1)] \, n/6 \qquad (1)$$

where τ_o is the lifetime of the donor in the absence of the acceptor; R_0 is the distance in Å between donor and acceptor molecules at which the transfer efficiency is 50%; r_1 is the average intermolecular distance of the triangular lattice; and n is the number of phospholipid molecules in each disc surrounding a given phospholipid molecule. Considering the random distribution of donor and acceptor molecules in the plane of the membrane, it is assumed that no change takes place in the orientation factor κ^2 (a parameter used in the calculation of R_0) in the passage from one lipid disc to the next [17].

Considering the rate of energy transfer, theoretical analyses were developed for a binary, partially mixed lipid bilayer undergoing lateral phase separation (Equation (6)), intended to represent a realistic condition met in biomembranes [17]. The root of this reasoning stems from the analysis of both an ideal mixture of lipids (Equation (2)) and a completely immiscible mixture of lipids (Equations (3) and (4)). In both cases, the experimental data were obtained from unilamellar vesicles, whereby the bilayer curvature was considered negligible.

$$k_T = [1 - N_A/(N_A + N_B)] \, f_a \, k_T(r_1) \qquad (2)$$

where N_A and N_B are the number of molecules of randomly distributed donor and acceptor lipids, respectively, and f_a is the fraction of B molecules.

$$k_T = [(2n + 6)/6n] \, f_a \, k_T(r_1) \tag{3}$$

where n is the number of lipid molecules in a cluster consisting of up to six molecules of the minority component in the lipid mixture, with completely immiscible A and B molecules, and

$$k_T = (6n)^{-1} \{6 + 12 \, [s + n_{exc}/6 \, (s + 1)]\} \, f_a \, k_T(r_1) \tag{4}$$

where s is the number of complete lipid shells of the cluster, which is an integer ≥ 1, and n_{exc} is the number of lipid molecules in the incomplete outer shell of the cluster.

Next, the rate of energy transfer for a binary partially mixed lipid bilayer undergoing lateral phase separation is calculated, as follows:

$$k_T = f_a \, k_T(r_1) \, \langle i \rangle^{-1} \, (\langle 1/i \rangle + 2 \langle s_i/i \rangle) \tag{5}$$

where i corresponds to lipid molecules of class A, and $\langle i \rangle$ and $\langle s_i/i \rangle$ are the average cluster size in terms of number of lipid molecules within and the ratio of cluster shells to lipid molecules in the cluster, respectively. Equation (5) can be reformulated by expressing the last term as $\langle (1 + 2s_i)/i \rangle = \frac{1}{2} \langle D_i/i \rangle$, where D_i is the diameter of the circular cluster i, and $\langle D_i/i \rangle = \langle D_i - 1 \rangle$. Thus,

$$k_T = \frac{1}{2} f_a \, k_T(r_1) \, \langle i \rangle^{-1} \, \langle D_i^{-1} \rangle \tag{6}$$

This allows one to calculate the average cluster size of the minority lipid (lipid A).

In summary, the average energy transfer efficiency provides a means to ascertain, directly from experimental observations, the average size of lipid clusters, correlating this information with the concentrations of both lipids in the mixture, within constrained molar fraction ranges. These novel contributions from Gutiérrez-Merino significantly contributed to enhancing our understanding of the thermodynamic principles governing lateral phase separation in lipid membranes [17].

The scope of this analysis was broadened to encompass additional conditions, in particular the inclusion of membrane proteins, as addressed in the second theoretical approach based on FRET, which Gutiérrez-Merino introduced more than forty years ago [18]. In this scenario, the assumption (a) of the first approach required modifications to incorporate the distribution and state of aggregation of integral membrane proteins. Again, FRET experiments conducted on these more complex biological systems were key to reaching the conclusion that the average rate of energy transfer could function as a quantitative ruler of the following, among other metrics of membrane properties: (a) transmembrane distances (i) between proteins or (ii) between proteins and lipids; (b) distances between sites within a single protein; (c) changes in protein aggregation; (d) lipid heterogeneities; and (e) random or non-random protein distribution. Measurements of the average rate of energy transfer between protein and phospholipid molecules, labeled with donor and acceptor molecules, respectively, were often used in these experiments. The ability to accurately characterize the above properties and processes strongly depends on the careful selection of donor and acceptor molecules. For example, in the examination of random and non-random protein distributions in a membrane, it is imperative to employ fluorescently labeled proteins for the donor–acceptor pair. To investigate protein lateral phase separation from lipids, it is usually necessary to resort to a donor-labeled protein and acceptor-labeled lipids. In the latter case, it is crucial to verify that the fluorescent label of the lipids does not exclude them from the immediate perimeter of the protein or induce non-preferential binding to the protein of interest [18].

The above theoretical approach was applied to the study of the (Ca^{2+}-Mg^{2+}) ATPase. In this case, ATPase labeled with a fluorescein tag at the ATP binding site served as the donor, and rhodamine-labeled lipids acted as acceptors. This configuration allowed the fluorescently labeled ATP binding site of the enzyme to sit at a distance from the lipid–water interface of the membrane. Moreover, this series of experiments made it possible to postulate that the (Ca^{2+}-Mg^{2+}) ATPase existed as a dimer, with the ATP binding sites of each monomer located close to the protein–protein interface [29]. Subsequently, using Co^{2+} as an acceptor for the fluorescence emitted by fluorescein and employing the same theoretical approach, it was possible to establish the location of functional binding sites, in particular the regulatory metal ion sites for free Co^{2+}, which likely correlate with Ca^{2+} sites (Figure 1A) [30].

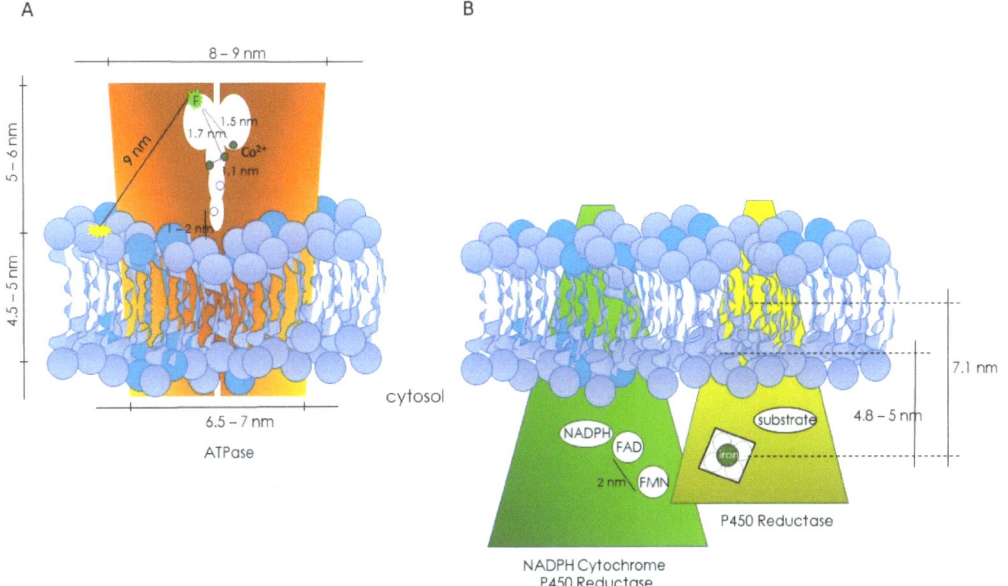

Figure 1. Diagrams depicting the hypothetical topographical relationships between the ATPase (**A**) and NADPH cytochrome P450 reductase and P450 reductase (**B**) with their respective lipid microenvironments. In both cases, information was obtained through FRET studies. (**A**) From Gutiérrez-Merino et al., refs. [29,30]. (**B**) From Centeno and Gutiérrez-Merino, ref. [31].

In 1994, Gutiérrez-Merino and colleagues [32] extensively discussed the utilization of FRET for measuring distances between donor and acceptor molecules, building upon their prior expertise [29–31,33]. As is now well established, this nonradiative process involves the transfer of excitation energy through long-range dipole–dipole coupling, a phenomenon affected by the distance between the two molecules and their orientation [28]. A significant cautionary note was issued regarding the precision of such measurements. Obtaining a single donor–acceptor pair in membrane systems is challenging unless very restrictive conditions are met, such as an R_0 value smaller than half the dimension of the protein diameter or a homogeneous dispersion of monomeric membrane proteins with substantial "dilution" in a lipid matrix. Hence, calculations of distances between two functional protein sites or a protein site and a lipid pose considerable uncertainty.

A similar reasoning was employed to investigate the positioning of functional centers in the microsomal cytochrome P450 system [31]. Energy-transfer studies enabled the determination of the locations of the two prosthetic groups (FAD and FMN) of NADPH-cytochrome P450 reductase, as well as the heme group and the substrate binding site of cytochrome P450 (Figure 1B). The estimated distance between the FAD and FMN groups (donor–acceptor pair) was approximately 2 nm. Using a lipid labeled with rhodamine (RPE) as an acceptor for the reductase's fluorescence, the position of the flavins was estimated to be more than 5 nm from the rhodamine group. Consequently, it was concluded that the FMN and FAD groups are not exposed to the enzyme's surface and are distant from the lipid–water interface, with FAD more deeply buried than FMN in the enzyme's 3D structure. In the case of cytochrome P450, two different donor–acceptor pairs were used: diphenylhexatriene (DPH)–heme and 4H7HC–heme, with DPH located deep inside the lipid bilayer, and the coumarin group of 4H7HC close to the polar headgroup. Distances of 7.1 nm between the heme and DPH groups and of approximately 4.8 nm from the heme group to the lipid–water interface were obtained. A third donor–acceptor pair was used (ethoxycoumarin–heme group). Ethoxycoumarin is a good substrate for these isoenzymes, and a distance of 5.3 nm between the heme group and 7-ethoxycoumarin could be calculated (Figure 1B) [31].

3. Gutiérrez-Merino's Incursions into the Field of Nicotinic Acetylcholine Receptor–Lipid Interactions

The influence of lipids on the conformation, function, and topography in the membrane of the nicotinic acetylcholine receptor (nAChR) has been the subject of intense study for the last 50 years [34]. Synthesis, assembly, and function of the nAChR strongly depend on the properties and characteristics of the membrane in which it is embedded. The layer of lipids in the immediate vicinity of the receptor has distinct properties relative to bulk lipids. Different experimental strategies have been used over the last decades to investigate receptor–lipid interactions. Fluorescence spectroscopy and fluorescence microscopy have occupied a central position in characterizing many of the properties of the nAChR that we now know of. Carlos Gutiérrez-Merino contributed to this endeavor during his collaboration with our laboratory in the early 1990s. In this Section, we will summarize some of these studies.

nAChRs are pentameric integral membrane proteins belonging to the Cys-loop superfamily of ligand-gated ion channels [35–38]. Each of its five subunits possesses a large extracellular region that harbors the agonist-binding site, a transmembrane region with extensive contacts with surrounding lipids through evolutionarily conserved structural motifs [34,39–41] and an intracellular region containing modulatory sites and determinants of channel conductance [42,43]. The transmembrane domain consists of four segments (TM1–TM4), with TM2 forming the walls of the ion channel pore and TM1, TM3, and TM4 being more externally located [34,44,45]. Among these, TM4, the most peripheral transmembrane domain, has the closest contact with membrane lipids and constitutes the lipid-sensing domain of the protein [46,47].

The nAChR is a typical transmembrane protein, and the properties and characteristics of the membrane in which it resides are therefore important influences on its function, biosynthesis, and proper assembly [36,46–50]. Reciprocally, the nAChR exerts influence on its neighboring lipids [51–53]. The muscle-type nAChR at the neuromuscular junction and the electric fish of electromotor synapses (electric eels and electric rays) is enveloped by a layer of interstitial lipids, relatively immobilized in the microsecond time-window of electron spin resonance (ESR) spectroscopy, with distinct features relative to bulk lipids [51]. Thus, the lipid molecules closely associated with the protein exhibit a slow exchange rate with bulk lipids. Mobile lipids interact with membrane proteins in a relatively less specific manner and exhibit a faster rate of exchange with bulk lipids [54–57]. It has been stressed that in contrast to other biological membranes, the postsynaptic membrane in which the nAChR is embedded is a unique system, whereby the amount of bulk lipid in the tight 2-dimensional lattice of receptor proteins is minimal, with only a few layers of interstitial lipid in between adjacent receptor molecules, and consequently with little, if any, "bulk" lipid [34].

Since lipid composition undergoes changes with aging and in response to various neurodegenerative diseases [58,59], and bearing in mind that lipid content varies across different tissues, it becomes imperative to comprehend how alterations in the nAChR lipid environment impact its structure, activity, and dysfunction.

One key aspect of biological membranes is their heterogeneity, which comprises both lateral and transbilayer asymmetries, two topographical properties that have an impact on integral membrane proteins. The aminophospholipids phosphatidylethanolamine (PE) and phosphatidylserine (PS), along with phosphatidylinositol, are primarily situated in the inner leaflet of the plasmalemma, while phosphatidylcholine (PC) and sphingomyelin (SM) are predominantly located in the outer leaflet in most mammalian cells [60,61]. In mouse synaptic plasma membranes, the outer monolayer exhibits greater fluidity than the inner leaflet [62,63], a phenomenon that correlates with the notable prevalence (88%) of cholesterol in the inner, cytoplasmic hemilayer in some biological membranes [64]. In one of Gutiérrez-Merino's visits to our laboratory, we explored lipid asymmetry in native nAChR-rich membranes from *Torpedo* electrocytes. The dimensions of a lipid bilayer, typically ranging from 4 to 5 nm [65,66], fall within the same range as the R_0 observed between different pairs of donor and acceptor fluorescent molecules commonly employed in biophysical studies of biological membranes. Hence, it was predicted that the efficiency of FRET between lipids labeled as donor and acceptor in opposite leaflets of the membrane bilayer would be significantly lower than the transfer between donor and acceptor molecules located on the same membrane hemilayer. We used lipids tagged with an NBD group as donor, labeled at various positions such as the headgroup, C6, and C12. The fluorescent probe rhodamine-PE (N-Rho-PE) was chosen as the acceptor. A calculated R_0 value of 5.58 nm for the donor–acceptor pair was determined [67]. We concluded that the phospholipids PC and PE were primarily located in the exofacial leaflet in nAChR-enriched membranes from *Torpedo*. Additionally, the evaluation of energy transfer efficiency reported deviations from a uniform distribution of the labelled lipids within this leaflet when high molar ratios of acceptor lipids were used in liposomes prepared with the endogenous PC fraction extracted from native nAChR-rich membrane samples.

In a subsequent study, we addressed the precise location of SM in native nAChR-rich membranes from *Torpedo marmorata*. At that time, the distribution of SM on the cell-surface membrane was not known, nor was it clear whether this lipid held any structural and/or functional significance relative to the major functional molecule in this membrane, the nAChR. Previous work had shown the enrichment of SM in membrane regions where nAChR clusters were present. The lipid composition of these regions differed from the bulk membrane composition [68]. In nAChR-rich membranes derived from the electric organ of Torpedinidae species, the primary phospholipids were PC (40%), PE (35%), and PS (13%), with a much lower SM content (~5% of the total phospholipid content) [69,70]. Using classical biochemical approaches, it was possible to conclude that SM in native nAChR-rich membranes from *T. marmorata* was enriched in the outer membrane hemilayer, confirming the transbilayer asymmetry of this lipid. However, this did not imply homogeneity in the distribution of SM in the external hemilayer. To address this question, N-[10-(1-pyrenyl)decanoyl] sphingomyelin (Py-SM) was used as a reporter group of the lipid physical state. FRET was also employed to assess the spatial relationship between the receptor protein and the fluorescent lipid analogue in the immediate vicinity of the nAChR protein as well as to determine its affinity for the receptor.

The ratio of excited-state pyrene dimer (excimer) to monomer Py-SM fluorescence (FE–FM) provides insight into the intermolecular collisional frequency of these fluorophores; hence, it constitutes a parameter directly affected by probe concentration. The increased rate in the FE–FM ratio as a function of Py-SM concentration was twofold higher under FRET conditions than under direct excitation of the probe. This observation suggested a preferential partitioning of the Py-SM analogue in the protein-adjacent region. Applying one of Gutiérrez-Merino's theoretical FRET approaches [17,18] to the experimental data enabled us to determine R_0. A value of 21 ± 2 Å was obtained, in good agreement with previous reports [71]. The new data permitted the calculation of the k_r for SM in the nAChR vicinity; a value of 0.55 relative to the average bulk lipid moiety in the membrane was obtained. This result suggested that Py-SM displayed a moderate affinity for the membrane-bound nAChR. Treatment of the membrane with sphingomyelinase converts SM into phosphorylcholine and ceramide (Cer). In intact membranes, enzymatic hydrolysis removes only outer leaflet SMs [72]. When nAChR-rich membranes were treated with sphingomyelinase and FRET efficiency was measured before and after enzymatic hydrolysis, a noticeable increase in FRET efficiency between the protein and the resulting Py-Cer was observed, indicating an enhanced affinity of Py-Cer for the donor protein and/or greater accessibility of this lipid to the lipid microenvironment of the nAChR relative to the Py-SM precursor. Additionally, a gradual decrease in the FE–FM ratio was observed during enzymatic digestion, reinforcing the idea that Py-Cer exhibits higher affinity and/or greater accessibility to the lipid–protein interface than Py-SM. This finding could be rationalized in terms of the structural similarity between Cer and free fatty acids (FFAs), since the latter exhibit approximately four times greater affinity for the membrane-bound *Torpedo* nAChR relative to PC [73,74]. Considering a total of 44 lipids comprising the nAChR vicinal lipid, only 2.2 molecules of SM were estimated to be at the nAChR–lipid interface [75]. If one considers that the conversion of SM to Cer, a process that occurs naturally and has significant functional consequences, could produce an increase in Cer molecules at the nAChR–lipid interface, it also implies a relative decrease in other lipids in the receptor microenvironment. These changes in the lipid–nAChR interface might entail functional consequences, given the well-known influence of lipids on the conformation and allosteric mechanisms of this receptor [34].

To learn about the physical characteristics of the membrane in which the nAChR is inserted and of the lipid belt region, we resorted to the amphiphilic fluorescent probe Laurdan (6-dodecanoyl-2-dimethylaminonaphthalene) [76]. Laurdan, one of the several solvatochromic probes conceived and synthesized by Gregorio Weber and colleagues, possesses an exquisite spectral sensitivity to the phase state of the membrane because of its capacity to sense the polarity and the molecular dynamics of dipoles in its surroundings, due to the effect of dipolar relaxation processes [77–79]. Laurdan localizes at the hydrophilic–hydrophobic interface of the lipid bilayer [80,81], with its lauric acid moiety at the phospholipid acyl chain region and its naphthalene moiety at the level of the phospholipid glycerol backbone. The so-called general polarization (GP) of Laurdan, a ratiometric fluorescence technique, exploits its advantageous spectral properties, as it was initially developed for time-resolved fluorescence emission spectral analysis in cuvette studies [76].

To learn about the physical state of the lipid microenvironment of the nAChR, we conceived a novel approach in Laurdan studies that relied on exploiting the Förster energy transfer from the intrinsic fluorescence of the nAChR (donor) to Laurdan as the acceptor, thus introducing FRET-GP in membrane biophysics [52]. As shown in Figure 2, the nAChR has 52 tryptophan residues, 51 at the transmembrane region and 1 at the extracellular domain. Using the structural data available at that time [82], we reasoned that the transmembrane Trp residues were arranged as an interconnected network in a ring-like three-dimensional structure with an outer radius of 32.5 Å. Furthermore, in view of the long-axis dimensions of the nAChR molecule and the width of the lipid bilayer [82], the height of the plane of nAChR tryptophan residues was allowed to vary between 0 and 50 Å (Figure 2). The nAChR cylinder was in turn assumed to be surrounded by a belt of lipid molecules of approximately 10 Å diameter each. The plane of acceptors was calculated assuming an area per lipid molecule of 0.75 nm^2 [83].

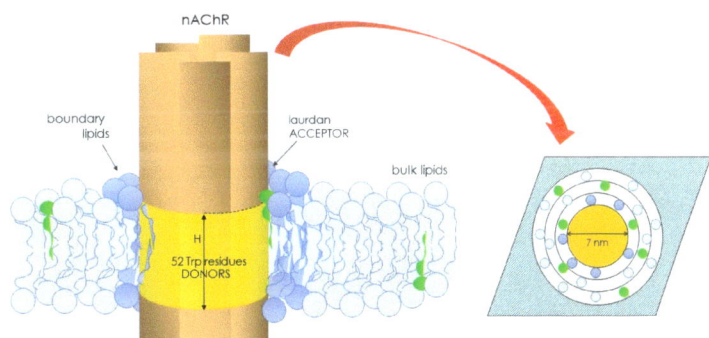

Figure 2. Illustration depicting the nAChR and its 52 Trp residues and the vicinal, boundary lipid of the Laurdan molecules' (green) partition. nAChR Trp residues act as donors, and the solvatochromic Laurdan molecules as acceptors. This pair constitutes the basis of the FRET-GP concept introduced in the field of biological membranes in 1996 (ref. [52]).

The parameter H was used as a measure of the distance between donor–acceptor planes normal to the membrane surface. Several conditions were considered [29]: (i) neighboring nAChR molecules did not generate an accessible surface area to acceptor molecules; (ii) the homotransfer of energy was allowed to occur between Trp residues; and (iii) a distance of closest approach (r) of 10 Å corresponding to the sum of the van der Waal radii of Trp and Laurdan was considered. The distribution (random or nonrandom) of Laurdan in the nAChR-vicinal lipid was calculated using the parameter α (Equation (7)), which considers the probability of occupancy of sites at the lipid belt region by Laurdan (L1) relative to unlabeled lipids (L2), as follows:

$$\alpha = (x_1/K_1)/(x_2/K_2) = (x_1/x_2) K_r^{-1} \tag{7}$$

where $x_1 + x_2 = 1$, and K_r is the apparent dissociation constant of Laurdan for the lipid belt region. A value of $K_r = 1$ implies random distribution of the probe in the membrane, whereas values less than or greater than 1 imply Laurdan´s preferential partition at the lipid belt region or Laurdan´s exclusion from this region, respectively. Theoretical fittings with varying R_0, r, and H were performed and compared with the experimental data using a set of curves with different K_r values (from 0.01 to 100) with a fixed R_0 (Figure 3) [52]. An R_0 value of 29 ± 1 Å for an intrinsic fluorescence protein–Laurdan donor–acceptor pair was calculated. With this value, an average value of r = 14 + 1 Å was chosen for H between 0 and 10 Å (Figure 3A,B). This value corresponds to the thickness of a single layer of phospholipid molecules (0.75 nm² in surface area; [83]), in agreement with the proposed location of Laurdan in the bilayer [78,80,81]. Finally, a value of K_r near 1 was obtained (Figure 3C), indicating a random distribution of Laurdan in the lipid bilayer, confirming previous observations that suggested that the location of Laurdan in the membrane was independent of the nature of the phospholipid polar headgroup [78].

In practice, theoretical and experimental FRET efficiency (E) are related as follows:

$$E = k_T/k_0 + k_T = 1 - \phi/\phi_D \approx 1 - I/I_D \tag{8}$$

where k_0 is the rate of energy transfer, and donor and acceptor molecules are separated by R_0; ϕ and ϕ_D are fluorescence quantum yields of the donor in the presence and absence of acceptor molecules, respectively; and I and I_D are the fluorescence emission intensity of the donor in the presence and absence of acceptor molecules, respectively.

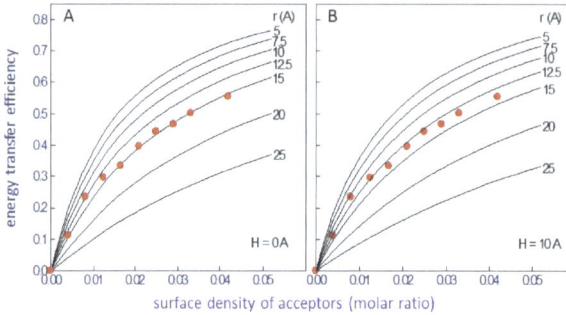
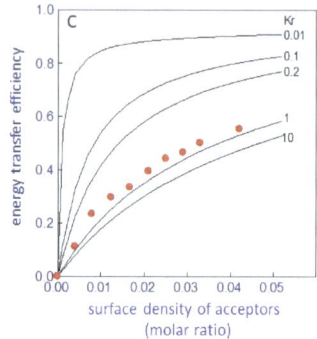

Figure 3. Efficacy of Förster resonance energy transfer (FRET) between the protein intrinsic fluorescence (nAChR) and Laurdan as a function of the surface density of energy transfer acceptors, in nAChR-rich membranes from *T. marmorata*. The continuous lines correspond to theoretical curves representing (**A**,**B**) minimal distances (r) between donor and acceptor, calculated utilizing the methodology proposed by Gutierrez-Merino [18], with R_0 = 29 Å and H set at 0 Å and 10 Å, respectively, and (**C**) different values of the apparent dissociation constant of Laurdan for the boundary lipids (Kr), calculated using the treatment of Gutiérrez-Merino et al. [29], with H = 0 Å, r = 15 Å, and R_0 = 29 Å. Data taken from ref. [52].

The knowledge gained through these studies on the precise localization of Laurdan at the first shell of lipids surrounding the nAChR and the observation that the convenient positioning of Laurdan made it possible to use this probe as an acceptor of the nAChR intrinsic fluorescence in FRET-GP prompted us to undertake a series of studies on nAChR–lipid interactions in native membranes. Using fluorescence spectroscopy, we could identify sites for free fatty acids, various sterols, and phospholipids in the nAChR [84]. These sites were found to be preserved after controlled proteolysis of the extracellular nAChR moiety and were masked during nAChR desensitization [53]. Additionally, we utilized this fluorescent donor–acceptor pair to study nAChR localization in liquid-ordered and/or liquid-disordered domains in membranes of various compositions and asymmetries [85,86].

4. Gutiérrez-Merino's Use of FRET in Imaging Studies of Biological Membranes

One of the most interesting aspects of FRET studies in membranes is the spatial selectivity, permitting the observation of phenomena restricted only to acceptor molecules that are just a few nanometers away from the donor molecule, thus providing high spatial resolution for the case of multiple acceptors per donor, a property that has been exploited in cell imaging.

Neuronal apoptosis is intimately related to oxidative stress [87], and a considerable amount of research has been undertaken in this field to understand not only physiological apoptosis but also that associated with pathophysiological conditions such as neurodegenerative diseases (i.e., Alzheimer disease [88]). Gutiérrez-Merino expanded the potential of FRET approaches by transitioning from cuvettes to the microscope, focusing on this challenging problem. Changes in the red/orange autofluorescence of flavoprotein cytochrome b5 reductase (Cb5R), a major component of the plasma membrane redox chain, and other flavoprotein oxidases also bound to membranes were observed under cellular oxidative stress conditions [89]. Thus, flavins were used as donor molecules to study their location in the plasma membrane. Two suitable acceptor molecules were *N*-(3-triethylammoniumpropyl)-4-(4-(4-(diethylamino)phenyl)butadienyl)-pyridinium dibromide (RH-414) and *N*-(3-triethylammoniumpropyl)-4-(6-(4-(diethylamino)phenyl)hexatrienyl) pyridinium dibromide (FM4-64), with the fluorescence of RH-414 homogeneously distributed in the plasma membrane [90], while FM4-64's fluorescence is concentrated in the actively recycling membrane at synaptic connections [91]. At cerebellar granule neurons (CGNs), R_0

values for both pairs of donor–acceptor molecules were in the range of 3.7–4.2 nm, with a FRET efficiency of 30–35% at 9 days of cell culture (mature CGN). Fluorescence microscopy images of CGN stained with FM4-64 obtained at the donor wavelength excitation showed that FM4-64 is distributed in clusters or discrete membrane domains 0.5–1 μm in diameter, largely present at inter-neuronal contact sites of the neuronal soma [92].

The membrane-bound isoform of Cb5R is a major protein component of the plasma membrane redox chain in rat liver cells [93], one of the five more abundant proteins of the caveolin–protein complex isolated from the vascular endothelial membrane [94], and a flavoprotein. Thus, working with CGN, FRET studies were conducted between CTB-Alexa488 and anti-caveolin-2/IgG-Alexa488 (as lipid raft markers) and anti-Cb5R/IgG-Cy3. The observed FRET between CTB-Alexa488 and anti-Cb5R/Cy3 indicates that Cb5R must be present in most "lipid raft" domains of the plasma [95]. More recently, FRET imaging with cerebellar cortex slices using Alexa488-cholera toxin B as the donor and the complex anti-Cb5R isoform 3/IgG-Cy3 as the acceptor confirms that a large part of Cb5R isoform 3 is located vicinal to lipid raft nanodomains [96]. Further FRET studies using CGNs in culture, with a methodological improvement based on the implementation of secondary fluorescent antibodies (Alexa488-IgG and Cy3-IgG) directed against primary antibodies for Cb5R and L-type calcium channels (L-VOCC), led to the suggestion that L-VOCC was anchored to raft domains through binding to caveolin complexes. This could occur at a distance between 10 and 100 nm from cytochrome b5 reductase [97]. Similar FRET experiments showed an enhanced clustering of cytochrome b5 reductase within caveolin-rich lipid raft microdomains in the early phase of apoptosis [98]. A contemporary study using a great variety of donor–acceptor pairs indicated that (a) L-VOCC and N-methyl D-aspartate receptors (NMDARs) are vicinal proteins in the plasma membrane, separated by less than 80 nm; (b) NMDARs also colocalize with neuronal nitric-oxide synthase (nNOS); (c) nNOS is closer to caveolin-2 than caveolin-1; and (d) CTB binding sites were located extracellularly and nNOS sites intracellularly. Together, these findings suggested the clustering of NMDARs, L-VOCC, and nNOS in caveolin-rich microdomains with dimensions <100 nm. Gutiérrez-Merino and colleagues named these domains "calcium-microchip-like structures" and speculated that they have a high degree of control over the neuronal excitability by calcium [99]. The donor–acceptor pairs used were anti-L-VOCC/IgG-Alexa488 and anti-NMDAR/IgG-Cy3; anti-NMDAR/IgG-Alexa488 and L-VOCC ligand ST-BODIPY dihydropyridine, a much smaller molecule; anti-nNOS/IgG-Alexa488 and anti-NMDAR/IgG-Cy3; and anti-nNOS/IgG-Alexa488 and CTB-Alexa555 as donors and anti-caveolin-1/IgG-Cy3 and anti-caveolin-2/IgGCy3 as acceptors [99].

Additionally, co-localization of the calcium extrusion systems (PMCA, plasma membrane calcium pump, and NCX, sodium–calcium exchanger) with the major calcium entry systems (L-VOCC and NMDAr) and the ROS/RNS enzymes (Cb5R and nNOS) was observed within lipid raft-associated sub-microdomains smaller than 200 nm [100]. From these studies, lipid rafts emerged as interesting markers of plasma membrane nanodomains, where cross-talk between redox and calcium signaling occurs.

Recently, and as a continuation of the same approach, Gutiérrez-Merino and colleagues initiated a series of studies on Alzheimer's disease, exploring the relationship between Aβ peptides, membrane lipids, and dysregulation of calcium homeostasis. FRET imaging was performed in mature CGN between the fluorescent derivative Aβ (1–42)-HiLyteTM Fluor555 and anti-CaM (calmodulin) conjugated with IgG-Alexa 488 (anti-CaM*A488) or anti-LTCC subunit 1C conjugated with IgG-Alexa 488 (anti-LTCCs*A488), and between anti-CaM*A488 and anti-HRas*Cy3. Several protein markers of lipid rafts were used as acceptors: anti-Cav-1 conjugated with IgG-Alexa 488 (anti-Cav1*A488), anti-HRas conjugated with IgG-Alexa 488 (anti-HRas*A488), and anti-PrPc conjugated with IgG-Alexa488 (anti-PrPc*A488). An extensive complexation of Aβ with CaM and LTCC with colocalization of CaM and HRas together with an Aβ association with lipid raft sub-microdomains was observed [101]. The dysregulation of calcium homeostasis observed in Alzheimer's disease was attributed to the inhibition of LTCC by CaM–Aβ complexes.

In a subsequent study, using the same fluorescence-labeled Aβ and Alexa488-labeled secondary antibodies for primary anti-PDI and anti-CaM or stromal interaction molecule 1 (STIM1) labeled with green fluorescent protein (STIM1-GFP), Gutiérrez-Merino and colleagues demonstrated that prior to the internal dysregulation of calcium homeostasis, a perturbation of store-operated calcium entry occurs through the internalization of Aβ and its inhibition of STIM1, along with partial activation of the ER Ca^{2+}-leak channels [102]. For these measurements, variations in donor fluorescence were analyzed, and the R_0 and the spectral overlap integral (J) values were obtained for the Aβ*555–SPM1-GFP donor–acceptor pair [102]. Recently, based on a similar formalism, Gutiérrez-Merino and colleagues showed that a short peptide of only six histidines binds with high affinity to Aβ(1–42) and also to Aβ(25–35), which still remains toxic, blocking the interaction of Aβ with CaM and calbindin-D28k [103]. This latest result opened an interesting line of research on the modulation of Aβ peptide toxicity.

5. Concluding Remarks and Future Prospects

In his "Zwischenmolekulare Energiewanderung und Fluoreszens (Intermolecular energy migration and fluorescence)" [28] and "Experimentelle und theoretische Untersuchung des zwischenmolekularen Übergangs von Elektronenanregungsenergie" [104] papers, Theodor Förster set the theoretical basis of what we currently know as the Förster resonance energy transfer (FRET) phenomenon, a non-radiative process through which a donor fluorophore in the excited state transfers energy to nearby acceptor molecules within nanometric distances. Lubert Stryer and Richard Haughland were among the first to qualify FRET as a "spectroscopic ruler" [105]. Gregorio Weber, another forefather of fluorescence spectroscopy in biological applications, considered FRET as the ultimate yardstick in intermolecular and intra-molecular measurements in solution. Carlos Gutiérrez-Merino made ample use of FRET in his many studies on biological systems and contributed to setting the theoretical basis for the application of FRET in biological membrane research. During our decade-long collaboration with Carlos Gutiérrez-Merino, we conceived the use of FRET in combination with the so-called general polarization of Laurdan, a solvatochromic fluorescent probe designed and synthesized by Gregorio Weber [106]. This combination resulted in FRET-GP, the first application of Laurdan as a sensor of a membrane-embedded protein's lipid microenvironment by excitation of the protein's intrinsic fluorophores [52].

The emergence of autofluorescent proteins and protein chimeras with spectroscopic characteristics suitable for FRET applications has opened the way to implement Förster resonance energy transfer in the light microscope. The study of four-dimensional (x,y,z,t) molecular-scale phenomena in live cells [107] is thus a reality that now projects beyond the optical diffraction barrier and into the realm of super-resolution light microscopy [108–114]. Furthermore, the ability to genetically manipulate the chemistry of donor and acceptor fluorescent proteins has expanded the spectral coverage of fluorescence microscopy in live-cell interrogation [110]. These advances are particularly relevant to the field of membrane biology. Hybrid FRET models that incorporate fluorescence spectroscopy concepts, optical microscopies, and artificial intelligence approaches (computational tools such as deep learning and neuronal networks) are now reaching atomistic structural levels and temporal resolutions relevant to cell phenomena. Additionally, a new dimension of FRET has been opened with hybrid/integrative modeling, where bio-macromolecular systems are studied simultaneously through a combination of experimental techniques (such as small-angle neutron and small-angle X-ray scatterings, along with NMR, EPR, and FRET spectroscopies), as reviewed in [115]. Single-molecule fluorescence spectroscopy is an emerging field in which FRET is a necessary partner, as demonstrated in a recent study characterizing the coexistence of stable oligomers of amyloid-β 42 within a heterogeneous and dynamic sample [116].

Author Contributions: Conceptualization, F.J.B. and S.S.A.; writing, S.S.A. and F.J.B.; illustrations, S.S.A.; review and editing, F.J.B. All authors have read and agreed to the published version of the manuscript.

Funding: The research work quoted in this review was supported by multiple grants from the National Council for Research and Technology of Argentina (CONICET) and the Ministry of Science, Technology and Innovative Production of Argentina (Mincyt) to F.J.B. and from ANPIDTYI (PICT 2019-02687) and Universidad Nacional del Sur (PGI 24/B282) to S.S.A.

Institutional Review Board Statement: Not applicable.

Informed Consent Statement: Not applicable.

Data Availability Statement: Not applicable.

Conflicts of Interest: The authors declare no conflicts of interest.

References

1. Singer, A.S.J.; Nicolson, G.L. The Fluid Mosaic Model of the Structure of Cell Membranes. *Science* **1972**, *175*, 720–731. [CrossRef]
2. Engelman, D.M. Membranes are more mosaic than fluid. *Nature* **2005**, *438*, 578–580. [CrossRef]
3. Bagatolli, L.A. Microscopy imaging of membrane domains. *Biochim. Biophys. Acta* **2010**, *1798*, 1285. [CrossRef]
4. Goñi, F.M. The basic structure and dynamics of cell membranes: An update of the Singer-Nicolson model. *Biochim. Biophys. Acta* **2014**, *1838*, 1467–1476. [CrossRef]
5. Nicolson, G.L. The fluid-mosaic model of membrane structure: Still relevant to understanding the structure, function and dynamics of biological membranes after more than 40 years. *Biochim. Biophys. Acta* **2014**, *1838*, 1451–1466. [CrossRef] [PubMed]
6. Tweet, A.G.; Bellamy, W.D.; Gaines, G.L. Fluorescence quenching and energy transfer in monomolecular films containing chlorophyll. *J. Chem. Phys.* **1964**, *41*, 2068. [CrossRef]
7. Vanderkooi, J.M.; Ierokomas, A.; Nakamura, H.; Martonosi, A. Fluorescence energy transfer between Ca^{2+} transport ATPase molecules in artificial membranes. *Biochemistry* **1977**, *16*, 1262–1267. [CrossRef] [PubMed]
8. Veatch, W.; Stryer, L. The dimeric nature of the Gramicidin A transmembrane channel: Conductance and fluorescence energy transfer studies of hybrid channels. *J. Mol. Biol.* **1977**, *113*, 89–102. [CrossRef] [PubMed]
9. Cantley, L.C.; Hammes, G.G. Investigation of quercetin binding sites on chloroplast coupling factor 1. *Biochemistry* **1976**, *15*, 1–8. [CrossRef] [PubMed]
10. Shaklai, N.; Yguerabide, J.; Ranney, H.M. Interaction of hemoglobin with red blood cell membranes as shown by a fluorescent chromophore. *Biochemistry* **1977**, *16*, 5585–5592. [CrossRef] [PubMed]
11. Shaklai, N.; Yguerabide, J.; Ranney, H.M. Classification and location of hemoglobin binding sites on red blood cell membranes. *Biochemistry* **1977**, *16*, 5593–5597. [CrossRef]
12. Fung, B.K.-K.; Stryer, L. Surface density determination in membranes by fluorescence energy transfer. *Biochemistry* **1978**, *17*, 5241–5248. [CrossRef] [PubMed]
13. Baird, B.; Pick, U.; Hammes, G.G. Structural investigation of reconstituted chloroplast ATPase with fluorescence measurements. *J. Bio. Chem.* **1979**, *254*, 3818–3825. [CrossRef]
14. Fleming, P.J.; Koppel, D.E.; Lau, A.L.Y.; Strittmatter, P. Intramembrane position of the fluorescent tyrptophanyl residue in the membrane-bound cytochrome b_5. *Biochemistry* **1979**, *18*, 5458–5464. [CrossRef] [PubMed]
15. Koppel, D.E.; Fleming, P.J.; Strittmatter, P. Intramembrane positions of membrane-bound chromophores determined by excitation energy transfer. *Biochemistry* **1979**, *18*, 5450–5457. [CrossRef] [PubMed]
16. Sklar, L.A.; Doody, M.C.; Gotto, A.M.; Pownall, H.J. Serum lipoprotein structure: Resonance energy transfer localization of fluorescent probes. *Biochemistry* **1980**, *19*, 1294–1301. [CrossRef] [PubMed]
17. Gutiérrez-Merino, C. Quantitation of the Forster energy transfer for two-dimensional systems. I. Lateral phase separation in unilamellar vesicles formed by binary phospholipid mixtures. *Biophys. Chem.* **1981**, *14*, 247–257.
18. Gutiérrez-Merino, C. Quantitation of the Forster energy transfer for two-dimensional systems. II. Protein distribution and aggregation state in biological membranes. *Biophys. Chem.* **1981**, *14*, 259–266. [CrossRef]
19. Snyder, B.; Freire, E. Fluorescence energy transfer in two dimensions. A numeric solution for random and nonrandom distributions. *Biophys. J.* **1982**, *40*, 137–148. [CrossRef]
20. Eisinger, J.; Flores, J. The relative locations of intramembrane fluorescent probes and the cytosol hemoglobin in erythrocytes, studied by transverse resonance energy transfer. *Biophys. J.* **1982**, *37*, 6–7. [CrossRef]
21. Doody, M.C.; Skalar, L.A.; Pownall, H.J.; Sparrow, J.T.; Gotto, A.M.; Smith, L.C. A simplified approach to resonance energy transfer in membranes, lipoproteins, and spatially restricted systems. *Biophys. Chem.* **1983**, *17*, 139–152. [CrossRef]
22. Holowka, D.; Baird, B. Structural studies on the membrane-bound immunoglobulin E-receptor complex 1. Characterization of large plasma membrane vesicles from rat basophilic leukemia cells and insertion of amphipathic fluorescent probes. *Biochemistry* **1983**, *22*, 3466–3474. [CrossRef]
23. Holowka, D.; Baird, B. Structural studies on the membrane-bound immunoglobulin E-receptor complex 2. Mapping the distance between sites on IgE and the membrane surface. *Biochemistry* **1983**, *22*, 3475–3484. [CrossRef]
24. Isaacs, B.S.; Husten, E.J.; Esmon, C.T.; Johnson, A.E. A domain of membrane-bound coagulation factor Va is located far from the phospholipid surface. A fluorescence energy transfer measurement. *Biochemistry* **1986**, *25*, 4958–4969. [CrossRef] [PubMed]

25. Gryczynski, I.; Wiczk, W.; Johnson, M.L.; Cheung, H.C.; Wang, C.K.; Lakowicz, J.R. Resolution of end-to-end distance distributions of flexible molecules using quenching-induced variations of the Forster distance for fluorescence energy transfer. *Biophys. J.* **1988**, *54*, 577–586. [CrossRef]
26. Lakowicz, J.R.; Gryczynski, I.; Cheung, H.C.; Wang, C.-K.; Johnson, M.L.; Joshi, N. Distance distributions in proteins recovered by using frequency-domain fluorometry. Applications to troponin I and its complex with troponin C. *Biochemistry* **1988**, *27*, 9149–9160. [CrossRef]
27. Trauble, H.; Sackmann, E. Studies of the crystalline-liquid crystalline phase transition of lipid model membranes. 3. Structure of a steroid-lecithin system below and above the lipid-phase transition. *J. Am. Chem. Soc.* **1972**, *94*, 4499–4510. [CrossRef]
28. Förster, T. Intermolecular energy migration and fluorescence. *Ann. Phys.* **1948**, *2*, 55–75. [CrossRef]
29. Gutiérrez-Merino, C.; Munkonge, F.; Mata, A.M.; East, J.M.; Levinson, B.L.; Napier, R.M.; Lee, A.G. The position of the ATP binding site on the (Ca^{2+} + Mg^{2+})-ATPase. *Biochim. Biophys. Acta* **1987**, *897*, 207–216. [CrossRef] [PubMed]
30. Cuenda, A.; Henao, F.; Gutiérrez-Merino, C. Distances between functional sites of the Ca^{2+} + $Mg^{2(+)}$-ATPase from sarcoplasmic reticulum using Co^{2+} as a spectroscopic ruler. *Eur. J. Biochem.* **1990**, *194*, 663–670. [CrossRef]
31. Centeno, F.; Gutiérrez-Merino, C. Location of functional centers in the microsomal cytochrome P450 system. *Biochemistry* **1992**, *31*, 8473–8481. [CrossRef]
32. Gutiérrez-Merino, C.; Centeno, F.; Garcia-Martin, E.; Merino, J.M. Fluorescence energy transfer as a tool to locate functional sites in membrane proteins. *Biochem. Soc. Trans.* **1994**, *22*, 784–788. [CrossRef]
33. Gutiérrez-Merino, C.; Molina, A.; Escudero, B.; Diez, A.; Laynez, J. Interaction of the Local Anesthetics Dibucaine and Tetracaine with Sarcoplasmic Reticulum Membranes. Differential Scanning Calorimetry and Fluorescence Studies. *Biochemistry* **1989**, *28*, 3398–3406. [CrossRef]
34. Barrantes, F.J. Structure and function meet at the nicotinic acetylcholine receptor-lipid interface. *Pharmacol. Res.* **2023**, *190*, 106729. [CrossRef]
35. Karlin, A.; Akabas, M.H. Toward a structural basis for the function of nicotinic acetylcholine receptors and their cousins. *Neuron* **1995**, *6*, 1231–1244. [CrossRef]
36. Le Novère, N.; Changeux, J.P. Molecular evolution of the nicotinic acetylcholine receptor: An example of multigene family in excitable cells. *J. Mol. Evol.* **1995**, *40*, 155–172. [CrossRef]
37. Changeux, J.P.; Edelstein, S.J. Allosteric receptors after 30 years. *Neuron* **1998**, *5*, 959–980. [CrossRef]
38. Paterson, D.; Nordberg, A. Neuronal nicotinic receptors in the human brain. *Prog. Neurobiol.* **2000**, *61*, 75–111. [CrossRef] [PubMed]
39. Unwin, N. Refined structure of the nicotinic acetylcholine receptor at 4A resolution. *J. Mol. Biol.* **2005**, *346*, 967–989. [CrossRef] [PubMed]
40. Baenziger, J.E.; Corringer, P.J. 3D structure and allosteric modulation of the transmembrane domain of pentameric ligand-gated ion channels. *Neuropharmacology* **2011**, *60*, 116–125. [CrossRef] [PubMed]
41. Baenziger, J.E.; daCosta, C.J.B. Molecular mechanisms of acetylcholine receptor-lipid interactions: From model membranes to human biology. *Biophys. Rev.* **2013**, *5*, 1–9. [CrossRef]
42. Corradi, J.; Bouzat, C. Understanding the bases of function and modulation of α7 nicotinic receptors: Implications for drug discovery. *Mol. Pharmacol.* **2016**, *90*, 288–299. [CrossRef]
43. Zarkadas, E.; Pebay-Peyroula, E.; Thompson, M.J.; Schoehn, G.; Uchański, T.; Steyaert, J.; Chipot, C.; Dehez, F.; Baenziger, J.E.; Nury, H. Conformational transitions and ligand-binding to a muscle-type nicotinic acetylcholine receptor. *Neuron* **2020**, *110*, 1358–1370. [CrossRef] [PubMed]
44. Absalom, N.L.; Schofield, P.R.; Lewis, T.M. Pore structure of the Cys-loop ligand gated ion channels. *Neurochem. Res.* **2009**, *34*, 1805–1815. [CrossRef] [PubMed]
45. Morales-Pérez, C.L.; Noviello, C.M.; Hibbs, R.E. X-ray structure of the human α4β2 nicotinic receptor. *Nature* **2016**, *538*, 411–415. [CrossRef] [PubMed]
46. Rahman, M.M.; Basta, T.; Teng, J.; Lee, M.; Worrell, B.T.; Stowell, M.H.B.; Hibbs, R.E. Structural mechanism of muscle nicotinic receptor desensitization and block by curare. *Nat. Struct. Mol. Biol.* **2022**, *29*, 386–394. [CrossRef]
47. daCosta, C.J.B.; Wagg, I.D.; McKay, M.E.; Baenziger, J.E. Phosphatidic acid and phosphatidylserine have distinct structural and functional interactions with the nicotinic acetylcholine receptor. *J. Biol. Chem.* **2004**, *279*, 14967–14974. [CrossRef]
48. Pediconi, M.F.; Gallegos, C.E.; Barrantes, F.J. Metabolic cholesterol depletion hinders cell-surface trafficking of the nicotinic acetylcholine receptor. *Neuroscience* **2004**, *128*, 239–249. [CrossRef]
49. Baier, C.J.; Barrantes, F.J. Sphingolipids are necessary for nicotinic acetylcholine receptor export in the early secretory pathway. *J. Neurochem.* **2007**, *101*, 1072–1084. [CrossRef]
50. Baenziger, J.E.; Hénault, C.M.; Therien, J.P.D.; Sun, J. Nicotinic acetylcholine receptor-lipid interactions: Mechanistic insight and biological function. *Biochim. Biophys. Acta Biomembr.* **2015**, *1848*, 1806–1817. [CrossRef] [PubMed]
51. Marsh, D.; Barrantes, F.J. Immobilized lipid in acetylcholine receptor-rich membranes from Torpedo marmorata. *Proc. Natl. Acad. Sci. USA* **1978**, *75*, 4329–4333. [CrossRef]
52. Antollini, S.S.; Soto, M.A.; Bonini de Romanelli, I.; Gutiérrez-Merino, C.; Sotomayor, P.; Barrantes, F.J. Physical state of bulk and protein associated lipid in nicotinic acetylcholine receptor-rich membrane studied by Laurdan generalized polarization and fluorescence energy transfer. *Biophys. J.* **1996**, *70*, 1275–1284. [CrossRef] [PubMed]

53. Fernández Nievas, G.A.; Barrantes, F.J.; Antollini, S.S. Conformation-sensitive steroid and fatty acid sites in the transmembrane domain of the nicotinic acetylcholine receptor. *Biochemistry* **2007**, *46*, 3503–3512. [CrossRef]
54. Lee, A.G. Lipid-protein interactions in biological membranes: A structural perspective. *Biochim. Biophys. Acta* **2003**, *1612*, 1–40. [CrossRef] [PubMed]
55. Bechara, C.; Robinson, C.V. Different modes of lipid binding to membrane proteins probed by mass spectrometry. *J. Am. Chem. Soc.* **2015**, *137*, 5240–5247. [CrossRef] [PubMed]
56. Landreh, M.; Marty, M.T.; Gault, J.; Robinson, C.V. A sliding selectivity scale for lipid binding to membrane proteins. *Curr. Opin. Struct. Biol.* **2016**, *39*, 54–60. [CrossRef]
57. Bolla, J.R.; Corey, R.A.; Sahin, C.; Gault, J.; Hummer, A.; Hopper, J.T.S.; Lane, D.P.; Drew, D.; Allison, T.M.; Stansfeld, P.J.; et al. A mass spectrometry-based approach to distinguish annular and specific lipid binding to membrane proteins. *Angew. Chem. Int. Ed. Engl.* **2020**, *59*, 3523–3528. [CrossRef]
58. Schaaf, C.P. Nicotinic acetylcholine receptors in human genetic disease. *Genet. Med.* **2014**, *16*, 649–656. [CrossRef]
59. Yadav, R.S.; Tiwari, N.K. Lipid integration in neurodegeneration: An overview of Alzheimer's disease. *Mol. Neurobiol.* **2014**, *50*, 168–176. [CrossRef]
60. Op den Kamp, J.A.F. Lipid asymmetry in membranes. *Annu. Rev. Biochem.* **1979**, *48*, 47–71. [CrossRef]
61. Devaux, P.F. Static and dynamic lipid asymmetry in cell membranes. *Biochemistry* **1991**, *30*, 1163–1173. [CrossRef]
62. Schroeder, F. *Methods for Studying Membrane Fluidity*; Alan, R., Ed.; Liss Inc.: New York, NY, USA, 1988; pp. 193–217.
63. Wood, W.G.; Gorka, C.; Schroeder, F. Acute and chronic effects of ethanol on transbilayer membrane domains. *J. Neurochem.* **1989**, *52*, 1925–1930. [CrossRef] [PubMed]
64. Wood, W.G.; Schroeder, F.; Hogy, L.; Rao, A.M.; Nemecz, G. Asymmetric distribution of a fluorescent sterol in synaptic plasma membranes: Effects of chronic ethanol consumption. *Biochim. Biophys. Acta* **1990**, *1025*, 243–246. [CrossRef] [PubMed]
65. Jain, M.K.; Wagner, R.C. *Introduction to Biological Membranes*; John Wiley and Sons: New York, NY, USA, 1980; p. 382.
66. Herbette, L.; DeFoor, P.; Fleischer, S.; Pascolini, D.; Scarpa, A.; Blasie, J.K. The separate profile structures of the functional calcium pump protein and the phospholipid bilayer within isolated sarcoplasmic reticulum membranes determined by X-ray and neutron diffraction. *Biochim. Biophys. Acta* **1985**, *817*, 103–122. [CrossRef] [PubMed]
67. Gutiérrez-Merino, C.; Pietrasanta, L.; Bonini de Romanelli, I.; Barrantes, F.J. Preferential distribution of fluorescent phospholipid probes NBD-phosphatidylcholine and Rhodamine-phosphatidylethanolamine in the exofacial leaflet of acetylcholine receptor-rich membranes from Torpedo marmorata. *Biochemistry* **1995**, *34*, 4846–4855. [CrossRef] [PubMed]
68. Scher, M.G.; Bloch, R.J. Phospholipid asymmetry in acetylcholine receptor clusters. *Exp. Cell Res.* **1993**, *208*, 485–491. [CrossRef] [PubMed]
69. González-Ros, J.M.; Llanillo, M.; Paraschos, A.; Martinez-Carrion, M. Lipid environment of acetylcholine receptor from Torpedo californica. *Biochemistry* **1982**, *21*, 3467–3474. [CrossRef] [PubMed]
70. Rotstein, N.P.; Arias, H.R.; Barrantes, F.J.; Aveldaño, M.I. Composition of lipids in elasmobranch electric organ and acetylcholine receptor membranes. *J. Neurochem.* **1987**, *49*, 1333–1340. [CrossRef]
71. Narayanaswami, V.; McNamee, M.G. Protein-lipid interactions and Torpedo californica nicotinic acetylcholine receptor function. 2. Membrane fluidity and ligand-mediated alteration in the accessibility of gamma subunit cysteine residues to cholesterol. *Biochemistry* **1993**, *32*, 12420–12427. [CrossRef]
72. Jansson, C.; Harmala, A.S.; Toivola, D.M.; Slotte, J.P. Effects of the phospholipids environment in the plasma membrane on receptor interaction with the adenylyl cyclase complex of intact cells. *Biochim. Biophys. Acta* **1993**, *1145*, 311–319. [CrossRef]
73. Ellena, J.F.; Blazing, M.A.; McNamee, M.G. Lipid-protein interactions in reconstituted membranes containing Acetylcholine receptor. *Biochemistry* **1983**, *22*, 5523–5535. [CrossRef]
74. Marsh, D.; Watts, A.; Barrantes, F.J. Phospholipid chain immobilization and steroid rotational immobilization in acetylcholine receptor-rich membranes from Torpedo marmorata. *Biochim. Biophys. Acta* **1981**, *645*, 97–101. [CrossRef]
75. Bonini, I.C.; Antollini, S.S.; Gutiérrez-Merino, C.; Barrantes, F.J. Sphingomyelin composition and physical asymmetries in native acetylcholine receptor-rich membranes. *Eur. Biophys. J.* **2002**, *31*, 417–427. [CrossRef]
76. Parasassi, T.; Conti, F.; Gratton, E. Time-resolved fluorescence emission spectra of laurdan in phospholipid vesicles by multifrequency phase and modulation fluorometry. *Cell. Mol. Biol.* **1986**, *32*, 103–108.
77. Parasassi, T.; De Stasio, G.; d'Ubaldo, A.; Gratton, E. Phase fluctuation in phospholipid membranes revealed by laurdan fluorescence. *Biophys. J.* **1990**, *57*, 1179–1186. [CrossRef] [PubMed]
78. Parasassi, T.; De Stasio, G.; Ravagnan, G.; Rusch, R.; Gratton, E. Quantitation of lipid phases in phospholipid vesicles by the GP of laurdan fluorescence. *Biophys. J.* **1991**, *60*, 179–189. [CrossRef] [PubMed]
79. Gunther, G.; Malacrida, L.; Jameson, D.M.; Gratton, E.; Sánchez, S.A. LAURDAN since Weber: The Quest for Visualizing Membrane Heterogeneity. *Acc. Chem. Res.* **2021**, *54*, 976–987. [CrossRef] [PubMed]
80. Chong, P.L.-G. Effect of hydrostatic pressure on the location of PRODAN in lipid bilayers and cellular membranes. *Biochemistry* **1988**, *27*, 399–404. [CrossRef] [PubMed]
81. Chong, P.L.-G. Interactions of PRODAN and laurdan with membranes at high pressure. *High Press. Res.* **1990**, *5*, 761–763. [CrossRef]
82. Unwin, N. Structure and action of the nicotinic acetylcholine receptor explored by electron microscopy. *FEBS Lett.* **2003**, *555*, 91–95. [CrossRef] [PubMed]

83. Rand, R.T. Interacting phospholipid bilayer: Measured forces and induced structural changes. *Annu. Rev. Biophys. Bioenerg.* **1981**, *10*, 277–314. [CrossRef]
84. Antollini, S.S.; Barrantes, F.J. Unique effects of different fatty acid species on the physical properties of the torpedo acetylcholine receptor membrane. *J. Biol. Chem.* **2002**, *277*, 1249–1254. [CrossRef] [PubMed]
85. Bermúdez, V.; Antollini, S.S.; Nievas, G.A.F.; Aveldaño, M.I.; Barrantes, F.J. Partition profile of the nicotinic acetylcholine receptor in lipid domains upon reconstitution. *J. Lipid Res.* **2010**, *51*, 2629–2641. [CrossRef]
86. Perillo, V.L.; Peñalva, D.A.; Vitale, A.J.; Barrantes, F.J.; Antollini, S.S. Transbilayer asymmetry and sphingomyelin composition modulate the preferential membrane partitioning of the nicotinic acetylcholine receptor in Lo domains. *Arch. Biochem. Biophys.* **2016**, *591*, 76–86. [CrossRef] [PubMed]
87. Franklin, J.L. Redox regulation of the intrinsic pathway in neuronal apoptosis. *Antioxid. Redox Signal.* **2011**, *14*, 1437–1448. [CrossRef]
88. Dhapola, R.; Beura, S.K.; Sharma, P.; Singh, S.K.; HariKrishnaReddy, D. Oxidative stress in Alzheimer's disease: Current knowledge of signaling pathways and therapeutics. *Mol. Biol. Rep.* **2024**, *51*, 48. [CrossRef]
89. Eide, L.; McMurray, C.T. Culture of adult mouse neurons. *BioTechniques* **2005**, *38*, 99–104. [CrossRef] [PubMed]
90. Schild, D.; Geiling, H.; Bischofberger, J. Imaging of Ltype Ca^{2+} channels in olfactory bulb neurones using fluorescent dihydropyridine and a styryl dye. *J. Neurosci. Methods* **1995**, *59*, 183–190. [CrossRef]
91. McKinney, R.A. Physiological roles of spinemotility: Development plasticity and disorders. *Biochem. Soc. Trans.* **2005**, *33*, 1299–1302. [CrossRef]
92. Samhan-Arias, A.K.; García-Bereguiaín, M.A.; Martín-Romero, F.J.; Gutiérrez-Merino, C. Regionalization of plasma membrane-bound flavoproteins of cerebellar granule neurons in culture by fluorescence energy transfer imaging. *J. Fluoresc.* **2006**, *16*, 393–401. [CrossRef]
93. Villalba, J.M.; Navarro, F.; Gómez-Díaz, C.; Arroyo, A.; Bello, R.I.; Navas, P. Role of cytochrome b_5 reductase on the antioxidant function of coenzyme Q in the plasma membrane. *Mol. Asp. Med.* **1997**, *18* (Suppl. S1), S7–S13. [CrossRef] [PubMed]
94. Chatenay-Rivauday, C.; Cakar, Z.P.; Jenö, P.; Kuzmenko, E.S.; Fiedler, K. Caveolae: Biochemical analysis. *Mol. Biol. Rep.* **2004**, *31*, 67–84. [CrossRef] [PubMed]
95. Samhan-Arias, A.K.; Garcia-Bereguiain, M.A.; Martin-Romero, F.J.; Gutiérrez-Merino, C. Clustering of plasma membrane-bound cytochrome b_5 reductase within 'lipid raft' microdomains of the neuronal plasma membrane. *Mol. Cell. Neurosci.* **2009**, *40*, 14–26. [CrossRef] [PubMed]
96. Samhan-Arias, A.K.; López-Sánchez, C.; Marques-da-Silva, D.; Lagoa, R.; Garcia-Lopez, V.; García-Martínez, V.; Gutiérrez-Merino, C. High expression of cytochrome b 5 reductase isoform 3/cytochrome b 5 system in the cerebellum and pyramidal neurons of adult rat brain. *Brain Struct. Funct.* **2015**, *221*, 2147–2162. [CrossRef] [PubMed]
97. Marques-da-Silva, D.; Samhan-Arias, A.K.; Tiago, T.; Gutiérrez-Merino, C. L-type calcium channels and cytochrome b_5 reductase are components of protein complexes tightly associated with lipid rafts microdomains of the neuronal plasma membrane. *J. Proteom.* **2010**, *73*, 1502–1510. [CrossRef] [PubMed]
98. Samhan-Arias, A.K.; Marques-da-Silva, D.; Yanamala, N.; Gutiérrez-Merino, C. Stimulation and clustering of cytochrome b_5 reductase in caveolin-rich lipid microdomains is an early event in oxidative stress-mediated apoptosis of cerebellar granule neurons. *J. Proteom.* **2012**, *75*, 2934–2949. [CrossRef]
99. Marques-da-Silva, D.; Gutiérrez-Merino, C. L-type voltage-operated calcium channels, N-methyl-D-aspartate receptors and neuronal nitric-oxide synthase form a calcium/redox nano-transducer within lipid rafts. *Biochem. Biophys. Res. Commun.* **2012**, *420*, 257–262. [CrossRef]
100. Marques-da-Silva, D.; Gutiérrez-Merino, C. Caveolin-rich lipid rafts of the plasma membrane of mature cerebellar granule neurons are microcompartments for calcium/reactive oxygen and nitrogen species cross-talk signaling. *Cell Calcium* **2014**, *56*, 108–123. [CrossRef]
101. Poejo, J.; Salazar, J.; Mata, A.M.; Gutiérrez-Merino, C. Binding of Amyloid-β (1–42)-Calmodulin Complexes to Plasma Membrane Lipid Rafts in Cerebellar Granule Neurons Alters Resting Cytosolic Calcium Homeostasis. *Int. J. Mol. Sci.* **2021**, *22*, 1984. [CrossRef]
102. Poejo, J.; Orantos-Aguilera, Y.; Martin-Romero, F.J.; Mata, A.M.; Gutiérrez-Merino, C. Internalized Amyloid-β (1–42) Peptide inhibits the store-operated calcium entry in HT-22 cells. *Int. J. Mol. Sci.* **2022**, *23*, 12678. [CrossRef]
103. Salazar, J.; Samhan-Arias, A.K.; Gutiérrez-Merino, C. Hexa-histidine, a peptide with versatile applications in the study of Amyloid-β (1–42) molecular mechanisms of action. *Molecules* **2023**, *28*, 7138. [CrossRef]
104. Förster, T. Experimentelle und theoretische Untersuchung des zwischenmolekularen Übergangs von Elektronenanregungsenergie. *Zeitschr. Natürforschung A* **1949**, *4*, 321–327. [CrossRef]
105. Stryer, L.; Haugland, R.P. Energy Transfer: A Spectroscopic Ruler. *Proc. Natl. Acad. Sci. USA* **1967**, *58*, 719–726. [CrossRef] [PubMed]
106. Weber, G.; Farris, F. Synthesis and spectral properties of a hydrophobic fluorescent probe: 6-propionyl-2-(dimethylamino)naphthalene. *Biochemistry* **1979**, *18*, 3075–3078. [CrossRef]
107. Hoppe, A.D.; Shorte, S.L.; Swanson, J.A.; Heintzmann, R. Three-dimensional FRET reconstruction microscopy for analysis of dynamic molecular interactions in live cells. *Biophys. J.* **2008**, *95*, 400–418. [CrossRef]

108. Ágnes, S.; Tímea, S.-S.; János, S.; Peter, N. Quo vadis FRET? Förster's method in the era of superresolution. *Methods Appl. Fluoresc.* **2020**, *8*, 032003.
109. Trumpp, M.; Oliveras, A.; Gonschior, H.; Ast, J.; Hodson, D.J.; Knaus, P.; Lehmann, M.; Birol, M.; Broichhagen, J. Enzyme self-label-bound ATTO700 in single-molecule and super-resolution microscopy. *Chem. Commun.* **2022**, *58*, 13724–13727. [CrossRef] [PubMed]
110. Tsien, R.Y.; Miyawaki, A. Seeing the machinery of live cells. *Science* **1998**, *280*, 1954–1955. [CrossRef]
111. Szalai, A.M.; Zaza, C.; Stefani, F.D. Super-resolution FRET measurements. *Nanoscale* **2021**, *13*, 18421–18433. [CrossRef] [PubMed]
112. Smith, J.T.; Sinsuebphon, N.; Rudkouskaya, A.; Michalet, X.; Intes, X.; Barroso, M. In vivo quantitative FRET small animal imaging: Intensity versus lifetime-based FRET. *Biophys. Rep.* **2023**, *3*, 100110. [CrossRef]
113. Carro, A.C.; Piccini, L.E.; Damonte, E.B. Blockade of dengue virus entry into myeloid cells by endocytic inhibitors in the presence or absence of antibodies. *PLoS. Negl. Trop. Dis.* **2018**, *12*, e0006685. [CrossRef] [PubMed]
114. Deng, S.; Chen, J.; Gao, Z.; Fan, C.; Yan, Q.; Wang, Y. Effects of donor and acceptor's fluorescence lifetimes on the method of applying Förster resonance energy transfer in STED microscopy. *J. Microsc.* **2018**, *269*, 59–65. [CrossRef]
115. Dimura, M.; Peulen, T.O.; Hanke, C.A.; Prakash, A.; Gohlke, H.; Seidel, C.A. Quantitative FRET studies and integrative modeling unravel the structure and dynamics of biomolecular systems. *Curr. Opin. Struct. Biol.* **2016**, *40*, 163–185. [CrossRef] [PubMed]
116. Meng, F.; Kim, J.-Y.; Gopich, I.V.; Chung, H.S. Single-molecule FRET and molecular diffusion analysis characterize stable oligomers of Amyloid-β 42 of extremely low population. *PNAS Nexus* **2023**, *2*, pgad253. [CrossRef] [PubMed]

Disclaimer/Publisher's Note: The statements, opinions and data contained in all publications are solely those of the individual author(s) and contributor(s) and not of MDPI and/or the editor(s). MDPI and/or the editor(s) disclaim responsibility for any injury to people or property resulting from any ideas, methods, instructions or products referred to in the content.

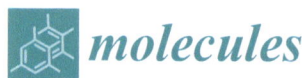
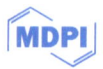

Review

Trabectedin and Lurbinectedin Modulate the Interplay between Cells in the Tumour Microenvironment—Progresses in Their Use in Combined Cancer Therapy

Adrián Povo-Retana [1,*], Rodrigo Landauro-Vera [1], Carlota Alvarez-Lucena [1], Marta Cascante [2,3] and Lisardo Boscá [1,4,*]

1. Instituto de Investigaciones Biomédicas Alberto Sols-Morreale (CSIC-UAM), Arturo Duperier 4, 28029 Madrid, Spain; rlandauro@iib.uam.es (R.L.-V.); clucena@iib.uam.es (C.A.-L.)
2. Department of Biochemistry and Molecular Biomedicine-Institute of Biomedicine (IBUB), Faculty of Biology, Universitat de Barcelona, 08028 Barcelona, Spain; martacascante@ub.edu
3. Department of Material Science and Physical Chemistry, Research Institute of Theoretical and Computational Chemistry (IQTCUB), University of Barcelona, 08028 Barcelona, Spain
4. Centro de Investigación Biomédica en Red de Enfermedades Cardiovasculares (CIBERCV), Institute of Health Carlos III (ISCIII), 28029 Madrid, Spain
* Correspondence: apovo@iib.uam.es (A.P.-R.); lbosca@iib.uam.es (L.B.); Tel.: +34-914975345 (A.P.-R.); +34-914972747 (L.B.)

Abstract: Trabectedin (TRB) and Lurbinectedin (LUR) are alkaloid compounds originally isolated from *Ecteinascidia turbinata* with proven antitumoral activity. Both molecules are structural analogues that differ on the tetrahydroisoquinoline moiety of the C subunit in TRB, which is replaced by a tetrahydro-β-carboline in LUR. TRB is indicated for patients with relapsed ovarian cancer in combination with pegylated liposomal doxorubicin, as well as for advanced soft tissue sarcoma in adults in monotherapy. LUR was approved by the FDA in 2020 to treat metastatic small cell lung cancer. Herein, we systematically summarise the origin and structure of TRB and LUR, as well as the molecular mechanisms that they trigger to induce cell death in tumoral cells and supporting stroma cells of the tumoral microenvironment, and how these compounds regulate immune cell function and fate. Finally, the novel therapeutic venues that are currently under exploration, in combination with a plethora of different immunotherapeutic strategies or specific molecular-targeted inhibitors, are reviewed, with particular emphasis on the usage of immune checkpoint inhibitors, or other bioactive molecules that have shown synergistic effects in terms of tumour regression and ablation. These approaches intend to tackle the complexity of managing cancer patients in the context of precision medicine and the application of tailor-made strategies aiming at the reduction of undesired side effects.

Keywords: trabectedin; lurbinectedin; macrophages; lymphocytes; ecteinascidins; combined therapies; innate immunity; adaptative immunity; molecular oncology

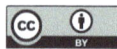

1. Introduction

Oceans and seas constitute 71% of the Earth's surface and account for 90% of biodiversity on our planet. Marine ecosystems are composed of complex communities of animals, plants, fungi, and microorganisms such as bacteria, protozoa, algae, and chromists [1]. Hence, the marine biosphere is rising as a fundamental potential source of bioactive molecules [2].

Thousands of marine natural products with biological therapeutic relevance are identified every year; in 2017, 1490 novel compounds were reported in 477 articles and 1544 were reported in 2018, which were vastly documented in 469 publications [3].

There is a growing interest within the pharmaceutical field for drug screening, discovery, and development in aquatic ecosystems due to the secondary metabolites that are generated by marine organisms.

2. Ascidians as a Source of Bioactive Molecules: *Ecteinascidia turbinata*

Ascidians are ancestral marine urochordates and tunicates that are considered filter-feeders [4]. This is the reason why they are considered pollution indicators and present unique characteristics in the animal kingdom; these organisms produce alternative proteins, such as specific oxidases and phytochelatins, and synthesize cellulose.

This enormous family is composed of more than 3000 different species whose reproduction is both sexual and asexual and, up-to-date, these organisms have directly been identified as a source of more than 1200 bioactive molecules [5].

Thus, ascidians have drawn the attention of the biomedical field due to their ability to synthesize secondary metabolites. Attending to the chemical nature and molecular structure of these biomolecules, there are three main groups: alkaloids, peptides, and polyketides [5–7].

Alkaloids are the most prominent family of compounds that exert antimicrobial [6] and anti-tumour activities [1,5,8]. Within this group it is relevant to mention saframycins, jorumycins, renieramycins, and ecteinascidins that share structural similarities within the bis-tetrahydroisoquinoline chemical moieties [9]. They inhibit essential kinases that regulate the cell cycle, such as protein kinase B (PKB) and cyclin-dependent kinases (CDKs), and alter the mitochondrial inner membrane potential [5]. Trabectedin and lurbinectedin, the anti-tumour compounds marketed by PharmaMar, belong to this category. Peptides from two to eighteen amino acids constitute a smaller subset (5% of bioactive molecules) distributed into linear peptides, cyclic peptides, and depsipeptides (peptides composed by ester and amide bonds). Finally, a third group has been identified, polyketides, which are complex molecules built from simple carboxylic acids and synthesized by polyketide synthetases [5,10].

This is a simplified overview as, not only are these molecules synthesized by ascidians, but their associated symbiont microorganisms have a pivotal role in the production of these defensive molecules that protect these marine creatures from their natural predators [5,7,11,12].

Ascidians show enhanced cellular plasticity within the Chordate phylum, and for this reason, are used as regenerative biology models [13].

Ecteinascidia turbinata is a tunicate that normally inhabits the Caribbean Sea, Gulf of Mexico, Bermuda, East Coast of Florida, and it has been seen in the Mediterranean Sea in the warmest periods [4] (Figure 1). This organism and a symbiont, *Candidatus Endoecteinascidia frumetensis*, are the natural sources of trabectedin [6,11], and it was the first ascidian compound with an anti-tumour activity to receive both EU (EMA) and US (FDA) approval [4].

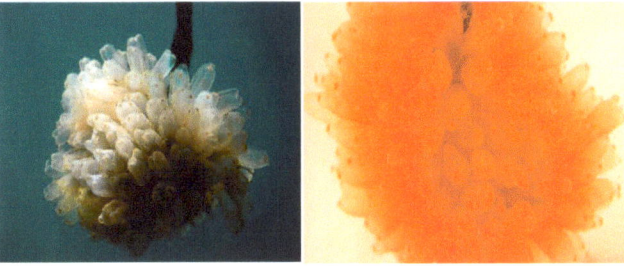

Figure 1. *Ecteinascidia turbinata*, the ascidian source for trabectedin and lurbinectedin (Courtesy of PharmaMar S.A., Madrid, Spain).

3. Trabectedin and Lurbinectedin Molecular Structures

Ecteinascidins' structures were first reported in 1987 by Rinehart et al., although the anti-tumour activity of these compounds was reported in 1969 from tunicate total extracts; however, due to the limited availability of the primary source, it took almost two decades to identify the molecular structure of the compounds that exerted the anti-tumour activity [14].

Trabectedin (ET-743 or TRB) was first isolated in 1990 and its X-ray crystallographic structure was resolved in 1992 [13]. It is a tetrahydroquinoline alkaloid with a molecular weight of 761.81 g/mol and a complex chemical structure composed of three fused tetrahydroisoquinoline rings (subunits A–C): a mono-bridged pentacyclic skeleton of two tetrahydroisoquinoline rings (subunits A and B) linked by a 10-member lactone bridge through a benzylic sulphide linkage attached to an additional ring by a -spyro ring to a third tetrahydroisoquinoline structure (Figure 2A). It is semi-synthetically produced and currently marketed as Yondelis® (Madrid, Spain) [15]. The complete synthesis of this compound by Ma and Chen's group has recently been reviewed by Gao et al. [9], along with other tetrahydroisoquinoline alkaloid compounds.

Lurbinectedin (PM01183 or LUR) is a structural derivative of the former molecule. TRB and LUR differ in the C-subunit; TRB presents a tetrahydroisoquinoline (circled in blue) which is replaced by a tetrahydro-β-carboline (circled in red; Figure 2B) [16,17]. As a consequence, there are important pharmacodynamic and pharmacokinetic modifications [17]; LUR exhibits a distribution volume four times lower than TRB and exhibits a three-fold higher tolerance dose (MTD), presenting a distinct profile [18]. The LUR molecular structure is slightly larger. The molecular weight for PM01183 is 784.87 g/mol, and it is commercialized as Zepzelca® (Madrid, Spain).

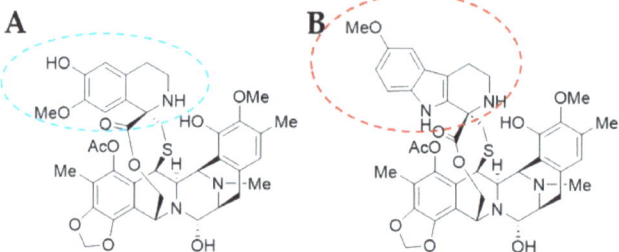

Figure 2. Molecular structure of trabectedin [14] (**A**) and lurbinectedin [18] (**B**).

4. Trabectedin and Lurbinectedin Uses in Oncology

TRB is indicated, in combination with pegylated liposomal doxorubicin, for patients with relapsed platinum-sensitive ovarian cancer [19–21], as well as for the treatment of advanced soft tissue sarcoma in adults [22–25] when ifosfamides and anthracyclines have failed [19,20].

TRB is applied for soft tissue sarcoma (STS) [26] and is applied in a phase III study of mesenchymal chondrosarcoma [27] as well as in a phase II study of extraskeletal myxoid chondrosarcoma. It is also used in non-operable liposarcomas and leiomyosarcomas [28–34] and it is applied for metastatic synovial sarcoma [35,36].

Recently, monocyte to lymphocyte ratio was demonstrated to be a prognostic tool in the treatment of STS with trabectedin. This ratio could be easily applied in clinical practice to assess TRB efficacy [37].

Lurbinectedin (LUR) was approved by the FDA in June 2020 after a phase II/III trial for the treatment of small cell lung carcinoma [38]. Additional assays were conducted for the treatment of ovarian cancer, breast cancer (ongoing in patients of BRCA1 loss of function), sarcoma, and acute myeloid leukaemia [39–43].

5. Mechanism of Action of Trabectedin and Lurbinectedin

Several mechanisms of action have been described for TRB and LUR. The most extensively documented mechanisms are related to their role as DNA-binding agents and transcriptional modulators. Still, there is mounting evidence suggesting that, apart from the well-known molecular mechanisms that are affected in tumoral cells (described below), the impact on the immune system compartment is of pivotal importance in the outcome of patients who are treated with these ecteinascidins [44,45].

5.1. TRB and LUR Act as DNA Intercalating Agents and Transcriptional Regulators

Both compounds bind to guanines in the DNA minor groove, specifically to the exocyclic N_2 amino moiety through an in situ iminium intermediate that is formed by the dehydration of the carbinolamine that is located in the A subunit. Thus, TRB and LUR act as intercalating DNA agents [45]. The DNA-TRB or LUR adduct is additionally stabilised by existing van der Waals interactions and hydrogen bonds between the A and B subunits. This covalent, newly formed interaction induces a DNA torsion towards the major groove; this feature seems to be unique to these families of compounds [17,46,47].

Combinatorial chemical substitutions revealed that the carbinolamine moiety is relevant to the pharmacological activity of these molecules since derived compounds (ET-745) lacking this functional group fail to bind to DNA. Both anti-tumour drugs induce transcription-dependent stress and genomic instability [48]. In addition, this interaction with the DNA interferes with the transcription of genes whose promoter regions contain CG-rich sequences. Moreover, this transcriptional regulation is implemented by the dephosphorylation, ubiquitination, and degradation of the RNA polymerase II (Pol II) on the DNA template [49].

5.2. TRB and LUR Affect Homologous Recombination (HR) and Nucleotide Excision Repair (NER) DNA Repair Mechanisms

The main DNA repairing mechanism that is affected by TRB and LUR is nucleotide excision repair (NER). When there is a lack of this process, the cytotoxic capacity of these molecules over tumour cells is diminished [50]. If the affected mechanism is homologous recombination (HR), as it occurs in decreased expression of BRCA1/2, the reported cytotoxic effect is higher. TRB and LUR inhibit both NER and HR in tumoral cells [51]. Two of the principal components of the NER mechanism are XPG (Xeroderma pigmentosum group G) and XPF (Xeroderma pigmentosum group F) endonucleases that cleave the damaged DNA double-strand and correct the lesion [52]. In vivo studies in the yeast *S. pombe* showed that Rad13, a homolog protein, forms a tertiary complex, Rad13-DNA-TRB, that induces double-strand breaks, leading to the activation of programmed cell death processes [53].

5.3. TRB and LUR Affect Transcription, Cell Cycle, and Induce Apoptosis in Tumour Cell Lines

The steric hindrance induced by the tertiary complex prevents transcription factor binding to conserved consensus DNA sequences where there is an enrichment in GC. A dose-dependent binding inhibition has been reported at low micromolar doses (50–300 µM) for TBP, E2F, SRF, and CCAAT transcription factors by gel shift assays, and at even lower concentrations for NF-Y (10–30 µM). TRB induced a decrease of nucleosomes at 100 nM [54,55].

NF-Y is a central transcription factor that mediates the activation of the human gene that codes for P-glycoprotein or MDR-1, which recruits histone acetyltransferase PCAF to the MDR-1 promoter. TRB abrogates its transcriptional activation [56,57] and in doing so, it prevents ABCB1 channel activity, and therefore, it avoids the multidrug resistance that is associated with the overexpression of this protein in tumour cells [58–60].

In the low nanomolar range, TRB inhibits B2 cyclin transcription which might explain G_2 cell cycle blockade [55,61]. It activates non-dependent P53 apoptosis and produces a cell cycle blockade in the late S and G_2-M phases [53,61].

These anti-tumour compounds trigger RNA polymerase dephosphorylation and facilitate RNA polymerase II degradation via ubiquitination [16,62–64], drastically modulating messenger RNA transcription [16,65].

TRB and LUR induce apoptosis by both the intrinsic and extrinsic pathways in lung cancer A549 cell lines [66], and in MCF-7 and MDA-MB-453 breast cancer cells [67] in a time- and concentration-dependent fashion. It has been proposed that lurbinectedin in monotherapy is more effective for relapsed SCLC than other approved therapies [68–70].

5.4. TRB and LUR Regulate Tumour Microenvironment

It has extensively been reported that these anti-tumour drugs impact the tumour microenvironment (TME), target human tumour-associated macrophages (hTAM) [46,71–73], and inhibit the transcription of pro-inflammatory cytokines such as CCL2 (chemokine ligand 2), IL-6 [74], VEGF [65], CCL3, CCL7, and CCL14 [53,75]. TRB and LUR are known to modulate the immune response within the tumour microenvironment by specifically targeting mononuclear phagocytes [44,65,73,76,77]. Furthermore, it has recently been shown that TRB and LUR modulate the macrophage electrophysiology and polarisation state towards a proinflammatory-like (M1) activation state in quiescent macrophages, suggesting that TAMs pro-inflammatory re-education occurs in murine peritoneal rodent macrophages [78]. Moreover, LUR effectively eliminates both cancer cells and cancer stem cells in preclinical models of uterine cervical cancer [79]. Human TAMs are functionally inhibited and depleted by TRB, which improves the anti-tumour adaptive response to anti-PD-1 therapy [80].

5.5. TRB and LUR Affect the Human Immune System

Both TRB and LUR exert a direct impact on all the immune cell subsets, which probably contributes to the therapeutic actions of these drugs. Nevertheless, adverse effects have occasionally been observed in oncological patients, constituting an exclusion criterion for patients undergoing treatment with these anti-tumour drugs [75,81–83]. At this point, the development of prognostic biomarkers associated with the appearance of adverse effects after treatment with these drugs is a relevant area of research. Additionally, both drugs have been proposed to be applied in combination with immune checkpoint inhibitors, along with a plethora of specific targeted therapies, as addressed in Section 7.

5.5.1. Impact on Phagocytes/Myeloid Compartment (Neutrophils, Monocyte/Macrophages, DCs)

The most common adverse effect of TRB or LUR administration is neutropenia, which is reported in one-third of cancer patients undergoing these treatments, and if it is severe, it constitutes a motive for withdrawal. Both drugs target the mononuclear phagocytic system, specifically, monocytes and macrophages. They can inhibit cytoskeleton dynamics and motility, phagocytosis, and efferocytosis, and trigger apoptosis, as well as the recruitment of monocytes to the tumour site and induce apoptosis [65,84–86].

There are no currently available studies on dendritic cells regarding TRB and LUR. It would be very interesting to evaluate the dual role of these cells in tumour immunity [87–92]. However, TRB antitumoral activity was assessed in an orthotopic xenograft murine model bearing a doxorubicin-resistant follicular dendritic cell sarcoma derived from a patient and it was concluded that this tumour was slightly sensitive to TRB, but it was not statistically significant [93].

It has been proposed, extensively studied, and reviewed that these anti-tumour molecules exert "tropism" for hTAM [44]. They inhibit angiogenesis by inhibiting the expression of VEGF, PDGF, FGF, and metastasis by regulating MMPs, and abolish the immunosuppression that is established within the TME. In this sense, LUR has been identified as an inhibitor of myeloid suppressor cells, both in vivo and in vitro [79,94].

The impact of TRB and LUR on human macrophages has been extensively reported: these antitumoral compounds induce programmed cell death in sensitive macrophages [86] and, in those that retain viability, it favours a pro-inflammatory-like activated state. These compounds upregulate HLA (MHC class I and II) transcripts, glycolysis, NF-κB, and P38 proinflammatory pathways, and induce mitochondrial biogenesis. Additionally, both antitumoral drugs activate PPP and increase NADPH-oxidase-dependent ROS production as well as O_2^- generation and induce a rupture of the TCA cycle at MDH and IDH, favouring the metabolic HIF-1α stabilisation. This metabolic reconfiguration leads to the canonical hMφ proinflammatory activation [95]. TNFα and IL-8 are augmented in the supernatant of primary hMφ [96] (Figure 3).

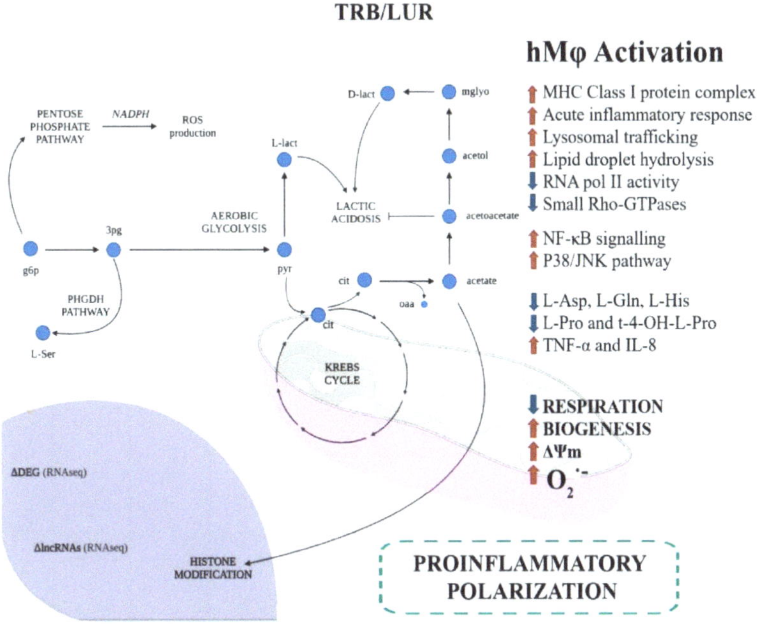

Figure 3. Immunometabolic and functional response of human macrophages to trabectedin and lurbinectedin. Glycolysis and the pentose phosphate pathway (PPP) are favoured, and serine production is predicted by RNAseq and fluxomic approaches [96].

Hence, not only do these ecteinascidins impact the tumour microenvironment and the tumour itself, but they also trigger a proinflammatory activation, at least in in vitro primary human macrophages' cell culture. Macrophage polarisation is driven by macrophage metabolism, and it regulates the biological function of these innate cells [95,97,98]. The understanding of these processes is crucial to comprehend the interplay between immune cells and the tumour and its microenvironment to design specific targeted therapies to improve oncologic patient outcomes and overall survival, as well as progression-free survival.

5.5.2. Impact on Lymphoid Subsets (T Cells, B Cells, NK Cells, and NKT Cells)

These molecules activate NK cells; TRB triggers direct and NK-mediated cytotoxicity in multiple myeloma [99], and both TRB and LUR exert a cytotoxic effect targeting B cells in Chronic Lymphocytic Leukaemia (CLL) [43,100]. TRB exhibited cytotoxic effects in diffuse large B cell leukaemia [101]. TRB and LUR have been shown to activate CD4[+] and CD8[+] T-cells as well, promoting the adaptive anti-tumour immune response, inducing their infiltration in vivo and the proliferation of activated effector T-cells in vitro [43,100,102,103].

Globally, TRB and LUR functionally/mechanistically exert three major roles: these drugs induce apoptosis in tumour cells and stromal supporting cells (TAMs), modulate the TME, and instruct both innate and adaptive immune cells towards an anti-tumour-activated phenotype. Thus, they directly kill tumour cells and prevent the immunosuppressive milieu that is established. These molecules potentiate the anti-tumour immune response to neutralise the tumour.

It has been suggested that the expression of TRAIL-R in the different leukocyte subsets is related to the mechanism of TRB-induced apoptosis and could be useful to explain the differential viability effects on cell viability of each of the myeloid and lymphoid subsets [44,100].

Figure 4 recapitulates the most extensively reported effects of TRB and LUR on tumour cells, the tumour microenvironment, and tumour-supporting cells, as well as immune cell activation, and is supported by experimental evidence [86,96].

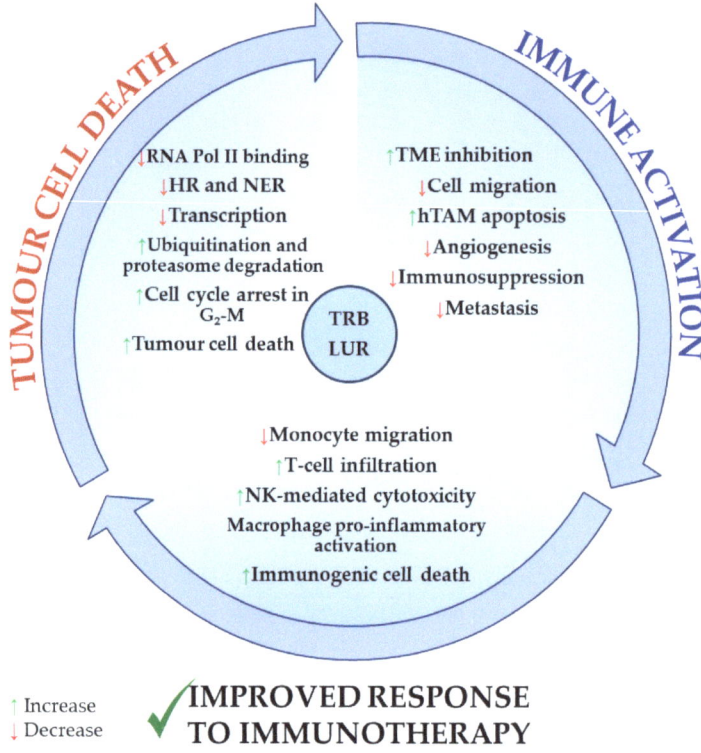

Figure 4. Reported molecular mechanisms for TRB and LUR in tumour cells, the tumour microenvironment, and immune cells. TRB and LUR are DNA intercalating molecules and transcriptional regulators. They impact human TAM biology acting as TME regulators and immunomodulate human immune response and activation.

Both drugs exert a direct cytotoxic effect in tumour cells by interfering with the transcription machinery and cell cycle and inducing immunogenic tumour cell death. As a result, they inhibit the immunosuppressive milieu that is normally established by the tumour and tumour supporting cells. TRB and LUR downregulate the expression of VEGF and several metalloproteases, preventing both tumour progression and metastasis and simultaneously activating NK-mediated cytotoxicity, T-cell infiltration (in vivo), and macrophage proinflammatory activation (in vitro). They reduce monocyte migration (Figure 4).

Taken together, these data strongly suggest that TRB and LUR elicit a higher immune response through two different paths: these drugs prevent the functional pro-tumoral immune suppression in the TME and favour immune cell activation, which explains tumour regression and overall patient improvement and makes these molecules great candidates for their combination with immunotherapy. Therefore, it is highly relevant to establish and explain how these ecteinascidins modulate the human adaptive immune response since mounting evidence demonstrates that, not only do these drugs induce tumour cell death, but they also instruct the immune system to activate and respond to neutralise the tumour.

6. Novel Functional and Molecular Targets for Trabectedin

Trabectedin induces ferroptosis via HIF-1α/IRP1/TFR1 and Keap1/Nrf2/GPX4 in non-small cell lung cancer cells (nSCLC) [104]. This biological process is proven to be essential in macrophage function and is arising as a novel target in oncology that is increasingly becoming a hot topic within the molecular oncology and immunotherapy field. NRF2 and redox biology seem to be regulated by the molecular mechanism of TRB [96,104], although this observation deserves further investigation.

It has additionally been nominated as a potential candidate for drug repositioning in the FDA for type II diabetes treatment by docking. It has been postulated as an α-glucosidase inhibitor with an in vitro IC_{50} of 1.2 ± 0.7 μM, alongside demeclocycline. Nonetheless, this repositioning needs to be further assessed due to its systemic toxicity, hence, a well-justified safety study ought to be conducted [105].

Recently, it has been shown that TRB inhibited therapy induced senescence in tumours by altering glutamine metabolism [106].

7. Combination Therapies Involving Trabectedin and Lurbinectedin

There is a pressing need to design combination treatments that may include conventional chemotherapeutic agents, immunologically targeted therapies such as immune checkpoint inhibitors (ICIs), or specific inhibitor molecules that target signaling or metabolic regulators, due to the complexity of tumoral biology and adaptation capacity, as well as resistance generation. In this sense, the field is experiencing a remarkable expansion: globally, TRB is assessed in combination with ICIs (antiPD-1/PD-L1 [107–110] and/or CTLA-4 [109]), monoclonal antibodies (-mAbs) that may act as either molecular inhibitors or activators, specific inhibitors of molecular targets (PARP [51,111–113], MDM2 [114], VEGF [115–117], CCR5 [118], m-TOR [119], IGF1-R [120], BCL2 [121], ATM/ATR [122],PPAR-γ [123], and CK-2/CLK2 [124]), recombinant proteins (shTRAIL [125]), topoisomerase inhibitors (irinotecan [126–131], topotecan [127], and camptothecin [132]), and immuno-modulatory biomolecules such as L19-mTNF [133] or dexamethasone [134], combined with propranolol [135], a β-adrenergic receptor inhibitor, or Wnt/β-catenin inhibitors [136] (PRI-724). It is combined with physical agents (hyperthermia [137] and radiation [138–141], among other strategies) as it is shown in Table 1, where it is indicated in which pathologies and cellular or murine models are applied.

Table 1. Combination therapies involving trabectedin.

Category	Treatment	Co-Treatment Function	Type of Cancer	Ref.
Monoclonal antibodies (mAb)	TRB + bevacizumab	Anti–VEGF	Partially platinum-sensitive recurrent ovarian cancer	[115]
	TRB + AVE1642	Anti–IGF1R	Ewing sarcoma	[120]
	TRB + VE-821 + KU-60019	Anti–ATR (VE-821) Anti–ATM (KU-60019)	Cervical carcinoma, ovarian carcinoma	[122]

Table 1. *Cont.*

Category	Treatment	Co-Treatment Function	Type of Cancer	Ref.
Immune checkpoint inhibitors (ICIs)	TRB + durvalumab	Anti–PD-L1	Platinum-refractory ovarian carcinoma	[107]
	TRB + avelumab	Anti–PD-L1	Advanced liposarcoma and leiomyosarcoma	[110]
	TRB + nivolumab + talimogene laherparepvec (TVEC)	Anti–PD-1 (nivolumab) Replication within tumours and production of GM-CSF (TVEC)	Advanced previously treated sarcomas	[108]
	TRB + ipilimumab + nivolumab	Anti–CTLA-4 (ipilimumab) Anti–PD-1 (nivolumab)	Advanced soft tissue sarcoma	[109]
	TRB + α-PD-1 mAb		Ovarian cancer	[142]
Inhibitors	TRB + olaparib	PARP inhibitor	Breast cancer	[111]
			Advanced and unresectable bone and soft-tissue sarcomas	[112]
			Ewing sarcoma	[113]
			Osteosarcoma, leiomyosarcoma	[143]
	TRB + RG7112	MDM2 antagonist	Soft tissue sarcoma	[114]
	TRB + rucaparib	PARP inhibitor	Soft tissue sarcoma, dedifferentiated liposarcoma	[51]
	TRB + PRI-724	Wnt/β-Catenin inhibitor	Soft tissue sarcoma	[136]
	TRB + ponatinib	Multi-tyrosine kinase inhibitor	Solitary fibrous tumour of the pleura	[116]
	TRB + propranolol	β-adrenergic receptors antagonist	Cervical cancer, ovarian cancer	[135]
	TRB + pioglitazone	PPARγ agonist	Myxoid liposarcoma	[123]
	TRB + topotecan	Topoisomerase I inhibitor	Ovarian clear cell carcinoma	[127]
	TRB + irinotecan	Topoisomerase I inhibitor	Ovarian clear cell carcinoma	[127]
			Rhabdomyosarcoma	[128]
			Cisplatin-resistant osteosarcoma	[129]
			Relapsed desmoplastic small round cell tumour	[131]
			Desmoplastic small round cell tumour	[130]
	TRB + everolimus	mTOR inhibition	Cisplatin-resistant and paclitaxel-resistant ovarian clear cell carcinoma	[119]
	TRB + maraviroc	CCR5 antagonist	Classical Hodgkin lymphoma-mesenchymal stromal cells	[118]
	TRB + metformin + CB-2	Hypoglycemic agent (metformin) MCT4 inhibitor (CB-2)	Diabetes-associated breast cancer	[144]
	TRB + camptothecin	Topoisomerase I inhibitor	Myxoid/round cell liposarcoma, undifferentiated pleomorphic sarcoma	[132]
	TRB + obatoclax	Bcl-2 inhibitor	Malignant pleural mesothelioma	[121]
	TRB + ABT-199	Bcl-2 inhibitor	Malignant pleural mesothelioma	[121]
	TRB + OSI-906	IGF1R inhibitor	Ewing sarcoma	[120]
	TRB + silmitasertib	CK2/CLK double-inhibitor	Uveal melanoma	[124]
	TRB + cabozantinib	c-MET/TAM (TYRO3, Axl, MERTK) receptor inhibitor	Uveal melanoma	[124]

Table 1. *Cont.*

Category	Treatment	Co-Treatment Function	Type of Cancer	Ref.
Biological agents	TRB + FOLFIRI (leucovorin + 5-fluorouracil + irinotecan)	Treatment of colorectal cancer	Colorectal cancer	[126]
	TRB + mitotane	Treatment of adrenocortical carcinoma	Adrenocortical carcinoma	[145]
	TRB + dexamethasone	Glucocorticoid medication	Advanced/metastatic soft tissue sarcoma	[134]
	TRB + gemcitabine	Treatment of advanced pancreatic cancer can disrupt DNA replication and activate the S phase checkpoint	Pancreatic cancer	[146]
	TRB + paclitaxel	Treatment of advanced solid tumours	Advanced solid tumours	[147]
	TRB + docetaxel	Treatment of ovarian and peritoneal cancer	Recurrent/persistent ovarian and peritoneal cancer	[148]
	TRB + enterolactone	Anti-angiogenic activity	Epithelial ovarian cancer	[117]
	TRB + cisplatin	Treatment of malignant pleural mesothelioma	Malignant pleural mesothelioma	[121]
	TRB + carboplatin	Treatment of advanced solid tumours	Advanced solid tumours	[149]
	TRB + shTRAIL	Targets cancer cells to induce apoptosis	Colon cancer	[125]
	TRB + pAXL × CD3ε	Redirects T-lymphocyte cytotoxicity to AXL-expressing cells	Osteosarcoma	[150]
	TRB + L19-mTNF	Pro-inflammatory cytokine	Fibrosarcoma	[133]
Physical agents	TRB + radiotherapy		Lung cancer, colon cancer	[138]
			Advanced soft tissue sarcoma	[139]
			Localized resectable myxoid liposarcoma	[140,141]
			Retroperitoneal leiomyosarcoma	[151]
	TRB + hyperthermia		Osteosarcoma, liposarcoma, synovial sarcoma	[137]

LUR has been evaluated in combination with ICIs (anti-PD-L1 and anti-CTLA-4 [152]) and in combination with irinotecan [153,154], ATR [122,155] alone or combined with ATM [156] and PARP [157] inhibitors, anti-VEGF [158] combined with cisplatin [83,159,160], paclitaxel [158], gemcitabine [161], capecitabine [162], doxorubicin [41,163,164], and immunomodulatory biomolecules such as antibody-drug complexes commonly referred to as ADCs (4C9-DM1 that targets c-Kit [165]).

TRB in combination with Anti-AXLxCD3ε has proven to be more effective than TRB alone in sarcoma cells [150]. TNT treatment (talimogene laherparepvec, nivolumab, and trabectedin) has shown to be synergistic against advanced sarcoma [108]. There is an ongoing phase I/II SAINT study using ipilimumab (CTLA-4 inhibitor), nivolumab (PD-1 inhibitor), and trabectedin, as a first-line treatment for advanced soft tissue sarcoma (ASTS) (NCT03138161) [109]. TRB + irinotecan has proven to be effective on a desmoplastic small round cell tumour patient-derived xenograft [130,131], cisplatin-resistant osteosarcoma [129], and rhabdomyosarcoma [128]. TRB + β-blocker propranolol combination has proven to be effective in vitro and ex vivo evaluations in cervical cancer in patient-derived organoids [135].

In the ovarian cancer cell model, TRB + anti-PD-1-mab showed synergistic efficacy [102], favouring the activation of effector $CD4^+$ and $CD8^+$ T-cells in vivo by the upregulation of IFN-γ and inducing a decrease of immunosuppressive MDSCs and regulatory T-cells [103,142]. Three dose levels of TRB + durvalumab (PD-L1 inhibitor) showed promising efficacy in a phase Ib multicentre trial (TRAMUNE) in relapsed platinum-refractory ovarian cancer [107,166].

A similar approach was conducted in murine osteosarcoma models where TRB inhibited osteosarcoma primary tumour growth and metastasis and enhanced the number of T-cell tumour-infiltrated cells (both $CD4^+$ and $CD8^+$). TRB induced the overexpression of PD-1 in vivo but it did not in vitro, and Chiara Ratti et al. proved that TRB + anti-PD-1 blocking antibody increased $CD8^+$ infiltrating cells and TRB efficacy, whereas anti-PD-1 alone did not reduce osteosarcoma growth. The combination further increased $CD4^+$ and $CD8^+$ recruitment, shifted $CD4^+$ naïve T cells to $CD4^+$ effector memory cells, and rendered a higher efficacy compared to TRB alone, preventing osteosarcoma progression. This combination enhanced the expression of CTLA-4, suggesting that it might be a third suitable partner for combined immunotherapy [167].

TRB + everolimus was synergistic in cisplatin and paclitaxel-resistant ovarian clear cell carcinoma cell lines and mice xenografts [119]. TRB + maraviroc (CCR5 antagonist) was effective in classical Hodgkin lymphoma mesenchymal stromal cells [118]. In a phase II clinical trial, TRB + dexamethasone improved safety in pre-treated soft tissue sarcoma patients [134]. TRB + mitotane reduced invasiveness and metastatic processes in adrenocortical carcinoma [145]. TRB + metformin + CB2 emerged as a novel venue for diabetes-associated breast cancer in cell lines and xenograft murine models [144]. TRB + PRI-724 [136] and TRB + RG7112 [114] were effective in human in vitro soft tissue sarcoma cell lines (in MDM2-amplified liposarcoma and fibrosarcoma cell lines [114] and STS cell lines and primary cultures [136]). TRB + radiotherapy combination has been assayed in A549 and HT-29 cell lines [138]. This approach has been identified as beneficial for STS patients, especially when tumour sinkage for symptomatic relief is required [139], and for phase I and phase II clinical trials for patients with myxoid liposarcoma. In the first one, there is an improvement in both safety and antitumoral activity [141]; in the second one, the primary endpoint was not achieved but the combination was well-tolerated and effective in terms of pathological response.

LUR has been combined with several agents as it is shown in Table 2 where, again, it is indicated in which pathologies/cellular or murine models the combinations are applied. LUR has been combined with irinotecan in ovarian cell clear carcinoma cell lines showing synergistic effects [154] and in a case report showing BRCA-mutated platinum-resistant ovarian cancer patients had exceptional clinical responses [153]. LUR + olaparib (PARP inhibitor), in a phase I clinical trial for advanced solid tumours, is feasible and exhibited a disease control rate of 72.6% [157]. LUR + doxorubicin improved safety in a phase III clinical trial of SCLC [164], and in a phase II clinical trial, a benefit was observed in several types of metastatic and unresectable sarcomas [41]. In an expanded phase I clinical trial for advanced endometrial cancer, this combination favoured a better response rate as its duration progressed [163].

Table 2. Combination therapies involving lurbinectedin.

Category	Treatment	Co-Treatment Function	Type of Cancer	Ref.
Monoclonal antibodies (mAb)	LUR + VE-821 + KU-60019	Anti–ATR (VE-821) Anti–ATM (KU-60019)	Cervical carcinoma, ovarian carcinoma	[122]
Immune checkpoint inhibitors (ICIs)	LUR + αPD-1 + αCTLA-4		Osteosarcoma, fibrosarcoma, lung cancer, breast cancer	[152]

Table 2. Cont.

Category	Treatment	Co-Treatment Function	Type of Cancer	Ref.
Inhibitors	LUR + irinotecan	Topoisomerase I inhibitor	Ovarian clear cell carcinoma	[154]
			BRCA-mutated platinum-resistant ovarian cancer patient	[153]
	LUR + olaparib	PARP inhibitor	Advanced solid tumours	[157]
	LUR + berzosertib	ATR inhibitor	Small-cell lung cancer	[155]
Biological agents	LUR + doxorubicin		Relapsed small-cell lung cancer	[164]
		Treatment of several sarcomas	Leiomyosarcoma, dedifferentiated liposarcoma, myxoid liposarcoma, synovial sarcoma, and desmoplastic small round cell tumour	[41]
			Recurrent advanced endometrial cancer	[163]
	LUR + capecitaine	Treatment of metastatic colorectal cancer (mCRC) and metastatic breast cancer (MBC)	Metastatic breast cancer	[162]
	LUR + paclitaxel	Treatment of several sarcoma	Small cell lung cancer, breast cancer, endometrial cancer	[158]
	LUR + paclitaxel + bevacizumab	Anti–VEGF (bevacizumab)	Epithelial ovarian cancer	[158]
	LUR + cisplatin		Mesothelioma	[160]
	LUR + gemcitabine	Treatment of advanced pancreatic cancer	Advanced solid tumours	[161]
	LUR + 4C9-DM1	Antibody-drug conjugate (ADC) that targets c-Kit	Small cell lung cancer	[165]

LUR + capecitabine was applied in a phase I trial for relapsed metastatic breast cancer (HR+) with promising results [162]. LUR + paclitaxel showed synergistic antitumoral activity and improved safety in a phase I trial in SCLC, breast and endometrial cancer patients, and in combination with bevacizumab (anti-VEGF) for epithelial ovarian cancer [158]. TRB or LUR + VE-821 + KU-60019 (anti-ATR and anti-ATM respectively) combinations were evaluated in ovarian and cervical cell lines and showed higher antitumoral activity, suggesting that this venue provided mechanistic evidence that could have potential therapeutic effects that need to be addressed [122]. For LUR in combination with ICIs: anti-PD-L1 and anti-CTLA-4 showed strong anti-neoplastic effects in osteosarcoma and fibrosarcoma cell lines, and breast cancer and fibrosarcoma murine models [152]. LUR + berzosertib (ATR inhibitor) showed synergy in SCLC in vivo, organoid, and in vitro models [155]. LUR + cisplatin showed promising activity in malignant pleural mesothelioma [160] but it was not feasible in advanced solid tumours due to toxicity issues [83]. TRB + gemcitabine was assessed in the phase I trial for several advanced tumour types showing well-tolerated results with higher antitumoral activity [161]. Finally, LUR + 4C9-DM1-ADC achieved a higher tumour growth inhibition rate compared to LUR alone in mice xenografts bearing human SCLC [165].

Interestingly, it has been proposed that these Ecteinascidins may be combined with specific antibodies forming antibody-drug complexes (ADC) [165] and nanoparticles [168]. These approaches might help to overcome unwanted collateral side effects and improve safety parameters, both locally in the vasculature at the injection site, and systemically.

8. Conclusions/Concluding Remarks

TRB and LUR induce apoptosis and immunogenic cell death in tumours through diverse molecular mechanisms that are still being identified.

TRB and LUR function as immune-modulatory drugs, both in the TME and over the innate immune cell compartment, as well as the adaptive compartment, irrespectively of the myeloid or lymphoid origin, although the most extensively characterised is the first one.

Both Ecteinascidins are being assessed in combination with a plethora of molecular targeted inhibitors, monoclonal antibodies, immune checkpoint blockades, as well as classical oncolytic treatments that include physical agents (radiotherapy or hyperthermia). and canonical chemotherapeutical drugs (i.e., irinotecan or topotecan) that synergise with TRB/LUR, enhancing their antitumoral activity and/or their safety profile.

Author Contributions: All authors provided intellectual input and improvements, discussed the information, and revised the manuscript. A.P.-R. and R.L.-V. wrote the paper, and L.B. provided funding and intellectual input. C.A.-L. and M.C. provided intellectual input and revised the manuscript. All authors have read and agreed to the published version of the manuscript.

Funding: This work has been supported by: PID2020-113238RB-I00 from MICIN/AEI 13039/501100011033, and Centro de Investigación Biomédica en Red en Enfermedades Cardiovasculares (CB16/11/00222) and Enfermedades Hepáticas y Digestivas (CB17/04/00023) from the Instituto de Salud Carlos III (co-financed by the European Development Regional Fund "A Way to Achieve Europe", by the "European Union" and by the "European Union NextGeneration EU/PRTR"); Comunidad de Madrid Programa Biociencias (S2022-BMD-7223).

Institutional Review Board Statement: Not applicable.

Acknowledgments: The authors would like to thank Álvar Povo Retana for his help in the design of Figures 3 and 4.

Conflicts of Interest: The authors declare no conflicts of interest.

References

1. Mauro, M.; Lazzara, V.; Punginelli, D.; Arizza, V.; Vazzana, M. Antitumoral Compounds from Vertebrate Sister Group: A Review of Mediterranean Ascidians. *Dev. Comp. Immunol.* **2020**, *108*, 103669. [CrossRef]
2. Dou, X.; Dong, B. Origins and Bioactivities of Natural Compounds Derived from Marine Ascidians and Their Symbionts. *Mar. Drugs* **2019**, *17*, 670. [CrossRef]
3. Casertano, M.; Menna, M.; Imperatore, C. The Ascidian-Derived Metabolites with Antimicrobial Properties. *Antibiotics* **2020**, *9*, 510. [CrossRef] [PubMed]
4. Watters, D.J. Ascidian Toxins with Potential for Drug Development. *Mar. Drugs* **2018**, *16*, 162. [CrossRef] [PubMed]
5. Conte, M.; Fontana, E.; Nebbioso, A.; Altucci, L. Marine-Derived Secondary Metabolites as Promising Epigenetic Bio-Compounds for Anticancer Therapy. *Mar. Drugs* **2020**, *19*, 15. [CrossRef] [PubMed]
6. Wang, E.; Sorolla, M.A.; Gopal Krishnan, P.D.; Sorolla, A. From Seabed to Bedside: A Review on Promising Marine Anticancer Compounds. *Biomolecules* **2020**, *10*, 248. [CrossRef] [PubMed]
7. Gao, Y.; Tu, N.; Liu, X.; Lu, K.; Chen, S.; Guo, J. Progress in the Total Synthesis of Antitumor Tetrahydroisoquinoline Alkaloids. *Chem. Biodivers.* **2023**, *20*, e202300172. [CrossRef] [PubMed]
8. Amoutzias, G.; Chaliotis, A.; Mossialos, D. Discovery Strategies of Bioactive Compounds Synthesized by Nonribosomal Peptide Synthetases and Type-I Polyketide Synthases Derived from Marine Microbiomes. *Mar. Drugs* **2016**, *14*, 80. [CrossRef]
9. Le, V.H.; Inai, M.; Williams, R.M.; Kan, T. Ecteinascidins. A Review of the Chemistry, Biology and Clinical Utility of Potent Tetrahydroisoquinoline Antitumor Antibiotics. *Nat. Prod. Rep.* **2015**, *32*, 328–347. [CrossRef]
10. Matos, A.; Antunes, A. Symbiotic Associations in Ascidians: Relevance for Functional Innovation and Bioactive Potential. *Mar. Drugs* **2021**, *19*, 370. [CrossRef]
11. Gordon, T.; Shenkar, N. Solitary Ascidians as Model Organisms in Regenerative Biology Studies. *Results Probl. Cell Differ.* **2018**, *65*, 321–336. [CrossRef]
12. Aune, G.J.; Furuta, T.; Pommier, Y. Ecteinascidin 743: A Novel Anticancer Drug with a Unique Mechanism of Action. *Anticancer Drugs* **2002**, *13*, 545–555. [CrossRef] [PubMed]
13. Sakai, R.; Rinehart, K.L.; Guan, Y.; Wang, A.H.J. Additional Antitumor Ecteinascidins from a Caribbean Tunicate: Crystal Structures and Activities in Vivo. *Proc. Natl. Acad. Sci. USA* **1992**, *89*, 11456–11460. [CrossRef] [PubMed]

14. D'Incalci, M.; Galmarini, C.M. A Review of Trabectedin (ET-743): A Unique Mechanism of Action. *Mol. Cancer Ther.* **2010**, *9*, 2157–2163. [CrossRef] [PubMed]
15. Cuevas, C.; Francesch, A. Development of Yondelis (Trabectedin, ET-743). A Semisynthetic Process Solves the Supply Problem. *Nat. Prod. Rep.* **2009**, *26*, 322–337. [CrossRef] [PubMed]
16. Soares, D.G.; Machado, M.S.; Rocca, C.J.; Poindessous, V.; Ouaret, D.; Sarasin, A.; Galmarini, C.M.; Henriques, J.A.P.; Escargueil, A.E.; Larsen, A.K. Trabectedin and Its C Subunit Modified Analogue PM01183 Attenuate Nucleotide Excision Repair and Show Activity toward Platinum-Resistant Cells. *Mol. Cancer Ther.* **2011**, *10*, 1481–1489. [CrossRef]
17. De Sanctis, R.; Jacobs, F.; Benvenuti, C.; Gaudio, M.; Franceschini, R.; Tancredi, R.; Pedrazzoli, P.; Santoro, A.; Zambelli, A. From Seaside to Bedside: Current Evidence and Future Perspectives in the Treatment of Breast Cancer Using Marine Compounds. *Front. Pharmacol.* **2022**, *13*, 909566. [CrossRef]
18. Markham, A. Lurbinectedin: First Approval. *Drugs* **2020**, *80*, 1345–1353. [CrossRef]
19. Pignata, S.; Pisano, C.; Di Napoli, M.; Cecere, S.C.; Tambaro, R.; Attademo, L. Treatment of Recurrent Epithelial Ovarian Cancer. *Cancer* **2019**, *125*, 4609–4615. [CrossRef]
20. Monk, B.J.; Herzog, T.J.; Wang, G.; Triantos, S.; Maul, S.; Knoblauch, R.; McGowan, T.; Shalaby, W.S.W.; Coleman, R.L. A Phase 3 Randomized, Open-Label, Multicenter Trial for Safety and Efficacy of Combined Trabectedin and Pegylated Liposomal Doxorubicin Therapy for Recurrent Ovarian Cancer. *Gynecol. Oncol.* **2020**, *156*, 535–544. [CrossRef]
21. D'Incalci, M. Trabectedin Mechanism of Action: What's New? *Future Oncol.* **2013**, *9*, 5–10. [CrossRef] [PubMed]
22. Sheng, J.Y.; Movva, S. Systemic Therapy for Advanced Soft Tissue Sarcoma. *Surg. Clin. N. Am.* **2016**, *96*, 1141–1156. [CrossRef] [PubMed]
23. Nakamura, T.; Sudo, A. The Role of Trabectedin in Soft Tissue Sarcoma. *Front. Pharmacol.* **2022**, *13*, 777872. [CrossRef]
24. Miwa, S.; Yamamoto, N.; Hayashi, K.; Takeuchi, A.; Igarashi, K.; Tsuchiya, H. Therapeutic Targets for Bone and Soft-Tissue Sarcomas. *Int. J. Mol. Sci.* **2019**, *20*, 170. [CrossRef] [PubMed]
25. Meyer, M.; Seetharam, M. First-Line Therapy for Metastatic Soft Tissue Sarcoma. *Curr. Treat. Options Oncol.* **2019**, *20*, 6. [CrossRef] [PubMed]
26. Andreeva-Gateva, P.; Chakar, S. The Place of Trabectedin in the Treatment of Soft Tissue Sarcoma: An Umbrella Review of the Level One Evidence. *Expert Opin. Orphan Drugs* **2019**, *7*, 105–115. [CrossRef]
27. Morioka, H.; Takahashi, S.; Araki, N.; Sugiura, H.; Ueda, T.; Takahashi, M.; Yonemoto, T.; Hiraga, H.; Hiruma, T.; Kunisada, T.; et al. Results of Sub-Analysis of a Phase 2 Study on Trabectedin Treatment for Extraskeletal Myxoid Chondrosarcoma and Mesenchymal Chondrosarcoma. *BMC Cancer* **2016**, *16*, 479. [CrossRef]
28. Rubio, M.J.; Lecumberri, M.J.; Varela, S.; Alarcón, J.; Ortega, M.E.; Gaba, L.; Espinós, J.; Calzas, J.; Barretina, P.; Ruiz, I.; et al. Efficacy and Safety of Trabectedin in Metastatic Uterine Leiomyosarcoma: A Retrospective Multicenter Study of the Spanish Ovarian Cancer Research Group (GEICO). *Gynecol. Oncol. Rep.* **2020**, *33*, 100594. [CrossRef]
29. Jones, R.L.; Maki, R.G.; Patel, S.R.; Wang, G.; McGowan, T.A.; Shalaby, W.S.; Knoblauch, R.E.; von Mehren, M.; Demetri, G.D. Safety and Efficacy of Trabectedin When Administered in the Inpatient versus Outpatient Setting: Clinical Considerations for Outpatient Administration of Trabectedin. *Cancer* **2019**, *125*, 4435–4441. [CrossRef]
30. Vincenzi, B.; Napolitano, A.; Comandone, A.; Sanfilippo, R.; Celant, S.; Olimpieri, P.P.; Di Segni, S.; Russo, P.; Casali, P.G. Trabectedin Use in Soft-Tissue Sarcoma Patients in a Real-World Setting: Data from an Italian National Drug-Access Registry. *Int. J. Cancer* **2023**, *152*, 761–768. [CrossRef]
31. Zhou, M.Y.; Bui, N.Q.; Charville, G.W.; Ganjoo, K.N.; Pan, M. Treatment of De-Differentiated Liposarcoma in the Era of Immunotherapy. *Int. J. Mol. Sci.* **2023**, *24*, 9571. [CrossRef] [PubMed]
32. Nassif, E.F.; Keung, E.Z.; Thirasastr, P.; Somaiah, N. Myxoid Liposarcomas: Systemic Treatment Options. *Curr. Treat. Options Oncol.* **2023**, *24*, 274–291. [CrossRef] [PubMed]
33. Thirasastr, P.; Lin, H.; Amini, B.; Wang, W.L.; Cloutier, J.M.; Nassif, E.F.; Keung, E.Z.; Roland, C.L.; Feig, B.; Araujo, D.; et al. Retrospective Evaluation of the Role of Gemcitabine-Docetaxel in Well-Differentiated and Dedifferentiated Liposarcoma. *Cancer Med.* **2023**, *12*, 4282–4293. [CrossRef] [PubMed]
34. Gutierrez-Sainz, L.; Martinez-Fdez, S.; Pedregosa-Barbas, J.; Peña, J.; Alameda, M.; Viñal, D.; Villamayor, J.; Martinez-Recio, S.; Perez-Wert, P.; Pertejo-Fernandez, A.; et al. Efficacy of Second and Third Lines of Treatment in Advanced Soft Tissue Sarcomas: A Real-World Study. *Clin. Transl. Oncol.* **2023**, *25*, 3519–3526. [CrossRef] [PubMed]
35. Patel, N.; Pokras, S.; Ferma, J.; Casey, V.; Manuguid, F.; Culver, K.; Bauer, S. Treatment Patterns and Outcomes in Patients with Metastatic Synovial Sarcoma in France, Germany, Italy, Spain and the UK. *Futur. Oncol.* **2023**, *19*, 1261–1275. [CrossRef] [PubMed]
36. Okazaki, M.; Katano, K.; Sugita, H.; Tokoro, T.; Gabata, R.; Takada, S.; Nakanuma, S.; Makino, I.; Yagi, S. Early Progression of a Pancreatic Metastasis of Synovial Sarcoma after Pancreatectomy. *Surg. Case Rep.* **2023**, *9*, 30. [CrossRef] [PubMed]
37. Fausti, V.; De Vita, A.; Vanni, S.; Ghini, V.; Gurrieri, L.; Riva, N.; Casadei, R.; Maraldi, M.; Ercolani, G.; Cavaliere, D.; et al. Systemic Inflammatory Indices in Second-Line Soft Tissue Sarcoma Patients: Focus on Lymphocyte/Monocyte Ratio and Trabectedin. *Cancers* **2023**, *15*, 1080. [CrossRef] [PubMed]
38. Farago, A.F.; Drapkin, B.J.; Lopez-Vilarino de Ramos, J.A.; Galmarini, C.M.; Núñez, R.; Kahatt, C.; Paz-Ares, L. ATLANTIS: A Phase III Study of Lurbinectedin/Doxorubicin versus Topotecan or Cyclophosphamide/Doxorubicin/Vincristine in Patients with Small-Cell Lung Cancer Who Have Failed One Prior Platinum-Containing Line. *Future Oncol.* **2019**, *15*, 231–239. [CrossRef]

39. Poveda, A.; Del Campo, J.M.; Ray-Coquard, I.; Alexandre, J.; Provansal, M.; Guerra Alía, E.M.; Casado, A.; Gonzalez-Martin, A.; Fernández, C.; Rodriguez, I.; et al. Phase II Randomized Study of PM01183 versus Topotecan in Patients with Platinum-Resistant/Refractory Advanced Ovarian Cancer. *Ann. Oncol.* **2017**, *28*, 1280–1287. [CrossRef]
40. Cruz, C.; Llop-Guevara, A.; Garber, J.E.; Arun, B.K.; Pérez Fidalgo, J.A.; Lluch, A.; Telli, M.L.; Fernández, C.; Kahatt, C.; Galmarini, C.M.; et al. Multicenter Phase II Study of Lurbinectedin in BRCA-Mutated and Unselected Metastatic Advanced Breast Cancer and Biomarker Assessment Substudy. *J. Clin. Oncol.* **2018**, *36*, 3134–3143. [CrossRef]
41. Cote, G.M.; Choy, E.; Chen, T.; Marino-Enriquez, A.; Morgan, J.; Merriam, P.; Thornton, K.; Wagner, A.J.; Nathenson, M.J.; Demetri, G.; et al. A Phase II Multi-Strata Study of Lurbinectedin as a Single Agent or in Combination with Conventional Chemotherapy in Metastatic and/or Unresectable Sarcomas. *Eur. J. Cancer* **2020**, *126*, 21–32. [CrossRef] [PubMed]
42. Benton, C.B.; Chien, K.S.; Tefferi, A.; Rodriguez, J.; Ravandi, F.; Daver, N.; Jabbour, E.; Jain, N.; Alvarado, Y.; Kwari, M.; et al. Safety and Tolerability of Lurbinectedin (PM01183) in Patients with Acute Myeloid Leukemia and Myelodysplastic Syndrome. *Hematol. Oncol.* **2019**, *37*, 96–102. [CrossRef] [PubMed]
43. Risnik, D.; Colado, A.; Podaza, E.; Almejún, M.B.; Elías, E.E.; Bezares, R.F.; Fernández-Grecco, H.; Seija, N.; Oppezzo, P.; Borge, M.; et al. Immunoregulatory Effects of Lurbinectedin in Chronic Lymphocytic Leukemia. *Cancer Immunol. Immunother.* **2020**, *69*, 813–824. [CrossRef] [PubMed]
44. Allavena, P.; Belgiovine, C.; Digifico, E.; Frapolli, R.; D'Incalci, M. Effects of the Anti-Tumor Agents Trabectedin and Lurbinectedin on Immune Cells of the Tumor Microenvironment. *Front. Oncol.* **2022**, *12*, 851790. [CrossRef] [PubMed]
45. Gadducci, A.; Cosio, S. Trabectedin and Lurbinectedin: Mechanisms of Action, Clinical Impact, and Future Perspectives in Uterine and Soft Tissue Sarcoma, Ovarian Carcinoma, and Endometrial Carcinoma. *Front. Oncol.* **2022**, *12*, 914342. [CrossRef] [PubMed]
46. D'Incalci, M.; Zambelli, A. Trabectedin for the Treatment of Breast Cancer. *Expert Opin. Investig. Drugs* **2016**, *25*, 105–115. [CrossRef]
47. Hurley, L.H.; Zewail-Foote, M. The Antitumor Agent Ecteinascidin 743: Characterization of Its Covalent DNA Adducts and Chemical Stability. *Adv. Exp. Med. Biol.* **2001**, *500*, 289–299. [CrossRef]
48. Tumini, E.; Herrera-Moyano, E.; San Martín-Alonso, M.; Barroso, S.; Galmarini, C.M.; Aguilera, A. The Antitumor Drugs Trabectedin and Lurbinectedin Induce Transcription-Dependent Replication Stress and Genome Instability. *Mol. Cancer Res.* **2019**, *17*, 773–782. [CrossRef]
49. Santamaría Nuñez, G.; Robles, C.M.G.; Giraudon, C.; Martínez-Leal, J.F.; Compe, E.; Coin, F.; Aviles, P.; Galmarini, C.M.; Egly, J.-M. Lurbinectedin Specifically Triggers the Degradation of Phosphorylated RNA Polymerase II and the Formation of DNA Breaks in Cancer Cells. *Mol. Cancer Ther.* **2016**, *15*, 2399–2412. [CrossRef]
50. Damia, G.; Silvestri, S.; Carrassa, L.; Filiberti, L.; Faircloth, G.T.; Liberi, G.; Foiani, M.; D'Incalci, M. Unique Pattern of ET-743 Activity in Different Cellular Systems with Defined Deficiencies in DNA-Repair Pathways. *Int. J. Cancer* **2001**, *92*, 583–588. [CrossRef]
51. Laroche, A.; Chaire, V.; Le Loarer, F.; Algéo, M.P.; Rey, C.; Tran, K.; Lucchesi, C.; Italiano, A. Activity of Trabectedin and the PARP Inhibitor Rucaparib in Soft-Tissue Sarcomas. *J. Hematol. Oncol.* **2017**, *10*, 84. [CrossRef] [PubMed]
52. Herrero, A.B.; Martín-Castellanos, C.; Marco, E.; Gago, F.; Moreno, S. Cross-Talk between Nucleotide Excision and Homologous Recombination DNA Repair Pathways in the Mechanism of Action of Antitumor Trabectedin. *Cancer Res.* **2006**, *66*, 8155–8162. [CrossRef] [PubMed]
53. Allavena, P.; Signorelli, M.; Chieppa, M.; Erba, E.; Bianchi, G.; Marchesi, F.; Olimpio, C.O.; Bonardi, C.; Garbi, A.; Lissoni, A.; et al. Anti-Inflammatory Properties of the Novel Antitumor Agent Yondelis (Trabectedin): Inhibition of Macrophage Differentiation and Cytokine Production. *Cancer Res.* **2005**, *65*, 2964–2971. [CrossRef] [PubMed]
54. Bonfanti, M.; La Valle, E.; Fernandez Sousa Faro, J.M.; Faircloth, G.; Caretti, G.; Mantovani, R.; D'Incalci, M. Effect of Ecteinascidin-743 on the Interaction between DNA Binding Proteins and DNA. *Anticancer Drug Des.* **1999**, *14*, 179–186.
55. D'Incalci, M.; Brunelli, D.; Marangon, E.; Simone, M.; Tavecchio, M.; Gescher, A.; Mantovani, R. Modulation of Gene Transcription by Natural Products—A Viable Anticancer Strategy. *Curr. Pharm. Des.* **2007**, *13*, 2744–2750. [CrossRef] [PubMed]
56. Jin, S.; Gorfajn, B.; Faircloth, G.; Scotto, K.W. Ecteinascidin 743, a Transcription-Targeted Chemotherapeutic That Inhibits MDR1 Activation. *Proc. Natl. Acad. Sci. USA* **2000**, *97*, 6775–6779. [CrossRef]
57. Barthomeuf, C.; Bourguet-Kondracki, M.-L.; Kornprobst, J.-M. Marine Metabolites Overcoming or Circumventing Multidrug Resistance Mediated by ATP-Dependent Transporters: A New Hope for Patient with Tumors Resistant to Conventional Chemotherapy. *Anticancer Agents Med. Chem.* **2012**, *8*, 886–903. [CrossRef] [PubMed]
58. Robey, R.W.; Pluchino, K.M.; Hall, M.D.; Fojo, A.T.; Bates, S.E.; Gottesman, M.M. Revisiting the Role of Efflux Pumps in Multidrug-Resistant Cancer. *Nat. Rev. Cancer* **2019**, *18*, 452–464. [CrossRef]
59. Kodan, A.; Futamata, R.; Kimura, Y.; Kioka, N.; Nakatsu, T.; Kato, H.; Ueda, K. ABCB1/MDR1/P-Gp Employs an ATP-Dependent Twist-and-Squeeze Mechanism to Export Hydrophobic Drugs. *FEBS Lett.* **2021**, *595*, 707–716. [CrossRef]
60. Bossennec, M.; Di Roio, A.; Caux, C.; Ménétrier-Caux, C. MDR1 in Immunity: Friend or Foe? *Oncoimmunology* **2018**, *7*, e1499388. [CrossRef]
61. Erba, E.; Cavallaro, E.; Damia, G.; Mantovani, R.; Di Silvio, A.; Di Francesco, A.M.; Riccardi, R.; Cuevas, C.; Faircloth, G.T.; D'Incalci, M. The Unique Biological Features of the Marine Product Yondelis (ET-743, Trabectedin) Are Shared by Its Analog ET-637, Which Lacks the C Ring. *Oncol. Res.* **2004**, *14*, 579–587. [CrossRef] [PubMed]

62. Larsen, A.K.; Galmarini, C.M.; D'Incalci, M. Unique Features of Trabectedin Mechanism of Action. *Cancer Chemother. Pharmacol.* **2016**, *77*, 663–671. [CrossRef] [PubMed]
63. Aune, G.J.; Takagi, K.; Sordet, O.; Guirouilh-Barbat, J.; Antony, S.; Bohr, V.A.; Pommier, Y. Von Hippel-Lindau-Coupled and Transcription-Coupled Nucleotide Excision Repair-Dependent Degradation of RNA Polymerase II in Response to Trabectedin. *Clin. Cancer Res.* **2008**, *14*, 6449–6455. [CrossRef] [PubMed]
64. Feuerhahn, S.; Giraudon, C.; Martínez-Díez, M.; Bueren-Calabuig, J.A.; Galmarini, C.M.; Gago, F.; Egly, J.-M. XPF-Dependent DNA Breaks and RNA Polymerase II Arrest Induced by Antitumor DNA Interstrand Crosslinking-Mimetic Alkaloids. *Chem. Biol.* **2011**, *18*, 988–999. [CrossRef] [PubMed]
65. Belgiovine, C.; Bello, E.; Liguori, M.; Craparotta, I.; Mannarino, L.; Paracchini, L.; Beltrame, L.; Marchini, S.; Galmarini, C.M.; Mantovani, A.; et al. Lurbinectedin Reduces Tumour-Associated Macrophages and the Inflammatory Tumour Microenvironment in Preclinical Models. *Br. J. Cancer* **2017**, *117*, 628–638. [CrossRef] [PubMed]
66. Martínez-Serra, J.; Maffiotte, E.; Martín, J.; Bex, T.; Navarro-Palou, M.; Ros, T.; Plazas, J.M.; Vögler, O.; Gutiérrez, A.; Amat, J.C.; et al. Yondelis® (ET-743, Trabectedin) Sensitizes Cancer Cell Lines to CD95-Mediated Cell Death: New Molecular Insight into the Mechanism of Action. *Eur. J. Pharmacol.* **2011**, *658*, 57–64. [CrossRef] [PubMed]
67. Atmaca, H.; Bozkurt, E.; Uzunoglu, S.; Uslu, R.; Karaca, B. A Diverse Induction of Apoptosis by Trabectedin in MCF-7 (HER2-/ER+) and MDA-MB-453 (HER2+/ER-) Breast Cancer Cells. *Toxicol. Lett.* **2013**, *221*, 128–136. [CrossRef]
68. Petty, W.J.; Paz-Ares, L. Emerging Strategies for the Treatment of Small Cell Lung Cancer: A Review. *JAMA Oncol.* **2023**, *9*, 419–429. [CrossRef]
69. Bhamidipati, D.; Subbiah, V. Lurbinectedin, a DNA Minor Groove Inhibitor for Neuroendocrine Neoplasms beyond Small Cell Lung Cancer. *Oncoscience* **2023**, *10*, 22–23. [CrossRef]
70. Fudio, S.; Pérez-Ramos, L.; Asín-Prieto, E.; Zeaiter, A.; Lubomirov, R. A Model-Based Head-to-Head Comparison of Single-Agent Lurbinectedin in the Pivotal ATLANTIS Study. *Front. Oncol.* **2023**, *13*, 1152371. [CrossRef]
71. Germano, G.; Mantovani, A.; Allavena, P. Targeting of the Innate Immunity/Inflammation as Complementary Anti-Tumor Therapies. *Ann. Med.* **2011**, *43*, 581–593. [CrossRef] [PubMed]
72. Céspedes, M.V.; Guillén, M.J.; López-Casas, P.P.; Sarno, F.; Gallardo, A.; Álamo, P.; Cuevas, C.; Hidalgo, M.; Galmarini, C.M.; Allavena, P.; et al. Lurbinectedin Induces Depletion of Tumor-Associated Macrophages, an Essential Component of Its in Vivo Synergism with Gemcitabine, in Pancreatic Adenocarcinoma Mouse Models. *Dis. Model. Mech.* **2016**, *9*, 1461–1471. [CrossRef] [PubMed]
73. Allavena, P.; Germano, G.; Belgiovine, C.; D'Incalci, M.; Mantovani, A. Trabectedin: A Drug from the Sea That Strikes Tumor-Associated Macrophages. *Oncoimmunology* **2013**, *2*, e24614. [CrossRef] [PubMed]
74. Colmegna, B.; Uboldi, S.; Frapolli, R.; Licandro, S.A.; Panini, N.; Galmarini, C.M.; Badri, N.; Spanswick, V.J.; Bingham, J.P.; Kiakos, K.; et al. Increased Sensitivity to Platinum Drugs of Cancer Cells with Acquired Resistance to Trabectedin. *Br. J. Cancer* **2015**, *113*, 1687–1693. [CrossRef]
75. Germano, G.; Frapolli, R.; Simone, M.; Tavecchio, M.; Erba, E.; Pesce, S.; Pasqualini, F.; Grosso, F.; Sanfilippo, R.; Casali, P.G.; et al. Antitumor and Anti-Inflammatory Effects of Trabectedin on Human Myxoid Liposarcoma Cells. *Cancer Res.* **2010**, *70*, 2235–2244. [CrossRef] [PubMed]
76. Germano, G.; Frapolli, R.; Belgiovine, C.; Anselmo, A.; Pesce, S.; Liguori, M.; Erba, E.; Uboldi, S.; Zucchetti, M.; Pasqualini, F.; et al. Role of Macrophage Targeting in the Antitumor Activity of Trabectedin. *Cancer Cell* **2013**, *23*, 249–262. [CrossRef] [PubMed]
77. Castelli, C.; Rivoltini, L.; Rodolfo, M.; Tazzari, M.; Belgiovine, C.; Allavena, P. Modulation of the Myeloid Compartment of the Immune System by Angiogenic- and Kinase Inhibitor-Targeted Anti-Cancer Therapies. *Cancer Immunol. Immunother.* **2015**, *64*, 83–89. [CrossRef] [PubMed]
78. Peraza, D.A.; Povo-Retana, A.; Mojena, M.; García-Redondo, A.B.; Avilés, P.; Boscá, L.; Valenzuela, C. Trabectedin Modulates Macrophage Polarization in the Tumor-Microenvironment. Role of KV1.3 and KV1.5 Channels. *Biomed. Pharmacother.* **2023**, *161*, 114548. [CrossRef]
79. Yokoi, E.; Mabuchi, S.; Shimura, K.; Komura, N.; Kozasa, K.; Kuroda, H.; Takahashi, R.; Sasano, T.; Kawano, M.; Matsumoto, Y.; et al. Lurbinectedin (PM01183), a Selective Inhibitor of Active Transcription, Effectively Eliminates Both Cancer Cells and Cancer Stem Cells in Preclinical Models of Uterine Cervical Cancer. *Investig. New Drugs* **2019**, *37*, 818–827. [CrossRef]
80. Belgiovine, C.; Frapolli, R.; Liguori, M.; Digifico, E.; Colombo, F.S.; Meroni, M.; Allavena, P.; D'Incalci, M. Inhibition of Tumor-Associated Macrophages by Trabectedin Improves the Antitumor Adaptive Immunity in Response to Anti-PD-1 Therapy. *Eur. J. Immunol.* **2021**, *51*, 2677–2686. [CrossRef]
81. Trigo, J.; Subbiah, V.; Besse, B.; Moreno, V.; López, R.; Sala, M.A.; Peters, S.; Ponce, S.; Fernández, C.; Alfaro, V.; et al. Lurbinectedin as Second-Line Treatment for Patients with Small-Cell Lung Cancer: A Single-Arm, Open-Label, Phase 2 Basket Trial. *Lancet Oncol.* **2020**, *21*, 645–654. [CrossRef] [PubMed]
82. Subbiah, V.; Paz-Ares, L.; Besse, B.; Moreno, V.; Peters, S.; Sala, M.A.; López-Vilariño, J.A.; Fernández, C.; Kahatt, C.; Alfaro, V.; et al. Antitumor Activity of Lurbinectedin in Second-Line Small Cell Lung Cancer Patients Who Are Candidates for Re-Challenge with the First-Line Treatment. *Lung Cancer* **2020**, *150*, 90–96. [CrossRef] [PubMed]
83. Metaxas, Y.; Kahatt, C.; Alfaro, V.; Fudio, S.; Zeaiter, A.; Plummer, R.; Sessa, C.; Von Moos, R.; Forster, M.; Stathis, A. A Phase I Trial of Lurbinectedin in Combination with Cisplatin in Patients with Advanced Solid Tumors. *Investig. New Drugs* **2022**, *40*, 91–98. [CrossRef]

84. Jones, J.D.; Sinder, B.P.; Paige, D.; Soki, F.N.; Koh, A.J.; Thiele, S.; Shiozawa, Y.; Hofbauer, L.C.; Daignault, S.; Roca, H.; et al. Trabectedin Reduces Skeletal Prostate Cancer Tumor Size in Association with Effects on M2 Macrophages and Efferocytosis. *Neoplasia* **2019**, *21*, 172–184. [CrossRef] [PubMed]
85. Sinder, B.P.; Zweifler, L.; Koh, A.J.; Michalski, M.N.; Hofbauer, L.C.; Aguirre, J.I.; Roca, H.; McCauley, L.K. Bone Mass Is Compromised by the Chemotherapeutic Trabectedin in Association With Effects on Osteoblasts and Macrophage Efferocytosis. *J. Bone Miner. Res.* **2017**, *32*, 2116–2127. [CrossRef] [PubMed]
86. Povo-Retana, A.; Mojena, M.; Stremtan, A.B.; Fernández-García, V.B.; Gómez-Sáez, A.; Nuevo-Tapioles, C.; Molina-Guijarro, J.M.; Avendaño-Ortiz, J.; Cuezva, J.M.; López-Collazo, E.; et al. Specific Effects of Trabectedin and Lurbinectedin on Human Macrophage Function and Fate—Novel Insights. *Cancers* **2020**, *12*, 3060. [CrossRef] [PubMed]
87. Gardner, A.; Ruffell, B. Dendritic Cells and Cancer Immunity. *Trends Immunol.* **2016**, *37*, 855–865. [CrossRef]
88. Gardner, A.; de Mingo Pulido, Á.; Ruffell, B. Dendritic Cells and Their Role in Immunotherapy. *Front. Immunol.* **2020**, *11*, 924. [CrossRef]
89. Wculek, S.K.; Cueto, F.J.; Mujal, A.M.; Melero, I.; Krummel, M.F.; Sancho, D. Dendritic Cells in Cancer Immunology and Immunotherapy. *Nat. Rev. Immunol.* **2020**, *20*, 7–24. [CrossRef]
90. Marciscano, A.E.; Anandasabapathy, N. The Role of Dendritic Cells in Cancer and Anti-Tumor Immunity. *Semin. Immunol.* **2021**, *52*, 101481. [CrossRef]
91. Mitchell, D.; Chintala, S.; Dey, M. Plasmacytoid Dendritic Cell in Immunity and Cancer. *J. Neuroimmunol.* **2018**, *322*, 63–73. [CrossRef] [PubMed]
92. Fu, C.; Jiang, A. Dendritic Cells and CD8 T Cell Immunity in Tumor Microenvironment. *Front. Immunol.* **2018**, *9*, 3059. [CrossRef] [PubMed]
93. Oshiro, H.; Tome, Y.; Kiyuna, T.; Miyake, K.; Kawaguchi, K.; Higuchi, T.; Miyake, M.; Zang, Z.; Razmjooei, S.; Barangi, M.; et al. Temozolomide Targets and Arrests a Doxorubicin-Resistant Follicular Dendritic-Cell Sarcoma Patient-Derived Orthotopic Xenograft Mouse Model. *Tissue Cell* **2019**, *58*, 17–23. [CrossRef] [PubMed]
94. Kuroda, H.; Mabuchi, S.; Kozasa, K.; Yokoi, E.; Matsumoto, Y.; Komura, N.; Kawano, M.; Hashimoto, K.; Sawada, K.; Kimura, T. PM01183 Inhibits Myeloid-Derived Suppressor Cells In Vitro and In Vivo. *Immunotherapy* **2017**, *9*, 805–817. [CrossRef] [PubMed]
95. Viola, A.; Munari, F.; Sánchez-Rodríguez, R.; Scolaro, T.; Castegna, A. The Metabolic Signature of Macrophage Responses. *Front. Immunol.* **2019**, *10*, 1462. [CrossRef]
96. Povo-Retana, A.; Fariñas, M.; Landauro-Vera, R.; Mojena, M.; Alvarez-Lucena, C.; Fernández-Moreno, M.A.; Castrillo, A.; de la Rosa Medina, J.V.; Sánchez-García, S.; Foguet, C.; et al. Immunometabolic Actions of Trabectedin and Lurbinectedin on Human Macrophages: Relevance for Their Anti-Tumor Activity. *Front. Immunol.* **2023**, *14*, 1211068. [CrossRef] [PubMed]
97. O'Neill, L.A.J.; Pearce, E.J. Immunometabolism Governs Dendritic Cell and Macrophage Function. *J. Exp. Med.* **2016**, *213*, 15–23. [CrossRef] [PubMed]
98. Povo-Retana, A.; Landauro-Vera, R.; Fariñas, M.; Sánchez-García, S.; Alvarez-Lucena, C.; Marin, S.; Cascante, M.; Boscá, L. Defining the Metabolic Signatures Associated with Human Macrophage Polarisation. *Biochem. Soc. Trans.* **2023**, *51*, 1429–1436. [CrossRef]
99. Cucè, M.; Gallo Cantafio, M.E.; Siciliano, M.A.; Riillo, C.; Caracciolo, D.; Scionti, F.; Staropoli, N.; Zuccalà, V.; Maltese, L.; Di Vito, A.; et al. Trabectedin Triggers Direct and NK-Mediated Cytotoxicity in Multiple Myeloma. *J. Hematol. Oncol.* **2019**, *12*, 32. [CrossRef]
100. Banerjee, P.; Zhang, R.; Ivan, C.; Galletti, G.; Clise-Dwyer, K.; Barbaglio, F.; Scarfò, L.; Aracil, M.; Klein, C.; Wierda, W.; et al. Trabectedin Reveals a Strategy of Immunomodulation in Chronic Lymphocytic Leukemia. *Cancer Immunol. Res.* **2019**, *7*, 2036–2051. [CrossRef]
101. Spriano, F.; Chung, E.Y.; Panini, N.; Cascione, L.; Rinaldi, A.; Erba, E.; Stathis, A.; D'Incalci, M.; Bertoni, F.; Gatta, R. Trabectedin Is a Novel Chemotherapy Agent for Diffuse Large B Cell Lymphoma. *Br. J. Haematol.* **2019**, *184*, 1022–1025. [CrossRef] [PubMed]
102. Bailly, C.; Thuru, X.; Quesnel, B. Survey and Summary: Combined Cytotoxic Chemotherapy and Immunotherapy of Cancer: Modern Times. *NAR Cancer* **2020**, *2*, zcaa002. [CrossRef] [PubMed]
103. Zhao, T.; Zhu, Y.; Morinibu, A.; Kobayashi, M.; Shinomiya, K.; Itasaka, S.; Yoshimura, M.; Guo, G.; Hiraoka, M.; Harada, H. HIF-1-Mediated Metabolic Reprogramming Reduces ROS Levels and Facilitates the Metastatic Colonization of Cancers in Lungs. *Sci. Rep.* **2014**, *4*, 3793. [CrossRef] [PubMed]
104. Cai, S.; Ding, Z.; Liu, X.; Zeng, J. Trabectedin Induces Ferroptosis via Regulation of HIF-1α/IRP1/TFR1 and Keap1/Nrf2/GPX4 Axis in Non-Small Cell Lung Cancer Cells. *Chem. Biol. Interact.* **2023**, *369*, 110262. [CrossRef]
105. Rashid, R.S.M.; Temurlu, S.; Abourajab, A.; Karsili, P.; Dinleyici, M.; Al-Khateeb, B.; Icil, H. Drug Repurposing of FDA Compounds against α-Glucosidase for the Treatment of Type 2 Diabetes: Insights from Molecular Docking and Molecular Dynamics Simulations. *Pharmaceuticals* **2023**, *16*, 555. [CrossRef] [PubMed]
106. Pacifico, F.; Mellone, S.; D'Incalci, M.; Stornaiuolo, M.; Leonardi, A.; Crescenzi, E. Trabectedin Suppresses Escape from Therapy-Induced Senescence in Tumor Cells by Interfering with Glutamine Metabolism. *Biochem. Pharmacol.* **2022**, *202*, 115159. [CrossRef] [PubMed]

107. Toulmonde, M.; Brahmi, M.; Giraud, A.; Chakiba, C.; Bessede, A.; Kind, M.; Toulza, E.; Pulido, M.; Albert, S.; Guégan, J.P.; et al. Trabectedin plus Durvalumab in Patients with Advanced Pretreated Soft Tissue Sarcoma and Ovarian Carcinoma (TRAMUNE): An Open-Label, Multicenter Phase Ib Study. *Clin. Cancer Res.* **2022**, *28*, 1765–1772. [CrossRef] [PubMed]
108. Chawla, S.P.; Tellez, W.A.; Chomoyan, H.; Valencia, C.; Ahari, A.; Omelchenko, N.; Makrievski, S.; Brigham, D.A.; Chua-Alcala, V.; Quon, D.; et al. Activity of TNT: A Phase 2 Study Using Talimogene Laherparepvec, Nivolumab and Trabectedin for Previously Treated Patients with Advanced Sarcomas (NCT# 03886311). *Front. Oncol.* **2023**, *13*, 1116937. [CrossRef]
109. Gordon, E.M.; Chawla, S.P.; Tellez, W.A.; Younesi, E.; Thomas, S.; Chua-Alcala, V.S.; Chomoyan, H.; Valencia, C.; Brigham, D.A.; Moradkhani, A.; et al. SAINT: A Phase I/Expanded Phase II Study Using Safe Amounts of Ipilimumab, Nivolumab and Trabectedin as First-Line Treatment of Advanced Soft Tissue Sarcoma. *Cancers* **2023**, *15*, 906. [CrossRef]
110. Wagner, M.J.; Zhang, Y.; Cranmer, L.D.; Loggers, E.T.; Black, G.; McDonnell, S.; Maxwell, S.; Johnson, R.; Moore, R.; De Viveiros, P.H.; et al. A Phase 1/2 Trial Combining Avelumab and Trabectedin for Advanced Liposarcoma and Leiomyosarcoma. *Clin. Cancer Res.* **2022**, *28*, 2306–2312. [CrossRef]
111. Ávila-Arroyo, S.; Nuñez, G.S.; García-Fernández, L.F.; Galmarini, C.M. Synergistic Effect of Trabectedin and Olaparib Combination Regimen in Breast Cancer Cell Lines. *J. Breast Cancer* **2015**, *18*, 329–338. [CrossRef] [PubMed]
112. Grignani, G.; D'Ambrosio, L.; Pignochino, Y.; Palmerini, E.; Zucchetti, M.; Boccone, P.; Aliberti, S.; Stacchiotti, S.; Bertulli, R.; Piana, R.; et al. Trabectedin and Olaparib in Patients with Advanced and Non-Resectable Bone and Soft-Tissue Sarcomas (TOMAS): An Open-Label, Phase 1b Study from the Italian Sarcoma Group. *Lancet Oncol.* **2018**, *19*, 1360–1371. [CrossRef] [PubMed]
113. Ordóñez, J.L.; Amaral, A.T.; Carcaboso, A.M.; Herrero-Martín, D.; Del Carmen García-Macías, M.; Sevillano, V.; Alonso, D.; Pascual-Pasto, G.; San-Segundo, L.; Vila-Ubach, M.; et al. The PARP Inhibitor Olaparib Enhances the Sensitivity of Ewing Sarcoma to Trabectedin. *Oncotarget* **2015**, *6*, 18875–18890. [CrossRef]
114. Obrador-Hevia, A.; Martinez-Font, E.; Felipe-Abrio, I.; Calabuig-Fariñas, S.; Serra-Sitjar, M.; López-Guerrero, J.A.; Ramos, R.; Alemany, R.; Martín-Broto, J. RG7112, a Small-Molecule Inhibitor of MDM2, Enhances Trabectedin Response in Soft Tissue Sarcomas. *Cancer Investig.* **2015**, *33*, 440–450. [CrossRef] [PubMed]
115. Colombo, N.; Zaccarelli, E.; Baldoni, A.; Frezzini, S.; Scambia, G.; Palluzzi, E.; Tognon, G.; Lissoni, A.A.; Rubino, D.; Ferrero, A.; et al. Multicenter, Randomised, Open-Label, Non-Comparative Phase 2 Trial on the Efficacy and Safety of the Combination of Bevacizumab and Trabectedin with or without Carboplatin in Women with Partially Platinum-Sensitive Recurrent Ovarian Cancer. *Br. J. Cancer* **2019**, *121*, 744–750. [CrossRef] [PubMed]
116. Ghanim, B.; Baier, D.; Pirker, C.; Müllauer, L.; Sinn, K.; Lang, G.; Hoetzenecker, K.; Berger, W. Trabectedin Is Active against Two Novel, Patient-Derived Solitary Fibrous Pleural Tumor Cell Lines and Synergizes with Ponatinib. *Cancers* **2022**, *14*, 5602. [CrossRef] [PubMed]
117. Zeng, Z.; Lin, C.; Zhang, M.C.; Kossinna, P.; Wang, P.; Cao, D.; Wang, J.; Xu, M.; Wang, X.; Li, Q.; et al. Enterolactone and Trabectedin Suppress Epithelial Ovarian Cancer Synergistically via Upregulating THBS1. *Phyther. Res.* **2023**, *37*, 4722–4739. [CrossRef]
118. Casagrande, N.; Borghese, C.; Aldinucci, D. In Classical Hodgkin Lymphoma the Combination of the CCR5 Antagonist Maraviroc with Trabectedin Synergizes, Enhances DNA Damage and Decreases Three-Dimensional Tumor-Stroma Heterospheroid Viability. *Haematologica* **2022**, *107*, 287–291. [CrossRef]
119. Mabuchi, S.; Hisamatsu, T.; Kawase, C.; Hayashi, M.; Sawada, K.; Mimura, K.; Takahashi, K.; Takahashi, T.; Kurachi, H.; Kimura, T. The Activity of Trabectedin as a Single Agent or in Combination with Everolimus for Clear Cell Carcinoma of the Ovary. *Clin. Cancer Res.* **2011**, *17*, 4462–4473. [CrossRef]
120. Amaral, A.T.; Garofalo, C.; Frapolli, R.; Manara, M.C.; Mancarella, C.; Uboldi, S.; Di Giandomenico, S.; Ordóñez, J.L.; Sevillano, V.; Malaguarnera, R.; et al. Trabectedin Efficacy in Ewing Sarcoma Is Greatly Increased by Combination with Anti-IGF Signaling Agents. *Clin. Cancer Res.* **2015**, *21*, 1373–1382. [CrossRef]
121. Hoda, M.A.; Pirker, C.; Dong, Y.; Schelch, K.; Heffeter, P.; Kryeziu, K.; Van Schoonhoven, S.; Klikovits, T.; Laszlo, V.; Rozsas, A.; et al. Trabectedin Is Active against Malignant Pleural Mesothelioma Cell and Xenograft Models and Synergizes with Chemotherapy and Bcl-2 Inhibition in Vitro. *Mol. Cancer Ther.* **2016**, *15*, 2357–2369. [CrossRef] [PubMed]
122. Lima, M.; Bouzid, H.; Soares, D.G.; Selle, F.; Morel, C.; Galmarini, C.M.; Henriques, J.A.; Larsen, A.K.; Escargueil, A.E. Dual Inhibition of ATR and ATM Potentiates the Activity of Trabectedin and Lurbinectedin by Perturbing the DNA Damage Response and Homologous Recombination Repair. *Oncotarget* **2016**, *7*, 25885–25901. [CrossRef] [PubMed]
123. Frapolli, R.; Bello, E.; Ponzo, M.; Craparotta, I.; Mannarino, L.; Ballabio, S.; Marchini, S.; Carrassa, L.; Ubezio, P.; Porcu, L.; et al. Combination of PPARg Agonist Pioglitazone and Trabectedin Induce Adipocyte Differentiation to Overcome Trabectedin Resistance in Myxoid Liposarcomas. *Clin. Cancer Res.* **2019**, *25*, 7565–7575. [CrossRef] [PubMed]
124. Glinkina, K.; Nemati, F.; Teunisse, A.F.A.S.; Gelmi, M.C.; Etienne, V.; Kuipers, M.J.; Alsafadi, S.; Jager, M.J.; Decaudin, D.; Jochemsen, A.G. Preclinical Evaluation of Trabectedin in Combination with Targeted Inhibitors for Treatment of Metastatic Uveal Melanoma. *Investig. Ophthalmol. Vis. Sci.* **2022**, *63*, 14. [CrossRef] [PubMed]
125. Wang, X.; Wang, L.; Liu, W.; Liu, X.; Jia, X.; Feng, X.; Li, F.; Zhu, R.; Yu, J.; Zhang, H.; et al. Dose-Related Immunomodulatory Effects of Recombinant TRAIL in the Tumor Immune Microenvironment. *J. Exp. Clin. Cancer Res.* **2023**, *42*, 216. [CrossRef] [PubMed]

126. Zhu, G.; Zhao, M.; Han, Q.; Tan, Y.; Sun, Y.; Bouvet, M.; Clary, B.; Singh, S.R.; Ye, J.; Hoffman, R.M. Combination of Trabectedin with Irinotecan, Leucovorin and 5-Fluorouracil Arrests Primary Colorectal Cancer in an Imageable Patient-Derived Orthotopic Xenograft Mouse Model. *Anticancer Res.* **2019**, *39*, 6463–6470. [CrossRef] [PubMed]
127. Kawano, M.; Mabuchi, S.; Kishimoto, T.; Hisamatsu, T.; Matsumoto, Y.; Sasano, T.; Takahashi, R.; Sawada, K.; Takahashi, K.; Takahashi, T.; et al. Combination Treatment with Trabectedin and Irinotecan or Topotecan Has Synergistic Effects against Ovarian Clear Cell Carcinoma Cells. *Int. J. Gynecol. Cancer* **2014**, *24*, 829–837. [CrossRef] [PubMed]
128. Riccardi, A.; Meco, D.; Ubezio, P.; Mazzarella, G.; Marabese, M.; Faircloth, G.T.; Jimeno, J.; D'Incalci, M.; Riccardi, R. Combination of Trabectedin and Irinotecan Is Highly Effective in a Human Rhabdomyosarcoma Xenograft. *Anticancer Drugs* **2005**, *16*, 811–815. [CrossRef]
129. Higuchi, T.; Miyake, K.; Oshiro, H.; Sugisawa, N.; Yamamoto, N.; Hayashi, K.; Kimura, H.; Miwa, S.; Igarashi, K.; Chawla, S.P.; et al. Trabectedin and Irinotecan Combination Regresses a Cisplatinum-Resistant Osteosarcoma in a Patient-Derived Orthotopic Xenograft Nude-Mouse Model. *Biochem. Biophys. Res. Commun.* **2019**, *513*, 326–331. [CrossRef]
130. Zuco, V.; Pasquali, S.; Tortoreto, M.; Percio, S.; Doldi, V.; Barisella, M.; Collini, P.; Dagrada, G.P.; Brich, S.; Gasparini, P.; et al. Effectiveness of Irinotecan plus Trabectedin on a Desmoplastic Small Round Cell Tumor Patient-Derived Xenograft. *DMM Dis. Model. Mech.* **2023**, *16*, dmm049649. [CrossRef]
131. Ferrari, A.; Chiaravalli, S.; Bergamaschi, L.; Nigro, O.; Livellara, V.; Sironi, G.; Gasparini, P.; Pasquali, S.; Zaffaroni, N.; Stacchiotti, S.; et al. Trabectedin-Irinotecan, a Potentially Promising Combination in Relapsed Desmoplastic Small Round Cell Tumor: Report of Two Cases. *J. Chemother.* **2023**, *35*, 163–167. [CrossRef] [PubMed]
132. Martinez-Cruzado, L.; Tornin, J.; Rodriguez, A.; Santos, L.; Allonca, E.; Fernandez-Garcia, M.T.; Astudillo, A.; Garcia-Pedrero, J.M.; Rodriguez, R. Trabectedin and Camptothecin Synergistically Eliminate Cancer Stem Cells in Cell-of-Origin Sarcoma Models. *Neoplasia* **2017**, *19*, 460–470. [CrossRef] [PubMed]
133. Corbellari, R.; Nadal, L.; Villa, A.; Neri, D.; De Luca, R. The Immunocytokine L19-TNF Eradicates Sarcomas in Combination with Chemotherapy Agents or with Immune Check-Point Inhibitors. *Anticancer Drugs* **2020**, *31*, 799–805. [CrossRef] [PubMed]
134. Paz-Ares, L.; López-Pousa, A.; Poveda, A.; Balañá, C.; Ciruelos, E.; Bellmunt, J.; Del Muro, J.G.; Provencio, M.; Casado, A.; Rivera-Herrero, F.; et al. Trabectedin in Pre-Treated Patients with Advanced or Metastatic Soft Tissue Sarcoma: A Phase II Study Evaluating Co-Treatment with Dexamethasone. *Investig. New Drugs* **2012**, *30*, 729–740. [CrossRef] [PubMed]
135. Di Fonte, R.; Strippoli, S.; Garofoli, M.; Cormio, G.; Serratì, S.; Loizzi, V.; Fasano, R.; Arezzo, F.; Volpicella, M.; Derakhshani, A.; et al. Cervical Cancer Benefits from Trabectedin Combination with the β-Blocker Propranolol: In Vitro and Ex Vivo Evaluations in Patient-Derived Organoids. *Front. Cell Dev. Biol.* **2023**, *11*, 1178316. [CrossRef] [PubMed]
136. Martinez-Font, E.; Pérez-Capó, M.; Ramos, R.; Felipe, I.; Garcías, C.; Luna, P.; Terrasa, J.; Martín-Broto, J.; Vögler, O.; Alemany, R.; et al. Impact of Wnt/β-Catenin Inhibition on Cell Proliferation through Cdc25a Downregulation in Soft Tissue Sarcomas. *Cancers* **2020**, *12*, 2556. [CrossRef] [PubMed]
137. Harnicek, D.; Kampmann, E.; Lauber, K.; Hennel, R.; Cardoso Martins, A.S.; Guo, Y.; Belka, C.; Mörtl, S.; Gallmeier, E.; Kanaar, R.; et al. Hyperthermia Adds to Trabectedin Effectiveness and Thermal Enhancement Is Associated with BRCA2 Degradation and Impairment of DNA Homologous Recombination Repair. *Int. J. Cancer* **2016**, *139*, 467–479. [CrossRef] [PubMed]
138. Manda, K.; Präkelt, T.; Schröder, T.; Kriesen, S.; Hildebrandt, G. Radiosensitizing Effects of Trabectedin on Human A549 Lung Cancer Cells and HT-29 Colon Cancer Cells. *Investig. New Drugs* **2020**, *38*, 967–976. [CrossRef]
139. Hindi, N.; García, I.C.; Sánchez-Camacho, A.; Gutierrez, A.; Peinado, J.; Rincón, I.; Benedetti, J.; Sancho, P.; Santos, P.; Sánchez-Bustos, P.; et al. Trabectedin plus Radiotherapy for Advanced Soft-Tissue Sarcoma: Experience in Forty Patients Treated at a Sarcoma Reference Center. *Cancers* **2020**, *12*, 3740; Erratum in *Cancers* **2021**, *13*, 1557. [CrossRef]
140. Sanfilippo, R.; Hindi, N.; Cruz Jurado, J.; Blay, J.-Y.; Lopez-Pousa, A.; Italiano, A.; Alvarez, R.; Gutierrez, A.; Rincón-Perez, I.; Sangalli, C.; et al. Effectiveness and Safety of Trabectedin and Radiotherapy for Patients With Myxoid Liposarcoma: A Nonrandomized Clinical Trial. *JAMA Oncol.* **2023**, *9*, 656–663. [CrossRef]
141. Gronchi, A.; Hindi, N.; Cruz, J.; Blay, J.Y.; Lopez-Pousa, A.; Italiano, A.; Alvarez, R.; Gutierrez, A.; Rincón, I.; Sangalli, C.; et al. Trabectedin and RAdiotherapy in Soft Tissue Sarcoma (TRASTS): Results of a Phase I Study in Myxoid Liposarcoma from Spanish (GEIS), Italian (ISG), French (FSG) Sarcoma Groups. *EClinicalMedicine* **2019**, *9*, 35–43. [CrossRef] [PubMed]
142. Guo, Z.; Wang, H.; Meng, F.; Li, J.; Zhang, S. Combined Trabectedin and Anti-PD1 Antibody Produces a Synergistic Antitumor Effect in a Murine Model of Ovarian Cancer. *J. Transl. Med.* **2015**, *13*, 247. [CrossRef] [PubMed]
143. Pignochino, Y.; Capozzi, F.; D'Ambrosio, L.; Dell'Aglio, C.; Basiricò, M.; Canta, M.; Lorenzato, A.; Vignolo Lutati, F.; Aliberti, S.; Palesandro, E.; et al. PARP1 Expression Drives the Synergistic Antitumor Activity of Trabectedin and PARP1 Inhibitors in Sarcoma Preclinical Models. *Mol. Cancer* **2017**, *16*, 86. [CrossRef] [PubMed]
144. Hao, Q.; Huang, Z.; Li, Q.; Liu, D.; Wang, P.; Wang, K.; Li, J.; Cao, W.; Deng, W.; Wu, K.; et al. A Novel Metabolic Reprogramming Strategy for the Treatment of Diabetes-Associated Breast Cancer. *Adv. Sci.* **2022**, *9*, 2102303. [CrossRef] [PubMed]
145. Abate, A.; Rossini, E.; Bonini, S.A.; Fragni, M.; Cosentini, D.; Tiberio, G.A.M.; Benetti, D.; Hantel, C.; Laganà, M.; Grisanti, S.; et al. Cytotoxic Effect of Trabectedin In Human Adrenocortical Carcinoma Cell Lines and Primary Cells. *Cancers* **2020**, *12*, 928. [CrossRef] [PubMed]
146. Miao, X.; Koch, G.; Ait-Oudhia, S.; Straubinger, R.M.; Jusko, W.J. Pharmacodynamic Modeling of Cell Cycle Effects for Gemcitabine and Trabectedin Combinations in Pancreatic Cancer Cells. *Front. Pharmacol.* **2016**, *7*, 421. [CrossRef] [PubMed]

147. Chu, Q.; Mita, A.; Forouzesh, B.; Tolcher, A.W.; Schwartz, G.; Nieto, A.; Soto-Matos, A.; Alfaro, V.; Lebedinsky, C.; Rowinsky, E.K. Phase I and Pharmacokinetic Study of Sequential Paclitaxel and Trabectedin Every 2 Weeks in Patients with Advanced Solid Tumors. *Clin. Cancer Res.* **2010**, *16*, 2656–2665. [CrossRef]
148. Monk, B.J.; Sill, M.W.; Hanjani, P.; Edwards, R.; Rotmensch, J.; De Geest, K.; Bonebrake, A.J.; Walker, J.L. Docetaxel plus Trabectedin Appears Active in Recurrent or Persistent Ovarian and Primary Peritoneal Cancer after up to Three Prior Regimens: A Phase II Study of the Gynecologic Oncology Group. *Gynecol. Oncol.* **2011**, *120*, 459–463. [CrossRef]
149. Vidal, L.; Magem, M.; Barlow, C.; Pardo, B.; Florez, A.; Montes, A.; Garcia, M.; Judson, I.; Lebedinsky, C.; Kaye, S.B.; et al. Phase i Clinical and Pharmacokinetic Study of Trabectedin and Carboplatin in Patients with Advanced Solid Tumors. *Investig. New Drugs* **2012**, *30*, 616–628. [CrossRef]
150. Polerà, N.; Mancuso, A.; Riillo, C.; Caracciolo, D.; Signorelli, S.; Grillone, K.; Ascrizzi, S.; Hokanson, C.A.; Conforti, F.; Staropoli, N.; et al. The First-In-Class Anti-AXL×CD3ε Pronectin™-Based Bispecific T-Cell Engager Is Active in Preclinical Models of Human Soft Tissue and Bone Sarcomas. *Cancers* **2023**, *15*, 1647. [CrossRef]
151. Tortorelli, I.; Navarria, F.; Di Maggio, A.; Banzato, A.; Lestuzzi, C.; Nicosia, L.; Chiusole, B.; Galiano, A.; Sbaraglia, M.; Zagonel, V.; et al. Trabectedin and Radiation Therapy for Cardiac Metastasis From Leiomyosarcoma: A Case Report and Review of the Literature. *Front. Oncol.* **2022**, *12*, 838114. [CrossRef] [PubMed]
152. Xie, W.; Forveille, S.; Iribarren, K.; Sauvat, A.; Senovilla, L.; Wang, Y.; Humeau, J.; Perez-Lanzon, M.; Zhou, H.; Martínez-Leal, J.F.; et al. Lurbinectedin Synergizes with Immune Checkpoint Blockade to Generate Anticancer Immunity. *Oncoimmunology* **2019**, *8*, e1656502. [CrossRef] [PubMed]
153. Cortesi, L.; Venturelli, M.; Barbieri, E.; Baldessari, C.; Bardasi, C.; Coccia, E.; Baglio, F.; Rimini, M.; Greco, S.; Napolitano, M.; et al. Exceptional Response to Lurbinectedin and Irinotecan in BRCA-Mutated Platinum-Resistant Ovarian Cancer Patient: A Case Report. *Ther. Adv. Chronic Dis.* **2022**, *13*, 20406223211063024. [CrossRef] [PubMed]
154. Takahashi, R.; Mabuchi, S.; Kawano, M.; Sasano, T.; Matsumoto, Y.; Kuroda, H.; Kozasa, K.; Hashimoto, K.; Sawada, K.; Kimura, T. Preclinical Investigations of PM01183 (Lurbinectedin) as a Single Agent or in Combination with Other Anticancer Agents for Clear Cell Carcinoma of the Ovary. *PLoS ONE* **2016**, *11*, e0151050. [CrossRef]
155. Schultz, C.W.; Zhang, Y.; Elmeskini, R.; Zimmermann, A.; Fu, H.; Murai, Y.; Wangsa, D.; Kumar, S.; Takahashi, N.; Atkinson, D.; et al. ATR Inhibition Augments the Efficacy of Lurbinectedin in Small-cell Lung Cancer. *EMBO Mol. Med.* **2023**, *15*, e17313. [CrossRef]
156. Porto, C.M.; Silva, V.D.L.; da Luz, J.S.B.; Filho, B.M.; da Silveira, V.M. Association between Vitamin D Deficiency and Heart Failure Risk in the Elderly. *ESC Heart Fail.* **2018**, *5*, 63–74. [CrossRef]
157. Poveda, A.; Lopez-Reig, R.; Oaknin, A.; Redondo, A.; Rubio, M.J.; Guerra, E.; Fariñas-Madrid, L.; Gallego, A.; Rodriguez-Freixinos, V.; Fernandez-Serra, A.; et al. Phase 2 Trial (POLA Study) of Lurbinectedin plus Olaparib in Patients with Advanced Solid Tumors: Results of Efficacy, Tolerability, and the Translational Study. *Cancers* **2022**, *14*, 915. [CrossRef]
158. Calvo, E.; Sessa, C.; Harada, G.; de Miguel, M.; Kahatt, C.; Luepke-Estefan, X.E.; Siguero, M.; Fernandez-Teruel, C.; Cullell-Young, M.; Stathis, A.; et al. Phase I Study of Lurbinectedin in Combination with Weekly Paclitaxel with or without Bevacizumab in Patients with Advanced Solid Tumors. *Investig. New Drugs* **2022**, *40*, 1263–1273. [CrossRef]
159. Metaxas, Y.; Früh, M.; Eboulet, E.I.; Grosso, F.; Pless, M.; Zucali, P.A.; Ceresoli, G.L.; Mark, M.; Schneider, M.; Maconi, A.; et al. Lurbinectedin as Second- or Third-Line Palliative Therapy in Malignant Pleural Mesothelioma: An International, Multi-Centre, Single-Arm, Phase II Trial (SAKK 17/16). *Ann. Oncol.* **2020**, *31*, 495–500. [CrossRef]
160. Metaxas, Y.; Cathomas, R.; Mark, M.; von Moos, R. Combination of Cisplatin and Lurbinectedin as Palliative Chemotherapy in Progressive Malignant Pleural Mesothelioma: Report of Two Cases. *Lung Cancer* **2016**, *102*, 136–138. [CrossRef]
161. Paz-Ares, L.; Forster, M.; Boni, V.; Szyldergemajn, S.; Corral, J.; Turnbull, S.; Cubillo, A.; Teruel, C.F.; Calderero, I.L.; Siguero, M.; et al. Phase I Clinical and Pharmacokinetic Study of PM01183 (a Tetrahydroisoquinoline, Lurbinectedin) in Combination with Gemcitabine in Patients with Advanced Solid Tumors. *Investig. New Drugs* **2017**, *35*, 198–206. [CrossRef] [PubMed]
162. Awada, A.H.; Boni, V.; Moreno, V.; Aftimos, P.; Kahatt, C.; Luepke-Estefan, X.E.; Siguero, M.; Fernandez-Teruel, C.; Cullell-Young, M.; Tabernero, J. Antitumor Activity of Lurbinectedin in Combination with Oral Capecitabine in Patients with Metastatic Breast Cancer. *ESMO Open* **2022**, *7*, 100651. [CrossRef] [PubMed]
163. Kristeleit, R.; Moreno, V.; Boni, V.; Guerra, E.M.; Kahatt, C.; Romero, I.; Calvo, E.; Basté, N.; López-Vilariño, J.A.; Siguero, M.; et al. Doxorubicin plus Lurbinectedin in Patients with Advanced Endometrial Cancer: Results from an Expanded Phase i Study. *Int. J. Gynecol. Cancer* **2021**, *31*, 1428–1436. [CrossRef] [PubMed]
164. Aix, S.P.; Ciuleanu, T.E.; Navarro, A.; Cousin, S.; Bonanno, L.; Smit, E.F.; Chiappori, A.; Olmedo, M.E.; Horvath, I.; Grohé, C.; et al. Combination Lurbinectedin and Doxorubicin versus Physician's Choice of Chemotherapy in Patients with Relapsed Small-Cell Lung Cancer (ATLANTIS): A Multicentre, Randomised, Open-Label, Phase 3 Trial. *Lancet. Respir. Med.* **2023**, *11*, 74–86. [CrossRef] [PubMed]
165. Kim, K.H.; Kim, J.O.; Park, J.Y.; Seo, M.D.; Park, S.G. Antibody-Drug Conjugate Targeting c-Kit for the Treatment of Small Cell Lung Cancer. *Int. J. Mol. Sci.* **2022**, *23*, 2264. [CrossRef]
166. Digklia, A.; Coukos, G.; Homicsko, K. Trabectedin and Durvalumab Combination Is Feasible and Active in Relapsing Ovarian Cancer. *Clin. Cancer Res.* **2022**, *28*, 1745–1747. [CrossRef]

167. Ratti, C.; Botti, L.; Cancila, V.; Galvan, S.; Torselli, I.; Garofalo, C.; Manara, M.C.; Bongiovanni, L.; Valenti, C.F.; Burocchi, A.; et al. Trabectedin Overrides Osteosarcoma Differentiative Block and Reprograms the Tumor Immune Environment Enabling Effective Combination with Immune Checkpoint Inhibitors. *Clin. Cancer Res.* **2017**, *23*, 5149–5161. [CrossRef]
168. Capasso Palmiero, U.; Morosi, L.; Bello, E.; Ponzo, M.; Frapolli, R.; Matteo, C.; Ferrari, M.; Zucchetti, M.; Minoli, L.; De Maglie, M.; et al. Readily Prepared Biodegradable Nanoparticles to Formulate Poorly Water Soluble Drugs Improving Their Pharmacological Properties: The Example of Trabectedin. *J. Control. Release* **2018**, *276*, 140–149. [CrossRef]

Disclaimer/Publisher's Note: The statements, opinions and data contained in all publications are solely those of the individual author(s) and contributor(s) and not of MDPI and/or the editor(s). MDPI and/or the editor(s) disclaim responsibility for any injury to people or property resulting from any ideas, methods, instructions or products referred to in the content.

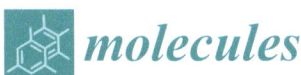

Review

Selenium—More than Just a Fortuitous Sulfur Substitute in Redox Biology

Luisa B. Maia [1,*], Biplab K. Maiti [2,*], Isabel Moura [1] and José J. G. Moura [1]

1. LAQV, REQUIMTE, Department of Chemistry, NOVA School of Science and Technology | NOVA FCT, 2829-516 Caparica, Portugal; isabelmoura@fct.unl.pt (I.M.); jose.moura@fct.unl.pt (J.J.G.M.)
2. Department of Chemistry, School of Sciences, Cluster University of Jammu, Canal Road, Jammu 180001, India
* Correspondence: luisa.maia@fct.unl.pt (L.B.M.); biplabmaiti@clujammu.ac.in (B.K.M.)

Abstract: Living organisms use selenium mainly in the form of selenocysteine in the active site of oxidoreductases. Here, selenium's unique chemistry is believed to modulate the reaction mechanism and enhance the catalytic efficiency of specific enzymes in ways not achievable with a sulfur-containing cysteine. However, despite the fact that selenium/sulfur have different physicochemical properties, several selenoproteins have fully functional cysteine-containing homologues and some organisms do not use selenocysteine at all. In this review, selected selenocysteine-containing proteins will be discussed to showcase both situations: (i) selenium as an obligatory element for the protein's physiological function, and (ii) selenium presenting no clear advantage over sulfur (functional proteins with either selenium or sulfur). Selenium's physiological roles in antioxidant defence (to maintain cellular redox status/hinder oxidative stress), hormone metabolism, DNA synthesis, and repair (maintain genetic stability) will be also highlighted, as well as selenium's role in human health. Formate dehydrogenases, hydrogenases, glutathione peroxidases, thioredoxin reductases, and iodothyronine deiodinases will be herein featured.

Keywords: selenium in biology; selenoproteins; formate dehydrogenases; hydrogenases; glutathione peroxidases; thioredoxin reductases; iodothyronine deiodinases; human health

Citation: Maia, L.B.; Maiti, B.K.; Moura, I.; Moura, J.J.G. Selenium—More than Just a Fortuitous Sulfur Substitute in Redox Biology. *Molecules* **2024**, *29*, 120. https://doi.org/10.3390/molecules29010120

Academic Editors: Manuel Aureliano, Carmen Lopez-Sanchez and Alejandro Samhan-Arias

Received: 30 November 2023
Revised: 19 December 2023
Accepted: 20 December 2023
Published: 24 December 2023

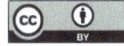

Copyright: © 2023 by the authors. Licensee MDPI, Basel, Switzerland. This article is an open access article distributed under the terms and conditions of the Creative Commons Attribution (CC BY) license (https://creativecommons.org/licenses/by/4.0/).

1. Introduction

Discovered in 1817, selenium was for long regarded as a toxic element [1–3] and only in the second half of the XX century was it demonstrated to be essential for all forms of life [4–10]. Living organisms have learned to harness the unique chemical features provided by selenium (over sulfur) and use this element mainly in the active site of oxidoreductases in the form of selenocysteine, an amino acid genetically encoded by a specific codon (UGA) that is considered the 21st amino acid.

Several selenocysteine-containing enzymes evolved to play essential roles in various biological processes. Still, some of those selenoproteins have fully functional cysteine-containing homologues and some organisms do not use selenocysteine at all. Hence, understanding the biological use of selenium is of considerable interest.

Herein, selected selenocysteine-containing enzymes will be described to highlight the biological versatility afforded by selenium, emphasizing the unique chemical features introduced by this element but also drawing attention to interesting cases where both selenium (selenocysteine) and sulfur (cysteine) are known to be catalytically competent. After briefly highlighting the chemical differences between selenium and sulfur (Section 2), formate dehydrogenase (FDH) (Section 3), one of the first enzymes demonstrated to contain selenium, will be discussed in a deeper detail, followed by hydrogenases (Hase) (Section 4). Concise accounts on glutathione peroxidases (GPx) (Section 5), thioredoxin reductases (TrxR) (Section 6), and iodothyronine deiodinases (Dios) (Section 7) will follow. A review of the relevance of selenium for human health will also be included (Section 8).

2. Selenium versus Sulfur

Selenium is a chemical element belonging to the chalcogens family of the Periodic Table (Group 16). It resembles the "lighter" sulfur in some chemical features and, in Biology, selenium can be found replacing sulfur in two amino acids: selenocysteine (Se-Cys) and selenomethionine (Se-Met). However, in spite of the similarities, many significant chemical differences exist between these two chalcogens [11–15]. As sulfur, selenium can display a wide range of oxidation states (from -2 to $+6$), but its preference for lower oxidation states and higher reactivity sets it apart from sulfur. Its reactions are often also faster than its sulfur counterparts because selenium is more polarizable (softer). Its larger spin—orbit coupling (compared to sulfur) probably facilitates spin-forbidden reactions, as the ones involved in the rapid oxidation of selenocysteine under air (compared to cysteine oxidation). Moreover, the selenocysteine selenol's lower pK_a value (5.2, compared to 8.3 of cysteine thiol) is expected to favor its deprotonation and nucleophilic character at physiological pH [16], while the weaker Se-H bond makes the selenocysteine less basic, compared to cysteine [17,18]. The biologically relevant redox chemistry is also significantly different in these two elements [19–21]. The selenocysteine one-electron oxidation-derived radical is more easily formed ($(RSe^{\bullet}/RSeH) = 0.43$ V versus $(RS^{\bullet}/RSH) = 0.92$ V [22]) and relatively more stable than the cisteine radical [22–24]. As a result, for example, while the cysteine radical can oxidize a tyrosine residue (to yield tyrosine radical), the selenocysteine radical can not [22]. Also noteworthy are the thiol/disulfide exchange reactions, where the selenocysteine reactions (Se-Cys/Cys-Se-Se-Cys) are faster than the cysteine ones [12,14,25,26].

This different chemistry suggests that the incorporation of a selenocysteine or a cysteine should modulate the enzyme catalytic activity, with a selenocysteine being able to perform roles that a "common" sulfur-containing cysteine can not. As such, selenium should not be just a fortuitous sulfur substitute in Biology. However, as will be discussed below, there are striking examples where the replacement of selenocysteine by cysteine does not affect the outcome of the biological reaction.

3. Formate Dehydrogenase

FDH was one of the first enzymes demonstrated to contain selenium and a selenocysteine-specific codon (TGA) in its gene sequence (*Clostridium thermoaceticum* and *E. coli* enzymes) [27,28]. Those seminal works were essential to overcome the prevailing idea that selenium was (only) a toxic substance and lead to its recognition as an essential element (also for mammals and humans by contemporary works).

In spite of being one of the most widely distributed selenoproteins (probably due to its extensive lateral gene transfer, together with the corresponding selenocysteine synthesis and incorporation system) [29], FDH constitutes a key example where, as far as is presently known, selenium does not present any clear advantage over sulfur. Contrary to other selenoenzymes, living organisms hold both active selenocysteine- and cysteine-containing FDH homologues and, thus, the selenium role in FDH catalysis remains, so far, elusive.

3.1. The Current Picture

3.1.1. Enzymatic Machinery

FDHs catalyze the two-electron interconversion of formate and carbon dioxide (Equation (1)) in diverse metabolic pathways, operating in different subcellular locations, such as C1 metabolism, carbon dioxide fixation (carbon assimilation), and to derive energy (coupling formate oxidation to the reduction of different terminal electron acceptors) [30–38]. Since each pathway requires a specific "FDH enzymatic machinery" to accomplish the respective biological function, FDHs evolved as a highly heterogeneous group of enzymes, displaying diverse structural (subunits) organization and composition of redox-active centers (Table 1) [39–48].

$$HCOO^- \rightleftharpoons CO_2 + 2e^- + H^+ \qquad (1)$$

Table 1. Key features of some representative FDHs.

Active Site [a]	Subunit Composition	Examples	Notes
no metal	α_2 no redox-active cofactors	*Candida boidinii* FDH	• NAD-dependent
W SeCys	α W, [4Fe-4S]	*Clostridium carboxidivorans* FDH	• cytoplasmic? • NAD-dependent
		Thermoanaerobacter kivui FDH	• hydrogen-dependent CO_2 reductase
	$\alpha\beta$ α: W, [4Fe-4S] β: 3 [4Fe-4S]	*Desulfovibrio gigas*, *Desulfovibrio alaskensis*, *Desulfovibrio vulgaris* FDHs	• periplasmic
	$(\alpha\beta)_2$ α: W, [4Fe-4S] β: 3 [4Fe-4S]	*Moorella thermoacetica* FDH	• cytoplasmic • NADP-dependent
	$(\alpha\beta\gamma)_2$ W, Fe	*Synthrobacter fumaroxidans* FDH	• periplasmic?
W Cys	$\alpha\beta$ α: W, $\geq$ 1 Fe/S β: [4Fe-4S], FMN	*Methylobacterium extorquens* FDH	• cytoplasmic • NAD-dependent
Mo SeCys	α Mo, [4Fe-4S]	*Escherichia coli* FDH H	• cytoplasmic • formate–hydrogen lyase system
		Acetobacterium woodii FDH	• hydrogen-dependent CO_2 reductase
	$\alpha\beta\gamma$ α: Mo, [4Fe-4S] β: 3 [4Fe-4S] γ: 4 *c* haems	*Desulfovibrio desulfuricans* FDH *Desulfovibrio vulgaris* FDH	• periplasmic
	$(\alpha\beta\gamma)_3$ α: Mo, [4Fe-4S] β: 4 [4Fe-4S] γ: 2 *b* haems	*E. coli* FDH N	• membrane-bound periplasm-faced • partner anaerobic nitrate–formate respir. system
		E. coli FDH O	• membrane-bound periplasm-faced • partner microaerobic nitrate–formate respir. syst.
Mo Cys	α Mo, [4Fe-4S]	*Pectobacterium atrosepticum*, *Corynebacterium glutamicum* FDHs	• cytoplasmic
	$\alpha\beta$ Mo, several Fe/S	*Clostridium pasteurianum* FDH	• cytoplasmic
	$\alpha\beta$ Mo, FAD, several Fe/S, Zn	*Methanobacterium formicicum* FDH	• cytoplasmic • F_{420}-dependent
	$\alpha\beta\gamma$ α: Mo, [4Fe-4S] β: 4 [4Fe-4S] γ: 4 *b* haems	*Wolinella succinogenes* FDH	• membrane-bound
	$(\alpha\beta\gamma)_2$ α: Mo, [2Fe-2S], 4 [4Fe-4S] β: [4Fe-4S], FMN γ: [2Fe-2S]	*Cupriavidus necator*, *Rhodobacter capsulatus*, *Methylosinus trichosporium*, *Pseudomonas oxalatus* FDHs	• cytoplasmic • NAD-dependent
	$(\alpha\beta\gamma\delta)_2$ Mo, $\geq$1 [2Fe–2S], $\geq$1 [4Fe-4S], FMN	*Methylosinus trichosporium* FDH	• cytoplasmic • NAD-dependent
	$(\alpha\beta\gamma\delta\epsilon\omega)_4$ α: 2 Zn β: Mo, [4Fe-4S] γ: 2 [4Fe-4S] γ: 4 *b* haems δ ϵ: 8 [4Fe-4S] ω	*Methanothermobacter wolfeiir* FMFDH	• cytoplasmic

[a] Metal (molybdenum or tungsten) and residue (selenocysteine or cysteine) present in the active site of metal-dependent FDHs and FMFDHs.

FDHs can be divided into two main classes. The metal-independent FDH class comprises enzymes, typically homodimers that have no metal ions or other redox-active centers, nor selenium [49–54]. These enzymes, found in bacteria, fungi, and plants, are NAD-dependent and belong to the D-specific dehydrogenases of the 2-oxyacids family. On the contrary, the metal-dependent FDH class, present only in prokaryotes, comprises enzymes that harbor different redox-active centers and display high structural diversity (Table 1) [41–43,45,46,48]. As the class name indicates, the active site of these enzymes holds one molybdenum or one tungsten ion in a very well conserved metal center (Figure 1). In its oxidized (6+) form, the metal (molybdenum or tungsten) is coordinated by the *cis*-dithiolene (–S–C=C–S–) group of two pyranopterin cofactor molecules, one terminal sulfido group (Mo^{6+}/W^{6+}=S), plus one selenium or one sulfur atom from a selenocysteine or cysteine residue (Mo^{6+}/W^{6+}-Se(Cys) or Mo^{6+}/W^{6+}-S(Cys)) (abbreviated as SeCys-Mo-FDH, SeCys-W-FDH, Cys-Mo-FDH, and Cys-W-FDH) [40,44,55,56]. Noteworthy, there is no apparent relation (as far as is presently known) between the metal (molybdenum or tungsten) and the presence of a selenocysteine or cysteine residue and catalytically efficient SeCys-Mo-FDH, SeCys-W-FDH, Cys-Mo-FDH, and Cys-W-FDH have been known for a long time.

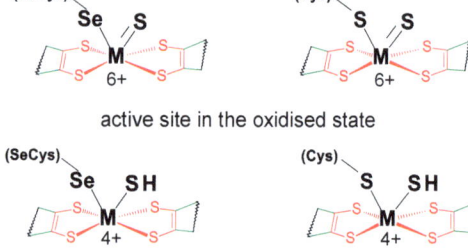

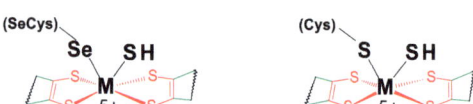

Figure 1. Active site structure of metal-dependent FDHs and FMFDHs. **Top**: Structure of the pyranopterin cofactor. The pyranopterin cofactor molecule is formed by pyrano(green)–pterin(blue)–dithiolene(red)–methylphosphate(black) moieties; in all so far characterized enzymes, the cofactor is found esterified with a guanosine monophosphate (dark gray). The dithiolene (–S–C=C–S–) group forms a five-membered ene-1,2-dithiolene chelate ring with the molybdenum or tungsten ion, here indicated as M (from metal). **Middle**: Structure of the active site in the oxidized and reduced state. **Bottom**: Active site structure supported by EPR data. In middle and bottom structures, for simplicity, only the dithiolene moiety of the pyranopterin cofactor is represented.

Similar to FDHs, selenocysteine-containing and cysteine-containing N-formyl-methanofuran dehydrogenases (SeCys-FMFDH and Cys-FMFDH) exist and selenium's role in FMFDH catalysis is unknown as well. FMFDHs are FDH-like enzymes that have two physically separated active sites: one catalyzes the reduction of carbon dioxide to formate, which is then intramolecularly transferred to the second active site, where it is condensed with methanofuran to form N-formyl-methanofuran [57–60]. The active site responsible for the carbon dioxide reduction is identical to the FDHs' one and harbors one molybdenum or tungsten ion coordinated by the cis-dithiolene group of two pyranopterin cofactor molecules, one terminal sulfido group (Mo^{6+}/W^{6+}=S), plus one selenium or one sulfur atom from a selenocysteine or cysteine residue (Figure 1).

3.1.2. Reaction Mechanism

Regardless of the physiological function and structural complexity, the reaction mechanism of the interconversion of formate and carbon dioxide (Equation (1)) is believed to be similar in all these selenocysteine- and cysteine-containing FDH and FMFDH enzymes. As originally proposed by Niks et al. [61] for formate oxidation and shortly after also for carbon dioxide reduction by Maia et al. [62], it is currently well established that formate oxidation and carbon dioxide reduction proceed through hydride transfer, with the oxidized and reduced active site sulfido group, Mo/W^{6+}=S and Mo/W^{4+}-SH, acting as the direct hydride acceptor and donor, respectively (Figure 2) [63–66] (even though other atomic details of the reaction mechanism are not yet consensual; see, for example [67]). It is noteworthy that no direct role in the chemical transformations is presently ascribed to the selenocysteine or cysteine residue, in accordance with the existence of catalytically efficient SeCys enzymes and Cys enzymes (a similar situation occurs with molybdenum and tungsten). Nevertheless, it is expected that the presence of a selenocysteine or cysteine should affect the active site properties and that each enzyme type has to cope with the intrinsic differences between selenium and sulfur (see Section 3.3).

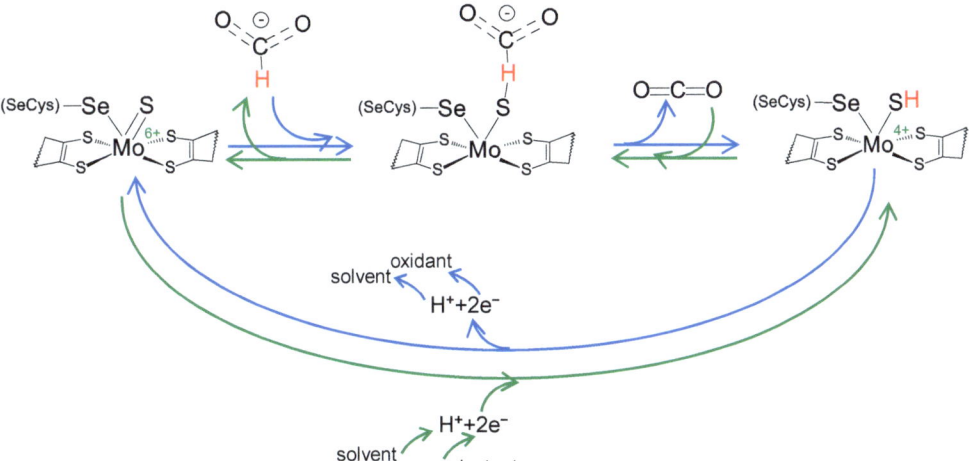

Figure 2. Reversible FDH and FMFDH reaction mechanism, as proposed by Maia et al. [62]. Reaction mechanism proposed for formate oxidation (blue arrows) and carbon dioxide reduction (green arrows) for both metal-dependent FDHs and FMFDHs. For simplicity, the mechanism is represented for a molybdenum, selenocysteine-containing enzyme, but it should be similar for tungsten and cysteine-containing enzymes. See text for details.

Briefly, formate oxidation (Figure 2, blue arrows) is initiated with the formate binding to the oxidized active site but not directly to the molybdenum/tungsten atom. Formate is suggested to bind in a binding pocket, where a conserved arginine residue "anchors" its oxygen atom(s) through hydrogen bond(s), and forces its Cα hydrogen to point towards the sulfido ligand (Mo^{6+}/W^{6+}=S). Subsequently, formate oxidation proceeds by a straightforward hydride transfer from formate to the sulfido group of the oxidized molybdenum/tungsten centre, leading to the formation of Mo/W^{4+}-SH and CO$_2$. The re-oxidation of Mo/W^{4+} to Mo/W^{6+} (via intramolecular electron transfer to the enzyme's other redox center(s) and, eventually, to the physiological partner) and the release of carbon dioxide close the catalytic cycle. The now oxidized Mo/W^{6+} favors the sulfido group deprotonation (dictated by the ligand pK_a [68–70]) and the initial oxidized metal centre, Mo/W^{6+}=S, is regenerated. Under non-steady-state catalytic conditions (such as the ones created in EPR experiments described below), the molybdenum/tungsten one-electron oxidation should be favored (Mo/W^{4+}→Mo/W^{5+}), leading to the formation of the EPR detectable species.

The carbon dioxide reduction is suggested to follow the reverse reaction mechanism (Figure 2, green arrows) but starting with a reduced active site, holding a protonated sulfido group, Mo/W^{6+}-SH (as is dictated by the ligands pK_a [68–70]). Carbon dioxide is suggested to bind to the same binding pocket, where the arginine residue is key to anchor it in the correct position to orient its carbon atom towards the protonated sulfido. Afterwards, the reaction proceeds through straightforward hydride transfer from the protonated sulfido group. This yields a formate moiety and Mo/W^{6+}=S. The subsequent re-reduction of Mo/W^{6+} to Mo/W^{4+} (via intramolecular electron transfer from the enzyme's physiological partner, through its redox center(s)) and formate release closes the catalytic cycle. The now reduced Mo/W^{4+} favors the sulfido group protonation and the initial reduced molybdenum/tungsten center, Mo/W^{4+}-SH, is regenerated.

3.2. How Was the Selenium Locus in Formate Dehydrogenases Established?

The presence and essentiality of selenium was demonstrated in pioneer works, mainly in the 1970s, following the incorporation in target enzymes of selenium-75 (present in the growth medium/feed). Actually, FDH was among the first enzymes shown to contain selenium [27,28].

The recognition of the presence of molybdenum or tungsten and selenium led to a series of spectroscopic studies that were decisive to the early characterization of the FDH active site. Electron paramagnetic resonance spectroscopy (EPR) was thoroughly explored (reviewed recently, for example, in [71–73]). In fact, the first evidence for the direct binding of selenium to a metal (molybdenum) active site center was obtained precisely with EPR [74,75]. The *E. coli* SeCys-Mo-FDH H was one of the first FDHs to be explored [75,76]. When reduced with formate, it gives rise to a nearly axial Mo^{5+} signal, with g_1 = 2.094 and $g_{2,3}$ = 2.001, 1.990, that displays coupling to one formate-derived solvent-exchangeable proton ($A_{1,2,3}$(^{1}H) = 7.5, 18.9, 20.9 MHz). When the EPR signal is generated from the ^{77}Se-enriched enzyme, a very strong and anisotropic interaction is observed ($A_{1,2,3}$(^{77}Se) = 13.2, 75, 240 MHz [77], values that are almost five times higher than the ones observed in Mo-Se model compounds [77,78]). This strong interaction, observed simultaneously with the expected ^{95,97}Mo hyperfine coupling, confirmed that the selenocysteine selenium atom is directly coordinated to the molybdenum (Figure 1) and suggested that the unpaired electron is delocalized 17–27% over the selenium (a finding in line with the expected covalency introduced by selenium in a Mo-Se bond) [77]. Moreover, photolysis assays showed that in the photo-converted enzyme, the interaction with ^{77}Se is not significantly affected, while the interaction with the solvent-exchangeable proton disappears, thus providing further evidence that the selenium remains bound to the molybdenum during the catalytic turnover [77]. These photolysis assays were also key in providing additional evidence that the selenocysteine residue could not be the hydrogen atom acceptor during catalysis, as is currently accepted (Figure 2) [61,62]. (Note: Studies with ^{2}H-labelled formate (in ^{1}H-water) showed that the coupled solvent-exchangeable proton originates from the substrate molecule and that the proton acceptor is located within magnetic contact to the molybdenum center [77]. Similar results were obtained with *D. desulfuricans* [79], *D. vulgaris* [80–83], and *C. necator* [61] enzymes, overall suggesting that the hydrogen atom is transferred from formate Cα to the molybdenum center in the course of the reaction and then exchanged with the solvent. Hence, the current general consensus is that the structure of the EPR signal-giving species is a Mo^{5+}-Se(Cys)(-SH) center that can arise from the one-electron oxidation/reduction of a catalytic intermediate (Figure 2) [61,62]).

These original studies with *E. coli* FDH H were supported and consolidated with other selenium-containing FDHs, including *Desulfovibrio desulfuricans* [79], *D. gigas* [84,85], *D. vulgaris* Hildenborough [80–83], and *Methylosinus trichosporium* [86] FDHs. These enzymes display rhombic Mo^{5+}/W^{5+} EPR signals with small anisotropy, a well-resolved hyperfine structure due to $^{95,97}Mo/^{183}W$, and interaction with a solvent-exchangeable proton (for example: *D. desulfuricans*: $g_{1,2,3}$ = 2.012, 1.996, 1.985, $A_{1,2,3}$(solvent-exchangeable ^1H) = 23.1, 29.9, 27.8 MHz [79]; *D. vulgaris* Hildenborough FDH 1: $g_{1,2,3}$ = 1.995, 1.881, 1.852, $A_{1,2,3}(^{183}W)$= 225, 129, 134 MHz [80]; *D. vulgaris* Hildenborough FDH 2 (main component): $g_{1,2,3}$ = 1.982, 1.876, 1.902, $A_{1,2,3}(^{183}W)$= 232, 119, 151 MHz [82]). The *D. desulfuricans* FDH displays also a hyperfine interaction with a second non-solvent-exchangeable proton (A_1 = 35.1 MHz, $A_{2,3}$ not detectable) that was assigned to the metal-bound selenocysteine Cβ hydrogen atoms [79]. Together, the EPR data suggest an FDH active site holding a stable selenocysteine–metal ligation. It also suggests that the active site holds a transient proton-accepting site (within the metal magnetic contact) that was assigned as the terminal sulfido group (please see Note above) [61,62]. Overall, the EPR clearly points to the FDH active site having a Mo^{5+}/W^{5+}-Se(Cys)(-SH) structure (Figure 1), formed from one-electron oxidation/reduction of a catalytic intermediate (Figure 2) or by chemical reduction.

The SeCys-FDH active site was also explored by X-ray absorption spectroscopy (XAS) since early times [87]. XAS at the molybdenum and selenium K-edges of the most explored model FDH, *E. coli* SeCys-Mo-FDH H, revealed four Mo-S ligands at 2.35 Å, one (originally not assigned) Mo=S at 2.1 Å, and one Mo-Se ligand at 2.62 Å, in both oxidized and reduced enzyme [88]. In the *D. desulfuricans* SeCys-Mo-FDH, the molybdenum and selenium K-edges data also showed a hexa-coordinated active site, with one Mo-Se ligand at 2.57 Å in both oxidized and reduced enzyme [89]. It is noteworthy that the replacement of the *E. coli* SeCys-Mo-FDH H selenocysteine by a cysteine residue abolished the Mo-Se fingerprint and gave rise to a spectrum consistent with five Mo-S ligands and one Mo=O at 1.7 Å [88]. Comparatively, XAS studies of native Cys-FDHs (for example, oxidized *Rhodobacter capsulatus* Cys-Mo-FDH [90,91]) confirmed that the cysteine residue is bound to the metal, as expected. Hence, the XAS results are in excellent agreement with the EPR proposed FDH active site structure, Mo^{5+}/W^{5+}-Se(Cys)(-SH) (Figure 1).

The crystallographic structure of different native SeCys- (and Cys-) FDHs entirely supports this active site structure. The first FDH 3D structure solved, in 1997, was the one of the model *E. coli* SeCys-Mo-FDH H [92] and this was the only one known for 5 years (2002), when the structure of two more enzymes were finally solved, the *E. coli* SeCys-Mo-FDH N [93] and *Desulfovibrio gigas* SeCys-W-FDH [94] (Figure 3). The first FMFDH structure (the *Methanothermobacter wolfeii* Cys-W-FMFDH) was revealed only 14 years after, in 2016 [59]. Presently, several structures are known [60,80,81,95–99] and the active site structure is firmly established to be the conserved Mo^{6+}-Se(Cys)(=S), W^{6+}-Se(Cys) (=S), Mo^{6+}-S(Cys)(=S), or W^{6+}-S(Cys)(=S) (Figure 1).

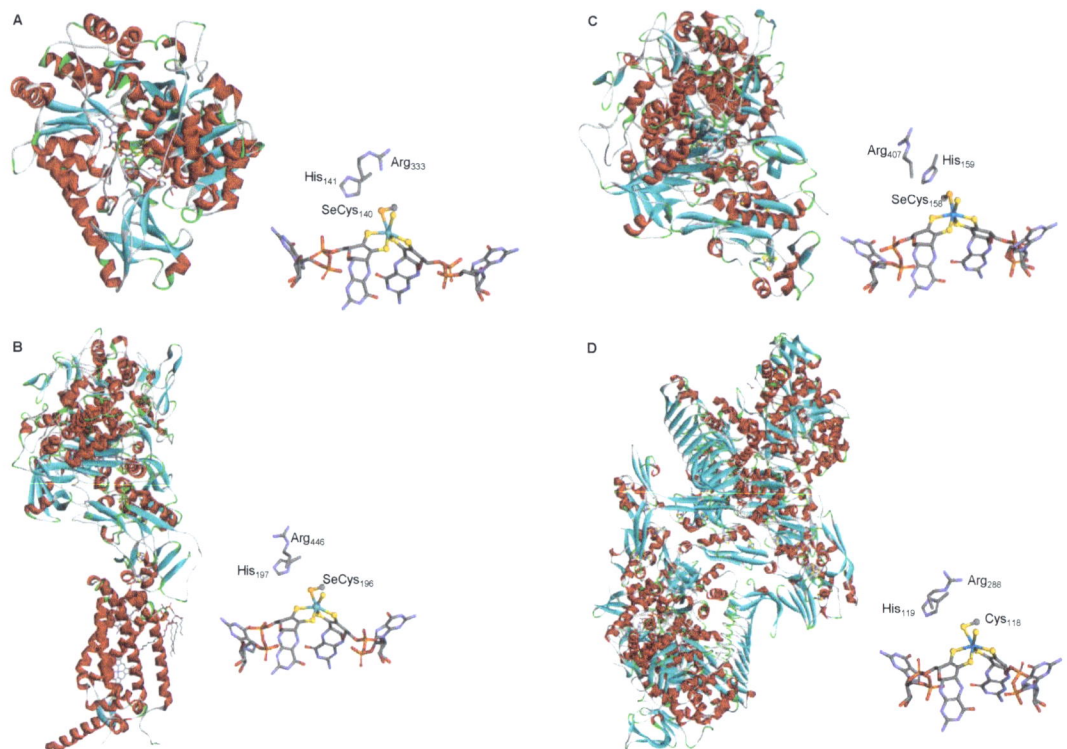

Figure 3. Three-dimensional structure view of some metal-dependent FDHs and FMFDHs and their active sites. (**A**) *E. coli* SeCys-Mo-FDH H [92]; (**B**) *E. coli* SeCys-Mo-FDH N [93]; (**C**) *D. gigas* SeCys-W-FDH [94]; (**D**) *M. wolfeii* Cys-W-FMFDH [59]. The structures shown are based on the PDB files 1FDO (**A**), 1KQF (**B**), 1H0H (**C**), and 5T5I (**D**) (α helices and β sheets are shown in red and cyan, respectively).

3.3. Why Do Some Formate Dehydrogenases Have a Selenocysteine and Not the Less "Expensive" Cysteine Residue?

Since its early identification as a selenium-containing enzyme, the role of selenium in FDH catalysis has intrigued the scientific community. A pioneer work in the late 1980s [100] with the model *E. coli* SeCys-Mo-FDH H showed that selenocysteine (SeCys$_{140}$) replacement with a cysteine residue resulted in significant lower FDH activity, while replacement with a serine residue rendered the enzyme inactive. In a subsequent, more comprehensive work by the Stadtman group [101], it was clearly shown that selenocysteine replacement with a cysteine resulted in a marked decrease in FDH activity ($k_{cat}/K_m^{formate}$ (SeCys-FDH) = 108 × 10^3 M^{-1}s^{-1} to $k_{cat}/K_m^{formate}$ (Cys-FDH) = 1 × 10^3 M^{-1}s^{-1}) and the Cys-FDH variant's slower kinetics was suggested to be due to a lower rate of the hydrogen atom transfer step (deuterium (formate) isotope effect on k_{cat}/K_m). Simultaneously, the pH-dependent alkylation-induced inactivation of the native SeCys-FDH and variant Cys-FDH (reaction with iodoacetamide in the presence of formate) was shown to follow the trend of the expected pK_a values of each amino acid (native SeCys-FDH was inactivated more than 80% at pH > 6 (pK_a (SeCys) ≈ 5.2), while variant Cys-FDH was inactivated more than 80% only at pH > 7 (pK_a (Cys) ≈ 8.2). Together, these results were taken to suggest that selenol (versus thiol) plays an essential role in catalysis. However, both native SeCys-FDH and variant Cys-FDH followed the same kinetic mechanism (ping-pong, bi-bi) and displayed similar pH dependencies with respect to activity and stability, which makes it difficult to reconcile with the hypothesis that a cysteine residue would render a catalytically incompetent enzyme because of its thiol features.

As other variant enzymes are studied, it is becoming clear that it is not surprising that variants are less active than wild types. Most relevant to the present discussion was the recognition that several "wild-type variants" (native Cys-FDH) exist that are as catalytically efficient as the native SeCys-FDHs (Table 1). In fact, several native Cys-FDHs were known for long, but they were overlooked by the groups studying FDH catalysis, which focused instead on a few model enzymes, mostly in *E. coli* SeCys-Mo-FDH H. In addition, coincidentally, those FDHs whose 3D structures were first solved (see Section 3.2) were all SeCys-FDHs and, thus, selenium acquired a highlighted role in FDH catalysis that is not consistent with the existence of native Cys-FDHs.

Presently, the accepted FDH reaction mechanism does not ascribe any direct role to the selenocysteine or cysteine residue (see Section 3.1.2), leaving open the question of why some formate dehydrogenases have a selenocysteine and not the common cysteine residue.

Selenocysteine incorporation is highly demanding ("expensive") for the cell. It requires additional energy and dedicated machinery to uptake selenium and to synthesize and orchestrate different biomolecules that lead to the recognition of target UGA-codon by specific *t*RNA molecules (and not as the "opal" stop-codon), culminating in selenocysteine being incorporated in the target protein [102–106]. Therefore, it is generally accepted that the presence of selenocysteine should constitute an intrinsic advantage for the cell [14,107–109]. Regarding FDHs, such an advantage was not yet proven. Among other hypothesis, we can think (as for other proteins, for example [110,111]) that the comparatively higher difficulty in forming higher oxidation states of selenium and the higher facility to non-enzymatically reduce them is an advantage for those organisms whose lifestyle makes their FDHs more prone to suffer oxidative modifications.

Regardless of the biological pressure behind the evolution of native SeCys-FDHs and native Cys-FDHs, it should be kept in mind that selenium is not a sulfur (see Section 2). Thus, it is reasonable that the presence of one or the other alters the reaction energy pattern, in spite of both enzyme types operating through the same general hydride transfer mechanism (same chemical transformations). Therefore, in order to be catalytically efficient, each enzyme type should have evolved a strategy to compensate for those Se/S physicochemical differences. Hence, more interesting and relevant than studying why some FDHs have selenium is to understand the strategies that allow both SeCys-FDH and Cys-FDH to be catalytically efficient. For example, it must be understood how the Cys-FDHs compensate for the presence of a less covalent Mo-S(Cys) bond, or, depending on the origin, how the SeCys-FDHs compensate for the more covalent selenium, because those Se/S-metal bond features are expected to influence the metal center reduction potential, which, in turn, modulates the electron transfer process (a step that even though it is not a chemical transformation is decisive for catalysis).

4. Hydrogenases

Hases are crucial role as an alternative energy source as they have potential applications in green hydrogen production [112,113]. Hydrogenases are a heterogeneous group of enzymes that differ in size, subunit composition, metal content, and cellular location (periplasmic, cytoplasmic, and cytoplasmic membrane-bound) and catalyze the reversible two electron oxidation of hydrogen (Equation (2)).

$$H_2 \rightleftharpoons 2H^+ + 2e^- \qquad (2)$$

4.1. Enzymatic Machineries

The metal-containing hydrogenases are subdivided into three classes: [Fe]-, [FeFe]-, and [NiFe]-hydrogenases (Figure 4) [112–117]. [Fe]-hydrogenases only contain one Fe ion in their active site and are designated as "Fe-only" hydrogenases. [FeFe]-hydrogenases contain an unusual iron-sulfur cluster termed the H-cluster that consists of an $[Fe_4S_4]$ subcluster bridged via a cysteine (Cys) thiolate to the binuclear iron subcluster, also coordinated by inorganic ligands: two S atoms and one CO or CN ligand. [NiFe]-hydrogenases are heterodimeric proteins constituted by a small and a large subunit (Figure 5). The small subunit accommodates three iron-sulfur clusters (two [4Fe-4S] clusters and one [3Fe-4S] cluster) involved in the electron transport to/from the active site ([NiFe] cluster); the large subunit contains the catalytic site: the nickel-iron center. In some [NiFe]-hydrogenases, one of the Ni-bound cysteines is replaced by a selenocysteine, and [NiFe]- and [NiFeSe]-hydrogenases represent a single superfamily, and the Ni-Fe core contains unusual ligands: carbon monoxide (CO) and cyanide (CN^-).

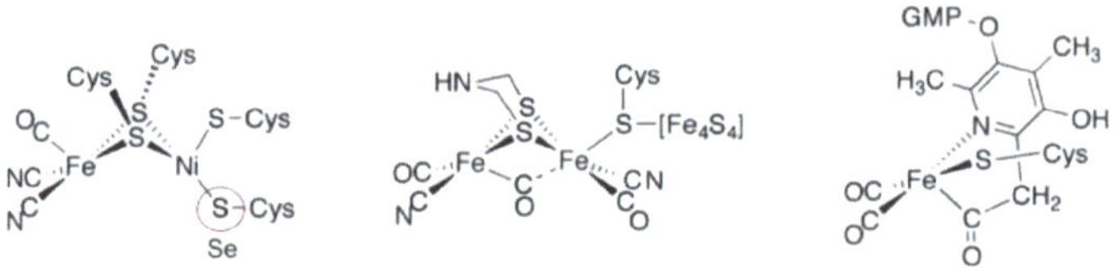

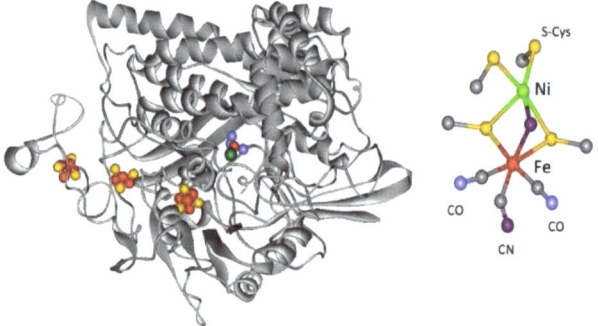

Figure 4. Active site structure of [NiFe]-, [FeFe]-, and [Fe]-hydrogenases [112].

Figure 5. Structure of the *D. gigas* hydrogenase enzyme and of its active site.

The [NiFe-Se] hydrogenases are found in some species of *Desulfovibrio* sp. The genes encoding the large and small subunits of the periplasmic hydrogenase from *Desulfovibrio (D.) baculatus* (DSM 1743) exhibit homology (40%) to the [NiFe] hydrogenases. The gene for the large subunit contains a codon (TGA) for selenocysteine in a position homologous to a codon (TGC) for cysteine in the [NiFe] hydrogenase. Spectroscopic studies support that selenium is a ligand to the nickel site (see below) [118–123].

As isolated, the active [NiFe] cluster contains a Ni(III) and a low-spin Fe(II) (diamagnetic) that remain unchanged during the enzyme mechanism. Different oxidized inactive states are attained by the enzyme. In general, the isolated states are mixtures of "unready" Ni-A and "ready" Ni-B states (Figure 6). These states show delocalized electron density between nickel and iron, attributed to a third bridging oxygenated ligand. Both oxidized states are paramagnetic and characterized by different EPR g-values. The bridging ligand in the Ni-B state has been assigned to an OH^- ligand and a water molecule is probably present in the Ni-A state [124–127]. After the reaction with the substrate (hydrogen), (Ni-C) develops with a bridging hydride (H^-) ligand. Other intermediates were denominated Ni-R and Ni-SI. In all states of standard hydrogenases, the nickel atom has a vacant or labile coordination site and, therefore, Ni represents the primary hydrogen binding site. The H_2 molecule can be accessed by the buried [NiFe] active site through hydrophobic tunnels leading to the Ni atom [128–131].

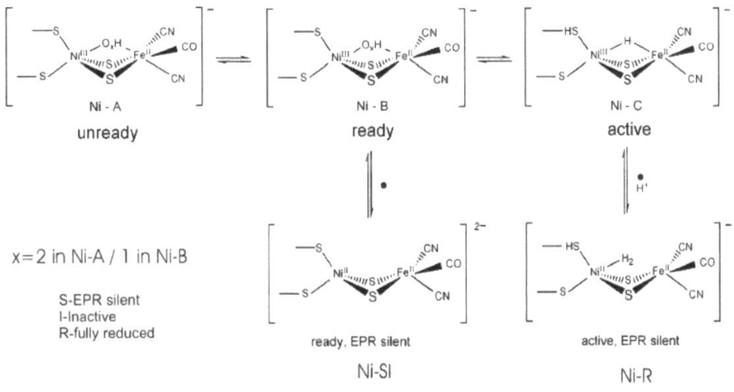

Figure 6. Redox and catalytic intermediates in [NiFe] hydrogenases. Adapted from [131].

The Ni site, in the [NiFeSe] cluster, is coordinated by three sulfur atoms from three cysteine residues and one Se atom from selenocysteine. The electron transfer pathway is similar to one described in [NiFe] enzymes, involving three iron–sulfur clusters present in the small subunit connecting the active site to the surface; however, the medial cluster is a [4Fe-4S] cluster instead of the [3Fe-4S] cluster present in [NiFe] hydrogenases [132–136].

The role of the selenocysteine has a remarkable influence on the catalytic properties of [NiFeSe] hydrogenases: (i) high catalytic activity in H_2 production direction is detected and is less sensitive to oxygen [118,137–139]; (ii) in general, the as-purified [NiFeSe] hydrogenases are almost EPR silent (Ni-A and Ni-B signals are not or are weakly detected). Upon reduction, the Ni-C EPR signals, assigned to active states of the fully developed enzyme, with spectral characteristics as observed in [NiFe] hydrogenases [135,140,141]; (iii) different oxygen permeation pathways in [NiFe] and [NiFeSe] hydrogenases have been described, based on computational studies [142].

4.2. Selenium and the Hydrogenase Reaction Mechanism

Isotopic substitutions are crucial for the identification of Ni and Se in hydrogenases. A ^{61}Ni isotope was used for assigning EPR signals to Ni (Figure 7) [143]. Selenium contains six isotopes, and five of them are stable (atomic numbers 74, 76, 77, 78, and 80). The sixth isotope, with an atom abundance of 8.73%, is selenium-82 (^{82}Se), a beta emitter which is weakly radioactive. The ^{77}Se isotope (7.5%) is a useful EPR marker, with an I = 1/2. ^{33}Se and ^{77}Se are useful markers for spectroscopic studies (EXAFS and EPR) (Table 2) [143–146].

Table 2. Comparison of the EPR properties of native and H_2-reduced states of [NiFe]- and [NiFeSe]-Hases [140].

Hase	SRB	Localization	EPR g-Values Native	EPR g-Values H_2 Red—Ni-C
[NiFe]	*D. gigas*	periplasm	2.31 2.23 2.02	2.19 2.14 2.02
[NiFe]	*D. desulfuricans* (ATCC 2774)	periplasm	2.32 2.16 2.02	2.19 2.14 2.02
[NiFeSe]	*D. desulfuricans* (Norway 4)	soluble	weak Ni(III) signals	2.20 2.15~2.0
[NiFeSe]	*D. salexigens*	periplasm	EPR silent	2.22 2.14 2.01
[NiFeSe]	*D. africanus*	soluble	EPR silent	2.21 2.17 2.01
[NiFeSe]	*D. baculatus*	soluble	weak Ni(III) signals	2.20 2.16 2.01

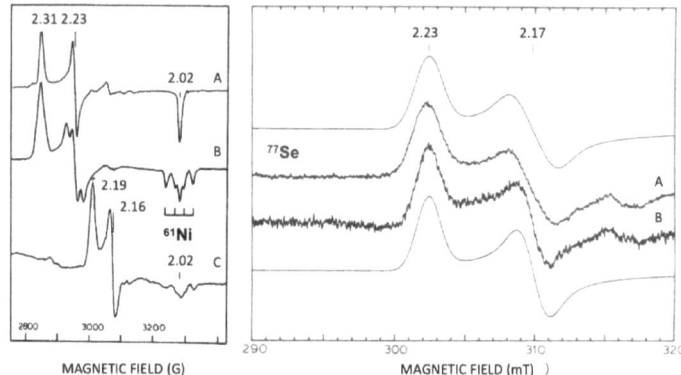

Figure 7. Revealing EPR, Ni, and Se at the active site of hydrogenases. Isotopic substitutions with ^{61}Ni and ^{77}Se. Left panel *D. gigas* [Ni-Fe] Hase. (**A**) Ni-A ^{61}Ni un-enriched; (**B**) Ni-A ^{61}Ni enriched; (**C**) Ni-C ^{61}Ni enriched. Right panel *D. baculatus* [Ni-Fe-Se] Hase. (**A**) Ni-C ^{77}Se enriched and (**B**) Ni-C ^{77}Se un-enriched; mooth lines are simulations of spectra A and B. Adapted from refs [143,145].

Proton–deuterium exchange measurements are quite appropriate to probe the influence of the Se–cysteine ligand in the mechanism of hydrogen handling. An important clue was the observation that the H_2/HD ratios were higher for [NiFeSe] hydrogenases than those observed for the [NiFe] ones, which is related to the activation of the hydrogen molecule (Figure 8).

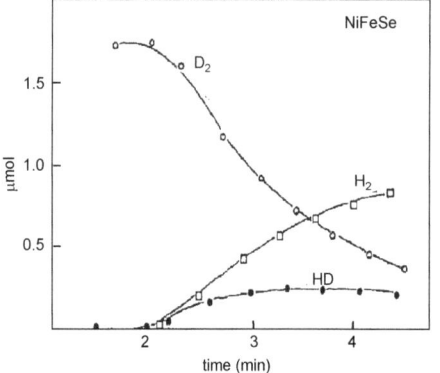
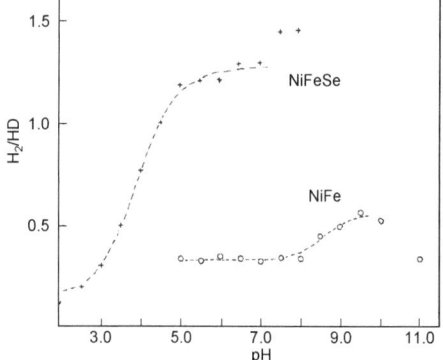

Figure 8. D_2/HD exchange activity of *D. salexigens* [NiFeSe] hydrogenase (**left panel**) and variation in the experimental ratios H_2/HD as a function of pH (**right panel**) of *D. baculatus* (cytoplasmic) [NiFeSe] hydrogenase and *D. gigas* [NiFe] (periplasmic). Left panel adapted from [140]; right panel adapted from [141].

Several studies on the role of transition metals in hydrogenation reactions describe the main processes for the activation of the H_2 molecule, catalyzed by transition metals, and the hydride–metal complex (rarely detected) has been indicated to be involved, with evidence mostly supporting kinetic studies of the reactional mechanisms involved [118,135,141,147].

$$\text{oxidative addition: } M^{n+} + H_2 \rightleftharpoons M^{n+} H_2 \tag{3}$$

$$\text{homolytic cleavage: } 2\, M^{n+} + H_2 \rightleftharpoons 2\, M^{n+1}\, H \tag{4}$$

$$\text{heterolyiyc cleavage: } M^{n+} + H_2 \rightleftharpoons M^{n+} H^- + H^+ \tag{5}$$

The exchange reaction with D_2/H^+ or H_2/D^+ gave important clues and was studied using whole cells, crude extracts, and purified enzymes, supporting the heterolytic cleavage mechanism since the first product of the reaction is HD. Also, by thermodynamic arguments, the heterolytic cleavage is favored in the homolytic process [148]. Isotopic exchange between D_2 and H^+ and the *ortho/para* hydrogen conversion is also consistent with the heterolytic cleavage of the hydrogen molecule. The presence of a metal–hydride complex and of a proton acceptor site for the stabilization of the proton by a base (external or a metal ligand) is a necessary requirement, as indicated in Equations (6) and (7) [118,135,141,147].

$$M + H_2 + B \rightleftharpoons M\text{-}H^- + B\text{-}H^+ \tag{6}$$

$$M...X + H_2 \rightleftharpoons M\text{-}H^- + X\text{-}H^+ \tag{7}$$

On the basis that the enzyme-bound H or D atoms exchange more rapidly with the solvent than the hydride, HD is the initial product, but D_2 (or H_2) is, however, the final product of the total exchange process since there occurs a secondary exchange step of the HD molecule. If the hydride and proton acceptor sites can exchange independently with the solvent, the amount of HD and D_2 produced depends on the relative exchange rates of both sites and, consequently, the ratio of products should be pH-dependent (as supported by the available experimental data). In reality, the alteration in the pK_a values of the proton acceptor at the active site will be reflected in the isotope ratios [149–151]. The [NiFeSe] hydrogenases have H_2/HD ratios greater than 1 (Figure 8). The [NiFe] hydrogenases isolated from *D. gigas*, *D. multispirans* n.sp., and *D. desulfuricans* (ATCC 27774) show a ratio of H_2/HD smaller than 1 (0.3) at pH 7.6, but maximal activity is generally attained at intermediate pH values. This trend is further evidence that a heterolytic process is operative by analogy with inorganic models such as the (Pd-salen) complex [151]. *D. baculatus* and *D. gigas* hydrogenases show pH-dependent H_2/HD ratios. The rate-limiting step for the cleavage process at acidic pH values is the protonation of the proton-accepting site. At basic pH values, the liming step is the reformation of the H_2 molecule since the proton-accepting site has been deprotonated [141,142]. The curve follows the profile of a normal titration curve reflecting the protonation of the proton acceptor site. In the pH range 5–11, the H2/HD ratio is always smaller than 1 for the *D. gigas* enzyme. The same ratio calculated for a *D. baculatus* cytoplasmic hydrogenase is greater than 1 at pH > 5. Substitution of one of the sulfur ligands to the nickel by the less electronegative selenium may have a direct effect on the destabilization of the hydride form of this hydrogenase.

4.3. Overview

Hydrogenases are a clear case study of the influence of Selenium (as a Se-Cys) on the modulating or fine-tuning of enzyme catalytic properties through an acid-base equilibrium at the proton acceptor site or at the hydride site and should be explored for protein design and molecular modelling [117].

The [NiFeSe] hydrogenases clearly emerge as a subgroup of [NiFe] and there is a structural homology between [NiFe] and [NiFeSe]. However, [NiFeSe] is distinct in terms of its catalytic and active-site composition. Electrochemical studies help to reveal the interplay between the catalytic intermediates [152]. These enzymes display very interesting catalytic properties for biological hydrogen production and bio-electrochemical applications: high H_2 production activity, low H_2 inhibition, and O_2 tolerance [153].

The direct role of selenocysteine in [NiFeSe] hydrogenase maturation and catalysis has also been discussed. An expression system for the production of recombinant [NiFeSe] hydrogenase from *Desulfovibrio vulgaris* Hildenborough and study of a selenocysteine–to-cysteine variant (Sec489Cys) in which, for the first time, a [NiFeSe] hydrogenase was converted to a [NiFe] type, reveal the direct involvement of this residue in the maturation process. It was proposed that selenium plays a crucial role in protecting against oxidative damage and the high catalytic activities of [NiFeSe] hydrogenases [133].

5. Glutathione Peroxidases

GPx is a multiple-isozyme family which protects the cellular organism from oxidative stress by the reductive transformation of hydroperoxide (H_2O_2) or organic hydroperoxide substrates (ROOH) to the product of H_2O or alcohol, respectively, using cellular glutathione (GSH) as an electron source [154,155]. In 1952, Mills and Co-workers first noticed that GP_X protected hemoglobin from oxidative degradation [156]. After that, in the 1960s, GP_X activity was also observed in the lungs and kidneys [157]. In the 1970s, GPx was characterized and discovered selenocysteine amino acid, which played a vital role in enzymatic activity [158–160]. In the GPx family, only one GPx_1 member was known until the 1980s. Then, this family grew to eight members [161]. In humans, five GPxs (GPx_{1-4} and GPx_6) are encoded with selenocysteine residue in their catalytic site, whereas the rest (GPx_5, GPx_7, and GPx_8) contain conventional Cys residue in their catalytic site [154,162–165]. The active site of GPxs possesses a conserved tetrad that is constructed by four amino acid residues including glutamine (Gln), asparagine (Asn), tryptophan (Trp), and either cysteine (Cys) or selenocysteine (Sec) [166,167]. For instance, the catalytic tetrad site of human GPx_4 possesses Sec_{46}, Gln_{81}, Trp_{136}, and Asn_{137} residues. The catalytic site is normally present at the N-terminal (Figure 9) [168]. The crystal structures of GPx_{1-3} and GPx_6 are homotetrameric enzymes with masses of ~22–25 kDa in each subunit, whereas GPx_4 is a monomeric enzyme with a mass of ~20–22 kDa (Figure 9) [169,170].

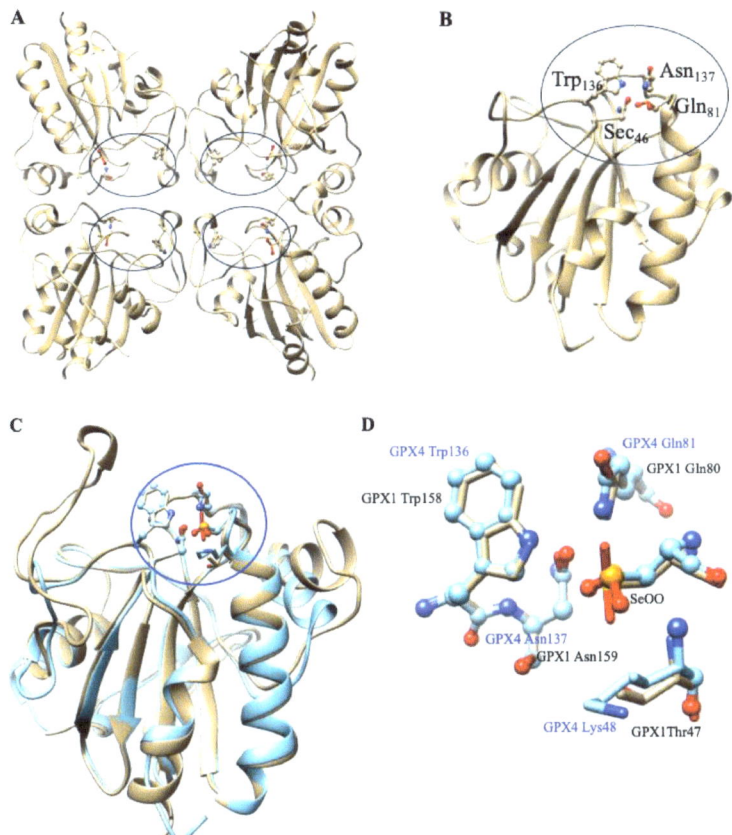

Figure 9. Crystal structure of GPxs. (**A**) Homo-tetramer of GPx1 (PDB file 1GP1) and (**B**) monomer of GPx4 (light blue; PDB file 6ELW). (**C**) Superimposed image of the crystal structures of GPx1 (one sub unit) and GPx4. (**D**) Highlighted is the conserved tetrad in the catalytic cycle of GPx1 and GPx4.

All GPxs display two steps of redox reactions in their catalytic cycle (Figure 10) [171,172]. In the first step, the selenocysteine (Sec-SeH) is oxidized to selenic acid (Sec-SeOH), which is a key intermediate product in the catalytic cycle. Simultaneously, the toxic hydroperoxide is reduced to the corresponding alcohol. In the second step, the reduction of oxidized Sec-SeOH proceeds into two subsequent 1 e$^-$ reduction steps. The Sec-SeOH is converted into GPx-SeGS by interacting with one equivalent reduced GSH, followed by the reduction of GPx-SeGS into GPx-Se by a second equivalent GSH for the next catalytic cycle [156,158,173–175]. The intermediate Sec-SeOH is stabilized by Gln and Trp, which are in the catalytic tetrad site [170], and additional Asn in tetrad contributes to the catalytic reaction [167]. Interestingly, the further oxidation product of Sec-SeH is seleninic acid (SeOO$^-$), which is found in the crystal structure of GPx4 (Figure 9), suggesting that selenium can shuttle between selenenic acid (RSeO$^-$) and seleninic acid (R-SeOO$^-$) redox states in the extended catalytic cycle. The highly oxidized R-SeOO$^-$ state in the enzyme may revert to the initial reduced state, R-Se$^-$ via RSeO$^-$, if suitable reducing species are available. This result may conclude that in a cellular redox state, the catalytic cycle of GPx4 may be mainly involved in R-Se$^-$ and R-SeO$^-$ redox states (low-oxidation cycle), but under oxidative stress, the catalytic cycle of GPx4 may be involved in R-SeO$^-$ and R-SeOO$^-$ redox states (high-oxidation cycle) [168]. The high-oxidation catalytic cycle may revert to a low-oxidation catalytic cycle if oxidative stress is overcome to the cellular redox state.

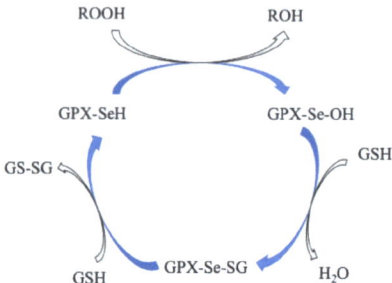

Figure 10. Proposed catalytic cycle of GPxs. Modified from [156].

6. Thioredoxin Reductases

TrxR belongs to the pyridine nucleotide–disulfide oxidoreductases family, of which some members are glutathione reductase, mercuric ion reductase, and lipoamide dehydrogenase [176]. A homodimeric flavoenzyme, it contains one redox-active dithiol/disulfide motif, FAD prosthetic group, and an NADPH binding site in each monomeric subunit [177]. TrxRs are distributed in all living systems and are generally classified into two major classes: (a) low molecular weight (LMW~35 kDa) TrxRs that are present in both lower eukaryotes and prokaryotes, and (b) high molecular weight (HMW~55 kDa) TrxRs that are present in higher eukaryotes [176,178]. Both classes of TrxR utilize NADPH as an electron source to reduce the oxidized state of TrxR that plays a vital role in cell proliferation. Due to large differences in structures, both classes of TrxRs have different catalytic paths to execute the same biochemical reaction. The LMW TrxRs have two redox centers such as an *N*-terminal dithiol/disulfide pair and an FAD prosthetic group [179,180], whereas HMW TrxRs contain three redox centers such as an *N*-terminal dithiol/disulfide pair and an FAD prosthetic group and sixteen additional amino acid residues with penultimate selenocysteine (Sec) in the catalytic site (-Cys-Secys-Gly sequence) at the end of the *C*-terminal [181–184].

There are three types of Mammals' TrxRs: (a) the cytosolic form, TrxR1 [185], (b) the mitochondrial form, TrxR2 [186,187], and (c) the testis-specific thioredoxin glutathione reductase (TGR) [188]. The overall protein fold of TrxR1 [189] is similar to other TrxR2 [190] and TGR [191]. Among them, TrxR1 is well-characterized. In 2001, the first three-dimensional (3D) structure of rat TrxR1 (Sec to Cys mutant) [189], followed by a large number of 3D structures (Sec-substituted mutants) of human TrxR1 [192] and mouse TrxR2 were published [190,193]. In 2009, the crystal structure of recombinant rat TrxR1 with Sec amino acid was reported by Cheng et al. [194]. However, the overall structure of rat TrxR1 is similar to human TrxR1. The 3D structure of rat TrxR1 reveals that it is a homodimeric protein and the two subunits arranged in a head-to-tail manner and each subunit consist of three domains which are the *N*-terminal, *C*-terminal, and interface domain. The *N*-terminal harbors FAD, NADPH, and the dithiol redox center (Cys59 and Cys64), and the *C*-terminal harbors a flexible sixteen amino acid extension with the selenolthiol redox centre (Cys497 and Secys498) (Figure 11) [194]. The two redox centers are far from to each other, but for the activity of TrxR, they come close to each other, forming a dimeric species where the *C*-terminal redox centre of one subunit directly interacts with the buried *N*-terminal redox centre of another subunit.

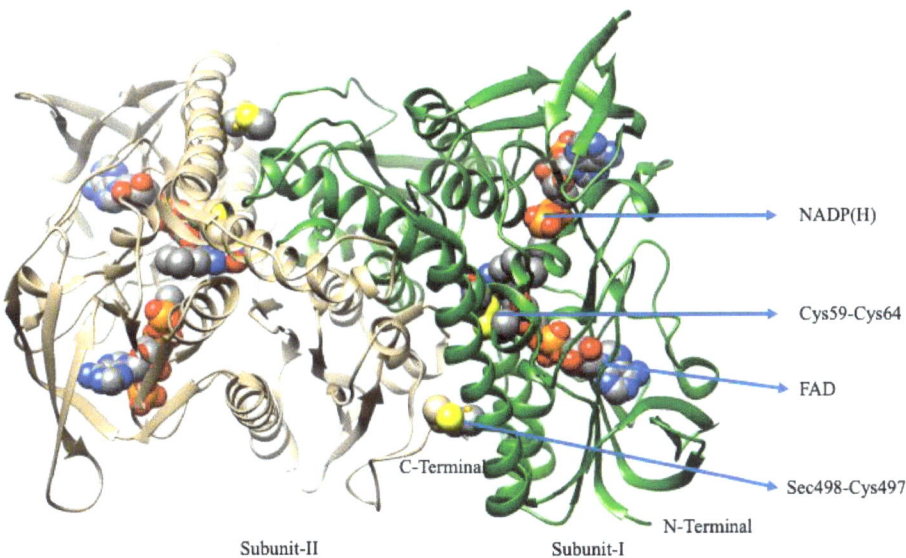

Figure 11. Crystal structure of dimer (subunit-I (green) and subunit-II (grey)) of recombinant rat selenocysteine TrXR 1 (PDB file 3EAO); highlighted are the redox centers in each subunit: *N*-terminal redox centre (Cys64 andCys59), FAD domain, and *C*-terminal redox centre (SeCys497 and Cys498).

TrxR is an important biological redox mediator for the two-electron reduction of substrates. The catalytic cycle of mammalian TrxR involves three redox centers: *N*-terminal dithiol (Cys_{59}–Cys_{64}), adjacent FAD/NADH, and *C*-terminal selenolthiol pair (Cys_{498}–Sec_{497}) in the other subunit), which relay e$^-$ from *N*-terminal dithiol to the substrate, thioredoxin via FAD/NADH. The human TrxR1 substrate–thioredoxin (Trx) complex is identified and the 3D structure of that complex reveals that the *C*-terminal arm binds with the substrate Trx through the disulphide bond (TrxR-Cys-S-S-Cys-Trx) [195]. A proposed mechanism of TrxR with Trx or small substrates (H_2O_2) is shown in Figure 12. The catalytic cycle starts by the 2e reduction of the Sec-Se-S-Cys to selenolate anion (Sec-Se$^-$) that reduces the Trx or substrate (like H_2O_2). For reduction, Cys-Se-S-Cys gains 2e electrons from NADPH via the FAD–dithiol (Cys_{59}–Cys_{64}) complex to produce Cys-SH and Sec-Se$^-$ at the *C*-terminal redox centre. The Sec-Se$^-$ ion is a relatively strong nucleophile over Cys-S$^-$. Therefore, Sec-Se$^-$ is more susceptible to oxidized selenenic acid (-SeOH) by H_2O_2 compared to Cys-S$^-$. Once it is formed, the adjacent cysteine thiol (Cys_{497}) reacts with selenenic acid to yield H_2O and selenenylsulfide that regenerates for the next cycle [196,197]. A similar catalytic mechanism is observed with Trx. The Sec-Se$^-$ nucleophilic attacks on the disulfide bond of oxidized Trx, yielding an enzyme–Trx complex through the selenenylsulfide bond, which is reopened by attacking the Cys497 of the selenolthiol pair (Cys_{498}–Sec_{497}), and subsequently forming selenenylsulfide (Sec498-Cys497) [196,198].

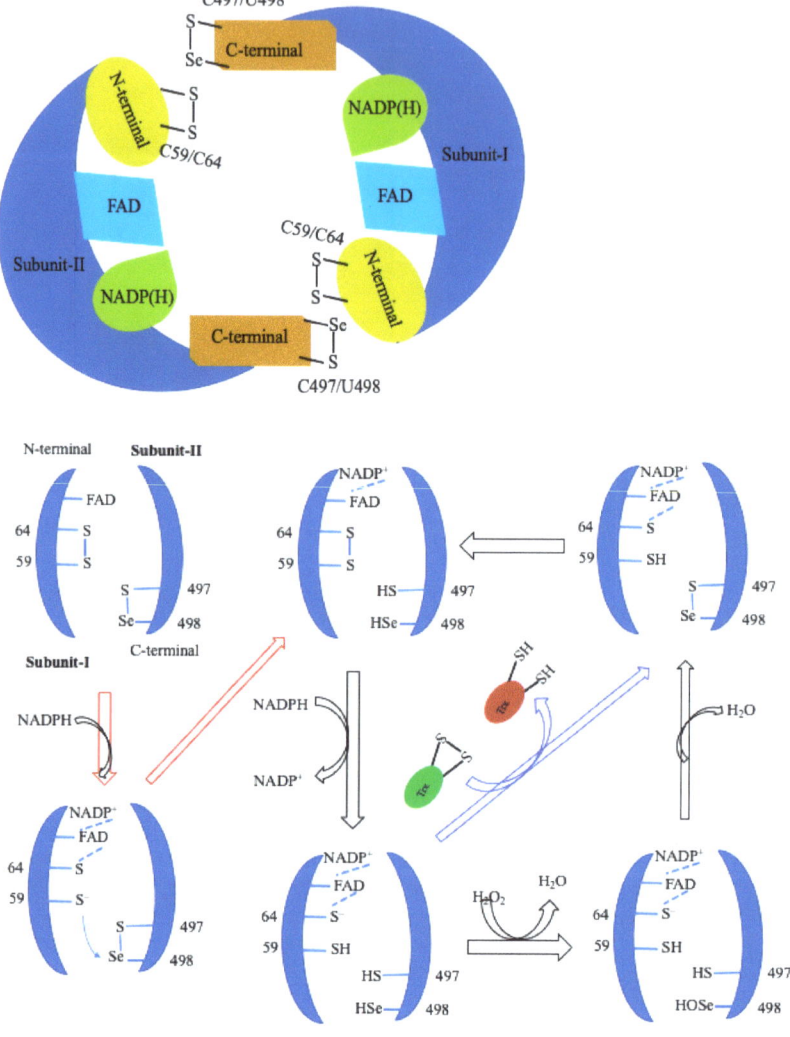

Figure 12. (**top**) Cartoon represents head-to-tail model of rat TrxR1 and (**bottom**) simplified possible mechanism for H_2O_2 or Trx reduction by TrxR. Modified from [196,197].

7. Iodothyronine Deiodinases

Dios are selenocysteine-dependent mammalian deiodinase enzymes that regulate thyroid hormones by deiodination of iodothyronine [199–202]. Dios have been classified into three isoforms, Dio1, Dio2, and Dio3, based on their sequence of amino acids and specificity of substrates. Dio1 enzymes non-selectively catalyze both inner- (phenolic group) and outer-ring (tyrosine group) deiodination of thyroid hormones, but Dio2 and Dio3 both selectively catalyze outer-ring and inner-ring deiodination (ORD and IRD) of thyroid hormones, respectively (Figure 13) [203–209]. For instance, Dio1 catalyzes the conversion of pro-hormone thyroxine (l-3,5,3′,5′-tetraiodothyronine; T4) to the biologically active hormone 3,5,3′-triiodothyronine (T3) or 3′,5′-triiodothyronine (rT3) by eliminating one iodine atom from ORD or IRD [210–213], whereas Dio3 (or Dio2) converts T3 (or rT3) into the biologically inactive hormone, 3,3′-T2. Therefore, Dio3 plays a vital role in protecting the cells from elevated thyroid hormones [203–209,214,215].

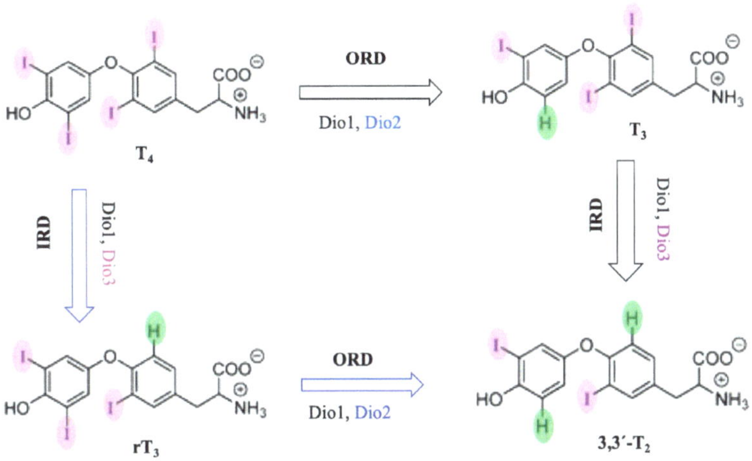

Figure 13. Probable mechanism of deiodination by deiodinase with thyroid hormone substrates.

8. Selenoproteins and Human Health

Selenoproteins (SePs) have been associated with many human health benefits but dysfunction of these proteins is associated with various human diseases such as diabetes, cancer, and viral infections [8,216–218]. SePs, particularly GPxs and TrxRs enzymes, participate in redox homeostasis and are believed to be a main contributing factor in the development and progression of various disease states [216].

8.1. Cancer

Compared to healthy cells, cancer cells generally harbor elevated reactive oxygen species (ROS), causing their abnormal growth with a high metabolic rate. To adjust the redox balance, cancer cells upregulate antioxidant systems to cope with the elevated ROS [197,219]. GPxs and TrxRs both can protect cancer cell development and progression by their antioxidant roles.

To date, several studies have attempted to analyze the role of GPxs, as well as changes in GPxs levels, in different types of tumors [216,220], but it remains controversial [221]. Indeed, GPx1 inhibits the oxidation of DNA mutations and, therefore, it may inhibit tumorigenesis [222], and overexpressed GPx1 reduces tumor growth, suggesting its protective effect in tumorigenesis [223]. However, reduced expression of GPx1 is detected in thyroid cancer [224], gastric cancer [225], and colorectal cancer [226], whereas GPx1 is highly expressed in kidney cancer [227] and pancreatic cancer [228]. Similar to GPx1, unusual expression of GPx2 is also observed in different tumors; for example, GPx2 is overexpressed in colorectal cancer [229], whereas a lower expression of GPx2 is detected in prostate intraepithelial neoplasia [230,231]. Regarding GPx3, it can be considered a novel tumor-suppressor gene [232,233] because hypermethylation is detected with down-regulation of GPx3 in tumor patients with Barrett's esophagus [234], prostate cancer [235], and endometrial adenocarcinoma [232,236]. Like GPx1-3, GPx4 is also a tumor suppressor due to its down-regulation in breast cancer [237] and pancreatic cancer [223]. In addition, overexpression of GPx4 reduces fibrosarcoma cell growth [238]. The role of other GPxs in tumorigenesis still remains controversial due to limited research [221].

Importantly, in excess, GPx may have detrimental effects due to a lack of necessary cellular oxidants [239,240] that can respond to cell growth, mitochondrial function, disulfide bond formation in protein, and cellular metabolism [241–244]. As GPx-1-4 are selenoproteins, these are readily affected by selenium levels in the cell. Several studies have shown that mixed results are observed in cancer after the administration of selenium supplements; therefore, selenium supplementation has a complex effect [245–247].

Polymorphism of human GPxs gene is a common phenomenon and it is associated with various diseases, especially tumors [248]. The GPx1 gene has various genetic polymorphisms and its most common polymorphism is the substitution of cytosine (C) to thymine (T) in DNA, resulting in the alteration of amino acid from proline (Pro) to leucine (Leu); thereby, the activity of GPx1 reduces by 5% [249]. Pro198Leu GPx1 polymorphism is associated with various types of cancer, mainly breast [250], prostate [251], lung [252], bladder [253], leukemia [254], and colon cancers [255]. However, the connection between GPx1 polymorphism and cancer vulnerability is controversial and inconclusive.

However, GPxs are overexpressed in several types of cancer/tumor cells and act as tumor promoters. Therefore, many studies are devoted to reducing the activity of GPxs by using suitable inhibitors for cancer therapy. Interestingly, several studies describe that the inactivation of GPx4 by the inhibitor of ferroptosis leads to oxidative destruction of the cancer cell via ferroptosis [256–258]. Therefore, GPx4 is considered to be a potential cancer therapy target. Several small-molecule drugs have been recognized as inhibitors of GPx4 that were originally pointed out as a modulator of ferroptosis in cancer/tumor cells. These small-molecule drugs are RSL3 [259], ML162, and ML210 [260]. The crystal structure of human GPx4 with an ML162 inhibitor (S enantiomer) (Figure 14) [261] reveals that ML162 is covalently bonded at the active site of GPx4, thus resulting in inactivation of the enzyme. GPx4 contains a selenocysteine in the catalytic site that affects redox regulation by consuming ROS [168]. Overall, GPxs have a dichotomous role as a tumor/cancer suppressor and in cancer progression. Therefore, more studies are needed to understand the dichotomous roles of GPxs in cancer.

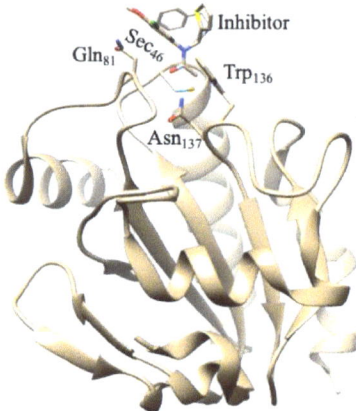

Figure 14. Crystal structure of human GPx4 with ML162 (inhibitor). PDB file 6HKQ.

Similar to GPxs, elevated TrxR levels are associated with the progression of tumor cells and increasing tumor drug resistance [197,262]. Several studies have reported that high levels of TrxR are observed in several human cancer cells, like the human A549 lung cancer cell line; thus, inhibiting TrxR function may be a promising strategy for cancer/tumor therapy [263–267]. TrxR contains two catalytic sites: $-Cys_{497}-Sece_{498}-$ and $-Cys_{59}-Cys_{64}-$ which reduce ROS, thus inhibiting its catalytic activity to halt cancer proliferation [268–271]. Therefore, several TrxR inhibitors have been reported to be anticancer agents and these are under pre-clinical and clinical trials [272]. Indeed, auranofin, a gold phosphine compound, can inhibit the catalytic activity of TrxR via interaction with a Sec amino acid residue at the catalytic site [271–275].

8.2. Diabetes

Diabetes mellitus (DM), a common human health problem around the globe, is a metabolic disorder and it is characterized by high levels of blood sugar (hyperglycemia), causing dysfunction in insulin secretion and/or sensitivity [276–280]. Insulin is a hormone synthesized in the β-cell of the pancreas and its action is also regulated by the pancreatic β-cell [280]. The most common type diabetes is Type 2 diabetes mellitus (T2DM) which is characterized by insulin resistance, caused by impairment of the pancreatic β-cell [280]. However, oxidative stress is believed to be the main cause of the onset and development of T2DM [281,282]. So, generation of ROS is a crucial factor in β-cell function [281]. Several studies have suggested that β-cells are highly susceptible to ROS because β-cells have lower antioxidant defenses, compared to other cells [281,283,284]. In addition, upon binding of its receptor, insulin commences a signaling cascade that elicits a mild oxidative burst of H_2O_2, which acts as a secondary messenger [285,286]. Many model studies have indicated that various antioxidant enzymes like selenoproteins are overexpressed in β-cells [281,285,287,288]. Indeed, high levels of GPx1 protect β-cells from H_2O_2, thus inhibiting insulin resistance in mice and human [287,288], but a deficiency of GPx1 raises insulin sensitivity in mice and human [289,290].

As oxidative stress is linked to the onset and progression of diabetes, antioxidant strategies would be a promising therapy for the treatment of diabetes.

8.3. Viral Infections

Viral infections occur when the human body is invaded by viruses, such as human immunodeficiency virus (HIV) and severe acute respiratory syndrome—coronavirus 2 (SARSCoV2), that lead to many diseases. Viral infection often alters the intracellular redox homeostasis in the host cell by increasing ROS production, which enhances the viral replication [291–294]. Several selenoproteins, like glutathione peroxidases (GPxs) and thioredoxin reductase (TrxR), are important host antioxidants that may play an important role against viral infections by consuming ROS.

8.3.1. Human Immunodeficiency Virus (HIV)

HIV, a single-stranded RNA virus, belongs to the lentivirus family [295] that infects human immune cells, causing a weakened immune system [295,296]. A large amount of experimental evidence has suggested that HIV infection triggers significant oxidative stress in host cells [297]. During virus entry into host cells, the glycoprotein-120 (gp120) of HIV interacts with cell surface receptor CD4 [298]. The conformational change of gp120 occurs due to the reduction of disulfide bonds to dithiol in gp120 [299–301], enabling cell fusion and resulting in HIV entry into the host cell [297]. Moreover, the dithiol/disulfide exchange form of CD4 is also a key factor for the interaction of CD4 and gp120 [302–305]. Therefore, the redox status in CD4 and gp120 is essential for HIV entry into the host cell, suggesting that the inhibition of thiol/disulfide exchange may be a promising target for the treatment of HIV [300,301,304–307].

After viral entry into host cell, HIV attempts replication, where Tat, a HIV-encoded trans-activating protein [308], is required. The primary structure of Tat contains 101 amino acids and its active site is located in the Cys-rich region (amino acids 20–39) [309,310]. However, the activity of Tat is markedly inhibited by the reducing agent, suggesting that the intramolecular disulfide bonds of Tat are crucial for Tat function [311]. Overall, during viral infection (entry and replication), both gp120 and Tat alter the host redox status, which is compensated by several host-detoxifying enzymes like glutathione, glutathione peroxidase, thioredoxin, and thioredoxin reductase [306,307]. These detoxifying enzymes are able to transfer electrons to gp120 and Tat, thus regulating the dithiol/disulfide exchange in structural conformations. Indeed, both gp120 and Tat suppress GSH levels, leading to an increase in the GSSG/GSH ratio [312–315]. GSSG/GSH supplies electrons to GPxs and TrxR, suggesting that HIV-1 infection changes the expression of selenoproteins [316].

As GPx and TrxR are selenoproteins, they are influenced by selenium levels in the cell. Several studies show that selenium supplementation suppresses the progression of HIV and improves CD4 counts [317].

Therefore, the inactivation of these enzymes might be a promising target for the treatment of HIV [300,301,304,305,307,318]. By inhibiting GPx or TrxR functions, the electrons supply to GSH or Trx1 might be frozen, thereby settling the reduction of disulfide bonds to dithiol in gp120 and Tat, which is crucial for HIV entry and replication [319]. Indeed, auranofin is a well-known TrxR1 inhibitor that can inhibit HIV infection by inhibiting the reduction of disulfide bonds in gp120 [320].

8.3.2. Coronavirus Disease-2019 (COVID-19)

The spread of Coronavirus Disease-2019 (COVID-19) caused a worldwide pandemic which has infected millions of people around the globe since 2019, caused by severe acute respiratory syndrome coronavirus-2 (SARS-CoV-2) [321–323]. The severity and mortality of COVID-19 are associated with various factors, including oxidative stress. The impairment of antioxidant defense is due to SARS-CoV-2 infection. Selenium and selenoproteins play a major role in combating oxidative stress in response to SARS-CoV-2 infections [324,325]. Several experiments from different countries have demonstrated that low serum levels are present in COVID-19 patients [326,327]. Interestingly, Se deficiency is also linked with the severity and mortality of other viral infections because deficiency of selenium reduces the activity of antioxidant enzymes leading to the amplification of ROS that induce viral replication [218,325,328–331]. However, currently, limited data on Se status in COVID-19 are available, and therefore further research is required to understand the role of Se in COVID-19.

The first step of SARS-CoV-2 entry into the host cell involves the binding of viral spike proteins onto a surface receptor enzyme, angiotensin-converting enzyme 2 (ACE 2) [332,333]. Both ACE2 and viral spike proteins have many cysteine residues that are responsible for the conformational modulation of viral spike proteins through thiol–disulfide exchange, enabling virus entry into host cells and the consequent depletion of intracellular redox homeostasis [334–336]. This thiol–disulfide equilibrium in the extracellular surface region is maintained by several host antioxidant enzymes including GSH and Trx [334–336].

Low levels of GSH enhance cellular oxidative stress associated with uncontrolled SARS-CoV-2 infection and with down-regulation of TrxR and GPx4 [337–339]. The homeostasis of GSH/GSSG (thiol-disulfide) depends on TrxR and GPx, seleno enzymes which catalyze the thiol–disulfide reaction, facilitating the reduction of the disulfide bonds of viral spike proteins and ACE2, thus resulting in impairment of virus-receptor adducts [335], but no experimental data are available.

In the process of virus replication, the main protease (Mpro), a highly conserved cysteine protease, cleaves polyproteins/peptides at multiple sites to produce multiple enzymatically active products [340,341]. Interestingly, the sequence of nsp13/14 junction (NVATLQ/A) of the Mpro cleavage site is similar to the GPx1 catalytic site sequence (NVASLU/G), wherein U (selenocysteine) lines up with Q (glutamine) in the Mpro sequence [342]. The U amino acid is not similar to the Q amino acid, but they are midrange in size and are polar amino acids in nature. The other two mismatched amino acid residues are S (serine) vs. T (threonine) and G (glycine) vs. A (alanine), both vary slightly by the presence of a methyl group [342,343]. Interestingly, GP_X1 significantly binds with the inactive Mpro mutant (C145A), but no interaction is observed between GPx1 and wild-type Mpro [342,343]. Based on this, Gallardo et al investigated experimentally the cleavage of the GPx1 10-mer peptide by Mpro, but no cleavage was observed [324]. It can be concluded that selenocysteine is significantly different from glutamine at the cleavage site. So, GPx1 can be considered at least as a potential Mpro substrate [344]. Gallardo et al. have also shown experimentally that Mpro can target the TrxR. The predicted cleavage was observed when the Sec498Ser mutant TrxR was incubated in Mpro, killing the C-terminal redox center of TrxR [324]. It is obvious that TrxR and GPx are disordered, resulting in increasing oxidative stress, which is associated with the severity and mortality of COVID-19.

8.4. Gestational Disorders

Selenium also plays an essential role in gestational health or during pregnancy, being one of the most important phases of a woman's life and human reproduction [345]. It is reported that during pregnancy, the mother and fetus both demand more oxygen, resulting in the formation of more ROS, which is associated with miscarriage, premature rupture of membranes, preeclampsia, and intrauterine growth restriction [346,347]. Se performs its antioxidant activity by including Se as selenocysteine in the active sites of selenoproteins such as GPx and TrxR. Many studies have reported that Se deficiency enables poor levels of GPx and TrxR expression, leading to gestational disorders [345,348,349]. Therefore, supplementation of Se during pregnancy can reduce oxidative stress, resulting in a decrease in pregnancy complications [350,351]. It has been suggested that selenoproteins play a key role in modulating the production of ROS during pregnancy, fostering maternal and fetal diseases; however, more experimental studies are needed to elucidate the gestational disorders in detail.

8.5. Overview

Overall, SePs are involved in human health and diseases such as diabetes, cancer, viral infections, and gestational disorders [8,216–218,345]. These diseases mainly enhance the production of harmful ROS that modulate redox homeostasis in cells. Cell-containing SePs, particularly GPxs and TrxRs, are the key enzymes for maintaining redox homeostasis, which is the main contributing factor in the development and progression of various disease states [216,345]. Figure 15 presents the connection between the production of ROS (during disease states) and the expression of SePs (GPxs and TrxRs). Numerous therapies have suggested that the expression level of GPxs and TrxRs can be modulated, which may halt the diseases. It is suggested that SePs play a key role in maintaining the redox balance during various disease states; however, more experimental studies are needed to elucidate the detailed mechanisms of these diseases.

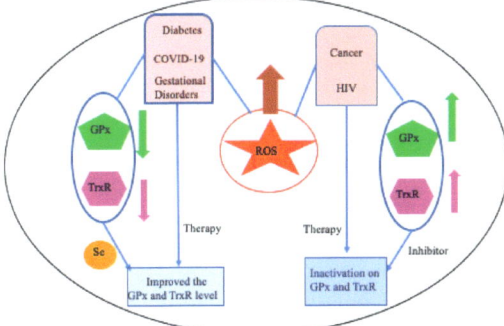

Figure 15. The cartoon illustrates all the connections between selenoproteins and various diseases. Arrows indicate up- and down-regulation.

9. Wrap-Up

Through the selenocysteine-containing enzymes above described, the following selected mechanistic and physiological roles of selenium were herein highlighted:

* Catalytic role in redox enzymes

The presence of one selenocysteine residue in an enzyme active site certainly introduces chemical features in the reaction mechanism which are not achievable with a "normal" cysteine. The selenocysteine selenol's lower pK_a value (5.2, compared to 8.3 of cysteine thiol) favors its deprotonation and nucleophilic character at a physiological pH (exploited, for example, in Hases). Selenium's preference for lower oxidation states and higher reactivity (compared to sulfur), as well as its ability to be easily regenerated (reduced back) from selenenic ($RSeO^-$) and seleninic ($R\text{-}SeOO^-$) forms and to participate in bridges with terminal sulfur atoms, represent other distinctive features (for example, to control cellular redox status and attain antioxidant activity). However, and remarkably, there are also striking examples, as is the case of FDHs, where replacing the selenium (selenocysteine) with sulfur (cysteine) does not affect at all the chemistry or the kinetics of the reaction.

* Physiological role in humans

Selenium is necessary for the conversion of the thyroid hormone thyroxine (T4) into its active form, triiodothyronine (T3), which is essential for regulating metabolism, growth, and development. Its role in immune system function is also key to enhancing the body's defence mechanisms against infections and other immune-related conditions. In addition, selenoproteins are involved in DNA synthesis and repair processes, contributing to the maintenance of genetic stability and prevention of mutations, as well as in sperm motility and function and in preventing complications during pregnancy. Some studies suggest that selenium may have a role in reducing the risk of certain cancers, such as prostate, lung, and colorectal cancer. However, more research is needed to confirm these potential benefits.

Funding: This work was supported by the PTDC/BTA-BTA/0935/2020 project and by the Associate Laboratory for Green Chemistry—LAQV (UIDB/50006/2020 and UIDP/50006/2020), which are financed by national funds from Fundação para a Ciência e a Tecnologia, MCTES (FCT/MCTES). FCT/MCTES is also acknowledged for the CEEC-Individual Program Contract (LBM). This work was also funded by DST–SERB for the CRG grant (file no CRG/2022/005673) and the Cluster University of Jammu for providing infrastructure facilities.

Data Availability Statement: The data presented in this study are available in article.

Conflicts of Interest: The authors declare no conflict of interest.

Abbreviations

ACE-2: angiotensin-converting enzyme 2; COVID-19, Coronavirus Disease-2019; Cys-FDH, cysteine-containing FDH; Cys-FMFDH, cysteine-containing FMFDH; Cys-Mo-FDH, cysteine and molybdenum-containing FDH; Cys-W-FDH, cysteine and tungsten-containing FDH; Dios, iodothyronine deiodinases; DM, diabetes mellitus; EPR, electron paramagnetic resonance spectroscopy; FDH, formate dehydrogenase; [Fe]-Hase, [Fe]-hydrogenase; [FeFe]-Hase, [FeFe]-hydrogenases; FMFDH, N-formyl-methanofuran dehydrogenases; GPx, glutathione peroxidase; GSH, glutathione; Hase, hydrogenases; HIV, human immunodeficiency virus; IRD, inner-ring deiodination; Mpro, main proteases; [NiFe]-Hase, [NiFe]-hydrogenase; [NiSeFe]-Hase, [NiSeFe]-hydrogenase; ORD, outer-ring deiodination; ROS, reactive oxygen species; R-SeOH, selenenic acid; R-SeOOH, seleninic acid; SARS-CoV-2, severe acute respiratory syndrome coronavirus 2; SeCys-FDH, selenocysteine-containing FDH; SeCys-FMFDH, selebocysteine-containing FMFDH; SeCys-Mo-FDH, selenocysteine and molybdenum-containing FDH; SeCys-W-FDH, selenocysteine and tungsten-containing FDH; SePs, selenoproteins; T2DM, Type 2 diabetes mellitus; TGR, thioredoxin glutathione reductase; Trx, thioredoxin; TrxR, thioredoxin reductase; XAS, X-ray absorption spectroscopy.

References

1. Painter, E.P. The Chemistry and Toxicity of Selenium Compounds, with Special Reference to the Selenium Problem. *Chem. Rev.* **1941**, *28*, 179–213. [CrossRef]
2. Hadrup, N.; Ravn-Haren, G. Acute human toxicity and mortality after selenium ingestion: A review. *J. Trace Elem. Med. Biol.* **2020**, *58*, 126435. [CrossRef] [PubMed]
3. Weekley, C.M.; Harris, H.H. Which form is that? The importance of selenium speciation and metabolism in the prevention and treatment of disease. *Chem. Soc. Rev.* **2013**, *42*, 8870–8894. [CrossRef] [PubMed]
4. Schwarz, K.; Foltz, C.M. Selenium as an integral part of factor 3 against dietary necrotic liver degeneration. *J. Am. Chem. Soc.* **1957**, *79*, 3292–3293. [CrossRef]
5. Fairweather-Tait, S.J.; Bao, Y.; Broadley, M.R.; Collings, R.; Ford, D.; Hesketh, J.E.; Hurst, R. Selenium in human health and disease. *Antioxid. Redox Signal.* **2011**, *14*, 1337–1383. [CrossRef] [PubMed]
6. Labunskyy, V.M.; Hatfield, D.L.; Gladyshev, V.N. Selenoproteins: Molecular pathways and physiological roles. *Physiol. Rev.* **2014**, *94*, 739–777. [CrossRef] [PubMed]
7. Kieliszek, M. Selenium–Fascinating Microelement, Properties and Sources in Food. *Molecules* **2019**, *24*, 1298. [CrossRef]
8. Roman, M.; Jitaru, p.; Barbante, C. Selenium biochemistry and its role for human health. *Metallomics* **2014**, *6*, 25–54. [CrossRef]
9. Driscoll, D.M.; Copeland, P.R. Mechanism and regulation of selenoprotein synthesis. *Annu. Rev. Nutr.* **2003**, *23*, 17–40. [CrossRef]

10. Hatfield, D.L.; Gladyshev, V.N. How selenium has altered our understanding of the genetic code. *Mol. Cell Biol.* **2002**, *22*, 3565–3576. [CrossRef]
11. Jacob, C.; Giles, G.I.; Giles, N.M.; Helmut Sies, H. Sulfur and Selenium: The Role of Oxidation State in Protein Structure and Function. *Angew. Chem. Int. Ed.* **2003**, *42*, 4742–4758. [CrossRef] [PubMed]
12. Wessjohann, L.A.; Schneider, A.; Abbas, M.; Brandt, W. Selenium in chemistry and biochemistry in comparison to sulfur. *Biol. Chem.* **2007**, *388*, 997–1006. [CrossRef]
13. Boyd, R. Selenium stories. *Nat. Chem.* **2011**, *3*, 570. [CrossRef] [PubMed]
14. Reich, H.J.; Hondal, R.J. Why Nature Chose Selenium. *ACS Chem. Biol.* **2016**, *11*, 821–841. [CrossRef] [PubMed]
15. Maiti, B.K. Cross-talk Between (Hydrogen)Sulfite and Metalloproteins: Impact on Human Health. *Chem.–A Eur. J.* **2022**, *28*, e202104342. [CrossRef] [PubMed]
16. Poole, L.B. The basics of thiols and cysteines in redox biology and chemistry. *Free Radic. Biol. Med.* **2015**, *80*, 148–157. [CrossRef]
17. Yukio Sugiura, Y.; Hojo, Y.; Tamai, Y.; Hisashi Tanaka, H. Selenium protection against mercury toxicity. Binding of methylmercury by the selenohydryl-containing ligand. *J. Am. Chem. Soc.* **1976**, *98*, 2339–2341. [CrossRef]
18. Huber, R.E.; Criddle, R.S. Comparison of the chemical properties of selenocysteine and selenocystine with their sulfur analogs. *Arch. Biochem. Biophys.* **1967**, *122*, 164–173. [CrossRef]
19. Bell, I.M.; Fisher, M.L.; Wu, Z.P.; Hilvert, D. Kinetic studies on the peroxidase activity of selenosubtilisin. *Biochemistry* **1993**, *32*, 3754–3762. [CrossRef]
20. Ruggles, E.L.; Snider, G.W.; Hondal, R.J. Chemical basis for the use of selenocysteine. In *Selenium: Its Molecular Biology and Role in Human Health*, 3rd ed.; Hatfield, D.L., Berry, M.J., Gladyshev, V.N., Eds.; Springer: New York, NY, USA, 2012; pp. 73–83.
21. Abdo, M.; Knapp, S. Biomimetic Seleninates and Selenonates. *J. Am. Chem. Soc.* **2008**, *130*, 9234–9235. [CrossRef]
22. Nauser, T.; Steinmann, D.; Grassi, G.; Koppenol, W.H. Why selenocysteine replaces cysteine in thioredoxin reductase: A radical hypothesis. *Biochemistry* **2014**, *53*, 5017–5022. [CrossRef] [PubMed]
23. Nauser, T.; Dockheer, S.; Kissner, R.; Koppenol, W.H. Catalysis of Electron Transfer by Selenocysteine. *Biochemistry* **2006**, *45*, 6038–6043. [CrossRef] [PubMed]
24. Nauser, T.; Steinmann, D.; Koppenol, W.H. Why do proteins use selenocysteine instead of cysteine? *Amino Acids* **2012**, *42*, 39–44. [CrossRef] [PubMed]
25. Joan, C.; Pleasants, J.C.; Guo, W.; Rabenstein, D.L. A comparative study of the kinetics of selenol/diselenide and thiol/disulfide exchange reactions. *J. Am. Chem. Soc.* **1989**, *111*, 6553–6558.
26. Hondal, R.J.; Marino, S.M.; Gladyshev, V.N. Selenocysteine in thiol/disulfide-like exchange reactions. *Antioxid Redox Signal.* **2013**, *18*, 1675–1689. [CrossRef] [PubMed]
27. Andreesen, J.R.; Ljungdahl, L.G. Formate dehydrogenase of Clostridium thermoaceticum: Incorporation of selenium-75, and the effects of selenite, molybdate, and tungstate on the enzyme. *J. Bacteriol.* **1973**, *116*, 867–873. [CrossRef] [PubMed]
28. Zinoni, F.; Birkmann, A.; Stadtman, T.C.; Böck, A. Nucleotide sequence and expression of the selenocysteine-containing polypeptide of formate dehydrogenase (formate-hydrogen-lyase-linked) from *Escherichia coli*. *Proc. Natl. Acad. Sci. USA* **1986**, *83*, 4650–4654. [CrossRef]
29. Zhang, Y.; Romero, H.; Salinas, G.; Gladyshev, V.N. Dynamic evolution of selenocysteine utilization in bacteria: A balance between selenoprotein loss and evolution of selenocysteine from redox active cysteine residues. *Genome Biol.* **2006**, *7*, R94.
30. Thauer, R.K.; Fuchs, G.; Jungermann, K. Role of iron-sulfur proteins in formate metabolism. In *Iron–Sulfur Proteins*; Lovenber, W., Ed.; Academic: New York, NY, USA, 1977; pp. 121–156.
31. Maden, B.; Edward, H. Tetrahydrofolate and tetrahydromethanopterin compared: Functionally distinct carriers in C1 metabolism. *Biochem. J.* **2000**, *350*, 609–629. [CrossRef]
32. Adams, M.W.W.; Mortenson, L.E. Mo reductases: Nitrate reductase and formate dehydrogenase. In *Molybdenum Enzymes*; Spiro, T.G., Ed.; Wiley Interscience: New York, NY, USA, 1985; pp. 519–593.
33. Ferry, J.G. Formate dehydrogenase. *FEMS Microbiol. Rev.* **1990**, *7*, 377–382. [CrossRef]
34. Unden, G.; Bongaerts, J. Alternative respiratory pathways of *Escherichia coli*: Energetics and transcriptional regulation in response to electron acceptors. *Biochim. Biophys. Acta* **1997**, *1320*, 217–234. [CrossRef] [PubMed]
35. Richardson, D.J. Bacterial respiration: A flexible process for a changing environment. *Microbiology* **2000**, *146*, 551–571. [CrossRef] [PubMed]
36. Richardson, D.; Sawers, G. Structural biology—PMF through the redox loop. *Science* **2002**, *295*, 1842–1843. [CrossRef] [PubMed]
37. Vorholt, J.A.; Thauer, R.K. Molybdenum and tungsten enzymes in C1 metabolism. *Met. Biol. Sys.* **2002**, *39*, 571–619.
38. Sawers, R.G. Formate and its role in hydrogen production in *Escherichia coli*. *Biochem. Soc. Trans.* **2005**, *33*, 42–46. [CrossRef] [PubMed]
39. Grimaldi, S.; Schoepp-Cothenet, B.; Ceccaldi, P.; Guigliarelli, B.; Magalon, A. The prokaryotic Mo/W-bisPGD enzymes family: A catalytic workhorse in bioenergetic. *Biochim. Biophys. Acta Bioenerg.* **2013**, *1827*, 1048–1085. [CrossRef] [PubMed]
40. Hille, R.; Hall, J.; Basu, P. The Mononuclear Molybdenum Enzymes. *Chem. Rev.* **2014**, *114*, 3963–4038. [CrossRef]
41. Maia, L.B.; Moura, J.J.; Moura, I. Molybdenum and tungsten-dependent formate dehydrogenases. *J. Biol. Inorg. Chem.* **2015**, *20*, 287–309. [CrossRef]
42. Hartmann, T.; Schwanhold, N.; Leimkühler, S. Assembly and catalysis of molybdenum or tungsten-containing formate dehydrogenases from bacteria. *Biochim. Biophys. Acta* **2015**, *1854*, 1090–1100. [CrossRef]

43. Maia, L.B.; Moura, I.; Moura, J.J. Molybdenum and tungsten-containing formate dehydrogenases: Aiming to inspire a catalyst for carbon dioxide utilization. *Inorg. Chim. Acta* **2017**, *455*, 350–363. [CrossRef]
44. Maia, L.B.; Moura, I.; Moura, J.J. Molybdenum and tungsten-containing enzymes: An overview. In *Molybdenum and Tungsten Enzymes: Biochemistry*; Hille, R., Schulzke, C., Kirk, M., Eds.; The Royal Society of Chemistry: Cambridge, UK, 2017; pp. 1–80.
45. Niks, D.; Hille, R. Reductive activation of CO_2 by formate dehydrogenases. *Methods Enzymol.* **2018**, *613*, 277–295. [PubMed]
46. Niks, D.; Hille, R. Molybdenum- and tungsten-containing formate dehydrogenases and formylmethanofuran dehydrogenases: Structure, mechanism, and cofactor insertion. *Prot. Sci.* **2019**, *28*, 111–122. [CrossRef] [PubMed]
47. Nielsen, C.F.; Lange, L.; Meyer, A.S. Classification and enzyme kinetics of formate dehydrogenases for biomanufacturing via CO_2 utilization. *Biotechnol. Adv.* **2019**, *37*, 107408. [CrossRef] [PubMed]
48. Maia, L.B.; Moura, I.; Moura, J.J.G. Carbon Dioxide Utilisation—The Formate Route. In *Enzymes for Solving Humankind's Problems*; Moura, J.J.G., Moura, I., Maia, L.B., Eds.; Springer International Publishing: Cham, Switzerland, 2021; pp. 29–81.
49. Kato, N. Formate dehydrogenase from methylotrophic yeasts. *Methods Enzymol.* **1990**, *188*, 459–462. [PubMed]
50. Vinals, C.; Depiereux, E.; Feytmans, E. Prediction of structurally conserved regions of D-specific hydroxy acid dehydrogenases by multiple alignment with formate dehydrogenase. *Biochem. Biophys. Res. Commun.* **1993**, *192*, 182–188. [CrossRef] [PubMed]
51. Popov, V.O.; Lamzin, V.S. NAD (+)-dependent formate dehydrogenase. *Biochem. J.* **1994**, *301*, 625–643. [CrossRef] [PubMed]
52. Filippova, E.V.; Polyakov, K.M.; Tikhonova, T.V.; Stekhanova, T.N.; Booeko, K.M.; Popov, V.O. Structure of a new crystal modification of the bacterial NAD-dependent formate dehydrogenase with a resolution of 2.1 Å. *Crystallogr. Rep.* **2005**, *50*, 796–800. [CrossRef]
53. Shabalin, I.G.; Polyakov, K.M.; Tishkov, V.I.; Popov, V.O. Atomic resolution crystal structure of nad+ dependent formate dehydrogenase from bacterium Moraxella sp. C-1. *Acta Nat.* **2009**, *1*, 89–93. [CrossRef]
54. Alekseeva, A.A.; Savin, S.S.; Tishkov, V.I. NAD+-dependent formate dehydrogenase from plants. *Acta Nat.* **2011**, *3*, 38–54. [CrossRef]
55. Hille, R. The mononuclear molybdenum enzymes. *Chem. Rev.* **1996**, *96*, 2757–2816. [CrossRef]
56. Johnson, M.K.; Rees, D.C.; Adams, M.W.W. Tungstoenzymes. *Chem. Rev.* **1996**, *96*, 2817–2839. [CrossRef] [PubMed]
57. Bertram, P.A.; Karrasch, M.; Schmitz, R.A.; Böcher, R.; Albracht, S.P.J.; Thauer, R.K. Formylmethanofuran dehydrogenases from methanogenic Archaea. Substrate specificity, EPR properties and reversible inactivation by cyanide of the molybdenum or tungsten iron-sulfur proteins. *Eur. J. Biochem.* **1994**, *220*, 477–484. [CrossRef] [PubMed]
58. Hochheimer, A.; Hedderich, R.; Thauer, R.K. The formylmethanofuran dehydrogenase isozymes in *Methanobacterium wolfeii* and *Methanobacterium terhmoautotrophicum*: Induction of the molybdenum isozyme by molybdate and constitutive synthesis of the tungsten isozyme. *Arch. Microbiol.* **1998**, *170*, 389–393. [CrossRef] [PubMed]
59. Wagner, T.; Ermler, U.; Shima, S. The methanogenic CO_2 reducing-and-fixing enzyme is bifunctional and contains 46 [4Fe-4S] clusters. *Science* **2016**, *354*, 114–117. [CrossRef] [PubMed]
60. Hemmann, J.L.; Wagner, T.; Shima, S.; Vorholt, J.A. Methylofuran is a prosthetic group of the formyltransferase/hydrolase complex and shuttles one-carbon units between two active sites. *Proc. Natl. Acad. Sci. USA* **2019**, *116*, 25583–25590. [CrossRef] [PubMed]
61. Niks, D.; Duvvuru, J.; Escalona, M.; Hille, R. Spectroscopic and Kinetic Properties of the Molybdenum-containing, NAD+-dependent Formate Dehydrogenase from *Ralstonia eutropha*. *J. Biol. Chem.* **2016**, *291*, 1162–1174. [CrossRef]
62. Maia, L.B.; Fonseca, L.; Moura, I.; Moura, J.J. Reduction of carbon dioxide by a molybdenum-containing formate dehydrogenase: A kinetic and mechanistic study. *J. Am. Chem. Soc.* **2016**, *138*, 8834–8846. [CrossRef] [PubMed]
63. Yu, X.; Niks, D.; Mulchandani, A.; Hille, R. Efficient reduction of CO_2 by the molybdenum-containing formate dehydrogenase from *Cupriavidus necator* (*Ralstonia eutropha*). *J. Biol. Chem.* **2017**, *292*, 16872–16879. [CrossRef]
64. Meneghello, M.; Oliveira, A.R.; Jacq-Bailly, A.; Pereira, I.A.C.; Léger, C.; Fourmond, V. Formate Dehydrogenases Reduce CO2 Rather than HCO_3^-: An Electrochemical Demonstration. *Angew. Chem.* **2021**, *60*, 9964–9967. [CrossRef]
65. Meneghello, M.; Uzel, A.; Broc, M.; Manuel, R.R.; Magalon, A.; Léger, C.; Pereira, I.A.C.; Walburger, A.; Fourmond, V. Electro-chemical Kinetics Support a Second Coordination Sphere Mechanism in Metal-Based Formate Dehydrogenase. *Angew. Chem.* **2023**, *62*, e202212224. [CrossRef]
66. Harmer, J.R.; Hakopian, S.; Niks, D.; Hille, R.; Bernhardt, P.V. Redox Characterization of the Complex Molybdenum Enzyme Formate Dehydrogenase from *Cupriavidus necator*. *J. Am. Chem. Soc.* **2023**, *145*, 25850–25863. [CrossRef] [PubMed]
67. Leimkühler, S. Metal-Containing Formate Dehydrogenases, a Personal View. *Molecules* **2023**, *28*, 5338. [CrossRef] [PubMed]
68. Stiefel, E.I. Proposed molecular mechanism for the action of molybedenum in enzymes: Coupled proton and electron transfer. *Proc. Natl. Acad. Sci. USA* **1973**, *70*, 988–992. [CrossRef] [PubMed]
69. Stiefel, E.I. The coordination and bioinorganic chemistry of molybdenum. *Prog. Inorg. Chem.* **1977**, *22*, 1–223.
70. Rajapakshe, A.; Snyder, R.A.; Astashkin, A.V.; Bernardson, P.; Evans, D.J.; Young, C.G.; Evans, D.H.; Enemark, J.H. Insights into the nature of Mo(V) species in solution: Modeling catalytic cycles for molybdenum enzymes. *Inorg. Chim. Acta* **2009**, *362*, 4603–4608. [CrossRef]
71. Maia, L.; Moura, I.; Moura, J.J.G. EPR spectroscopy on mononuclear molybdenum-containing enzymes. In *Future Directions in Metalloprotein and Metalloenzyme Research, Biological Magnetic Resonance*; Hanson, G., Berliner, L.J., Eds.; Springer International Publishing: Cham, Switzerland, 2017; Volume 33, pp. 55–101.
72. Kirk, M.L.; Hille, R. Spectroscopic Studies of Mononuclear Molybdenum Enzyme Centers. *Molecules* **2022**, *27*, 4802. [CrossRef]

73. Hille, R.; Niks, D. Application of EPR and related methods to molybdenum-containing enzymes. *Methods Enzymol.* **2022**, *666*, 373–412.
74. Gladyshev, V.N.; Khangulov, S.V.; Stadtman, T.C. Nicotinic acid hydroxylase from Clostridium barkeri: Electron paramagnetic resonance studies show that selenium is coordinated with molybdenum in the catalytically active selenium-dependent enzyme. *Proc. Natl. Acad. Sci. USA* **1994**, *91*, 232–236. [CrossRef]
75. Gladyshev, V.N.; Khangulov, S.V.; Axley, M.J.; Stadtman, T.C. Coordination of selenium to molybdenum in formate dehydrogenase H from *Escherichia coli*. *Proc. Natl. Acad. Sci. USA* **1994**, *91*, 7708–7711. [CrossRef]
76. Gladyshev, V.N.; Boyington, J.C.; Khangulov, S.V.; Grahame, D.A.; Stadtman, T.C.; Sun, P.D. Characterization of crystalline formate dehydrogenase H from *Escherichia coli*: Stabilization, EPR spectroscopy, and preliminary crystallographic analysis. *J. Biol. Chem.* **1996**, *271*, 8095–8100. [CrossRef]
77. Khangulov, S.V.; Gladyshev, V.N.; Dismukes, G.C.; Stadtman, T.C. Selenium-containing formate dehydrogenase H from *Escherichia coli*: A molybdopterin enzyme that catalyzes formate oxidation without oxygen transfer. *Biochemistry* **1998**, *37*, 3518–3528. [CrossRef] [PubMed]
78. Hanson, G.R.; Wilson, G.L.; Bailey, T.D.; Pilbrow, J.R.; Wedd, A.G. Multifrequency electron spin resonance of molybdenum (V) and tungsten (V) compounds. *J. Am. Chem. Soc.* **1987**, *109*, 2609–2616. [CrossRef]
79. Rivas, M.G.; González, P.J.; Brondino, C.D.; Moura, J.J.; Moura, I. EPR characterization of the molybdenum (V) forms of formate dehydrogenase from *Desulfovibrio desulfuricans* ATCC 27774 upon formate reduction. *J. Inorg. Biochem.* **2007**, *101*, 1617–1622. [CrossRef] [PubMed]
80. Oliveira, A.R.; Mota, C.; Klymanska, K.; Biaso, F.; Romão, M.J.; Guigliarelli, B.; Pereira, I.C. Spectroscopic and Structural Characterization of Reduced *Desulfovibrio vulgaris* Hildenborough W-FdhAB Reveals Stable Metal Coordination during Catalysis. *ACS Chem. Biol.* **2022**, *17*, 1901–1909. [CrossRef] [PubMed]
81. Oliveira, A.R.; Mota, C.; Mourato, C.; Domingos, R.M.; Santos, M.F.; Gesto, D.; Pereira, I.A. Toward the mechanistic understanding of enzymatic CO2 reduction. *ACS Catal.* **2020**, *10*, 3844–3856. [CrossRef]
82. Graham, J.E.; Niks, D.; Zane, G.M.; Gui, Q.; Hom, K.; Hille, R.; Raman, C.S. How a formate dehydrogenase responds to oxygen: Unexpected O_2 insensitivity of an enzyme harboring tungstopterin, selenocysteine, and [4Fe–4S] clusters. *ACS Catal.* **2022**, *12*, 10449–10471. [CrossRef]
83. Raman, C.S. Reply to Comment on 'How a Formate Dehydrogenase Responds to Oxygen: Unexpected O_2 Insensitivity of an Enzyme Harboring Tungstopterin, Selenocysteine, and [4Fe–4S] Clusters'. *ACS Catal.* **2023**, *13*, 9629–9632. [CrossRef]
84. Almendra, M.J.; Brondino, C.D.; Gavel, O.; Pereira, A.S.; Tavares, P.; Bursakov, S.; Moura, I. Purification and characterization of a tungsten-containing formate dehydrogenase from *Desulfovibrio gigas*. *Biochemistry* **1999**, *38*, 16366–16372. [CrossRef]
85. Raaijmakers, H.; Teixeira, S.; Dias, J.M.; Almendra, M.J.; Brondino, C.D.; Moura, I.; Romão, M.J. Tungsten-containing formate dehydrogenase from *Desulfovibrio gigas*: Metal identification and preliminary structural data by multi-wavelength crystallography. *J. Biol. Inorg. Chem.* **2001**, *6*, 398–404. [CrossRef]
86. Jollie, D.R.; Lipscomb, J.D. Formate dehydrogenase from Methylosinus trichosporium OB3b. Purification and spectroscopic characterization of the cofactors. *J. Biol. Chem.* **1991**, *266*, 21853–21863. [CrossRef]
87. Cramer, S.P.; Liu, C.L.; Mortenson, L.E.; Spence, J.T.; Liu, S.M.; Yamamoto, I.; Ljungdahl, L.G. Formate dehydrogenase molybdenum and tungsten sites—Observation by EXAFS of structural differences. *J. Inorg. Biochem.* **1985**, *23*, 119–124. [CrossRef]
88. George, G.N.; Colangelo, C.M.; Dong, J.; Scott, R.A.; Khangulov, S.V.; Gladyshev, V.N.; Stadtman, T.C. X-ray absorption spectroscopy of the molybdenum site of *Escherichia coli* formate dehydrogenase. *J. Am. Chem. Soc.* **1998**, *120*, 1267–1273. [CrossRef]
89. George, G.N.; Costa, C.; Moura, J.J.G.; Moura, I. Observation of ligand-based redox chemistry at the active site of a molybdenum enzyme. *J. Am. Chem. Soc.* **1999**, *121*, 2625–2626. [CrossRef]
90. Schrapers, P.; Hartmann, T.; Kositzki, R.; Dau, H.; Reschke, S.; Schulzke, C.; Haumann, M. Sulfido and cysteine ligation changes at the molybdenum cofactor during substrate conversion by formate dehydrogenase (FDH) from *Rhodobacter capsulatus*. *Inorg. Chem.* **2015**, *54*, 3260–3271. [CrossRef] [PubMed]
91. Duffus, B.R.; Schrapers, P.; Schuth, N.; Mebs, S.; Dau, H.; Leimkühler, S.; Haumann, M. Anion binding and oxidative modification at the molybdenum cofactor of formate dehydrogenase from *Rhodobacter capsulatus* studied by X-ray absorption spectroscopy. *Inorg. Chem.* **2020**, *59*, 214–225. [CrossRef] [PubMed]
92. Boyington, J.C.; Gladyshev, V.N.; Khangulov, S.V.; Stadtman, T.C.; Sun, P.D. Crystal structure of formate dehydrogenase H: Catalysis involving Mo, molybdopterin, selenocysteine, and an Fe4S4 cluster. *Science* **1997**, *275*, 1305–1308. [CrossRef] [PubMed]
93. Jormakka, M.; Tornroth, S.; Byrne, B.; Iwata, S. Molecular basis of proton motive force generation: Structure of formate dehydrogenase-N. *Science* **2002**, *295*, 1863–1868. [CrossRef] [PubMed]
94. Raaijmakers, H.; Macieira, S.; Dias, J.M.; Teixeira, S.; Bursakov, S.; Huber, R.; Moura, I.; Moura, M.J.; Romão, M.J. Gene sequence and the 1.8 Å crystal structure of the tungsten-containing formate dehydrogenase from *Desulfovibrio gigas*. *Structure* **2002**, *10*, 1261–1272. [CrossRef]
95. Radon, C.; Mittelstädt, G.; Duffus, B.R.; Burger, J.; Hartmann, T.; Mielke, T.; Teutloff, C.; Leimkuhler, S.; Wendler, P. Cryo-EM structures reveal intricate Fe-S cluster arrangement and charging in *Rhodobacter capsulatus* formate dehydrogenase. *Nat. Commun.* **2020**, *11*, 1912. [CrossRef]

96. Young, T.; Niks, D.; Hakopian, S.; Tam, T.K.; Yu, X.; Hille, R.; Blaha, G.M. Crystallographic and kinetic analyses of the FdsBG subcomplex of the cytosolic formate dehydrogenase FdsABG from *Cupriavidus necator*. *J. Biol. Chem.* **2020**, *295*, 6570–6585. [CrossRef]
97. Dietrich, H.M.; Righetto, R.D.; Kumar, A.; Wietrzynski, W.; Trischler, R.; Schuller, S.K.; Schuller, J.M. Membrane-anchored HDCR nanowires drive hydrogen-powered CO_2 fixation. *Nature* **2022**, *607*, 823–830. [CrossRef] [PubMed]
98. Yoshikawa, T.; Makino, F.; Miyata, T.; Suzuki, Y.; Tanaka, H.; Namba, K.; Kano, K.; Sowa, K.; Kitazumi, Y.; Shirai, O. Multiple electron transfer pathways of tungsten-containing formate dehydrogenase in direct electron transfer-type bioelectrocatalysis. *Chem. Commun.* **2022**, *58*, 6478–6481. [CrossRef] [PubMed]
99. Vilela-Alves, G.; Manuel, R.R.; Oliveira, A.R.; Pereira, I.C.; Romão, M.J.; Mota, C. Tracking W-Formate Dehydrogenase Structural Changes during Catalysis and Enzyme Reoxidation. *Int. J. Mol. Sci.* **2022**, *24*, 476. [CrossRef] [PubMed]
100. Zinoni, F.; Birkmann, A.; Leinfelder, W.; Bock, A. Cotranslational insertion of selenocysteine into formate dehydrogenase from *Escherichia coli* directed by a UGA codon. *Proc. Natl. Acad. Sci. USA* **1987**, *84*, 3156–3160. [CrossRef] [PubMed]
101. Axley, M.J.; Böck, A.; Stadtman, T.C. Catalytic properties of an *Escherichia coli* formate dehydrogenase mutant in which sulfur replaces selenium. *Proc. Natl. Acad. Sci. USA* **1991**, *88*, 8450–8454. [CrossRef] [PubMed]
102. Berry, M.J.; Martin, G.W.; Tujebajeva, R.; Grundner-Culemann, E.; Mansell, J.B.; Morozova, N.; Harney, J.W. Selenocysteine Insertion Sequence Element Characterization and Selenoprotein Expression. *Methods Enzymol.* **2002**, *347*, 17–24.
103. Hatfield, D.L.; Carlson, B.A.; Xu, X.M.; Mix, H.; Gladyshev, V.N. Selenocysteine Incorporation Machinery and the Role of Selenoproteins in Development and Health. *Prog. Nucleic Acid Res. Mol. Biol.* **2006**, *81*, 97–142.
104. Allmang, C.; Wurth, L.; Krol, A. The Selenium to Selenoprotein Pathway in Eukaryotes: More Molecular Partners than Anticipated. *Biochim. Biophys. Acta Gen. Subj.* **2009**, *1790*, 1415–1423. [CrossRef]
105. Yoshizawa, S.; Böck, A. The Many Levels of Control on Bacterial Selenoprotein Synthesis. *Biochim. Biophys. Acta Gen. Subj.* **2009**, *1790*, 1404–1414. [CrossRef]
106. Bulteau, A.-L.; Chavatte, L. Update on Selenoprotein Biosynthesis. *Antioxid. Redox Signal.* **2015**, *23*, 775–794. [CrossRef]
107. Arnér, E.S. Selenoproteins—What unique properties can arise with selenocysteine in place of cysteine? *Exp. Cell Res.* **2010**, *316*, 1296–1303. [CrossRef] [PubMed]
108. Brigelius-Flohe, R. The Evolving Versatility of Selenium in Biology. *Antioxid. Redox Signal.* **2015**, *23*, 757–760. [CrossRef] [PubMed]
109. Bortoli, M.; Torsello, M.; Bickelhaupt, F.M.; Orian, L. Role of the Chalcogen (S, Se, Te) in the Oxidation Mechanism of the Glutathione Peroxidase Active Site. *ChemPhysChem* **2017**, *18*, 2990–2998. [CrossRef] [PubMed]
110. Maroney, M.J.; Hondal, R.J. Selenium Versus Sulfur: Reversibility of Chemical Reactions and Resistance to Permanent Oxidation in Proteins and Nucleic Acids. *Free Radic. Biol. Med.* **2018**, *127*, 228–237. [CrossRef]
111. Ingold, I.; Berndt, C.; Schmitt, S.; Doll, S.; Poschmann, G.; Buday, K.; Roveri, A.; Peng, X.; Porto Freitas, F.; Seibt, T.; et al. Selenium Utilization by GPx4 Is Required to Prevent Hydroperoxide-Induced Ferroptosis. *Cell* **2018**, *172*, 409–422. [CrossRef]
112. Lubitz, W.; Ogata, H.; Rüdiger, O.; Reijerse, E. Hydrogenases. *Chem. Rev.* **2014**, *114*, 4081–4148. [CrossRef]
113. Ogata, H.; Nishikawa, K.; Lubitz, W. Hydrogens detected by subatomic resolution protein crystallography in a [NiFe] hydrogenase. *Nature* **2015**, *520*, 571–574. [CrossRef]
114. Fauque, G.; Peck, H.D., Jr.; Moura, J.J.G.; Huynh, B.H.; Berlier, Y.; DerVartanian, D.V.; Teixeira, M.; Przybyla, A.E.; Lespinat, P.A.; Moura, I. The three classes of hydrogenases from sulfate-reducing bacteria of the genus Desulfovibrio. *FEMS Microbiol. Rev.* **1988**, *4*, 299–344. [CrossRef]
115. Pereira, A.S.; Tavares, P.; Moura, I.; Moura, J.J.; Huynh, B.H. Mössbauer characterization of the iron-sulfur clusters in *Desulfovibrio vulgaris* hydrogenase. *J. Am. Chem. Soc.* **2001**, *123*, 2771–2782. [CrossRef]
116. Patil, D.S.; Moura, J.J.; He, S.H.; Teixeira, M.; Prickril, B.C.; DerVartanian, D.V.; Peck, H.D., Jr.; LeGall, J.; Huynh, B.H. EPR-detectable redox centers of the periplasmic hydrogenase from *Desulfovibrio vulgaris*. *J. Biol. Chem.* **1988**, *263*, 18732–18738. [CrossRef]
117. Moura, J.J.G.; Teixeira, M.; Moura, I. The role of nickel and iron-sulfur centers in the bioproduction of hydrogen. *Pure Appl. Chem.* **1989**, *61*, 915–921. [CrossRef]
118. Wombwell, C.; Caputo, C.A.; Reisner, E. [NiFeSe]-Hydrogenase Chemistry. *Acc. Chem. Res.* **2015**, *48*, 2858–2865. [CrossRef] [PubMed]
119. Barbosa, T.M.; Baltazar, C.S.A.; Cruz, D.R.; Lousa, D.; Soares, C.M. Studying O2 pathways in [NiFe]- and [NiFeSe]-hydrogenases. *Sci. Rep.* **2020**, *10*, 10540. [CrossRef] [PubMed]
120. Happe, R.P.; Roseboom, W.; Pierik, A.J.; Albracht, S.P.; Bagley, K.A. Biological Activation of Hydrogen. *Nature* **1997**, *385*, 126. [CrossRef] [PubMed]
121. Bleijlevens, B.; van Broekhuizen, F.A.; De Lacey, A.L.; Roseboom, W.; Fernandez, V.M.; Albracht, S.P. The Activation of the [NiFe]-Hydrogenase from Allochromatium Vinosum. An Infrared Spectro-Electrochemical Study. *J. Biol. Inorg. Chem.* **2004**, *9*, 743–752. [CrossRef] [PubMed]
122. Fichtner, C.; Laurich, C.; Bothe, E.; Lubitz, W. Spectroelectrochemical Characterization of the [NiFe] Hydrogenase of *Desulfovibrio vulgaris* Miyazaki F. *Biochemistry* **2006**, *5*, 9706–9716. [CrossRef] [PubMed]
123. Frey, M.; Fontecilla-Camps, J.C.; Volbeda, A. Nickel–Iron Hydrogenases. In *Handbook of Metalloproteins*; Messerschmidt, A., Huber, R., Poulos, T., Wieghardt, K., Eds.; John Wiley & Sons, Ltd.: Chichester, UK, 2001; p. 880.

124. LeGall, J.; Ljungdahl, P.O.; Moura, I.; Peck, H.D., Jr.; Xavier, A.V.; Moura, J.J.G.; Teixera, M.; Huynh, B.H. DerVartanian DV. The presence of redox-sensitive nickel in the periplasmic hydrogenase from *Desulfovibrio gigas*. *Biochem. Biophys. Res. Commun.* **1982**, *106*, 610–616. [CrossRef] [PubMed]
125. Higuchi, Y.; Yagi, T.; Yasuoka, N. Unusual Ligand Structure in Ni-Fe Active Center and an Additional Mg Site in Hydrogenase Revealed by High Resolution X-Ray Structure Analysis. *Structure* **1997**, *5*, 1671–1680. [CrossRef]
126. Volbeda, A.; Garcin, E.; Piras, C.; deLacey, A.L.; Fernandez, V.M.; Hatchikian, E.C.; Frey, M.; FontecillaCamps, J.C. Structure of the [NiFe] Hydrogenase Active Site: Evidence for Biologically Uncommon Fe Ligands. *J. Am. Chem. Soc.* **1996**, *118*, 12989–12996. [CrossRef]
127. Carepo, M.; Tierney, D.L.; Brondino, C.D.; Yang, T.C.; Pamplona, A.; Telser, J.; Moura, I.; Moura, J.J.; Hoffman, B.M. ^{17}O ENDOR detection of a solvent-derived Ni-(OH(x))-Fe bridge that is lost upon activation of the hydrogenase from *Desulfovibrio gigas*. *J. Am. Chem. Soc.* **2002**, *124*, 281–286. [CrossRef]
128. Teixeira, M.; Moura, I.; Xavier, A.V.; Huynh, B.H.; DerVartanian, D.V.; Peck, H.D., Jr.; LeGall, J.; Moura, J.J. Electron paramagnetic resonance studies on the mechanism of activation and the catalytic cycle of the nickel-containing hydrogenase from *Desulfovibrio gigas*. *J. Biol. Chem.* **1985**, *260*, 8942–8950. [CrossRef] [PubMed]
129. Teixeira, M.; Moura, I.; Xavier, A.V.; Moura, J.J.; LeGall, J.; DerVartanian, D.V.; Peck, H.D., Jr.; Huynh, B.H. Redox intermediates of *Desulfovibrio gigas* [NiFe] hydrogenase generated under hydrogen. Mössbauer and EPR characterization of the metal centers. *J. Biol. Chem.* **1989**, *264*, 16435–16450. [CrossRef] [PubMed]
130. Foerster, S.; van Gastel, M.; Brecht, M.; Lubitz, W. An Orientation-Selected ENDOR and HYSCORE Study of the Ni-C Active State of *Desulfovibrio vulgaris* Miyazaki F Hydrogenase. *J. Biol. Inorg. Chem.* **2005**, *10*, 51–62. [CrossRef] [PubMed]
131. Yang, X.; Darensbourg, M.Y. The roles of chalcogenides in O_2 protection of H_2ase active sites. *Chem. Sci.* **2020**, *11*, 9366–9377. [CrossRef] [PubMed]
132. Marques, M.C.; Coelho, R.; De Lacey, A.L.; Pereira, I.A.; Matias, P.M. The Three-Dimensional Structure of [NiFeSe] Hydrogenase from *Desulfovibrio vulgaris* Hildenborough: A Hydrogenase without a Bridging Ligand in the Active Site in its Oxidised, "As-Isolated" State. *J. Mol. Biol.* **2010**, *396*, 893–907. [CrossRef]
133. Marques, M.C.; Tapia, C.; Gutierrez-Sanz, O.; Ramos, A.R.; Keller, K.L.; Wall, J.D.; De Lacey, A.L.; Matias, P.M.; Pereira, I.A.C. The Direct Role of Selenocysteine in [NiFeSe] Hydrogenase Maturation and Catalysis. *Nat. Chem. Biol.* **2017**, *13*, 544–550. [CrossRef]
134. Baltazar, C.S.A.; Marques, M.C.; Soares, C.M.; DeLacey, A.M.; Pereira, I.A.C.; Matias, P.M. Nickel–iron–selenium hydrogenases—An overview. *Eur. J. Inorg. Chem.* **2011**, *2011*, 948–962. [CrossRef]
135. Teixeira, M.; Moura, I.; Fauque, G.; Dervartanian, D.V.; Legall, J.; Peck, H.D., Jr.; Moura, J.J.; Huynh, B.H. The iron-sulfur centers of the soluble [NiFeSe] hydrogenase, from *Desulfovibrio baculatus* (DSM 1743). EPR and Mossbauer Characterization. *Eur. J. Biochem.* **1990**, *189*, 381–386. [CrossRef]
136. Parkin, A.; Goldet, G.; Cavazza, C.; Fontecilla-Camps, J.C.; Armstrong, F.A. The Difference a se Makes? Oxygen-Tolerant Hydrogen Production by the [NiFeSe]-Hydrogenase from *Desulfomicrobium baculatum*. *J. Am. Chem. Soc.* **2008**, *130*, 13410–13416. [CrossRef]
137. Rüdiger, O.; Gutiérrez-Sánchez, C.; Olea, D.; Pereira, I.A.C.; Vélez, M.; Fernández, V.M.; De Lacey, A.L. Enzymatic Anodes for Hydrogen Fuel Cells Based on Covalent Attachment of Ni-Fe Hydrogenases and Direct Electron Transfer to SAM-Modified Gold Electrodes. *Electroanalysis* **2010**, *22*, 776–783. [CrossRef]
138. Valente, F.M.A.; Oliveira, A.S.F.; Gnadt, N.; Pacheco, I.; Coelho, A.V.; Xavier, A.V.; Teixeira, M.; Soares, C.M.; Pereira, I.A.C. Hydrogenases in *Desulfovibrio vulgaris* Hildenborough: Structural and Physiologic Characterisation of the Membrane-Bound [NiFeSe] Hydrogenase. *J. Biol. Inorg. Chem.* **2005**, *10*, 667–682. [CrossRef] [PubMed]
139. Medina, M.; Claude Hatchikian, E.; Cammack, R. Studies of Light-Induced Nickel EPR Signals in Hydrogenase: Comparison of Enzymes with and without Selenium. *Biochim. Biophys. Acta* **1996**, *1275*, 227–236. [CrossRef]
140. Teixeira, M.; Fauque, G.; Moura, I.; Lespinat, P.A.; Berlier, Y.; Prickril, B.; Peck, H.D., Jr.; Xavier, A.V.; LeGall, J.; Moura, J.J.G. Nickel-[iron-sulfur]-selenium-containing hydrogenases from *Desulfovibrio baculatus* (DSM 1743). Redox centers and catalytic properties. *Eur. J. Biochem.* **1987**, *167*, 47–58. [CrossRef] [PubMed]
141. Teixeira, M.; Moura, I.; Fauque, G.; Czechowski, M.; Berlier, Y.; Lespinat, P.A.; Le Gall, J.; Xavier, A.V.; Moura, J.J.G. Redox properties and activity studies on a nickel-containing hydrogenase isolated from a halophilic sulfate reducer *Desulfovibrio salexigens*. *Biochimie* **1986**, *68*, 75–84. [CrossRef] [PubMed]
142. Lespinat, P.A.; Berlier, Y.; Fauque, G.; Czechowski, M.H.; Dimon, B.; LeGall, J. The pH dependence of proton-deuterium exchange, hydrogen production and uptake catalyzed by hydrogenases from sulfate-reducing bacteria. *Biochimie* **1986**, *68*, 55–61. [CrossRef] [PubMed]
143. Moura, J.J.G.; Moura, I.; Huynh, B.H.; Krüger, H.J.; Teixeira, M.; DuVarney, R.C.; DerVartanian, D.V.; Xavier, A.V.; Peck, H.D., Jr.; LeGall, J. Unambiguous identification of the nickel EPR signal in ^{61}Ni-enriched *Desulfovibrio gigas* hydrogenase. *J. Biochem. Biophys. Res. Commun.* **1982**, *108*, 1388–1393. [CrossRef] [PubMed]
144. Gutierrez-Sanz, O.; Marques, M.C.; Baltazar, C.S.; Fernandez, V.M.; Soares, C.M.; Pereira, I.A.C.; De Lacey, A.L. Influence of the Protein Structure Surrounding the Active Site on the Catalytic Activity of [NiFeSe] Hydrogenases. *J. Biol. Inorg. Chem.* **2013**, *18*, 419–427. [CrossRef] [PubMed]

145. He, S.H.; Teixeira, M.; LeGall, J.; Patil, D.S.; Moura, I.; Moura, J.J.; DerVartanian, D.V.; Huynh, B.H.; Peck, H.D., Jr. EPR studies with 77Se-enriched (NiFeSe) hydrogenase of *Desulfovibrio baculatus*. Evidence for a selenium ligand to the active site nickel. *J. Biol. Chem.* **1989**, *264*, 2678–2682. [CrossRef]
146. Eidsness, M.K.; Scott, R.A.; Prickril, B.C.; DerVartanian, D.V.; LeGall, J.; Moura, I.; Moura, J.J.; Peck, H.D., Jr. Evidence for selenocysteine coordination to the active site nickel in the [NiFeSe] hydrogenases from *Desulfovibrio baculatus*. *Proc. Natl. Acad. Sci. USA* **1989**, *86*, 147–151. [CrossRef]
147. Moura, J.J.G.; Teixeira, M.; Moura, I.; LeGall, J. [Ni-Fe] hydrogenases from sulfate reducing bacteria: Nickel catalytic and regulatory roles. In *Nickel in Biochemistry*; Lancaster, J.R., Ed.; VCH Publishers: New York, NY, USA, 1988; Chapter 9; pp. 191–224.
148. van der Zwaan, J.W.; Albracht, S.P.J.; Fontijn, R.D.; Slater, E.C. Monovalent nickel in hydrogenase from *Chromatium vinosum*. *FEBS Lett.* **1985**, *179*, 271–277. [CrossRef]
149. Fauque, G.D.; Barton, L.L.; LeGall, J. Oxidative Phosphorylation Linked to the Dissimilatory Reduction of Elemental Sulphur by Desulfovibrio. *Ciba Found. Symp.* **1980**, *72*, 71–86.
150. Fischer, H.F.; Krasna, A.I.; Rittenberg, D. The interaction of hydrogenase with oxygen. *J. Biol. Chem.* **1954**, *209*, 569–578. [CrossRef]
151. Olive, H.; Olive, S. Hydrogenation catalysts: A synthetic hydrogenase model. *J. Mol. Catal.* **1976**, *1*, 121–125. [CrossRef]
152. Moura, I.; Cordas, C.; Moura, J.J.G. Direct electrochemistry study of the multiple redox centers of hydrogenase from *Desulfovibrio gigas*. *Bioelectrochemistry* **2008**, *74*, 83–89.
153. Zacarias, S.; Vélez, M.; Pita, M.; De Lacey, A.L.; Matias, P.M.; Pereira, I.A.C. Characterization of the [NiFeSe] hydrogenase from *Desulfovibrio vulgaris* Hildenborough. *Methods Enzymol.* **2018**, *613*, 169–201. [PubMed]
154. Stolwijk, J.M.; Garje, R.; Sieren, J.C.; Buettner, G.R.; Zakharia, Y. Understanding the Redox Biology of Selenium in the Search of Targeted Cancer Therapies. *Antioxidants* **2020**, *9*, 420. [CrossRef] [PubMed]
155. Weaver, K.; Skouta, R. The Selenoprotein Glutathione Peroxidase 4: From Molecular Mechanisms to Novel Therapeutic Opportunities. *Biomedicines* **2022**, *10*, 891. [CrossRef] [PubMed]
156. Mills, G.C. *Hemoglobin catabolism*. I. *Glutathione peroxidase*, an erythrocyte enzyme which protects hemoglobin from oxidative breakdown. *J. Biol. Chem.* **1957**, *229*, 189–197. [CrossRef]
157. Little, C.; Olinescu, R.; Reid, K.G.; O'Brien, P.J. Properties and Regulation of *Glutathione peroxidase*. *J. Biol. Chem.* **1970**, *245*, 3632–3636. [CrossRef]
158. Flohe, L.; Günzler, W.A.; Schock, H.H. *Glutathione peroxidase*: A selenoenzyme. *FEBS Lett.* **1973**, *32*, 132–134. [CrossRef]
159. Rotruck, J.T.; Pope, A.L.; Ganther, H.E.; Swanson, A.B.; Hafeman, D.G.; Hoekstra, W.G. Selenium: Biochemical role as a component of glutathione peroxidase. *Science* **1973**, *179*, 588–590. [CrossRef] [PubMed]
160. Forstrom, J.W.; Zakowski, J.J.; Tappel, A.L. Identification of the catalytic site of rat liver glutathione peroxidase as selenocysteine. *Biochemistry* **1978**, *17*, 2639–2644. [CrossRef] [PubMed]
161. Trenz, T.S.; Delaix, C.L.; Turchetto-Zolet, A.C.; Zamocky, M.; Lazzarotto, F.; Margis-Pinheiro, M. Going Forward and Back: The Complex Evolutionary History of the GPx. *Biology* **2021**, *10*, 1165. [CrossRef] [PubMed]
162. Herbette, S.; Roeckel-Drevet, P.; Drevet, J.R. Seleno-independent glutathione peroxidases. More than simple antioxidant scavengers. *FEBS J.* **2007**, *274*, 2163–2180. [CrossRef]
163. Mariotti, M.; Ridge, P.G.; Zhang, Y.; Lobanov, A.V.; Pringle, T.H.; Guigo, R.; Hatfield, D.L.; Gladyshev, V.N. Composition and evolution of the vertebrate and mammalian selenoproteomes. *PLoS ONE* **2012**, *7*, e33066. [CrossRef]
164. Toppo, S.; Vanin, S.; Bosello, V.; Tosatto, S.C.E. Evolutionary and structural insights into the multifaceted glutathione peroxidase (Gpx) superfamily. *Antioxid. Redox Signal.* **2008**, *10*, 1501–1514. [CrossRef]
165. Kryukov, G.V.; Castellano, S.; Novoselov, S.V.; Lobanov, A.V.; Zehtab, O.; Guigó, R.; Gladyshev, V.N. Characterization of mammalian selenoproteomes. *Science* **2003**, *300*, 1439–1443. [CrossRef]
166. Janowski, R.; Scanu, S.; Niessing, D.; Madl, T. Crystal and solution structural studies of mouse phospholipid hydroperoxide glutathione peroxidase 4. *Acta Crystallogr. Sect. F Struct. Biol. Commun.* **2016**, *72*, 743–749. [CrossRef]
167. Tosatto, S.C.E.; Bosello, V.; Fogolari, F.; Mauri, P.; Roveri, A.; Toppo, S.; Flohe, L.; Ursini, F.; Maiorino, M. The Catalytic Site of Glutathione Peroxidases. *Antioxid. Redox Signal.* **2008**, *10*, 1515–1526. [CrossRef]
168. Borchert, A.; Kalms, J.; Roth, S.R.; Rademacher, M.; Schmidt, A.; Holzhutter, H.-G.; Hartmut Kuhn, H.; Scheerer, P. Crystal structure and functional characterization of selenocysteine-containing glutathione peroxidase 4 suggests an alternative mechanism of peroxide reduction. *Biochim. Biophys. Acta Mol. Cell Biol. Lipids* **2018**, *1863*, 1095–1107. [CrossRef]
169. Takahashi, K.; Avissar, N.; Whitin, J.; Cohen, H. Purification and characterization of human plasma glutathione peroxidase: A selenoglycoprotein distinct from the known cellular enzyme. *Arch. Biochem. Biophys.* **1987**, *256*, 677–686. [CrossRef] [PubMed]
170. Epp, O.; Ladenstein, R.; Wendel, A. The refined structure of the selenoenzyme glutathione peroxidase at 0.2-nm resolution. *Eur. J. Biochem.* **1983**, *133*, 51–69. [CrossRef] [PubMed]
171. Brigelius-Flohé, R.; Flohé, L. Regulatory Phenomena in the Glutathione Peroxidase Superfamily. *Antioxid. Redox Signal.* **2020**, *33*, 498–516. [CrossRef] [PubMed]
172. Labrecque, C.L.; Fuglestad, B. Electrostatic Drivers of GPx4 Interactions with Membrane, Lipids, and DNA. *Biochemistry* **2021**, *60*, 2761–2772. [CrossRef] [PubMed]
173. Kraus, R.J.; Foster, S.J.; Ganther, H.E. Identification of selenocysteine in glutathione peroxidase by mass spectroscopy. *Biochemistry* **1983**, *22*, 5853–5858. [CrossRef] [PubMed]

174. Gladyshev, V.N.; Factor, V.M.; Housseau, F.; Hatfield, D.L. Contrasting patterns of regulation of the antioxidant selenoproteins, thioredoxin reductase, and glutathione peroxidase, in cancer cells. *Biochem. Biophys. Res. Commun.* **1998**, *251*, 488–493. [CrossRef] [PubMed]
175. Masuda, R.; Kimura, R.; Karasaki, T.; Sase, S.; Goto, K. Modeling the Catalytic Cycle of Glutathione Peroxidase by Nuclear Magnetic Resonance Spectroscopic Analysis of Selenocysteine Selenenic Acids. *J. Am. Chem. Soc.* **2021**, *143*, 6345–6350. [CrossRef] [PubMed]
176. Mustacich, D.; Powis, G. Thioredoxin reductase. *Biochem. J.* **2000**, *346*, 1–8. [CrossRef]
177. Williams, C.H., Jr. *Chemistry and Biochemistry of Flavoenzymes*; Müller, F., Ed.; CRC: Boca Raton, FL, USA, 1992; Volume III, pp. 121–211.
178. Arscott, L.D.; Gromer, S.; Schirmer, R.H.; Williams, C.H., Jr. The mechanism of thioredoxin reductase from human placenta is similar to the mechanisms of lipoamide dehydrogenase and glutathione reductase and is distinct from the mechanism of thioredoxin reductase from *Escherichia coli*. *Proc. Natl. Acad. Sci. USA* **1997**, *94*, 3621–3626. [CrossRef]
179. Williams, C.H.; Arscott, L.D.; Müller, S.; Lennon, B.W.; Ludwig, M.L.; Wang, P.F.; Veine, D.M.; Becker, K.; Schirmer, R.H. Thioredoxin reductase two modes of catalysis have evolved. *Eur. J. Biochem.* **2000**, *267*, 6110–6117. [CrossRef]
180. Williams, C.H., Jr. Mechanism and structure of thioredoxin reductase from *Escherichia coli*. *FASEB J.* **1995**, *9*, 1267–1276. [CrossRef] [PubMed]
181. Zhong, L.; Arnér, E.S.; Ljung, J.; Aslund, F.; Holmgren, A. Rat and calf thioredoxin reductase are homologous to glutathione reductase with a carboxyl-terminal elongation containing a conserved catalytically active penultimate selenocysteine residue. *J. Biol. Chem.* **1998**, *273*, 8581–8591. [CrossRef]
182. Gladyshev, V.N.; Jeang, K.T.; Stadtman, T.C. Selenocysteine, identified as the penultimate C-terminal residue in human T-cell thioredoxin reductase, corresponds to TGA in the human placental gene. *Proc. Natl. Acad. Sci. USA* **1996**, *93*, 6146–6151. [CrossRef] [PubMed]
183. Miranda-Vizuete, A.M.; Damdimopoulos, A.E.; Pedrajas, J.R.; Gustafsson, J.-Å.; Spyrou, G. Human mitochondrial thioredoxin reductase. *Eur. J. Biochem.* **1999**, *261*, 405–412. [CrossRef]
184. Lee, S.R.; Bar-Noy, S.; Kwon, J.; Levine, R.L.; Stadtman, T.C.; Rhee, S.G. Mammalian thioredoxin reductase: Oxidation of the C-terminal cysteine/selenocysteine active site forms a thioselenide, and replacement of selenium with sulfur markedly reduces catalytic activity. *Proc. Natl Acad. Sci. USA* **2000**, *97*, 2521–2526. [CrossRef] [PubMed]
185. Holmgren, A.; Björnstedt, M. Thioredoxin and thioredoxin reductase. *Methods Enzymol.* **1995**, *252*, 199–208.
186. Lee, S.R.; Kim, J.R.; Kwon, K.S.; Yoon, H.W.; Levine, R.L.; Ginsburg, A.; Rhee, S.G. Molecular cloning and characterization of a mitochondrial selenocysteine-containing thioredoxin reductase from rat liver. *J. Biol. Chem.* **1999**, *274*, 4722–4734. [CrossRef]
187. Turanov, A.A.; Su, D.; Gladyshev, V.N. Characterization of alternative cytosolic forms and cellular targets of mouse mitochondrial thioredoxin reductase. *J. Biol. Chem.* **2006**, *281*, 22953–22963. [CrossRef]
188. Arnér, E.S.J. Focus on mammalian thioredoxin reductases--important selenoproteins with versatile functions. *Biochim. Biophys. Acta* **2009**, *1790*, 495–526. [CrossRef]
189. Sandalova, T.; Zhong, L.; Lindqvist, Y.; Holmgren, A.; Schneider, G. Three-dimensional structure of a mammalian thioredoxin reductase: Implications for mechanism and evolution of a selenocysteine-dependent enzyme. *Proc. Natl Acad. Sci. USA* **2001**, *98*, 9533–9538. [CrossRef]
190. Biterova, E.I.; Turanov, A.A.; Gladyshev, V.N.; Barycki, J.J. Crystal structures of oxidized and reduced mitochondrial thioredoxin reductase provide molecular details of the reaction mechanism. *Proc. Natl. Acad. Sci. USA* **2005**, *102*, 15018–15023. [CrossRef] [PubMed]
191. Karplus, P.A.; Schulz, G.E. Refined structure of glutathione reductase at 1.54 A resolution. *J. Mol. Biol.* **1987**, *195*, 701–729. [CrossRef] [PubMed]
192. Fritz-Wolf, K.; Urig, S.; Becker, K. The structure of human thioredoxin reductase 1 provides insights into C-terminal rearrangements during catalysis. *J. Mol. Biol.* **2007**, *370*, 116–127. [CrossRef] [PubMed]
193. Eckenroth, B.; Harris, K.; Turanov, A.A.; Gladyshev, V.N.; Raines, R.T.; Hondal, R.J. Semisynthesis and characterization of mammalian thioredoxin reductase. *Biochemistry* **2006**, *45*, 5158–5170. [CrossRef] [PubMed]
194. Cheng, Q.; Sandalova, T.; Lindqvist, Y.; Arnér, E.S.J. Crystal structure and catalysis of the selenoprotein thioredoxin reductase 1. *J. Biol. Chem.* **2009**, *284*, 3998–4008. [CrossRef] [PubMed]
195. Fritz-Wolf, K.; Kehr, S.; Stumpf, M.; Rahlfs, S.; Becker, K. Crystal structure of the human thioredoxin reductase-thioredoxin complex. *Nat. Commun.* **2011**, *2*, 383. [CrossRef] [PubMed]
196. Zhong, L.; Arnér, E.S.; Holmgren, A. Structure and mechanism of mammalian thioredoxin reductase: The active site is a redox-active selenolthiol/selenenylsulfide formed from the conserved cysteine-selenocysteine sequence. *Proc. Natl. Acad. Sci. USA* **2000**, *97*, 5854–5859. [CrossRef]
197. Zhang, J.; Li, X.; Han, X.; Liu, R.; Fang, J. Targeting the Thioredoxin System for Cancer Therapy. *Trends Pharmacol. Sci.* **2017**, *38*, 794–808. [CrossRef]
198. Besse, D.; Siedler, F.; Diercks, T.; Kessler, H.; Moroder, L. The redox potentials of selenocystine in unconstrained cyclic peptides. *Angew. Chem. Int. Ed. Engl.* **1997**, *36*, 883–885. [CrossRef]
199. Marsan, E.S.; Bayse, C.A. A Halogen Bonding Perspective on Iodothyronine Deiodinase Activity. *Molecules* **2020**, *25*, 1328. [CrossRef]

200. Behne, D.; Kyriakopoulos, A.; Meinhold, H.; Köhrle, J. Identification of type I iodothyronine 5′-deiodinase as a selenoenzyme. *Biochem. Biophys. Res. Commun.* **1990**, *173*, 1143–1149. [CrossRef] [PubMed]
201. Berry, M.J.; Banu, L.; Larsen, P.R. Type I iodothyronine deiodinase is a selenocysteine-containing enzyme. *Nature* **1991**, *349*, 438–440. [CrossRef] [PubMed]
202. Larsen, P.R.; Berry, M.J. Nutritional and hormonal regulation of thyroid hormone deiodinases. *Annu. Rev. Nutr.* **1995**, *15*, 323–352. [CrossRef] [PubMed]
203. Bianco, A.C.; Salvatore, D.; Gereben, B.; Berry, M.J.; Larsen, P.R. Biochemistry, Cellular and Molecular Biology, and Physiological Roles of the Iodothyronine Selenodeiodinases. *Endocr. Rev.* **2002**, *23*, 38–89. [CrossRef] [PubMed]
204. Köhrle, J. Iodothyronine deiodinases. *Methods Enzymol.* **2002**, *347*, 125–167. [PubMed]
205. Koehrle, J.; Auf'mkolk, M.; Rokos, H.; Hesch, R.D.; Cody, V. Rat liver iodothyronine monodeiodinase. Evaluation of the iodothyronine ligand-binding site. *J. Biol. Chem.* **1986**, *261*, 11613–11622. [CrossRef] [PubMed]
206. Kuiper, G.G.J.M.; Kester, M.H.A.; Peeters, R.P.; Visser, T.J. Biochemical mechanisms of thyroid hormone deiodination. *Thyroid* **2005**, *15*, 787–798. [CrossRef]
207. Visser, T.J.; Schoenmakers, C.H. Characteristics of type III iodothyronine deiodinase. *Acta Med. Austriaca* **1992**, *19*, 18–21.
208. Köhrle, J. Local activation and inactivation of thyroid hormones: The deiodinase family. *Mol. Cell Endocrinol.* **1999**, *151*, 103–119. [CrossRef]
209. Köhrle, J.; Jakob, F.; Contempré, B.; Dumont, J.E. Selenium, the thyroid, and the endocrine system. *Endocr. Rev.* **2005**, *26*, 944–984. [CrossRef]
210. Gentile, F.; DiLauro, R.; Salvatore, G. Biosynthesis and Secretion of Thyroid Hormones. In *Endocrinology*, 3rd ed.; DeGroot, L.J., Ed.; WB Saunders Company: Philadelphia, PA, USA, 1995; pp. 517–542.
211. Taurog, A. Hormone synthesis. In *The Thyroid*; Braverman, L.E., Utiger, R., Eds.; Lippincott Williams & Wilkins: Philadelphia, PA, USA, 2000; pp. 61–85.
212. Brent, G.A. Mechanisms of thyroid hormone action. *J. Clin. Investig.* **2012**, *122*, 3035–3043. [CrossRef] [PubMed]
213. Mullur, R.; Liu, Y.-Y.; Brent, G.A. Thyroid hormone regulation of metabolism. *Physiol. Rev.* **2014**, *94*, 355–382. [CrossRef] [PubMed]
214. Bianco, A.C.; Kim, B.W. Deiodinases: Implications of the local control of thyroid hormone action. *J. Clin. Investig.* **2006**, *116*, 2571–2579. [CrossRef] [PubMed]
215. Debasish Manna, D.; Mugesh, G. Regioselective Deiodination of Thyroxine by Iodothyronine Deiodinase Mimics: An Unusual Mechanistic Pathway Involving Cooperative Chalcogen and Halogen Bonding. *J. Am. Chem. Soc.* **2012**, *134*, 4269–4279. [CrossRef]
216. Handy, D.E.; Loscalzo, J. The role of glutathione peroxidase-1 in health and disease. *Free Radic. Biol. Med.* **2022**, *188*, 146–161. [CrossRef]
217. Hu, Y.J.; Diamond, A.M. Role of glutathione peroxidase 1 in breast cancer: Loss of heterozygosity and allelic differences in the response to selenium. *Cancer Res.* **2003**, *63*, 3347–3351.
218. Rayman, M.P. Selenium and human health. *Lancet* **2012**, *379*, 1256–1268. [CrossRef]
219. Dagnell, M.; Schmidt, E.E.; Arnér, E.S.J. The A to Z of modulated cell patterning by mammalian thioredoxin reductases. *Free Radic. Biol. Med.* **2018**, *115*, 484–496. [CrossRef]
220. Lubos, E.; Loscalzo, J.; Handy, D.E. Glutathione Peroxidase-1 in Health and Disease: From Molecular Mechanisms to Therapeutic Opportunities. *Antioxid. Redox Signal.* **2011**, *15*, 1957–1997. [CrossRef]
221. Zhang, M.-L.; Wu, H.-T.; Chen, W.-J.; Xu, Y.; Ye, Q.-Q.; Shen, J.-X.; Liu, J. Involvement of glutathione peroxidases in the occurrence and development of breast cancers. *J. Transl. Med.* **2020**, *18*, 247. [CrossRef]
222. Baliga, M.S.; Wang, H.; Zhuo, P.; Schwartz, J.L.; Diamond, A.M. Selenium and GPx-1 overexpression protect mammalian cells against UV-induced DNA damage. *Biol. Trace. Elem. Res.* **2007**, *115*, 227–242. [CrossRef] [PubMed]
223. Liu, J.; Du, J.; Zhang, Y.; Sun, W.; Smith, B.J.; Oberley, L.W.; Cullen, J.J. Suppression of the malignant phenotype in pancreatic cancer by overexpression of phospholipid hydroperoxide glutathione peroxidase. *Hum. Gene Ther.* **2006**, *17*, 105–116. [CrossRef] [PubMed]
224. Metere, A.; Frezzotti, F.; Graves, C.E.; Vergine, M.; De Luca, A.; Pietraforte, D.P.; Giacomelli, L. A possible role for selenoprotein glutathione peroxidase (GPx1) and thioredoxin reductases (TrxR1) in thyroid cancer: Our experience in thyroid surgery. *Cancer Cell Int.* **2018**, *18*, 7. [CrossRef] [PubMed]
225. Min, S.Y.; Kim, H.S.; Jung, E.J.; Jung, E.J.; Jee, C.D.; Kim, W.H. Prognostic significance of glutathione peroxidase 1 (GPX1) down-regulation and correlation with aberrant promoter methylation in human gastric cancer. *Anticancer Res.* **2012**, *32*, 3169–3175. [PubMed]
226. Nalkiran, I.; Turan, S.; Arikan, S.; Kahraman, Ö.T.; Acar, L.; Yaylim, I.; Ergen, A. Determination of Gene Expression and Serum Levels of MnSOD and GPX1 in Colorectal Cancer. *Anticancer Res.* **2015**, *35*, 255–259. [PubMed]
227. Cheng, Y.; Xu, T.; Li, S.; Ruan, H. GPX1, a biomarker for the diagnosis and prognosis of kidney cancer, promotes the progression of kidney cancer. *Aging* **2019**, *11*, 12165–12176. [CrossRef]
228. Meng, Q.; Xu, J.; Liang, C.; Liu, J.; Hua, J.; Zhang, Y.; Ni, Q.; Shi, S.; Yu, X. GPx1 is involved in the induction of protective autophagy in pancreatic cancer cells in response to glucose deprivation. *Cell Death Dis.* **2018**, *9*, 1187. [CrossRef] [PubMed]
229. Al-Taie, O.H.; Uceyler, N.; Eubner, U.; Jakob, F.; Mork, H.; Scheurlen, M.; Brigelius-Flohe, R.; Schottker, K.; Abel, J.; Thalheimer, A.; et al. Expression Profiling and Genetic Alterations of the Selenoproteins GI-GPx and SePP in Colorectal Carcinogenesis. *Nutr. Cancer* **2004**, *48*, 6–14. [CrossRef]

230. Woenckhaus, M.; Klein-Hitpass, L.; Grepmeier, U.; Merk, J.; Pfeifer, M.; Wild, P.; Bettstetter, M.; Wuensch, P.; Blaszyk, H.; Hartmann, A.; et al. Smoking and cancer-related gene expression in bronchial epithelium and non-small-cell lung cancers. *J. Pathol.* **2006**, *210*, 192–204. [CrossRef]
231. Banning, A.; Kipp, A.; Schmitmeier, S.; Löwinger, M.; Florian, S.; Krehl, S.; Thalmann, S.; Thierbach, R.; Steinberg, P.; Brigelius-Flohé, R. Glutathione Peroxidase 2 Inhibits Cyclooxygenase-2–Mediated Migration and Invasion of HT-29 Adenocarcinoma Cells but Supports Their Growth as Tumors in Nude Mice. *Cancer Res.* **2008**, *68*, 9746–9753. [CrossRef]
232. Jiao, Y.; Wang, Y.; Guo, S.; Wang, G. Glutathione peroxidases as oncotargets. *Oncotarget* **2017**, *8*, 80093–80102. [CrossRef] [PubMed]
233. Chang, C.; Worley, B.L.; Phaëton, R.; Hempel, N. Extracellular Glutathione Peroxidase GPx3 and Its Role in Cancer. *Cancers* **2020**, *12*, 2197. [CrossRef] [PubMed]
234. Lee, O.-J.; Schneider-Stock, R.; McChesney, P.A.; Kuester, D.; Roessner, A.; Vieth, M.; Moskaluk, C.A.; El-Rifai, W. Hypermethylation and Loss of Expression of Glutathione Peroxidase-3 in Barrett's Tumorigenesis1. *Neoplasia* **2005**, *7*, 854–861. [CrossRef] [PubMed]
235. Yu, Y.P.; Yu, G.; Tseng, G.; Cieply, K.; Nelson, J.; Defrances, M.; Zarnegar, R.; Michalopoulos, G.; Luo, J.-H. Glutathione peroxidase 3, deleted or methylated in prostate cancer, suppresses prostate cancer growth and metastasis. *Cancer Res.* **2007**, *67*, 8043–8050. [CrossRef] [PubMed]
236. Eva Falck, E.; Karlsson, S.; Carlsson, J.; Helenius, G.; Karlsson, M.; Klinga-Levan, K. Loss of glutathione peroxidase 3 expression is correlated with epigenetic mechanisms in endometrial adenocarcinoma. *Cancer Cell Int.* **2010**, *10*, 46. [CrossRef] [PubMed]
237. Cejas, P.; García-Cabezas, M.A.; Casado, E.; Belda-Iniesta, C.; De Castro, J.; Fresno, J.A.; Sereno, M.; Barriuso, J.; Espinosa, E.; Zamora, P.; et al. Phospholipid hydroperoxide glutathione peroxidase (PHGPx) expression is downregulated in poorly differentiated breast invasive ductal carcinoma. *Free Radic. Res.* **2007**, *41*, 681–687. [CrossRef] [PubMed]
238. Heirman, I.; Ginneberge, D.; Brigelius-Flohé, R.; Hendrickx, N.; Agostinis, P.; Brouckaert, P.; Rottiers, P.; Grooten, J. Blocking tumor cell eicosanoid synthesis by GP x 4 impedes tumor growth and malignancy. *Free Radic. Biol. Med.* **2006**, *40*, 285–294. [CrossRef] [PubMed]
239. Handy, D.E.; Lubos, E.; Yang, Y.; Galbraith, J.D.; Kelly, N.; Zhang, Y.-Y.; Leopold, J.A.; Loscalzo, J. Glutathione peroxidase-1 regulates mitochondrial function to modulate redox-dependent cellular responses. *J. Biol. Chem.* **2009**, *284*, 11913–11921. [CrossRef]
240. McClung, J.P.; Roneker, C.A.; Mu, W.; Lisk, D.J.; Langlais, P.; Liu, F.; Lei, X.G. Development of insulin resistance and obesity in mice overexpressing cellular glutathione peroxidase. *Proc. Natl. Acad. Sci. USA* **2004**, *101*, 8852–8857. [CrossRef]
241. Rajasekaran, N.S.; Connell, P.; Christians, E.S.; Yan, L.-J.; Taylor, R.P.; Orosz, A.; Zhang, X.Q.; Stevenson, T.J.; Peshock, R.M.; Leopold, J.A.; et al. Human alpha B-crystallin mutation causes oxido-reductive stress and protein aggregation cardiomyopathy in mice. *Cell* **2007**, *130*, 427–439. [CrossRef]
242. Kim, J.-W.; Gao, P.; Dang, C.V. Effects of hypoxia on tumor metabolism. *Cancer Metastasis Rev.* **2007**, *26*, 291–298. [CrossRef]
243. Nyengaard, J.R.; Ido, Y.; Kilo, C.; Williamson, J.R. Interactions Between Hyperglycemia and Hypoxia: Implications for Diabetic Retinopathy. *Diabetes* **2004**, *53*, 2931–2938. [CrossRef] [PubMed]
244. Tilton, R.G. Diabetic vascular dysfunction: Links to glucose-induced reductive stress and VEGF. *Microsc. Res. Technol.* **2002**, *57*, 390–407. [CrossRef] [PubMed]
245. Clark, L.C.; Combs, G.F., Jr.; Turnbull, B.W.; Slate, E.H.; Chalker, D.K.; Chow, J.; Davis, L.S.; Glover, R.A.; Graham, G.F.; Gross, E.G.; et al. Effects of selenium supplementation for cancer prevention in patients with carcinoma of the skin. A randomized controlled trial. Nutritional Prevention of Cancer Study Group. *JAMA* **1996**, *276*, 1957–1963. [CrossRef] [PubMed]
246. Short, S.P.; Williams, C.S. Selenoproteins in Tumorigenesis and Cancer Progression. *Adv. Cancer Res.* **2017**, *136*, 49–83. [PubMed]
247. Combs, G.F., Jr. Status of selenium in prostate cancer prevention. *Br. J. Cancer* **2004**, *91*, 195–199. [CrossRef]
248. Imyanitov, E.N.; Togo, A.V.; Hanson, K.P. Searching for cancer-associated gene polymorphisms: Promises and obstacles. *Cancer Lett.* **2004**, *204*, 3–14. [CrossRef]
249. Jablonska, E.; Gromadzinska, J.; Peplonska, B.; Fendler, W.; Reszka, E.; Krol, M.B.; Wieczorek, E.; Bukowska, A.; Gresner, P.; Galicki, M.; et al. Lipid peroxidation and glutathione peroxidase activity relationship in breast cancer depends on functional polymorphism of GPX1. *BMC Cancer* **2015**, *15*, 657. [CrossRef]
250. Hu, J.; Zhou, G.-W.; Wang, N.; Wang, Y.-J. GPX1 Pro198Leu polymorphism and breast cancer risk: A meta-analysis. *Breast Cancer Res. Treat.* **2010**, *124*, 425–431. [CrossRef]
251. Arsova-Sarafinovska, Z.; Matevska, N.; Eken, A.; Petrovski, D.; Banev, S.; Dzikova, S.; Georgiev, V.; Sikole, A.; Erdem, O.; Sayal, A.; et al. Glutathione peroxidase 1 (GPX1) genetic polymorphism, erythrocyte GPX activity, and prostate cancer risk. *Int. Urol. Nephrol.* **2009**, *41*, 63–70. [CrossRef]
252. Raaschou-Nielsen, O.; Sørensen, M.; Hansen, R.D.; Frederiksen, K.; Tjønneland, A.; Overvad, K.; Vogel, U. GPX1 Pro198Leu polymorphism, interactions with smoking and alcohol consumption, and risk for lung cancer. *Cancer Lett.* **2007**, *247*, 293–300. [CrossRef] [PubMed]
253. Men, T.; Zhang, X.; Yang, J.; Shen, B.; Li, X.; Chen, D.; Wang, J. The rs1050450 C > T polymorphism of GPX1 is associated with the risk of bladder but not prostate cancer: Evidence from a meta-analysis. *Tumor Biol.* **2014**, *35*, 269–275. [CrossRef] [PubMed]
254. Bănescu, C.; Trifa, A.P.; Voidăzan, S.; Moldovan, V.G.; Macarie, I.; Lazar, E.B.; Dima, D.; Duicu, C.; Dobreanu, M. CAT, GPX1, MnSOD, GSTM1, GSTT1, and GSTP1 Genetic Polymorphisms in Chronic Myeloid Leukemia: A Case-Control Study. *Oxid. Med. Cell. Longev.* **2014**, *2014*, 875861. [CrossRef] [PubMed]

255. Hansen, R.; Saebø, M.; Skjelbred, C.F.; Nexø, B.A.; Hagen, P.C.; Bock, G.; Lothe, I.M.B.; Johnson, E.; Aase, S.; Hansteen, I.-L.; et al. GPX Pro198Leu and OGG1 Ser326Cys polymorphisms and risk of development of colorectal adenomas and colorectal cancer. *Cancer Lett.* **2005**, *229*, 85–91. [CrossRef] [PubMed]
256. Yang, W.S.; SriRamaratnam, R.; Welsch, M.E.; Shimada, K.; Skouta, R.; Viswanathan, V.S.; Cheah, J.H.; Clemons, P.A.; Shamji, A.F.; Clish, C.B.; et al. Regulation of ferroptotic cancer cell death by GPX4. *Cell* **2014**, *156*, 317–331. [CrossRef] [PubMed]
257. Viswanathan, V.S.; Ryan, M.J.; Dhruv, H.D.; Gill, S.; Eichhoff, O.M.; Seashore-Ludlow, B.; Kaffenberger, S.D.; Eaton, J.K.; Shimada, K.; Aguirre, A.J.; et al. Dependency of a therapy-resistant state of cancer cells on a lipid peroxidase pathway. *Nature* **2017**, *547*, 453–457. [CrossRef] [PubMed]
258. Hangauer, M.J.; Viswanathan, V.S.; Ryan, M.J.; Bole, D.; Eaton, J.K.; Matov, A.; Galeas, J.; Dhruv, H.D.; Berens, M.E.; Schreiber, S.L.; et al. Drug-tolerant persister cancer cells are vulnerable to GPX4 inhibition. *Nature* **2017**, *551*, 247–250. [CrossRef] [PubMed]
259. Yang, W.S.; Stockwell, B.R. Synthetic lethal screening identifies compounds activating iron-dependent, nonapoptotic cell death in oncogenic-RAS-harboring cancer cells. *Chem. Biol.* **2008**, *15*, 234–245. [CrossRef]
260. Weïwer, M.; Bittker, J.A.; Lewis, T.A.; Shimada, K.; Yang, W.S.; MacPherson, L.; Dandapani, S.; Palmer, M.; Stockwell, B.R.; Schreiber, S.L.; et al. Development of small-molecule probes that selectively kill cells induced to express mutant RAS. *Bioorg. Med. Chem. Lett.* **2012**, *22*, 1822–1826. [CrossRef]
261. Moosmayer, D.; Hilpmann, A.; Hoffmann, J.; Schnirch, L.; Zimmermann, K.; Badock, V.; Furst, L.; Eaton, J.K.; Viswanathan, V.S.; Schreiber, S.L.; et al. Crystal structures of the selenoprotein glutathione peroxidase 4 in its apo form and in complex with the covalently bound inhibitor ML162. *Acta Crystallogr. D Struct. Biol.* **2021**, *77*, 237–248. [CrossRef]
262. Lincoln, D.T.; Emadi, E.M.A.; Tonissen, K.F.; Clarke, F.M. The thioredoxin-thioredoxin reductase system: Over-expression in human cancer. *Anticancer Res.* **2003**, *23*, 2425–2433. [PubMed]
263. Smart, D.K.; Ortiz, K.L.; Mattson, D.; Bradbury, C.M.; Bisht, K.S.; Sieck, L.K.; Brechbiel, M.W.; Gius, D. Thioredoxin Reductase as a Potential Molecular Target for Anticancer Agents That Induce Oxidative Stress. *Cancer Res.* **2004**, *64*, 6716–6724. [CrossRef] [PubMed]
264. di Bernardo, D.; Thompson, M.J.; Gardner, T.S.; Chobot, S.E.; Eastwood, E.L.; Wojtovich, A.P.; Elliott, S.J.; Schaus, S.E.; Collins, J.J. Chemogenomic profiling on a genome-wide scale using reverse-engineered gene networks. *Nat. Biotechnol.* **2005**, *23*, 377–383. [CrossRef] [PubMed]
265. He, L.; Chen, T.; You, Y.; Hu, H.; Zheng, W.; Kwong, W.-L.; Zou, T.; Che, C.-M. A cancer-targeted nanosystem for delivery of gold(III) complexes: Enhanced selectivity and apoptosis-inducing efficacy of a gold(III) porphyrin complex. *Angew. Chem. Int. Ed. Engl.* **2014**, *53*, 12532–12536. [CrossRef] [PubMed]
266. Li, X.; Hou, Y.; Meng, X.; Ge, C.; Ma, H.; Li, J.; Fang, J. Selective Activation of a Prodrug by Thioredoxin Reductase Providing a Strategy to Target Cancer Cells. *Angew. Chem. Int. Ed. Engl.* **2018**, *57*, 6141–6145. [CrossRef]
267. Wang, K.; Zhu, C.; He, Y.; Zhenqin Zhang, Z.; Zhou, W.; Muhammad, N.; Guo, Y.; Wang, X.; Guo, Z. Restraining Cancer Cells by Dual Metabolic Inhibition with a Mitochondrion-Targeted Platinum(II) Complex. *Angew. Chem. Int. Ed. Engl.* **2019**, *58*, 4638–4643. [CrossRef]
268. Gromer, S.; Arscott, L.D.; Williams, C.H., Jr.; Schirmer, R.H.; Becker, K. Human placenta thioredoxin reductase. Isolation of the selenoenzyme, steady state kinetics, and inhibition by therapeutic gold compounds. *J. Biol. Chem.* **1998**, *273*, 20096–20101. [CrossRef]
269. Sasada, T.; Nakamura, H.; Ueda, S.; Sato, N.; Kitaoka, Y.; Gon, Y.; Takabayashi, A.; Spyrou, G.; Holmgren, A.; Yodoi, J. Possible involvement of thioredoxin reductase as well as thioredoxin in cellular sensitivity to cis-diamminedichloroplatinum (II). *Free Radic. Biol. Med.* **1999**, *27*, 504–514. [CrossRef]
270. Tibodeau, J.D.; Benson, L.M.; Isham, C.R.; Owen, W.G.; Bible, K.C. The Anticancer Agent Chaetocin Is a Competitive Substrate and Inhibitor of Thioredoxin Reductase. *Antioxid. Redox Signal.* **2008**, *11*, 1097–1106. [CrossRef]
271. Cai, W.; Zhang, B.; Duan, D.; Wu, J.; Fang, J. Curcumin targeting the thioredoxin system elevates oxidative stress in HeLa cells. *Toxicol. Appl. Pharmacol.* **2012**, *262*, 341–348. [CrossRef]
272. Jin-Jing Jia, J.-J.; Geng, W.-S.; Wang, Z.-Q.; Chen, L.; Zeng, X.-S. The role of thioredoxin system in cancer: Strategy for cancer therapy. *Cancer Chemother. Pharmacol.* **2019**, *84*, 453–470.
273. Liang, Y.-W.; Zheng, J.; Li, X.; Zheng, W.; Chen, T. Selenadiazole derivatives as potent thioredoxin reductase inhibitors that enhance the radiosensitivity of cancer cells. *Eur. J. Med. Chem.* **2014**, *84*, 335–342. [CrossRef] [PubMed]
274. Zhang, B.; Zhang, J.; Peng, S.; Liu, R.; Li, X.; Hou, Y.; Han, X.; Fang, J. Thioredoxin reductase inhibitors: A patent review. *Expert Opin. Ther. Pat.* **2017**, *27*, 547–556. [CrossRef] [PubMed]
275. Onodera, T.; Momose, I.; Kawada, M. Potential Anticancer Activity of Auranofin. *Chem. Pharm. Bull.* **2019**, *67*, 186–191. [CrossRef] [PubMed]
276. Zachary Bloomgarden, Z. Evolution of type 2 diabetes mellitus treatment approaches: 2. *J. Diabetes Res.* **2019**, *11*, 4–6. [CrossRef] [PubMed]
277. Jetton, T.L.; Lausier, J.; LaRock, K.; Trotman, W.E.; Larmie, B.; Habibovic, A.; Peshavaria, M.; Leahy, J.L. Mechanisms of compensatory beta-cell growth in insulin-resistant rats: Roles of Akt kinase. *Diabetes* **2005**, *54*, 2294–2304. [CrossRef] [PubMed]
278. Italiani, P.; Boraschi, D. From Monocytes to M1/M2 Macrophages: Phenotypical vs. Functional Differentiation. *Front. Immunol.* **2014**, *4*, 514. [CrossRef]

279. Evren Okur, M.E.; Karantas, I.D.; Siafaka, P.I. Diabetes Mellitus: A Review on Pathophysiology, Current Status of Oral Pathophysiology, Current Status of Oral Medications and Future Perspectives. *ACTA Pharm. Sci.* **2017**, *55*, 61–82.
280. Chatterjee, S.; Khunti, K.; Davies, M.J. Type 2 diabetes. *Lancet* **2017**, *389*, 2239–2251. [CrossRef]
281. Burgos-Morón, E.; Abad-Jiménez, Z.; de Marañón, A.M.; Iannantuoni, F.; Escribano-López, I.; López-Domènech, S.; Salom, C.; Jover, A.; Mora, V.; Roldan, I.; et al. Relationship Between Oxidative Stress, ER Stress, and Inflammation in Type 2 Diabetes: The Battle Continues. *J. Clin. Med.* **2019**, *8*, 1385. [CrossRef]
282. Karunakaran, U.; Park, K.-G. A systematic review of oxidative stress and safety of antioxidants in diabetes: Focus on islets and their defense. *Diabetes Metab. J.* **2013**, *37*, 106–112. [CrossRef] [PubMed]
283. Lenzen, S.; Drinkgern, J.; Tiedge, M. Low antioxidant enzyme gene expression in pancreatic islets compared with various other mouse tissues. *Free Radic. Biol. Med.* **1996**, *20*, 463–466. [CrossRef] [PubMed]
284. Robertson, R.P.; Harmon, J.; Tran, P.O.; Tanaka, Y.; Takahashi, H. Glucose toxicity in beta-cells: Type 2 diabetes, good radicals gone bad, and the glutathione connection. *Diabetes* **2003**, *52*, 581–587. [CrossRef] [PubMed]
285. Steinbrenner, H.; Speckmann, B.; Pinto, A.; Sies, H. High selenium intake and increased diabetes risk: Experimental evidence for interplay between selenium and carbohydrate metabolism. *J. Clin. Biochem. Nutr.* **2011**, *48*, 40–45. [CrossRef] [PubMed]
286. May, J.M.; de Haën, C. Insulin-stimulated intracellular hydrogen peroxide production in rat epididymal fat cells. *J. Biol. Chem.* **1979**, *254*, 2214–2220. [CrossRef] [PubMed]
287. Wang, X.D.; Vatamaniuk, M.Z.; Wang, S.K.; Roneker, C.A.; Simmons, R.A.; Lei, X.G. Molecular mechanisms for hyperinsulinaemia induced by overproduction of selenium-dependent glutathione peroxidase-1 in mice. *Diabetologia* **2008**, *51*, 1515–1524. [CrossRef] [PubMed]
288. Hawkes, W.C. Association of Glutathione Peroxidase Activity with Insulin Resistance and Dietary Fat Intake during Normal Pregnancy. *J. Clin. Endocrinol. Metab.* **2004**, *89*, 4772–4773. [CrossRef]
289. Loh, K.; Deng, H.; Fukushima, A.; Cai, X.; Boivin, B.; Galic, S.; Bruce, C.; Shields, B.J.; Skiba, B.; Ooms, L.M.; et al. Reactive oxygen species enhance insulin sensitivity. *Cell Metab.* **2009**, *10*, 260–272. [CrossRef]
290. Schoenmakers, E.; Agostini, M.; Mitchell, C.; Schoenmakers, N.; Papp, L.; Rajanayagam, O.; Padidela, R.; Ceron-Gutierrez, L.; Doffinger, R.; Prevosto, C.; et al. Mutations in the selenocysteine insertion sequence-binding protein 2 gene lead to a multisystem selenoprotein deficiency disorder in humans. *J. Clin. Investig.* **2010**, *120*, 4220–4235. [CrossRef]
291. Molteni, C.G.; Principi, N.; Esposito, S. Reactive oxygen and nitrogen species during viral infections. *Free Radic. Res.* **2014**, *48*, 1163–1169. [CrossRef]
292. Khomich, O.A.; Kochetkov, S.N.; Bartosch, B.; Ivanov, A.V. Redox Biology of Respiratory Viral Infections. *Viruses* **2018**, *10*, 392. [CrossRef] [PubMed]
293. Seet, R.C.S.; Lee, C.-Y.J.; Lim, E.C.H.; Quek, A.M.L.; Yeo, L.L.L.; Huang, S.-H.; Halliwell, B. Oxidative damage in dengue fever. *Free Radic. Biol. Med.* **2009**, *47*, 375–380. [CrossRef] [PubMed]
294. Korenaga, M.; Wang, T.; Li, Y.; Showalter, L.A.; Chan, T.; Sun, J.; Weinman, S.A. Hepatitis C virus core protein inhibits mitochondrial electron transport and increases reactive oxygen species (ROS) production. *J. Biol. Chem.* **2005**, *280*, 37481–37488. [CrossRef] [PubMed]
295. Ferguson, M.R.; Rojo, D.R.; von Lindern, J.J.; O'Brien, W.A. HIV-1 replication cycle. *Clin. Lab. Med.* **2002**, *22*, 611–635. [CrossRef] [PubMed]
296. Freed, E.O.; Martin, M.A. HIVs and their replication. In *Fields Virology*; Knipe, D.M., Howley, P.M., Eds.; Lippincott Williams & Wilkins: Philadelphia, PA, USA, 2007; pp. 2107–2185.
297. Ryser, H.J.-P.; Flückiger, R. Progress in targeting HIV-1 entry. *Drug Discov. Today* **2005**, *10*, 1085–1194. [CrossRef] [PubMed]
298. Chan, D.C.; Kim, P.S. HIV Entry and Its Inhibition. *Cell* **1998**, *93*, 681–684. [CrossRef] [PubMed]
299. Barbouche, R.; Miquelis, R.; Jones, I.M.; Fenouillet, E. Protein-disulfide isomerase-mediated reduction of two disulfide bonds of HIV envelope glycoprotein 120 occurs post-CXCR4 binding and is required for fusion. *J. Biol. Chem.* **2003**, *278*, 3131–3136. [CrossRef]
300. Gallina, A.; Hanley, T.M.; Mandel, R.; Trahey, M.; Broder, C.C.; Viglianti, G.A.; Ryser, H.J.-P. Inhibitors of protein-disulfide isomerase prevent cleavage of disulfide bonds in receptor-bound glycoprotein 120 and prevent HIV-1 entry. *J. Biol. Chem.* **2002**, *277*, 50579–50588. [CrossRef]
301. Markovic, I.; Stantchev, T.S.; Fields, K.H.; Tiffany, L.J.; Tomiç, M.; Weiss, C.D.; Broder, C.C.; Strebel, K.; Clouse, K.A. Thiol/disulfide exchange is a prerequisite for CXCR4-tropic HIV-1 envelope-mediated T-cell fusion during viral entry. *Blood* **2004**, *103*, 1586–1594. [CrossRef]
302. Cerutti, N.; Killick, M.; Jugnarain, V.; Papathanasopoulos, M.; Capovilla, A. Disulfide reduction in CD4 domain 1 or 2 is essential for interaction with HIV glycoprotein 120 (gp120), which impairs thioredoxin-driven CD4 dimerization. *J. Biol. Chem.* **2014**, *289*, 10455–10465. [CrossRef]
303. Matthias, L.J.; Azimi, I.; Tabrett, C.A.; Hogg, P.J. Reduced monomeric CD4 is the preferred receptor for HIV. *J. Biol. Chem.* **2010**, *285*, 40793–40799. [CrossRef] [PubMed]
304. Matthias, L.J.; Yam, P.T.W.; Jiang, X.-M.; Vandegraaff, N.; Li, P.; Poumbourios, P.; Donoghue, N.; Hogg, P.J. Disulfide exchange in domain 2 of CD4 is required for entry of HIV-1. *Nat. Immunol.* **2002**, *3*, 727–732. [CrossRef] [PubMed]
305. Moolla, N.; Killick, M.; Papathanasopoulos, M.; Capovilla, A. Thioredoxin (Trx1) regulates CD4 membrane domain localization and is required for efficient CD4-dependent HIV-1 entry. *Biochim. Biophys. Acta* **2016**, *1860*, 1854–1863. [CrossRef] [PubMed]

306. Auwerx, J.; Isacsson, O.; Söderlund, J.; Balzarini, J.; Johansson, M.; Lundberg, M. Human glutaredoxin-1 catalyzes the reduction of HIV-1 gp120 and CD4 disulfides and its inhibition reduces HIV-1 replication. *Int. J. Biochem. Cell Biol.* **2009**, *41*, 1269–1275. [CrossRef] [PubMed]
307. Ryser, H.J.; Levy, E.M.; Mandel, R.; DiSciullo, G.J. Inhibition of human immunodeficiency virus infection by agents that interfere with thiol-disulfide interchange upon virus-receptor interaction. *Proc. Natl. Acad. Sci. USA* **1994**, *91*, 4559–4563. [CrossRef] [PubMed]
308. Karn, J. Tackling Tat. *J. Mol. Biol.* **1999**, *293*, 235–254. [CrossRef] [PubMed]
309. Kuppuswamy, M.; Subramanian, T.; Srinivasan, A.; Chinnadurai, G. Multiple functional domains of Tat, the trans-activator of HIV-1, defined by mutational analysis. *Nucleic Acids Res.* **1989**, *17*, 3551–3561. [CrossRef] [PubMed]
310. Frankel, A.D.; Pabo, C.O. Cellular uptake of the tat protein from human immunodeficiency virus. *Cell* **1988**, *55*, 1189–1193. [CrossRef]
311. Koken, S.E.; Greijer, A.E.; Verhoef, K.; van Wamel, J.; Bukrinskaya, A.G.; Berkhout, B. Intracellular analysis of in vitro modified HIV Tat protein. *J. Biol. Chem.* **1994**, *269*, 8366–8375. [CrossRef]
312. Price, T.O.; Ercal, N.; Nakaoke, R.; Banks, W.A. HIV-1 viral proteins gp120 and Tat induce oxidative stress in brain endothelial cells. *Brain Res.* **2005**, *1045*, 57–63. [CrossRef]
313. Banerjee, A.; Zhang, X.; Manda, K.R.; Banks, W.A.; Nuran Ercal, N. HIV proteins (gp120 and Tat) and methamphetamine in oxidative stress-induced damage in the brain: Potential role of the thiol antioxidant N-acetylcysteine amide. *Free Radic. Biol. Med.* **2010**, *48*, 1388–1398. [CrossRef] [PubMed]
314. Samikkannu, T.; Ranjith, D.; Rao, K.V.K.; Atluri, V.S.R.; Pimentel, E.; El-Hage, N.; Nair, M.P.N. HIV-1 gp120 and morphine induced oxidative stress: Role in cell cycle regulation. *Front. Microbiol.* **2015**, *6*, 614. [CrossRef] [PubMed]
315. Richard, M.-J.; Guiraud, P.; Didier, C.; Seve, M.; Flores, S.C.; Favier, A. Impairs Selenoglutathione Peroxidase Expression and Activity by a Mechanism Independent of Cellular Selenium Uptake: Consequences on Cellular Resistance to UV-A Radiation. *Arch. Biochem. Biophys.* **2001**, *386*, 213–220. [CrossRef] [PubMed]
316. Gladyshev, V.N.; Stadtman, T.C.; Hatfield, D.L.; Jeang, K.T. Levels of major selenoproteins in T cells decrease during HIV infection and low molecular mass selenium compounds increase. *Proc. Natl. Acad. Sci. USA* **1999**, *96*, 835–839. [CrossRef] [PubMed]
317. Hurwitz, B.E.; Klaus, J.R.; Llabre, M.M.; Gonzalez, A.; Lawrence, P.J.; Maher, K.J.; Greeson, J.M.; Baum, M.K.; Shor-Posner, G.; Skyler, J.S.; et al. Suppression of human immunodeficiency virus type 1 viral load with selenium supplementation: A randomized controlled trial. *Arch. Intern. Med.* **2007**, *167*, 148–154. [CrossRef] [PubMed]
318. Lundberg, M.; Mattsson, Å.; Reiser, K.; Holmgren, A.; Curbo, S. Inhibition of the thioredoxin system by PX-12 (1-methylpropyl 2-imidazolyl disulfide) impedes HIV-1 infection in TZM-bl cells. *Sci. Rep.* **2019**, *9*, 5656. [CrossRef] [PubMed]
319. Reiser, K.; Mathys, L.; Curbo, S.; Pannecouque, C.; Noppen, S.; Liekens, S.; Engman, L.; Lundberg, M.; Balzarini, J.; Karlsson, A. The Cellular Thioredoxin-1/Thioredoxin Reductase-1 Driven Oxidoreduction Represents a Chemotherapeutic Target for HIV-1 Entry Inhibition. *PLoS ONE* **2016**, *11*, e0147773. [CrossRef]
320. Reiser, K.; François, K.O.; Schols, D.; Bergman, T.; Jörnvall, H.; Balzarini, J.; Karlsson, A.; Lundberg, M. Thioredoxin-1 and protein disulfide isomerase catalyze the reduction of similar disulfides in HIV gp120. *Int. J. Biochem. Cell Biol.* **2012**, *44*, 556–562. [CrossRef]
321. Wu, F.; Zhao, S.; Yu, B.; Chen, Y.-M.; Wang, W.; Song, Z.-G.; Hu, Y.; Tao, Z.-W.; Tian, J.-H.; Pei, Y.-Y.; et al. A new coronavirus associated with human respiratory disease in China. *Nature* **2020**, *579*, 265–269. [CrossRef]
322. Li, Q.; Guan, X.; Wu, P.; Wang, X.; Zhou, L.; Tong, Y.; Ren, R.; Leung, K.S.; Lau, E.H.; Wong, J.Y.; et al. Early Transmission Dynamics in Wuhan, China, of Novel Coronavirus-Infected Pneumonia. *N. Engl. J. Med.* **2020**, *382*, 1199–1207. [CrossRef]
323. Maiti, B.K. Can Papain-like Protease Inhibitors Halt SARS-CoV-2 Replication? *ACS Pharmacol. Transl. Sci.* **2020**, *3*, 1017–1019. [CrossRef] [PubMed]
324. Gallardo, I.A.; Todd, D.A.; Lima, S.T.; Jonathan, R.; Chekan, J.R.; Chiu, N.H.; Taylor, E.W. SARS-CoV-2 Main Protease Targets Host Selenoproteins and Glutathione Biosynthesis for Knockdown via Proteolysis, Potentially Disrupting the Thioredoxin and Glutaredoxin Redox Cycles. *Antioxidants* **2023**, *12*, 559. [CrossRef] [PubMed]
325. Tomo, S.; Saikiran, G.; Banerjee, M.; Paul, S. Selenium to selenoproteins—Role in COVID-19. *EXCLI J.* **2021**, *20*, 781–791. [PubMed]
326. Moghaddam, A.; Heller, R.A.; Sun, Q.; Seelig, J.; Cherkezov, A.; Seibert, L.; Hackler, J.; Seemann, P.; Diegmann, J.; Pilz, M.; et al. Selenium Deficiency Is Associated with Mortality Risk from COVID-19. *Nutrients* **2020**, *12*, 2098. [CrossRef] [PubMed]
327. Zhang, J.; Taylor, E.W.; Bennett, K.; Saad, R.; Rayman, M.P. Association between regional selenium status and reported outcome of COVID-19 cases in China. *Am. J. Clin. Nutr.* **2020**, *111*, 1297–1299. [CrossRef] [PubMed]
328. Zhang, J.; Saad, R.; Taylor, E.W.; Rayman, M.P. Selenium and selenoproteins in viral infection with potential relevance to COVID-19. *Redox Biol.* **2020**, *37*, 101715. [CrossRef] [PubMed]
329. Beck, M.A.; Kolbeck, P.C.; Rohr, L.H.; Shi, Q.; Morris, V.C.; Levander, O.A. Benign human enterovirus becomes virulent in selenium-deficient mice. *J. Med. Virol.* **1994**, *43*, 166–170. [CrossRef]
330. Avery, J.C.; Hoffmann, P.R. Selenium, Selenoproteins, and Immunity. *Nutrients* **2018**, *10*, 1203. [CrossRef]
331. Barchielli, G.; Capperucci, A.; Tanini, D. The Role of Selenium in Pathologies: An Updated Review. *Antioxidants* **2022**, *11*, 251. [CrossRef]
332. Lan, J.; Ge, J.; Yu, J.; Shan, S.; Zhou, H.; Fan, S.; Zhang, Q.; Shi, X.; Wang, Q.; Zhang, L.; et al. Structure of the SARS-CoV-2 spike receptor-binding domain bound to the ACE2 receptor. *Nature* **2020**, *581*, 215–220. [CrossRef]

333. Maiti, B.K. Potential Role of Peptide-Based Antiviral Therapy against SARS-CoV-2 Infection. *ACS Pharmacol. Transl. Sci.* **2020**, *3*, 783–785. [CrossRef] [PubMed]
334. Shi, Y.; Zeida, A.; Edwards, C.E.; Mallory, M.L.; Sastre, S.; Machado, M.R.; Pickles, R.J.; Fu, L.; Liu, K.; Yang, J.; et al. Thiol-based chemical probes exhibit antiviral activity against SARS-CoV-2 via allosteric disulfide disruption in the spike glycoprotein. *Proc. Natl. Acad. Sci. USA* **2022**, *119*, e2120419119. [CrossRef] [PubMed]
335. Hati, S.; Sudeep Bhattacharyya, S. Impact of Thiol-Disulfide Balance on the Binding of COVID-19 Spike Protein with Angiotensin-Converting Enzyme 2 Receptor. *ACS Omega* **2020**, *5*, 16292–16298. [CrossRef] [PubMed]
336. Giustarini, D.; Santucci, A.; Bartolini, D.; Galli, F.; Rossi, R. The age-dependent decline of the extracellular thiol-disulfide balance and its role in SARS-CoV-2 infection. *Redox Biol.* **2021**, *41*, 101902. [CrossRef] [PubMed]
337. Polonikov, A. Endogenous Deficiency of Glutathione as the Most Likely Cause of Serious Manifestations and Death in COVID-19 Patients. *ACS Infect. Dis.* **2020**, *6*, 1558–1562. [CrossRef] [PubMed]
338. Soria-Castro, E.; Soto, M.E.; Guarner-Lans, V.; Rojas, G.; Perezpeña-Diazconti, M.; Críales-Vera, S.A.; Manzano Pech, L.; Pérez-Torres, I. The kidnapping of mitochondrial function associated with the SARS-CoV-2 infection. *Histol. Histopathol.* **2021**, *36*, 947–965.
339. Yang, M.; Lai, C.L. SARS-CoV-2 infection: Can ferroptosis be a potential treatment target for multiple organ involvement? *Cell Death Discov.* **2020**, *6*, 130. [CrossRef]
340. Jin, Z.; Du, X.; Xu, Y.; Deng, Y.; Liu, M.; Zhao, Y.; Zhang, B.; Li, X.; Zhang, L.; Peng, C.; et al. Structure of Mpro from SARS-CoV-2 and discovery of its inhibitors. *Nature* **2020**, *582*, 289–293. [CrossRef]
341. Zhang, L.; Lin, D.; Sun, X.; Curth, U.; Drosten, C.; Sauerhering, L.; Becker, S.; Rox, K.; Hilgenfeld, R. Crystal structure of SARS-CoV-2 main protease provides a basis for design of improved α-ketoamide inhibitors. *Science* **2020**, *368*, 409–412. [CrossRef]
342. Taylor, E.W.; Radding, W. Understanding Selenium and Glutathione as Antiviral Factors in COVID-19: Does the Viral Mpro Protease Target Host Selenoproteins and Glutathione Synthesis? *Front. Nutr.* **2020**, *7*, 143. [CrossRef]
343. Li, F.; Leier, A.; Liu, Q.; Wang, Y.; Xiang, D.; Akutsu, T.; Webb, G.I.; Smith, A.I.; Marquez-Lago, T.; Li, J.; et al. Procleave: Predicting Protease-specific Substrate Cleavage Sites by Combining Sequence and Structural Information. *Genom. Proteom. Bioinform.* **2020**, *18*, 52–64. [CrossRef] [PubMed]
344. Gordon, D.E.; Jang, G.M.; Bouhaddou, M.; Xu, J.; Obernier, K.; White, K.M.; O'Meara, M.J.; Rezelj, V.V.; Guo, J.Z.; Swaney, D.L.; et al. A SARS-CoV-2 protein interaction map reveals targets for drug repurposing. *Nature* **2020**, *583*, 459–468. [CrossRef]
345. Hogan, C.; Perkins, A.V. Selenoproteins in the Human Placenta: How Essential Is Selenium to a Healthy Start to Life? *Nutrients* **2022**, *14*, 628. [CrossRef] [PubMed]
346. Hussain, T.; Murtaza, G.; Metwally, E.; Kalhoro, D.H.; Kalhoro, M.S.; Rahu, B.A.; Sahito, R.G.A.; Yin, Y.; Yang, H.; Chughtai, M.I.; et al. The Role of Oxidative Stress and Antioxidant Balance in Pregnancy. *Mediat. Inflamm.* **2021**, *2021*, 9962860. [CrossRef] [PubMed]
347. Chiarello, D.I.; Abad, C.; Rojas, D.; Toledo, F.; Vázquez, C.M.; Mate, A.; Sobrevia, L.; Marín, R. Oxidative stress: Normal pregnancy versus preeclampsia. *Biochim. Biophys. Acta (BBA)-Mol. Basis Dis.* **2020**, *1866*, 165354. [CrossRef] [PubMed]
348. Scaife, P.J.; Simpson, A.; Kurlak, L.O.; Briggs, L.V.; Gardner, D.S.; Broughton Pipkin, F.; Jones, C.J.P.; Mistry, H.D. Increased Placental Cell Senescence and Oxidative Stress in Women with Pre-Eclampsia and Normotensive Post-Term Pregnancies. *Int. J. Mol. Sci.* **2021**, *22*, 7295. [CrossRef] [PubMed]
349. Farzin, L.; Sajadi, F. Comparison of serum trace element levels in patients with or without pre-eclampsia. *J. Res. Med. Sci.* **2012**, *17*, 938–941.
350. Khera, A.; Vanderlelie, J.J.; Perkins, A.V. Selenium supplementation protects trophoblast cells from mitochondrial oxidative stress. *Placenta* **2013**, *34*, 594–598. [CrossRef]
351. Biswas, K.; McLay, J.; Campbell, F.M. Selenium Supplementation in Pregnancy-Maternal and Newborn Outcomes. *J. Nutr. Metab.* **2022**, *2022*, 4715965. [CrossRef]

Disclaimer/Publisher's Note: The statements, opinions and data contained in all publications are solely those of the individual author(s) and contributor(s) and not of MDPI and/or the editor(s). MDPI and/or the editor(s) disclaim responsibility for any injury to people or property resulting from any ideas, methods, instructions or products referred to in the content.

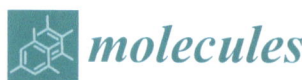

Review

Mediterranean Shrub Species as a Source of Biomolecules against Neurodegenerative Diseases

Natividad Chaves *, Laura Nogales, Ismael Montero-Fernández, José Blanco-Salas and Juan Carlos Alías

Department of Plant Biology, Ecology and Earth Sciences, Faculty of Science, Universidad de Extremadura, 06080 Badajoz, Spain; lnogalesg@unex.es (L.N.); ismonterof@unex.es (I.M.-F.); blanco_salas@unex.es (J.B.-S.); jalias@unex.es (J.C.A.)
* Correspondence: natchalo@unex.es

Abstract: Neurodegenerative diseases are associated with oxidative stress, due to an imbalance in the oxidation-reduction reactions at the cellular level. Various treatments are available to treat these diseases, although they often do not cure them and have many adverse effects. Therefore, it is necessary to find complementary and/or alternative drugs that replace current treatments with fewer side effects. It has been demonstrated that natural products derived from plants, specifically phenolic compounds, have a great capacity to suppress oxidative stress and neutralize free radicals thus, they may be used as alternative alternative pharmacological treatments for pathological conditions associated with an increase in oxidative stress. The plant species that dominate the Mediterranean ecosystems are characterized by having a wide variety of phenolic compound content. Therefore, these species might be important sources of neuroprotective biomolecules. To evaluate this potential, 24 typical plant species of the Mediterranean ecosystems were selected, identifying the most important compounds present in them. This set of plant species provides a total of 403 different compounds. Of these compounds, 35.7% are phenolic acids and 55.6% are flavonoids. The most relevant of these compounds are gallic, vanillic, caffeic, chlorogenic, *p*-coumaric, and ferulic acids, apigenin, kaempferol, myricitrin, quercetin, isoquercetin, quercetrin, rutin, catechin and epicatechin, which are widely distributed among the analyzed plant species (in over 10 species) and which have been involved in the literature in the prevention of different neurodegenerative pathologies. It is also important to mention that three of these plant species, *Pistacea lentiscus*, *Lavandula stoechas* and *Thymus vulgaris*, have most of the described compounds with protective properties against neurodegenerative diseases. The present work shows that the plant species that dominate the studied geographic area can provide an important source of phenolic compounds for the pharmacological and biotechnological industry to prepare extracts or isolated compounds for therapy against neurodegenerative diseases.

Keywords: natural antioxidants; neuroprotective compounds; phenols; Mediterranean species

Citation: Chaves, N.; Nogales, L.; Montero-Fernández, I.; Blanco-Salas, J.; Alías, J.C. Mediterranean Shrub Species as a Source of Biomolecules against Neurodegenerative Diseases. *Molecules* 2023, 28, 8133. https://doi.org/10.3390/molecules28248133

Academic Editors: Alejandro Samhan-Arias, Manuel Aureliano and Carmen Lopez-Sanchez

Received: 16 November 2023
Revised: 12 December 2023
Accepted: 14 December 2023
Published: 16 December 2023

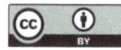

Copyright: © 2023 by the authors. Licensee MDPI, Basel, Switzerland. This article is an open access article distributed under the terms and conditions of the Creative Commons Attribution (CC BY) license (https://creativecommons.org/licenses/by/4.0/).

1. Introduction

1.1. Brief Description of Neurodegenerative Diseases and Their Causes

Neurodegenerative diseases, diabetes, cardiovascular diseases, sarcopenia, and cancer are associated with the "free radical theory" of aging [1–3]. This theory is based on the structural damage-based hypothesis claiming that tissue dysfunction due to aging can be attributed to the accumulation of oxidative damage of macromolecules by free radicals [1]. Oxidative stress results from an imbalance in reduction and oxidation reactions at the cellular level. The consequence of this imbalance is the formation of reactive oxygen or nitrogen species (ROS/RNS) and sometimes it can be attributed to a decrease in the level of antioxidant defense [4,5]. In particular, the excessive production of ROS contributes to oxidative stress leading to neuronal cell death and an alteration of brain function [2,6]. The central nervous system is vulnerable to oxidative stress since it has a large requirement for oxygen and has a lower amount of antioxidant enzymes, compared with other tissues [7,8].

Harman et al. [1] extended the "free radical theory" of aging to the "mitochondrial theory of aging", which states that ROS accumulation induces mitochondrial dysfunction, which contributes to aging and the development of related diseases [9–11]. Over the last decade, a connection between mitochondria and longevity has become increasingly evident. Mitochondria are also regulators of some types of cell death, such as apoptosis, and thus, their mitochondrial dysfunction might affect the lifespan of individuals presenting defects in this organelle [11].

Neurodegenerative diseases are frequently associated with neuroinflammation, which is a process related to oxidative and nitrosative stress. The inflammatory response is further propagated by the activation of glial cells and the modulation of constitutively expressed extracellular matrix proteins [12,13].

Many neurodegenerative diseases have been described to be highly prevalent in the population and have a high socioeconomic impact. Alzheimer's disease (AD), Parkinson's disease (PD), Huntington's disease (HD), amyotrophic lateral sclerosis, and frontotemporal dementia are some examples [14,15]. All these diseases, specifically AD and PD, are associated with high morbidity and mortality and represent a primary health problem, especially in the aged population [16]. These disorders share common pathological characteristics, such as the induction of oxidative stress, abnormal protein aggregation, perturbed Ca^{2+} homeostasis, excitotoxicity, inflammation and apoptosis [17,18].

AD is a progressive neurological condition and the world's most common form of dementia [19]. The pathological characteristics include extracellular deposits of amyloid β, (Aβ), intracellular formation of neurofibrillary tangles and loss of neuronal synapses and pyramidal neurons [20]. Aβ deposits derive from amyloid precursor protein and the neurofibrillary tangles containing an abnormally phosphorylated form of tau, which is a microtubule-associated protein [21]. A growing body of research supports that Aβ aggregation and decreased Aβ clearance are the leading causes of this disease onset.

Different studies indicate that oxidative stress plays a fundamental role in the development and evolution of AD. For example, elevated ROS production has been shown to initiate toxic amyloid beta precursor protein processing, thereby triggering Aβ generation [22]. These ROS are primarily generated via NADPH oxidase 2, which is well associated with inflammation and amyloid plaque deposition, leading to mitochondrial dysfunction and decreased glutathione levels. Neurons contain a high amount of polyunsaturated fatty acids that can interact with ROS, leading to a self-propagating cascade of lipid peroxidation and molecular destruction [23]. Products of lipid peroxidation have also been shown to be elevated in blood samples and brains of AD patients at autopsy [24]. It has also been correlated with the initial stage of the disease DNA oxidative damage in the AD brains, due to increased expression of ERCC-80 and 89 genes related to DNA repair activity [25].

On the other hand, the "cholinergic hypothesis of AD" is based on acetylcholine deficiency [26,27]. This neurotransmitter is involved in cognition and memory processes that are known to be decreased in AD. Thus, cholinesterase inhibitors are the first line of therapy for the management of AD [28,29].

PD is the second most common age-related neurodegenerative disorder in the central nervous system. This disease is a clinical syndrome characterized by motor impairments, including bradykinesia, resting tremor, muscle rigidity, loss of postural reflexes, freezing phenomenon and flexed posture. PD involves the loss of dopaminergic neurons of the pars compacta region of the substantia nigra and the accumulation of intracellular proteins (synucleins), leading to cognitive and motor deterioration in people who suffer from it [30–33].

It is possible that processes, such as oxidation, may be responsible for the gradual dysfunction that can be manifested throughout the disease. Previous publications have reported evidence of this oxidative stress through the detection of oxidized DNA, lipids, and proteins in the brain tissues of PD patients [34]. Dopaminergic neurons contain large amounts of ROS derived from dopamine's enzymatic and non-enzymatic metabolism.

Dopamine may be catabolized by monoamine oxidase (MAO) in a process that generates 3,4-dihydroxyphenyl-acetaldehyde, ammonia and H_2O_2, which reacts with Fe^{2+} to form hydroxyl radical. In addition, dopamine oxidation may spontaneously generate 6-hydroxydopamine, which is subsequently transformed into reactive electrophilic molecules in the presence of oxygen [35]. On the other hand, several studies suggest that the overexpression or misfolding of α-synuclein increases ROS production and cell susceptibility to oxidative stress [36,37].

In general, the treatments for neurodegenerative diseases tend to be limited in their therapeutic approach, due to their symptom management but non-curative nature [38], and the continuous use of certain conventional drugs generates many adverse effects, such as nausea, diarrhea, eating disorders and kidney and liver affectations [39]. Therefore, it is necessary to find complementary and/or alternative treatments. Several clinical trials have proved the implication of natural products as antioxidant agents (e.g., ferulic and *p*-coumaric acids, resveratrol, catechin, epi-catechin, quercetin, ginsenosides.) [40–43] and, given the role of oxidative stress in the pathogenesis of neurodegenerative diseases, these compounds can be a good therapeutic alternative against these diseases.

1.2. Phenolic Compounds: Their Importance and Implication in Neurodegenerative Diseases

Many studies have focused on natural phytocomponents as important bioactive molecules against aging-related chronic diseases, including neurodegenerative diseases [44–46]. The wide and countless number of natural compounds from plants, animals, fungi and microorganisms provide a rich and unique source for new drug search [47], with plants being the main source of these compounds. In most cases, the biological activity attributed to plant extracts derives from secondary metabolites, which include two extensive categories: nitrogen-containing and non-nitrogen-containing compounds [48,49]. In the latter category, phenols are one of the most extensive groups of secondary metabolites in the plant kingdom [50]. Structurally, they are characterized by the presence of at least one hydroxyl functional group (-OH) linked to an aromatic ring [51]. Polyphenol classification is based on the number of phenol rings in the molecule, and the main subgroups include phenolic acids, coumarins, stilbenes, flavonoids, tannins and lignans [50]. These compounds exert different biological activities, including antioxidant, antiallergic, anti-inflammatory, antiviral, antiproliferative and anticarcinogenic effects [52,53].

One of the most remarkable functions of phenols is their capacity to suppress oxidative stress and neutralize free radicals. They can act as reducing agents, metal chelators, free-radical scavengers, enzyme modulators and regulators of diverse proteins and transcriptional factors (Figure 1) [54,55]. The antioxidant potential of these compounds confers therapeutic activities for a wide variety of diseases, such as cardiovascular diseases, cancer, liver diseases, diabetes and neurodegenerative disorders [56,57].

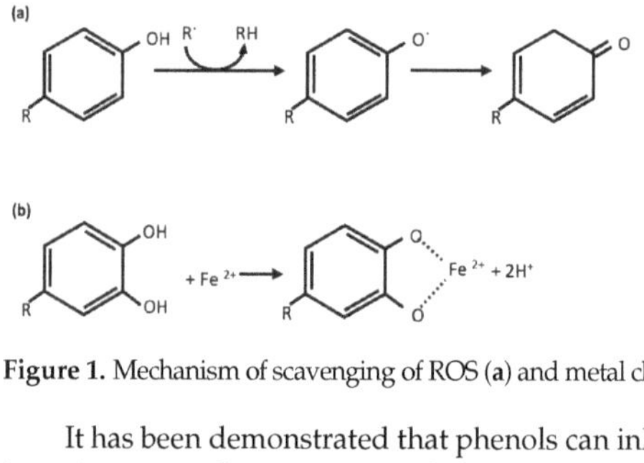

Figure 1. Mechanism of scavenging of ROS (**a**) and metal chelation (**b**) by phenolic compounds antioxidants.

It has been demonstrated that phenols can inhibit the aggregation of proteins involved in various neurodegenerative pathologies in which cognitive deterioration occurs, including AD, PD, dementia with Lewy bodies, and multiple system atrophy [58]. In fact, studies conducted with flavonoids show that these compounds would be involved in preventing neurodegeneration [59]. Their bioactivity is attributed to their antioxidant effect and their capacity to inhibit acetylcholinesterase (AChE)/butyrylcholinesterase (BChE) [19] and the GABA receptor [60], alleviate mitochondrial dysfunction [61], modulate neuronal signaling pathways critical for the control of neuronal resistance to neurotoxic oxidants, inhibition inflammatory mediators [62] and chelation of transition metal ions [59].

It has been shown that the interaction of flavonoids with these receptors depends on the structure [63], implying that not all phenols have the same activity and importance as agents to prevent or treat neurodegenerative diseases. It has been suggested that B-ring hydroxylation is a differentiating element in the action exerted by flavonoids, particularly the positive contribution of 5-dehydroxylation and $3',4'$-ortho-dihydroxylation on the B-ring [64]. Furthermore, a study on flavonoid-PI3-kinase interaction has further confirmed the pivotal role of B-ring hydroxylation [65], and highly sensitive allosteric modulation has been proposed [60].

Other studies have reported the direct involvement of phenolic compounds in preventing various pathologies associated with oxidative stress. One of these compounds is resveratrol, a phenol that can directly target multiple signaling cascades involved in neurodegenerative diseases, such as anti-inflammatory activity and inhibiting the aggregation of toxic Aβ amyloid protein [66]. Another example is 3,4,5–trihydroxybenzoic acid, a phenol that inhibits the plasma membrane Pdr5p efflux pump in AD124567 yeast strain overexpressing the PDR5 gene [67]. Another study demonstrated that 4-hydroxy-3-methoxybenzaldehyde represses translation in yeast, as concluded by the accumulation of processing bodies and stress granules composed of non-translating mRNAs and proteins after 4-hydroxy-3-methoxybenzaldehyde exposure [68].

In studies conducted in *Saccharomyces*, Sunthonkun et al. [69] observed the positive effects of 3,4-dihydroxybenzoic acid against aging. In this sense, 3,4-dihydroxybenzoic acid positively modulated the life span of *Saccharomyces* by reducing ROS, conferring cells greater resistance against free radicals. According to these authors, regarding the reduction of ROS levels, 3,4-dihydroxybenzoic acid seems to imitate the effect of the inactivation of proteins such as Sir2 (silent information regulator 2), Tor1 (protein kinase) or Sch9 (protein kinase).

Considering all this information and the multifactor origin of neurodegenerative disorders, it is interesting and necessary to delve into the study of natural multitarget compounds and their bioavailability [70,71].

Mediterranean ecosystems show a great diversity of plant species derived from the specific climatic conditions and the heterogeneity of their habitats [72]. The species that dominate these habitats endure harsh conditions due to the frequency of wild fires, high temperatures, water stress in summer and herbivory [73]. These unfavorable conditions stimulate the production of compounds derived from secondary metabolism, specifically phenolic compounds [74,75], which play an important ecological role in the adaptive response to these unfavorable conditions. Therefore, the species of these ecosystems may constitute an important and diverse source of compounds that should be studied.

This work aimed to evaluate the potential of Mediterranean shrub species as a source of phenolic compounds. To this end, we selected the shrub species that dominate a particular geographic area of the Iberian Peninsula.

2. Description of the Study Area and Article Search Strategy

The study area selected was Extremadura, a region of the Western Iberian Peninsula with a surface of 41,635 km^2. From a biogeographic perspective, it is in the Mediterranean region and is characterized by a diverse set of plant associations that result from the interaction of its biotic and abiotic factors. The bioclimatic floors and levels that may be found in the region of Extremadura are mesomediterranean, supramediterranean and orosubmediterranean [76], and they are associated with a rainfall of 200–2000 mm/year and an average annual temperature of 4–19 °C. These conditions are responsible for the wide variability of the plant landscape of this region, which is represented by the vegetation sets described in "Plant Landscape and Dynamics in Extremadura" [77], with the following dominating shrub formations: orophilous laburnum and creeping juniper, heath and rock rose, broom and rotem, thyme and cantuesar, gorse and basophilic rock rose, wild olive and mastic, strawberry tree, arborescent juniper, kermes oaks, and garrigues and thorny bushes (brambles and thorns). These groupings are characterized and dominated by the following 24 species: *Cistus ladanifer, Cistus salviifolius, Cistus monspeliensis, Cistus crispus, Cistus albidus, Cistus populifoius, Cytisus multiflorus, Cytisus scoparius, Cytisus striatus, Erica multiflora, Erica scoparia, Erica australis, Calluna vulgaris, Myrtus communis, Pistacea lentiscus, Pistacea terebinthus, Rosmarinus officinalis, Quercus ilex, Quercus suber, Arbutus unedo, Lavandula stoechas, Thymus mastichina, Thymus vulgaris* and *Rubus ulmifolius*.

In this study, we reviewed the works conducted on the identification of phenolic compounds in the 24 selected species. The data reflect the compounds identified in studies published between 1996 and 2022 in the Pubmed, ScienceDirect and Scopus databases. We selected the articles where the identification of these compounds was supported, at least, by techniques such as high-performance liquid chromatography (HPLC)–photodiode array detection (DAD)–mass spectrometry (MS), which provide reliable information about the constitution of phenolic compounds. Articles that were not available in full-text were not considered. Moreover, articles without a clear experimental procedure were also excluded.

3. Description and Classification of the Phenolic Compounds Present in the Selected Species

Table 1 presents the list of phenolic compounds that have been identified by different authors in the 24 species selected for this study. A total of 403 different phenolic compounds can be found in this entire set of species. These compounds belong to different classes or groups: phenolic acids, flavonoids, other polyphenols, lignans and stilbenes. Each of these groups accounts for 35.7%, 55.6%, 5.7%, 2% and 0.7%, respectively (Table 2). As can be observed, the largest group is constituted by flavonoids; thus, these species are an important and diverse source of these phenols.

Table 1. Phenolic compounds identified in the 24 species selected in this study.

	Species																							
	Cl	Cs	Cm	Cc	Ca	Cp	Cym	Cys	Cyst	Em	Es	Ea	Cv	Mc	Pl	Pt	Ro	Qi	Qs	Au	Ls	Tm	Tv	Ru
Class: Phenolic acid. Sub Class:																								
Hydroxybenzoic acids																								
Acetovanillone	+																							
Anisic acid	+						+										+			+				
Benzoic acid	+																							
Benzyl benzoate	+																							
Methyl benzoate	+																							
Castalagin	+					+														+				
Cornusiin	+	+																						
3-hydroxybenzoic acid																					+	+	+	
4-hydroxybenzoic acid	+														+		+			+	+		+	+
4-hydroxybenzoic acid glucuronide																	+			+			+	
Glucose p-hydroxy benzoate																+					+			
Dihydroxy-methoxybenzoic acid																					+			
Dihydroxybenzoic acid di-pentoside																+								
Dihydroxybenzoic acid hexoside																				+				
Ducheside A	+																							
3,4'-dihydroxypropiofenone-3-glucoside	+	+																		+				
3-O-galloylquinic acid (Theogallin)		+													+					+				
3-O-galloylshikimic acid															+					+				
3,4-Di-O-galloylquinic acid		+														+				+				
5-O-galloylquinic acid														+						+				
5-O-galloylshikimic acid																				+				
Galloyl arbutin	+	+														+				+				
Galloyl glucose																				+				
Galloyl glucuronide																				+				
Galloyl hexoside																				+				
Galloyl-bis-HHDP glucose																							+	
Galloyl-HHDP-DHHDP-hexoside																				+				
Galloyl-HHDP-hexoside															+					+				
Digallic acid	+																							
Digalloyl glucose																				+				
Digalloyl shikimic acid																				+				
Digalloyl-HHDP-hexoside																				+				
Digalloylarbutin																				+				
Digalloylquinic shikimic acid																				+				
Tetra-galloyl-hexoside																				+				
Trigalloylquinic acid																		+						
Trigalloylshikimic acid																				+				
Pentagalloyl glucose															+						+			
Ellagic acid	+											+								+	+			+

Table 1. Cont.

	Species																							
	Cl	Cs	Cm	Cc	Ca	Cp	Cym	Cys	Cyst	Em	Es	Ea	Cv	Mc	Pl	Pt	Ro	Qi	Qs	Au	Ls	Tm	Tv	Ru
Ellagic acid-7-xyloside	+																							
Ellagic acid arabinoside		+			+	+																		
Ellagic acid diglucoside																				+				+
Ellagic acid glucoside																				+				+
Ellagic acid glucuronide																								+
Ellagic acid hexoside																				+				
Ellagic acid mannopyranoside																				+				+
Ellagic acid pentoside																				+				+
Ellagic acid xylofuranoside																				+				
Ellagitannin																								
Methylellagic acid rhamnoside																								
3,3'-di-O-Methylellagic acid			+																					
4-O-β-D-(2''-acetyl) glucoside																								
Gallic acid (3,4,5-trihydroxybenzoic acid)	+	+	+		+	+	+								+	+	+	+	+	+	+		+	+
Gallic acid dihexoside																				+				
Gallic acid glucoside																				+				
Gallic acid hexoside																				+				
Gallotannin																								
Ethyl gallate		+				+																		
Methyl gallate						+																		
Gentisic acid																		+						
Gentisoyl glucoside	+		+														+				+		+	
Gentisoyl hexoside	+																							
Glucogallin	+														+									
Hexahydroxydiphenoyl-glucose	+		+	+																				
Isoeugenol																	+							
Lambertianin C																						+		
Methoxysalicylic acid								+																
Protocatechualdehyde (3,4-dihidroxy-benzaldehyde)																								
Protocatechuic acid (3,4-dihydroxy-benzoic acid)								+																
Protocatechuic acid glucoside															+	+		+		+	+		+	+
Punicalagin		+	+			+																		
Punicalin		+	+			+																		
Punicalagin-gallate																								
Sanguin H-10																								
Sanguin H-10 isomer		+		+																+				
Shikimic acid gallate		+	+																					
Shikimic acid dimer																+	+			+				
Strictinin ellagitannin																				+				
Syringic acid	+																			+				
Syringyl-shikimic acid		+			+																		+	+

Table 1. Cont.

	Species																							
	Cl	Cs	Cm	Cc	Ca	Cp	Cym	Cys	Cyst	Em	Es	Ea	Cv	Mc	Pl	Pt	Ro	Qi	Qs	Au	Ls	Tm	Tv	Ru
TriGG-dehydrohexahydroxydiphenoyl (DHHDP)-glucose	+																							
Uralenneoside																				+				
Vanillic acid		+					+					+			+	+	+	+		+	+		+	+
Vanillic acid sulfoquinovoside																					+			
Class: Phenolic acid. Sub Class: Hydroxycinnamic acids																								
Caffeic acid (3,4-dihydroxycinnamic acid)		+					+								+			+		+		+	+	+
caffeic acid 4-O-glucoside												+											+	
Caffeic acid derivate																				+		+	+	
Caffeic acid hexoside																								+
Caffeic acid trimer																							+	
Dihydrocaffeic acid																					+		+	
Caffeoyl arbutin																				+				
Caffeoyl ferulic acid		+																						
Caffeoyl feruloyl tartaric acid																					+			
Caffeoyl hexoside																					+			+
Caffeoyl hexoside derivative																					+			
4-O-Caffeoyl quinic acid										+														+
Caffeoyl quinic acid glucoside			+		+																			
Caffeoyl quinic acid derivative		+			+												+							
Caffeoyl tartaric acid (caftaric acid)							+																	
Dicaffeoyl shikimic acid		+																						
1,4-dicaffeoyl quinic acid															+									+
3,5-dicaffeoyl quinic acid																								+
6-Caffeoyl sucrose																					+			
Chlorogenic acid (3-O-caffeoylquinic acid)		+		+			+	+			+				+	+	+			+	+	+	+	+
Methyl caffeate																					+			
Cinnamic acid	+														+	+				+				
Cinnamic acid derivative																				+				
Methoxycinnamic acid															+									
Cinnamic acid-O xylosyl hexoside																				+				
Hydrocinnamic acid	+																							
Hydrocinnamic acid glucoside																					+			
Hydroxycinnamoyl-quinic acid																						+		
p-Coumaric acid		+													+		+			+			+	+
p-Coumaricacid derivate																								+
Coumaroyl quinic acid		+	+																					
Coumaroyl quinic acid derivative		+			+																			
Coumaric acid hexoside																				+	+			
Chicoric acid																					+			

87

Table 1. Cont.

	Cl	Cs	Cm	Cc	Ca	Cp	Cym	Cys	Cyst	Em	Es	Ea	Cv	Mc	Pl	Pt	Ro	Qi	Qs	Au	Ls	Tm	Tv	Ru
Ferulic acid	+	+													+	+		+	+	+	+		+	+
Ferulic acid derivative		+																		+	+		+	+
3-O-Feruloylquinic acid		+	+																	+				
Feruloylquinic glucoside			+		+																			
Feruloyl-1-glucoside																								
Hydroxy-ferulic acid hexoside			+														+							
Hydroxy-ferulic acid rhamnoside			+		+																			
Feruloyl tartaric acid (fertaric acid)		+	+		+																+			
6′-O-Sinapoylsucrose																					+			
3,4-Dihydroxyphenyllactic acid hexoside																					+			
3-(3,4-Dihydroxyphenyl)-2-hydroxypropanoic acid																								
Rosmarinic acid			+	+	+												+				+	+	+	
Rosmarinic acid hexoside			+	+																	+		+	
Rosmarinic acid-3-O-glucoside					+												+							
Dihydroxy-dihydro feruloyl methyl rosmarinic acid		+	+																					
Methylrosmaric acid			+	+													+				+		+	
p-Hydroxybenzylrosmarinic acid																					+			
Isosalvianolic acid A																					+			
Methyl melitrate																								
Salvianolic acid A																					+			
Salvianolic acid B																					+			
Salvianolic acid C																					+			
Sinapaldehyde																					+			
3-Sinapoylquinic acid			+																					
Sinapic acid																					+		+	
Yunnaneic acid F																							+	
Verbascoside															+									
Class: Phenolic acid. Sub Class: Hydroxyphenylacetic acids																								
p-Hydroxyphenylacetic acid															+									
3,4-Dihydroxyphenylacetic acid																				+	+		+	
3,4-dihydroxyphenyllactic acid hexoside																					+			
Class: Flavonoid. Sub Class: Flavanones																								
Eriodictyol																					+		+	
Eriodictyol 7-O-rutinoside																	+						+	
Eriodictyol 7-O-glucuronide																						+	+	
Eriodictyol-O-di-hexoside																							+	+
Eriodictyol-O-hexoside																						+		
Eriodictyol-O-hexuronide																+								
Glucodistylin																								

Table 1. Cont.

												Species												
	Cl	Cs	Cm	Cc	Ca	Cp	Cym	Cys	Cyst	Em	Es	Ea	Cv	Mc	Pl	Pt	Ro	Qi	Qs	Au	Ls	Tm	Tv	Ru
Glucodistylin isomer																+								
Hesperetin 7-O-rutinoside (Hesperidin)																	+					+	+	+
Methyleriodictyol-O-pentosylhexoside																						+	+	+
Naringenin					+											+								
Naringenin-di-hexoside																						+		
Naringenin 7-O-glucoside (Naringin-Prunina)		+			+			+									+						+	+
Pinocembrin																								+
Class: Flavonoid. Sub Class: Flavones																								
Apigenin	+	+	+				+		+								+				+	+	+	
Apigenin 7-O-glucuronide																					+	+	+	
Apigenin glucuronide hexoside							+															+	+	
Apigenin 6,8-di-C-glucoside	+		+		+											+	+				+	+	+	
Apigenin 7-O-glucoside							+														+			
Apigenin C-hexoside							+																	
Apigenin pentoside		+																						
Apigenin-7-O-rutinoside							+													+				
Apigenin-O-hexoside							+																	
Apigenin-O-hexoside derivative																	+			+				
Isovitexin 7-O-glucoside																				+				
Apigenin 8-C-glucoside (Vitexin)							+										+							
2″-O-pentosyl-6-C-hexosyl-apigenin							+																	
2″-O-Pentosyl-8-C-hexoside apigenin isomer I							+																	
2″-O-Pentosyl-8-C-hexoside apigenin isomer II							+																	
2″-O-pentosyl-8-C-hexosyl-apigenin							+																	
2″-O-Pentoxide-8-C-hexoside apigenin							+																	
4'-O-Rutinoside of 7-O-methylated apigenin																							+	
6″-O-(3-hydroxy-3-methylglutaroyl)-2″-O-pentosyl-C-hexosyl-apigenin							+																	
Apigenin 4'-methyl ether																	+				+			
Apigenin 7-methyl ether (Genkwanin)			+																			+		
Apigenin 4',7-dimethyl ether			+														+				+			
Chalcone															+									
Chrysin derivative							+																	
Chrysin-7-O-glucoside							+																	
Circimaritin																								
Hispidulin (Scutellarein 6-methyl ether)																	+							
Hispidulin 7-O-glucose (homoplantaginin)																	+						+	
6″-O-(E)-feruloylhomoplantaginin																	+							
Hispidulin-rutinoside																								
Hypolaetin di-glucuronide																					+			
Hypolaetin 8-O-glucuronide																					+			
Isoscutellarein 7-O-glucoside																	+							

Table 1. Cont.

Compound	Cl	Cs	Cm	Cc	Ca	Cp	Cym	Cys	Cyst	Em	Es	Ea	Cv	Mc	Pl	Pt	Ro	Qi	Qs	Au	Ls	Tm	Tv	Ru
Isoscutellarein 8-O-glucuronide																					+			
Ladanein (5,6-dihydroxy-7,4′-dimethoxyflavone)																	+							+
Luteolin (3′,4′,5,7-Tetrahydroxyflavone)		+							+						+	+	+				+	+	+	+
Chrysoeriol-O-hexoside (Luteolin 3′-methyl ether)																						+	+	
Diosmetin (Luteolin 4′-methyl ether)																	+							
Cirsilineol (6-Methoxyluteolin 3′,7-dimethyl ether)																							+	
Luteolin 7,3-dimethyl ether																					+			
Luteolin 3′-O-glucuronide																	+							
Luteolin 7-O-glucuronide																	+				+		+	+
Luteolin 7,4′-di-glucuronide																	+				+		+	+
Luteolin 4-O-glucoside																	+							
Luteolin 7-O-glucoside														+							+		+	
Luteolin 5-O-glucoside																	+							
Luteolin 8-C-glucoside (Orientin)								+																
Luteolin 6-C-glucoside (Isoorientin)															+		+						+	
Luteolin-O-hexoronide																						+		
Luteolin-7-O-rutinoside		+															+					+	+	
Luteolin-hexoside		+	+														+							
Luteolin 6-hydroxy-7-O-glucoside		+	+																					
Luteolin-O-malonyl-hexoside)							+																	
2″-O-Pentosyl-8-C-hexoside luteolin							+																	
2″-O-pentosyl-6-C-hexosyl-luteolin							+																	
2″-O-pentosyl-8-C-hexosyl-luteolin							+																	
6″-O-(3-hydroxy-3-methylglutaroyl)-2″-O-pentosyl-C-hexosyl-luteolin																								
Nepitrin (Nepetin 7-O-glucoside)																	+							
6″-O-(E)-feruloylhepitrin																	+							
Salvigenin (5-Hydroxy-6,7,4′-trimethoxyflavone)																	+							
Techtochrysin																+								
Class: Flavonoid. Sub Class: Flavonols																								
Isorhamnetin																								
Isorhamnetin 3-O-glucoside																	+	+		+				
Isorhamnetin 3-O-rutinoside																	+			+				
Isorhamnetin-3-O-hexoside							+																	
Isorhamnetin-O-(6″-caffeoyl)hexoside										+														
Isorhamnetin-O-deoxyhexosyl-hexoside							+				+													
Isorhamnetin-O-hexoside-O-rhamnoside											+													
Galangin (3,5,7-Trihydroxyflavone)	+																							+

Table 1. *Cont.*

	Species																							
	Cl	Cs	Cm	Cc	Ca	Cp	Cym	Cys	Cyst	Em	Es	Ea	Cv	Mc	Pl	Pt	Ro	Qi	Qs	Au	Ls	Tm	Tv	Ru
Kaempferol	+				+			+		+	+	+			+	+	+				+	+	+	+
6-Hydroxykaempferol																				+				
Dihydrokaempferol 3-O-glucoside																								+
Kaempferol 3-methyl ether	+	+			+																		+	
Kaempferol 3,4'-dimethyl ether	+	+																						
Kaempferol 3,7-dimethyl ether	+	+																						
Kaempferol 3,7,4'-trimethyl ether	+		+																				+	
kaempferol methylether O-rutinoside																							+	
Kaempferol dimethylether hexoside	+																							
Kaempferol 3-O-(6''-galloyl) glucoside											+							+		+				
kaempferol-3-O-(6''-feruloyl)-β-D-glucopyranoside																								+
Kaempferol 3-O-(6''-p-coumaroyl) glucoside isomers					+													+		+				
Kaempferol-3-O-(2'',6''-di-p-coumaroyl)glucoside																		+						
kaempferol-3-O-(2'',6''-di-E-p-coumaroyl)-glucopyranoside																		+						
kaempferol-3-O-(3''-acetyl-2'',6''-di-p-coumaroyl)glucoside																		+						
Kaempferol-3-O-(3'',4''-diacetyl-2'',6''-di-p-coumaroyl)glucoside isomers					+								+					+						+
kaempferol-3-O-(6''-p-coumaroyl) glucopyranoside (Tiliroside)																								+
Kaempferol-3-galactoside-6''-rhamnoside-3'''-rhamnoside																				+				
kaempferol malonyl glucoside																				+				
kaempferol 3-O-ramnopyranoside																				+				+
Kaempferol-O-rhamnoside		+			+		+													+				
Kaempferol 7-O-(6''-rhamnosyl) glucoside		+								+														
kaempferol-3-O-arabinofuranoside															+									
kaempferol-3-O-arabinopyranoside							+			+														
Kaempferol 3-O-glucoside (Astragalin)	+	+																		+				+
Kaempferol 3-O-rutinoside	+	+																		+				+
Kaempferol-acetyl-O-rutinoside		+					+																	
Kaempferol-acetyl-O-rahmnoside		+																		+				+
Kaempferol O-glucuronide																				+				+
Kaempferol 7-O-hexuronide		+																		+				
Kaempferol 3-O-pentoside							+																	
Kaempferol O-hexoside							+																	+

Table 1. Cont.

	Species																							
	Cl	Cs	Cm	Cc	Ca	Cp	Cym	Cys	Cyst	Em	Es	Ea	Cv	Mc	Pl	Pt	Ro	Qi	Qs	Au	Ls	Tm	Tv	Ru
Kaempferol O-pentosyl hexoside		+																						
Kaempferol-3-O-hydroxybenzoyl glucoside																								+
kaempferol-3-O-galactoside																								+
Kaempferol xyloside	+																							
Kaempferol-O-di-hexoside																				+				+
Morin		+																		+				
Myricetin	+											+			+					+				
(3,3′,4′,5,5′,7-Hexahydroxyflavone)					+													+						
Myricetin 3-O-(6″-rhamnosyl) glucoside			+																	+				
Myricetin-O-(6″-benzoyl) hexoside											+													
Myricetin-O-(6″-cinnamoyl) hexoside											+													
Myricetin-O-(6″-p-coumaroyl) hexoside											+													
Myricetin-O-(galloyl) hexoside		+																		+				
Methoxy-myricetin-O-rhamnoside											+													
Myricetin 3,7,4′,5′-tetramethyl ether			+																					
Myricetin-3-arabinoside																				+				
myricetin 3-O-arabinofuranoside														+										
Myricetin-3-O-galactoside					+							+								+				
Myricetin-3-O-glucoside		+													+	+								
Myricetin-3-O-glucuronide		+												+	+	+								
Myricetin 3-O-hexoside													+											
Myricetin 7-O-hexuronide					+															+				
Myricetin 3-O-pentoside													+							+				
Myricetin 7-O-pentoside											+	+								+				
Myricetin-O-rhamnoside (Myricitrin)	+	+			+						+	+		+	+	+		+						
Myricitrin-2″-O-gallate (Desmanthin)		+													+	+								
Myricetin-O-rutinoside		+			+										+									
Myricetin 3-O-xyloside																				+				
Pinobanksin (bioflavonoide)																	+							+
Quercetin (3,3′,4′,5,7-Pentahydroxyflavone)	+	+			+					+		+			+	+		+		+				+
Quercetin (acetyl) rutinoside		+				+																		
Quercetin (acetyl) hexoside		+																						
Quercetin (acetyl)-O-rhamnoside							+																	
Quercetin-O-(6″-cinnamoyl) hexoside												+												
quercetin 3-O-(2′-coumaroyl) rutinoside		+								+														
Quercetin 3-O-(6″-p-coumaroyl) hexoside																				+	+	+	+	
Quercetin-3-O-(6″-galloyl) hexoside																				+				
Quercetin-O-(6″-p-hydroxybenzoyl) hexoside											+													
Quercetin-O-(malonyl) hexoside																+								
Quercetrin-O-gallate		+																						
Quercertin methyl ether-3-O-galactoside									+															
Quercetin 4′,5′-dimethyl ether																								
Quercetin 3,7,4′,5′-tetramethyl ether			+																					
Quercetin 3-O-arabinoside																				+				

Table 1. Cont.

	Cl	Cs	Cm	Cc	Ca	Cp	Cym	Cys	Cyst	Em	Es	Ea	Cv	Mc	Pl	Pt	Ro	Qi	Qs	Au	Ls	Tm	Tv	Ru
quercetin 3-O-arabinofuranoside	+														+					+				+
Quercetin 3-O-galactoside (Hyperoside)		+	+												+					+	+		+	+
Quercetin 3-O-glucoside (Isoquercetin)	+	+	+	+		+	+					+						+		+	+	+	+	+
Quercetin 3-O-glucuronide	+															+				+				
Quercetin 3-O-hexoside			+				+			+		+								+		+		
Quercetin 3-O-hexuronide											+									+				
Quercetin hexose protocatechuic acid	+																							
Quercetin-O-rhamnoside (Quercetrin)	+	+	+		+					+		+		+	+						+			+
Quercetin-O-rutinoside (Rutin)	+	+			+	+	+			+		+		+	+	+	+	+		+	+		+	+
Quercetin 3-O-pentoside	+																			+				
Quercetin 3-O-xyloside													+											
Quercetin 3-O-rhamnoside-7-O-glucoside																								
Quercetin 3,4-diglucoside	+		+		+										+									+
Quercetin-O-deoxyhexosyl-hexoside	+						+																	
Quercetin-O-dihexoside	+						+																	
Quercetin-pentosyl-hexoside	+																							
Taxifolin (dihydroquercetin)		+													+	+							+	+
Taxifolin-3-O-glucoside																+								
Taxifolin 3-O-rhamnoside																				+				
Taxifolin-O-hexoside											+													
Taxifolin pentoside																							+	+
Class: Flavonoid. Sub Class: Flavanols																								
Catechin	+	+										+			+	+		+	+	+	+		+	+
Catechin 3-gallate																			+	+				
4,3',4'-Trimethylcatechin			+																	+				
Catechin derivates					+							+												
Catechin glucose																				+				
Catechin-(4α→8)-Catechin (Procyanidin B3)																		+	+	+				
Dehydrodicatechin A																		+						
Epicatechin		+			+							+			+			+	+	+	+		+	+
Epicatechin derivatives			+																	+				
Epicatechin methyl gallate			+															+			+			
Epicatechin gallate		+													+	+				+				
epicatechin-4,6-catechin																				+				
epicatechin-4,8-catechin																				+				
epicatechin-4,8-epicatechin-4,8-catechin																				+				
epicatechin-4,8-epicatechin-4,8-Epicatechin																+				+				+
Epicatechin-A-epicatechin																				+				+
Epicatechin-B-epicatechin-A-epicatechin																				+				
Epicatechin-epicatechin 3-O gallate				+																+				
Epicatechin-epigallocatechin				+	+															+				

Table 1. Cont.

	Cl	Cs	Cm	Cc	Ca	Cp	Cym	Cys	Cyst	Em	Es	Ea	Cv	Mc	Pl	Pt	Ro	Qi	Qs	Au	Ls	Tm	Tv	Ru
Epigallocatechin	+																							+
Epigallocatechin gallate(Teatannin II)		+		+																+				
Epigallocatechin-catechin																+								
Epigallocatechin-epicatechin																				+				
Epigallocatechin-epigallocatechin	+				+																			
Fzelechin-catechin-3-O-rhamnoside (proanthocyanidin)																		+						
Gallocatechin																+				+				
Gallocatechin-4,8-catechin																	+			+				
Procyanidin B2		+																						
Tannic acid															+									
Class: Flavonoid. Sub Class: Anthocyanins																								
Cyanidin 3-O-arabinoside															+					+				+
Cyanidin-3-galactoside		+																		+				
Cyanidin 3-O-glucoside			+											+						+				+
Cyanidin 3-O-rutinoside																				+				+
Cyanidin 3-O-xyloside																								+
Cyanidin dihexoside																								+
Cyanidin-3,5-diglucoside																				+				
Delphinidin 3-O-galactoside														+						+				
Delphinidin 3-O-glucoside														+	+					+				
Malvidin-3-O-glucoside/Oenin														+										
Pelargonidin 3-O-(6″-malonyl) glucoside		+		+										+										
Pelargonidin-3-O-glucoside		+		+													+							+
Pelargonidin 3-rutinoside		+																						+
Peonidin 3-O-(6″-p-coumaroyl) glucoside					+									+										
Peonidin-3-O-glucoside		+																						
Petunidin					+									+										
Petunidin-3-O-glucoside		+													+									
Class: Flavonoid. Sub Class: Isoflavonoids																								
Daidzein										+														
3′-Hydroxydaidzein										+														
Genistein										+														
2′-Hydroxygenistein																								
Glycitin 6″-O-malonate			+			+																		
Class: Other polyphenols. Sub Class: Hydroxybenzaldehydes																								
4-hydroxybenzaldehyde																					+			
4-hydroxybenzoic acid																	+				+			
4-(6-O-sulfo)glucoside								+																
Syringaldehyde																								+

Table 1. *Cont.*

	Cl	Cs	Cm	Cc	Ca	Cp	Cym	Cys	Cyst	Em	Es	Ea	Cv	Mc	Pl	Pt	Ro	Qi	Qs	Au	Ls	Tm	Tv	Ru
Vanillin	+																						+	
Class: Other polyphenol. Sub Class: Hydroxycoumarins																								
4-methylumbelliferone																								+
6,7-Dihydroxycoumarin 3O-glucoside (Aesculin)																				+				
Coumarin																	+							
Class: Other polyphenol. Sub Class: Tyroslos																								
Oleuropein		+																						
Class: Lignans. Sub Class: Lignans																								
Carnosic acid																	+					+	+	
Carnosol																	+						+	
Isolariciresinol 3-glucoside																					+			
Methyl carnosic acid																	+				+		+	
Pinoresinol																	+							
Rosmanol																	+							
Rosmanol derivate																								
Sagerinic acid																					+			
Thymol																							+	
Class: Other polyphenols. Sub Class: Other polyphenols																								
5-Nonadecylresorcinol																					+			
Arbutin																				+				+
Catechol																		+	+					
Coniferaldehyde																				+				
Hydroquinone derivative																				+				
Salvianolic acid																					+	+	+	
Salvianolic acid A																					+	+	+	
salvianolic acid B (lithospermic acid B)																					+	+	+	
Salvianolic acid B/E/L																					+			
Salvianolic acid C																					+			
Salvianolic acid C isomer																						+		
Salvianolic acid F																						+		
Salvianolic acid K																						+		
Salvianolic acid I																								
Sculetin																					+			
Class: Stilbenes. Sub Class: Stilbenes																								

Table 1. Cont.

	Cl	Cs	Cm	Cc	Ca	Cp	Cym	Cys	Cyst	Em	Es	Ea	Cv	Mc	Pl	Pt	Ro	Qi	Qs	Au	Ls	Tm	Tv	Ru
Piceid																				+				
Resveratrol																+				+				+
Stilbericoside																				+				
References	[75, 78–86]	[81, 87, 88]	[81, 83, 88–90]	[81]	[81, 88, 91]	[81, 82]	[92–96]	[97–99]	[100]	[100]	[101]	[102, 103]	[101]	[83, 104]	[105–107]	[108, 109]	[110–115]	[116–118]	[117]	[119–133]	[134–139]	[140–142]	[143–152]	[92, 153–162]

Cl: *C. ladanifer*; Cs: *C. salviifolius*; Cm: *C. monspeliensis*; Cc: *C. crispus*; Ca: *C. albidus*; Cp: *C. populifolius*; Cym: *C. multiflorus*; Cys: *C. scoparius*; Cyst: *C. striatus*; Em: *E. multiflora*; Es: *E. scoparia*; Ea: *E. australis*; Cv: *C. vulgaris*; Mc: *M. communis*; Pl: *P. lentiscus*; Pt: *P. terebinthus*; Ro: *R. officinalis*; Qi: *Q. ilex*; Qs: *Q. suber*; Au: *A. unedo*; Ls: *L. stoechas*; Tm: *T. mastichina*; Tv: *T. vulgaris*; Ru: *R. ulmifolius*.

Table 2. Number and percentage of phenolic compounds, grouped by class and subclass, found in the 24 species selected in this study.

	N° Compound	Percentage (%)
Class: Phenolic acid	144	35.72%
Sub Class: Hydroxybenzoic acids	82	20.34%
Sub Class: Hydroxycinnamic acids	59	14.64%
Sub Class: Hydroxyphenylacetic acids	3	0.74%
Class: Flavonoid	224	55.56%
Sub Class: Flavanones	13	3.22%
Sub Class: Flavones	59	14.64%
Sub Class: Flavonols	103	25.55%
Sub Class: Flavanols	28	6.94%
Sub Class: Anthocyanins	16	3.97%
Sub Class: Isoflavonoids	5	1.24%
Class: Other polyphenols	23	5.69%
Sub Class: Hydroxybenzaldehydes	4	0.99%
Sub Class: Hydroxycoumarins	3	0.74%
Sub Class: Tyrosols	1	0.24%
Sub Class: Other polyphenols	15	3.72%
Class: Lignans. Sub Class: Lignans	9	2.23%
Class: Stilbenes. Sub Class: Stilbenes	3	0.74%

There is a clear difference in the number of compounds identified in each species. The species with the largest number of compounds is *A. unedo* (142 compounds), whereas only 5 to 8 compounds have been identified in *C. crispus*, *C. striatus* and *C. vulgaris*. The identification of more or fewer compounds in a species is due to the number of studies conducted on each, which is determined by their commercial interest. Some of them, such as *A. unedo*, have a high commercial interest, which explains the existence of many studies on this species and, therefore, a larger number of compounds identified in it.

Furthermore, the compounds are unequally represented. Some phenols have only been cited in one species, while others have been reported in many species (Table 1). Considering the compounds that appear in more than 5 species (Table 3), 38 phenolic compounds are found in these species, 15 of which are phenolic acids and 23 are flavonoids.

Table 3. Identified phenolic compounds in more than 5 species among the 24 species selected in this study. The percentage of representation in these species is also shown.

Phenolic Compound	Species in Which It Appears	Percentage (%)
Class: Phenolic acid. Sub Class: Hydroxybenzoic acids		
4-hydroxybenzoic acid	7	29.16%
Ellagic acid	8	33.33%
Gallic acid (3,4,5-trihydroxybenzoic acid)	17	70.83%
Hexahydroxydiphenoyl-glucose	6	25.00%
Protocatechuic acid (3,4-dihydroxy-benzoic acid)	9	37.50%
Syringic acid	8	33.33%
Vanillic acid	10	41.66%
Class: Phenolic acid. Sub Class: Hydroxycinnamic acids		
Caffeic acid (3,4-dihydroxycinnamic acid)	12	50.00%
Chlorogenic acid (3-O-caffeoylquinic acid)	13	54.16%
Cinnamic acid	7	29.16%
p-Coumaric acid	10	41.66%

Table 3. Cont.

Phenolic Compound	Species in Which It Appears	Percentage (%)
Coumaroyl quinic acid	5	20.83%
Ferulic Acid	12	50.00%
Rosmarinic acid	5	20.83%
Methylrosmaric acid	6	25.00%
Class: Flavonoid. Sub Class: Flavanones		
Hesperetin 7-O-rutinoside (Hesperidin)	5	20.83%
Naringenin	8	33.33%
Naringenin 7-O-glucoside (Naringin-Prunina)	9	37.50%
Class: Flavonoid. Sub Class: Flavones		
Apigenin	11	45.83%
Apigenin 7-O-glucoside	6	25.00%
Luteolin (3′.4′.5.7-Tetrahydroxyflavone)	9	37.50%
Luteolin 7-O-glucoside	5	20.83%
Luteolin-7-O-rutinoside	6	25.00%
Class: Flavonoid. Sub Class: Flavonols		
Kaempferol	13	54.16%
Kaempferol O-hexoside	5	20.83%
Myricetin (3.3′.4′.5.5′.7-Hexahydroxyflavone)	9	37.50%
Myricetin 3-O-hexoside	6	25.00%
Myricetin-O-rhamnoside (Myricitrin)	12	50.00%
Myricetin-O-rutinoside	5	20.83%
Quercetin (3.3′.4′.5.7-Pentahydroxyflavone)	15	62.50%
Quercetin 3-O-glucoside (Isoquercetin)	16	66.66%
Quercetin-O-hexoside	8	33.33%
Quercetin-O-rhamnoside (Quercetrin)	11	45.83%
Quercetin 3-O-rutinoside (Rutin)	16	66.66%
Class: Flavonoid. Sub Class: Flavanols		
Catechin	11	45.83%
Epicatechin	10	41.66%
Epicatechin gallate	5	20.83%
Class: Flavonoid. Sub Class: Anthocyanins		
Cyanidin 3-O-glucoside	6	25.00%

4. Neuroprotective Effect of the Most Represented Phenolic Compounds in the Selected Species

The most distributed phenolic compounds among the selected species belong to two classes (Table 3): phenolic acids and flavonoids. Activity against neurodegenerative disorders has been attributed to most of these compounds. In fact, one of the activities most strongly associated with phenolic acids is their antioxidant capacity. This activity depends on the number of hydroxyl moieties attached to the aromatic ring of benzoic or cinnamic acid molecules. For example, Rice-Evans et al. [163] reported that the total antioxidant activity of phenolic acids, in decreasing order, is gallic > p-coumaric > ferulic > vanillic > syringic > caffeic > m-coumaric > protocatechuic > gentisic > o-coumaric >

salicylic > *p*-hydroxybenzoic. Free-radical scavenging is the activity that confers them with the protective function against neurodegenerative disorders.

Six phenolic acids (gallic, chlorogenic, ferulic, caffeic, vanillic and *p*-coumaric acids) are represented in more than 40% of the species studied. These compounds have been assigned neuroprotective functions (Figure 2). Some of the properties attributed to them are described below.

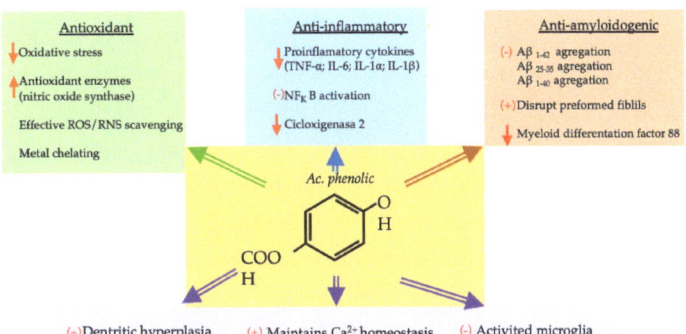

Figure 2. Diagram with neuroprotective mechanisms of phenolic acid. ↑: increase, ↓: decrease, (+): activation, (−): inhibition, ROS: reactive oxygen species, RNS: reactive nitrogen species, TNF-α: tumor necrosis factor-alfa, IL: interleukin, NF$_k$B: nuclear factor kappa B, AB: amyloid beta-peptide.

Gallic acid (GA) is present in 70% of the species that dominate the ecosystems of Extremadura. GA is a well-known 5,4,3-trihydroxybenzoic acid found abundantly in free and conjugated (hydrolyzable tannins) or esterified forms in many plants [164]. It is a phenol with great interest for the treatment of patients with AD and PD, due to its antioxidant, anti-inflammatory, and anti-amyloidogenic properties [165]. Different studies have shown its application as a therapy to interact with amyloid (Aβ) monomers and fibrils. These studies have proved that GA-loaded transferrin-functionalized liposomes could inhibit Aβ$_{1-42}$ aggregation and fibrillation and disrupt preformed fibrils, and thus it could be considered for AD therapy [166]. GA has been demonstrated to reduce memory deficit and cerebral oxidative stress in a unilateral 6-hydroxydopamine-induced PD model in rats [167]. Moreover, its neuroprotective effect has been shown in models of traumatic brain injury [168] and glutamate-induced neurotoxicity in rats [169], due to the improvement in the antioxidant profile and the inhibition of proinflammatory cytokine generation [168,169].

The mechanisms by which GA exerts its prophylactic action in these processes have been analyzed in several studies. For instance, refs. [170,171] reported that, in animals with multiple sclerosis (MS), the administration of GA improved the oxidative and inflammatory response and induced dendritic hyperplasia. This causes an increase in the number of dendritic spines, which could explain the positive response in the dendritic morphology of the three regions (CA1-CA3-DG) of the rat hippocampus with MS. It has been indicated that GA inhibits Aβ-induced neurotoxicity via suppressing microglial-mediated neuroinflammation and decreasing cytokine generation [172]. Studies conducted by [173] show that GA treatment maintains Ca^{2+} homeostasis and insulin-like growth factor 1 (IGF-1) expression and protects neurons from glutamate-induced neurotoxicity.

A recent study conducted by [174] estimated the neuroprotective effects of (GA) against aluminum chloride-induced AD in adult Wistar rats. The trials performed showed that there was a significant decrease in antioxidant enzymes, serum electrolyte and neurotransmitter levels with a corresponding increase in stress markers (MDA, H$_2$O$_2$ and NO) among the rats treated with aluminum, which were restored to nearly normal levels after GA administration. Histological observation showed neurofibrillary tangles and amyloid plaques in the external granular layer of the rats treated with aluminum, although this effect disappeared after GA administration [174].

These studies suggest that structural and functional alterations in the neurons of animals with neurodegenerative diseases are reverted after GA treatment; consequently, neurochemical processes are restored, improving recognition memory [175].

Chlorogenic acid (CGA) is another type of polyphenol that has demonstrated potent anti-inflammatory and antioxidant activities [176]. CGA is present in 54.1% of the species analyzed in this study. Its mechanism of action could be related to the attenuation of mRNA and protein expression levels of proinflammatory and profibrotic mediators, and the reduction of the levels of serum proinflammatory cytokines, such as TNF-α (tumor necrosis factor-alfa) IL-6 (interleukin-6) and IL-1β, as is reported in studies conducted in female rats [177]. CGA treatment also suppressed CCl_4-induced NF-κB (nuclear factor kappa-B) activation and reduced the expression levels of Toll-like receptor 4, myeloid differentiation factor 88, inducible nitric oxide synthase and cyclooxygenase in rats exposed to CCl_4 [178].

Ferulic acid (FA) is present in 50% of the 24 species selected in this study. This compound has been reported to increase neuronal survival, enhance antioxidant enzyme function, modulate multiple neuronal signal transduction, and impair cholinesterase activity (ChAT) [179].

FA has been identified as an effective ROS and RNS scavenger, reducing the likelihood of attack of radicals on proteins and thereby preventing oxidative changes. The antioxidant and anti-inflammatory potential of FA could be due to its ability to suppress leukotriene synthesis and reduce oxidative stress in the brain [180].

Several studies have highlighted the anti-inflammatory effects of FA [181,182]. Particularly, FA has been shown to reduce the neuroinflammation induced by chronic unpredictable mild stress in the prefrontal cortex through the inhibition of NF-κB activation [183].

The potential role of FA against AD has also been investigated in cell models. In particular, Kikugawa et al. [184] showed that the pretreatment of primary cerebral cortical neurons with FA exerted a protective effect toward $Aβ_{25-35}$-induced cytotoxicity; moreover, FA was able to inhibit the aggregation of $Aβ_{25-35}$, $Aβ_{1-40}$ and $Aβ_{1-42}$ and to destabilize pre-aggregated Aβ.

It is worth highlighting that the potential usefulness of FA in AD has also been investigated in in vivo studies [185]. Yan et al. [186] reported that IL-1β production, neuroinflammation and gliosis, induced by the intracerebroventricular injection of Aβ in the mouse hippocampus, were counteracted by pretreatment with FA, and this phenolic acid was able to improve memory loss. Kim et al. [41] also showed that FA prevented the $Aβ_{1-42}$-induced increase in endothelial nitric oxide synthase and 3-nitrotyrosine and suppressed IL-1α immunoreactivity in the hippocampus [187]. Along with the amelioration of Aβ plaque deposition, Wang et al. [188] recently found that FA prevented the reduction in the density and diameter of hippocampal capillaries, thus favoring the oxygen and nutrient supply and the removal of metabolic wastes from the brain, which finally led to improved spatial memory.

Caffeic acid (CA) is another phenol that is present among 50% of the selected species. It has been shown that CA reduces elevated oxidative stress and neuroinflammation and improves synaptic/memory dysfunctions in AD mice [189]. Studies conducted in mice have reported that CA has strong antioxidative and anti-inflammatory properties and prevents the mice brain from Aβ-induced oxidative stress and neuroinflammation [190]. These findings suggest that CA significantly reduces activated microglia and astrocytes in the brains of AD mice.

There are markers clearly related to neurodegenerative conditions and memory dysfunctions, such as phosphatidylinositol 3-kinase /protein kinase b signaling pathway, and downregulation of neuronal growth factors, such as brain-derived neurotrophic factor [191–193]. It has been proved that CA considerably upregulates the expression of these markers in the brains of Aβ-injected mice, and a significant improvement was observed with CA treatment [194].

Vanillic acid (VA) is present in 42% of the species analyzed in this study, and this phenolic acid has been reported to have a clear anti-inflammatory function [195]. Studies conducted with VA have shown that this compound significantly increases neurite outgrowth after 48 h in culture. This compound significantly reduces the expression of cyclooxygenase-2, NF-κB, tenascin-C, chondroitin sulfate proteoglycans and glial fibrillary acidic protein in astrocytes in the LPC-induced model of inflammation. This study supports the hypothesis that VA has anti-inflammatory activities, and, since axonal and synaptic damage is present in most and possibly all neurodegenerative diseases, including AD, PD, and HD [196], the effects of VA on neurite outgrowth make it a potential candidate to encourage the regeneration of neurites after demyelination.

p-coumaric acid (PCA) is present in over 40% of the studied species. In recent years, this compound has been the focus of numerous studies due to its wide variety of biological activities: antioxidant [197], anti-inflammatory [198], neuroprotective [199] and memory-ameliorating effects [200]. Authors such as Rashno et al. [201] explored the effects of oral administration of PCA on passive avoidance memory function, LTP (long-term potentiation) induction in the hippocampal dentate gyrus and hippocampal Aβ plaque formation following $AlCl_3$ exposure in male rats, a condition that resembles the symptoms of AD. The results obtained by this group demonstrated that treatment with PCA alleviated passive avoidance deficit, improved hippocampal LTP impairment and prevented Aβ plaque formation in the $AlCl_3$-exposed rats. Cognitive-improving effects of PCA have been reported in various neuropathological conditions, such as cerebral ischemia [202], lipopolysaccharide-induced neurological changes [200] and scopolamine-induced neurotoxicity [42].

In addition to the group of phenolic acids, the other group of phenols widely distributed among these species is that of flavonoids. Of the 224 different flavonoids that can be found in the entire set of species selected in this study, 23 are present in over 20% of them. Within this group, quercetin and its derivatives quercetin 3-O-rutinoside and quercetin 3-O-glucoside (isoquercetin) stand out, as they are present in over 60% of the selected species. Other flavonols and flavones that are also widely distributed include quercetin-O-rhamnoside (quercetrin), apigenin, kaempferol and myricetin-O-rhamnoside (myricitrin), being present in 45–55% of the selected species.

Different in vitro and in vivo experiments found that these polyphenols may exert a beneficial effect in the prevention and treatment of neurodegenerative diseases associated with oxidative stress, shown in Figure 3, and that the activity of flavonoids such as galangin, kaempferol, quercetin, myricetin, fisetin, apigenin, luteolin and rutin was correlated with the number of OH groups and their side on their phenyl ring [63,203]. It is worth highlighting that these phenolic compounds and their metabolites can enter the brain at detectable levels in mammals, which supports their direct neurological action [204].

Flavonoids, depending on the degree of oxidation and saturation in the heterocyclic C-ring, can be divided into different subclasses, varying in their bioavailability. Thus, flavanols, flavanones and flavonol glycosides have intermediate rates of absorption and bioavailability, while proanthocyanidins, flavanol gallates and anthocyanins have the lowest absorption [205]. According to different studies, epicatechin metabolites seem to reach the brain of rodents at levels that might be physiologically effective [206], and some conjugated forms of quercetin can also accumulate in the brain after oral administration [207,208].

Among flavonoids, flavonols and flavones constitute the largest group and have been associated with a clear neuroprotective role [70,209–213]. It has been demonstrated in numerous studies that flavonols such as quercetin, myricetin and kaempferols, as well as their derivatives, have strong antioxidant activity [209] and also demonstrate that their glucosylated derivatives have greater activity than the corresponding aglycones [213]. The radical scavenging and metal chelating activity of flavonols contribute to ameliorating oxidative stress [167,214]; in turn, this activity depends on the number of the hydroxyl and the sugar moiety associated [213,215].

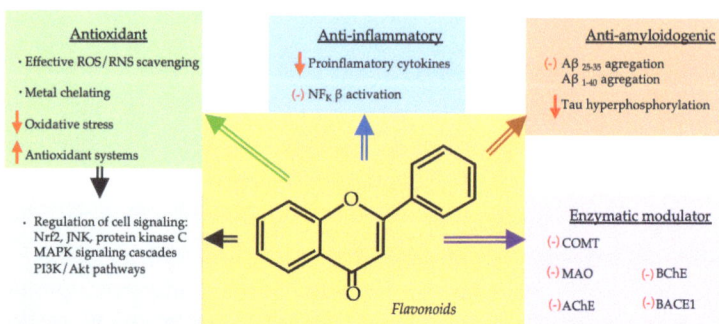

Figure 3. Diagram with neuroprotective mechanisms of flavonoids. ↑: increase, ↓: decrease, (−): inhibition, ROS: reactive oxygen species, RNS: reactive nitrogen species, NF$_k$B: nuclear factor kappa B, Aβ: amyloid beta-peptide, Nrf2: nuclear factor erythroid-derived 2, JNK (Jun-NH$_2$-terminal kinase), MAPK (the mitogen-activated protein kinase), PI3K/Akt (phosphoinositide 3-kinase), COMT (catechol-O-methyltransferase), MAO (monoamine oxidase), AChE (acetylcholinesterase), BchE (butyrylcholinesterase), BACE1 (amyloid precursor protein cleaving enzyme I).

In addition to the antioxidant capacity of these compounds as free-radical scavengers, the mechanisms involved in the neuroprotector effect of these compounds would be associated with their capacity to inhibit Aβ aggregation, the amyloid precursor protein cleaving enzyme (BACE1) [216] and AChE [217]. Studies on AChE inhibition in the brain of oxidative stress-induced rats report that AChE activity significantly decreases [218,219]. Specifically, treatment with flavonol quercetin in hippocampal neurons has resulted in the elevation of neurogenesis, synaptogenesis, and cell proliferation, as well as restoration of Aβ-induced synaptic loss [220]. This flavonol also exerts positive effects on PD, as it can inhibit the activity of catechol-O-methyltransferase and monoamine oxidase enzymes, which can lead to an increase in the bioavailability of L-dopa in the brain [4]. Quercetin has also been attributed to the capacity to act through different signaling pathways, including regulation of cytokines via Nrf2 (nuclear factor erythroid-derived 2), JNK (Jun-NH$_2$-terminal kinase), protein kinase C, MAPK (the mitogen-activated protein kinase) signaling cascades, and PI3K/Akt (phosphoinositide 3-kinase) pathways [221].

Another flavonoid with clear antioxidant functions is flavan-3-ol catechin [222], which, along with its isomers and/or conjugates of gallic acid, is a naturally occurring constituent in plants [223]. This has been observed among the studied species, as this flavonoid is present in 46% of the species. Different studies report the neuroprotective properties of catechins, mostly through antioxidative and anti-inflammatory effects, mainly involving Nrf2 and NF-kB signaling pathways [222,224,225]. One in vivo study has revealed that it can improve cognitive impairment induced by doxorubicin via increasing antioxidant defense, preventing neuroinflammation and inhibiting AChE [226]. Catechin has also been indicated to inhibit the late stages of Aβ-soluble aggregate growth change in the fibrillar form of Aβ [227]. It has also prevented neurotoxin-induced dopamine neuron loss in substantia nigra in a mouse model of PD [228]. The other flavanol with a high representation among the studied species is epicatechin, which is present in 42% of them. It has been demonstrated that epicatechin treatment prevents oxidative damage to the hippocampus induced by Aβ$_{25-35}$ [229]. This flavanol may reduce Tau hyperphosphorylation, downregulate BACE1 and Aβ$_{1-42}$ expression and boost AD rats' antioxidant system, as well as their cognition and memory [230,231].

5. Main Species with Neuroprotective Activity

As can be observed, the species considered in this study can be an important source of phenolic compounds with activity against neurodegenerative diseases. However, focusing on the most represented compounds (in over 40% of the analyzed species) and the species that contain all or most of these compounds (Table 4), 7 of these species stand out: *C. multiflorus*, *P. lentiscus*, *A. unedo*, *L. stoechas*, *R. ulmifolius* and *T. vulgaris* contain the 6 most frequent phenolic acids (gallic, chlorogenic, ferulic, caffeic, vanillic and *p*-coumaric acids) and *C. salviifolius* and *P. lentiscus* contain the main flavonoids.

Table 4. Species with the most represented phenolic compounds (present in over 10 of the 24 analyzed species).

	GA	VA	CA	CHA	p-CA	FA	Ap	K	MOR	Q	QOG	QOR	QORU	Ca	Epi
C. ladanifer	+	+				+	+		+	+	+	+	+		
C. salviifolius	+		+	+	+	+	+		+	+	+	+	+	+	+
C. monspeliensis	+						+		+	+	+	+	+		
C. crispus	+			+							+				
C. albidus	+			+				+	+	+		+	+		+
C. populifolius	+									+					
C. multiflorus	+	+	+	+	+	+	+			+	+		+		
C. scoparius	+		+	+			+	+		+	+		+		
C. striatus							+								
E. multiflora			+					+		+			+		
E. scoparia								+	+						
E. australis		+		+				+	+		+	+		+	+
C. vulgaris			+						+		+				
M. communis									+			+	+		
P. lentiscus	+	+	+	+	+	+		+	+	+	+		+	+	+
P. terebinthus	+		+		+	+		+	+	+		+	+		
R. officinalis	+	+	+		+	+	+	+		+			+		
Q. ilex	+	+	+			+			+	+	+		+	+	+
Q. suber	+					+								+	+
A. unedo	+	+	+	+	+	+		+	+		+	+	+	+	+
L. stoechas	+	+	+	+	+	+	+	+		+	+		+	+	+
T. mastichina			+	+			+	+		+	+				
T. vulgaris	+	+	+	+	+	+	+		+	+			+	+	+
R. ulmifolius	+	+	+	+	+	+	+		+	+	+	+	+	+	+

GA: Gallic acid; VA: Vallic acid; CA: Caffeic acid; CHA: Chlorogenic acid; *p*-CA: *p*-coumaric acid; FA: Ferulic acid; Ap: Apigenin; K: Kaemferol; MOR: Myricetin-O-rhamnoside; Q: Quercetin; QOG: Quercetin-O-glucoside; QORU: Quercetin-O-rutinoside; Ca: Catechin; Epi: Epicatechin.

Of these 7 species, studies have been conducted with extracts of *P. lentiscus*, *L. stoechas* and *T. vulgaris* to demonstrate their activity against neurodegenerative diseases [107,136,138,151,232]. These studies have reported the in vitro AChE inhibitory activity of *P. lentiscus* and its extract exhibited a significant dose-related AChE inhibitory activity. This extract also showed the ability to prevent neurodegeneration and improve memory and cognitive function. This indicates that *P. lentiscus* inhibited Al-induced neurodegeneration of neurons in the brain cortex, which is known to be susceptible in AD and to play an important role in learning and memory functions [107,233,234]. These findings explain the protective effects of *P. lentiscus* on cognitive deficit. Moreover, the capability of the extract to correct the in vivo disorders may be explained by its ability to inhibit oxidative stress and lipid oxidation induced by Al [213,235].

The extracts of *L. stoechas* also significantly ($p < 0.001$) enhanced the retention power and learning capacity of mice brains. Similarly, treatment of animals with extracts of lavender showed a significant ($p < 0.001$) reduction in the level of AChE and relieved the patient of memory loss [136,139].

On their part, studies conducted with the extract of *T. vulgaris* also indicate that this species can present neuroprotective effects [151,152]. The results obtained by [236] suggest that the antiamnesic effect of *T. vulgaris* extract on scopolamine-induced memory impairment may be related to the antioxidant activity of the extract or mediation of the cholinergic nervous system [148,150].

The protective activities attributed to these species can be inherent to the presence of these phenolic compounds (flavonoids and phenolic acids), where the presence of all of them may exert a synergistic effect as neuroprotective agents.

6. Conclusions

This review highlights the relevance of the species of Mediterranean ecosystems as a diverse source of phenolic compounds. Among these compounds, phenolic acids and flavonoids stand out. The most represented compounds among the species studied are gallic, vanillic, caffeic, chlorogenic, *p*-coumaric and ferulic acids, apigenin, kaempferol, myricitrin, quercetin, isoquercetin, quercetrin, rutin, catechin and epicatechin, which have been attributed neuroprotective functions. Given this information, these Mediterranean scrub species could be considered as sources of compounds for use in therapy against neurodegenerative diseases such as AD and PD.

Author Contributions: Conceptualization, N.C., L.N., I.M.-F., J.B.-S. and J.C.A.; methodology, N.C.; validation, N.C., L.N., I.M.-F., J.B.-S. and J.C.A.; investigation, N.C.; data curation, N.C. and J.C.A.; writing—original draft preparation, N.C. and J.C.A.; writing—review and editing, N.C., L.N., I.M.-F., J.B.-S. and J.C.A.; visualization, N.C., L.N., I.M.-F., J.B.-S. and J.C.A.; supervision, N.C.; project administration, N.C.; funding acquisition, N.C., J.B.-S. and J.C.A. All authors have read and agreed to the published version of the manuscript.

Funding: This research has been financed by the project titled "Direct subsidy to the University of Extremadura for the implementation of the LA4 lines of action of the I+D+i program in the area of Biodiversity. LIA4:Evaluation and mitigation of the impact of global change on biodiversity—FEDER Funds"/LIA4 Complementary Plan, co-financed by the Ministry of Economy, Science and Digital Agenda of the Government of Extremadura and by the European Regional Development Fund (FEDER) of Extremadura corresponding to the 2021–2027 programming period.

Institutional Review Board Statement: Not applicable.

Informed Consent Statement: Not applicable.

Data Availability Statement: No new data were created or analyzed in this study. Data sharing is not applicable to this article.

Conflicts of Interest: The authors declare no conflict of interest.

References

1. Harman, D. Aging: A theory based on free radical and radiation chemistry. *J. Gerontol.* **1956**, *11*, 298–300. [CrossRef] [PubMed]
2. Liguori, I.; Russo, G.; Curcio, F.; Bulli, G.; Aran, L.; Della-Morte, D.; Gargiulo, G.; Testa, G.; Cacciatore, F.; Bonaduce, D. Oxidative stress, aging, and diseases. *Clin. Interv. Aging* **2018**, *13*, 757–772. [CrossRef] [PubMed]
3. Costanzo, P.; Oliverio, M.; Maiuolo, J.; Bonacci, S.; De Luca, G.; Masullo, M.; Arcone, R.; Procopio, A. Novel hydroxytyrosol-donepezil hybrids as potential antioxidant and neuroprotective agents. *Front. Chem.* **2021**, *9*, 741444. [CrossRef] [PubMed]
4. Singh, E.; Devasahayam, G. Neurodegeneration by oxidative stress: A review on prospective use of small molecules for neuroprotection. *Mol. Biol. Rep.* **2020**, *47*, 3133–3140. [CrossRef] [PubMed]
5. Dilberger, B.; Weppler, S.; Eckert, G.P. Phenolic acid metabolites of polyphenols act as inductors for hormesis in *C. elegans*. *Mech. Ageing Dev.* **2021**, *198*, 111518. [CrossRef] [PubMed]
6. Singh, A.; Kukreti, R.; Saso, L.; Kukreti, S. Oxidative stress: A key modulator in neurodegenerative diseases. *Molecules* **2019**, *24*, 1583. [CrossRef]
7. Bouayed, J.; Rammal, H.; Dicko, A.; Younos, C.; Soulimani, R. Chlorogenic acid, a polyphenol from *Prunus domestica* (Mirabelle), with coupled anxiolytic and antioxidant effects. *J. Neurol. Sci.* **2007**, *262*, 77–84. [CrossRef]
8. Kanazawa, I.; Inaba, M.; Inoue, D.; Uenishi, K.; Saito, M.; Shiraki, M.; Suzuki, A.; Takeuchi, Y.; Hagino, H.; Fujiwara, S.; et al. Executive summary of clinical practice guide on fracture risk in lifestyle diseases. *J. Bone Miner. Metab.* **2020**, *38*, 746–758. [CrossRef]
9. Harman, D. The Biologic Clock: The Mitochondria? *J. Am. Geriatr. Soc.* **1972**, *20*, 145–147. [CrossRef]
10. Marzetti, E.; Csiszar, A.; Dutta, D.; Balagopal, G.; Calvani, R.; Leeuwenburgh, C. Role of mitochondrial dysfunction and altered autophagy in cardiovascular aging and disease: From mechanisms to therapeutics. *Am. J. Physiol. Heart Circ. Physiol.* **2013**, *305*, H459–H476. [CrossRef]

11. Dilberger, B.; Baumanns, S.; Schmitt, F.; Schmiedl, T.; Hardt, M.; Wenzel, U.; Eckert, G.P. Mitochondrial oxidative stress impairs energy metabolism and reduces stress resistance and longevity of *C. elegans*. *Oxid. Med. Cell. Longev.* **2019**, *2019*, 6840540. [CrossRef] [PubMed]
12. Kumar, A.; Mehta, V.; Raj, U.; Varadwaj, P.K.; Udayabanu, M.; Yennamalli, R.M.; Singh, T.R. Computational and in-vitro validation of natural molecules as potential acetylcholinesterase inhibitors and neuroprotective agents. *Curr. Alzheimer Res.* **2019**, *16*, 116–127. [CrossRef] [PubMed]
13. Khazdair, M.R.; Anaeigoudari, A.; Hashemzehi, M.; Mohebbati, R. Neuroprotective potency of some spice herbs, a literature review. *J. Tradit. Complement. Med.* **2019**, *9*, 98–105. [CrossRef] [PubMed]
14. Maher, P. The Potential of Flavonoids for the Treatment of Neurodegenerative Diseases. *Int. J. Mol. Sci.* **2019**, *20*, 3056. [CrossRef] [PubMed]
15. Prince, M.; Bryce, R.; Albanese, E.; Wimo, A.; Ribeiro, W.; Ferri, C.P. The global prevalence of dementia: A systematic review and metaanalysis. *Alzheimer's Dement.* **2013**, *9*, 63–75.e62. [CrossRef] [PubMed]
16. Chung, S.-C.; Providencia, R.; Sofat, R.; Pujades-Rodriguez, M.; Torralbo, A.; Fatemifar, G.; Fitzpatrick, N.K.; Taylor, J.; Li, K.; Dale, C.; et al. Incidence, morbidity, mortality and disparities in dementia: A population linked electronic health records study of 4.3 million individuals. *Alzheimer's Dement.* **2023**, *19*, 123–135. [CrossRef] [PubMed]
17. Zhuang, J.; Chen, Z.; Cai, P.; Wang, R.; Yang, Q.; Li, L.; Yang, H.; Zhu, R. Targeting microRNA-125b promotes neurite outgrowth but represses cell apoptosis and inflammation via blocking PTGS2 and CDK5 in a FOXQ1-dependent way in Alzheimer disease. *Front. Cell. Neurosci.* **2020**, *14*, 587744. [CrossRef]
18. Sharma, C.; Kim, S.R. Linking oxidative stress and proteinopathy in Alzheimer's disease. *Antioxidants* **2021**, *10*, 1231. [CrossRef]
19. Orhan, I.E.; Senol, F.S.; Ercetin, T.; Kahraman, A.; Celep, F.; Akaydin, G.; Sener, B.; Dogan, M. Assessment of anticholinesterase and antioxidant properties of selected sage (*Salvia*) species with their total phenol and flavonoid contents. *Ind. Crops Prod.* **2013**, *41*, 21–30. [CrossRef]
20. Serrano-Pozo, A.; Frosch, M.P.; Masliah, E.; Hyman, B.T. Neuropathological alterations in Alzheimer disease. *Cold Spring Harb. Perspect. Med.* **2011**, *1*, a006189. [CrossRef]
21. Iqbal, K.; Alonso, A.d.C.; Chen, S.; Chohan, M.O.; El-Akkad, E.; Gong, C.-X.; Khatoon, S.; Li, B.; Liu, F.; Rahman, A. Tau pathology in Alzheimer disease and other tauopathies. *Biochim. Biophys. Acta Mol. Basis Dis.* **2005**, *1739*, 198–210. [CrossRef] [PubMed]
22. Tamagno, E.; Parola, M.; Bardini, P.; Piccini, A.; Borghi, R.; Guglielmotto, M.; Santoro, G.; Davit, A.; Danni, O.; Smith, M. β-Site APP cleaving enzyme up-regulation induced by 4-hydroxynonenal is mediated by stress-activated protein kinases pathways. *J. Neurochem.* **2005**, *92*, 628–636. [CrossRef] [PubMed]
23. Nunomura, A.; Castellani, R.J.; Zhu, X.; Moreira, P.I.; Perry, G.; Smith, M.A. Involvement of oxidative stress in Alzheimer disease. *J. Neuropathol. Exp. Neurol.* **2006**, *65*, 631–641. [CrossRef] [PubMed]
24. Jeandel, C.; Nicolas, M.B.; Dubois, F.; Nabet-Belleville, F.; Penin, F.; Cuny, G. Lipid peroxidation and free radical scavengers in Alzheimer's disease. *Gerontology* **1989**, *35*, 275–282. [CrossRef] [PubMed]
25. Gabbita, S.P.; Lovell, M.A.; Markesbery, W.R. Increased nuclear DNA oxidation in the brain in Alzheimer's disease. *J. Neurochem.* **1998**, *71*, 2034–2040. [CrossRef] [PubMed]
26. Craig, L.A.; Hong, N.S.; McDonald, R.J. Revisiting the cholinergic hypothesis in the development of Alzheimer's disease. *Neurosci. Biobehav. Rev.* **2011**, *35*, 1397–1409. [CrossRef]
27. Hampel, H.; Mesulam, M.-M.; Cuello, A.C.; Khachaturian, A.S.; Vergallo, A.; Farlow, M.; Snyder, P.; Giacobini, E.; Khachaturian, Z.; Cholinergic System Working Group, and for the Alzheimer Precision Medicine Initiative (APMI). Revisiting the cholinergic hypothesis in Alzheimer's disease: Emerging evidence from translational and clinical research. *J. Prev. Alzheimer's Dis.* **2019**, *6*, 2–15.
28. Dou, K.-X.; Tan, M.-S.; Tan, C.-C.; Cao, X.-P.; Hou, X.-H.; Guo, Q.-H.; Tan, L.; Mok, V.; Yu, J.-T. Comparative safety and effectiveness of cholinesterase inhibitors and memantine for Alzheimer's disease: A network meta-analysis of 41 randomized controlled trials. *Alzheimer's Res.Ther.* **2018**, *10*, 126. [CrossRef]
29. Marucci, G.; Buccioni, M.; Ben, D.D.; Lambertucci, C.; Volpini, R.; Amenta, F. Efficacy of acetylcholinesterase inhibitors in Alzheimer's disease. *Neuropharmacology* **2021**, *190*, 108352. [CrossRef]
30. Poewe, W.; Seppi, K.; Tanner, C.M.; Halliday, G.M.; Brundin, P.; Volkmann, J.; Schrag, A.E.; Lang, A.E. Parkinson disease. *Nat. Rev. Dis. Primers* **2017**, *3*, 17013. [CrossRef]
31. González-Casacuberta, I.; Juárez-Flores, D.L.; Morén, C.; Garrabou, G. Bioenergetics and Autophagic Imbalance in Patients-Derived Cell Models of Parkinson Disease Supports Systemic Dysfunction in Neurodegeneration. *Front. Neurosci.* **2019**, *13*, 894. [CrossRef] [PubMed]
32. Cacabelos, R. Parkinson's Disease: From pathogenesis to pharmacogenomics. *Int. J. Mol. Sci.* **2017**, *18*, 551. [CrossRef] [PubMed]
33. Naveen, K.; Bhattacharjee, A. Medicinal herbs as neuroprotective agents. *WJPPS* **2021**, *10*, 675–689.
34. Nakabeppu, Y.; Tsuchimoto, D.; Yamaguchi, H.; Sakumi, K. Oxidative damage in nucleic acids and Parkinson's disease. *Neurosci. Res.* **2007**, *85*, 919–934. [CrossRef]
35. Graves, S.M.; Xie, Z.; Stout, K.A.; Zampese, E.; Burbulla, L.F.; Shih, J.C.; Kondapalli, J.; Patriarchi, T.; Tian, L.; Brichta, L.; et al. Dopamine metabolism by a monoamine oxidase mitochondrial shuttle activates the electron transport chain. *Nat. Neurosci.* **2020**, *23*, 15–20. [CrossRef]

36. Junn, E.; Mouradian, M.M. Human alpha-synuclein over-expression increases intracellular reactive oxygen species levels and susceptibility to dopamine. *Neurosci. Lett.* **2002**, *320*, 146–150. [CrossRef]
37. Perfeito, R.; Ribeiro, M.; Rego, A.C. Alpha-synuclein-induced oxidative stress correlates with altered superoxide dismutase and glutathione synthesis in human neuroblastoma SH-SY5Y cells. *Arch. Toxicol.* **2017**, *91*, 1245–1259. [CrossRef]
38. Gómez, L.A.; Tovar, H.C.; Agudelo, C. Utilización de servicios de salud y perfiles epidemiológicos como parámetros de adecuación del Plan Obligatorio de Salud en Colombia. *Rev. Salud Pública* **2003**, *5*, 246–262. [CrossRef]
39. López Locanto, Ó. Tratamiento farmacológico de la enfermedad de Alzheimer y otras demencias. *Arch. Med. Interna* **2015**, *37*, 61–67.
40. Blesa, J.; Lanciego, J.; Obeso, J.A. Editorial: Parkinson's disease: Cell vulnerability and disease progression. *Front. Neuroanat.* **2015**, *9*, 125. [CrossRef]
41. Kim, H.-S.; Cho, J.-y.; Kim, D.-H.; Yan, J.-J.; Lee, H.-K.; Suh, H.-W.; Song, D.-K. Inhibitory Effects of Long-Term Administration of Ferulic Acid on Microglial Activation Induced by Intracerebroventricular Injection of β-Amyloid Peptide (1—42) in Mice. *Biol. Pharm. Bull.* **2004**, *27*, 120–121. [CrossRef] [PubMed]
42. Kim, H.-B.; Lee, S.; Hwang, E.-S.; Maeng, S.; Park, J.-H. p-Coumaric acid enhances long-term potentiation and recovers scopolamine-induced learning and memory impairments. *Biochem. Biophys. Res. Commun.* **2017**, *492*, 493–499. [CrossRef] [PubMed]
43. Kim, K.H.; Lee, D.; Lee, H.L.; Kim, C.E.; Jung, K.; Kang, K.S. Beneficial effects of Panax ginseng for the treatment and prevention of neurodegenerative diseases: Past findings and future directions. *J. Ginseng Res.* **2018**, *42*, 239–247. [CrossRef] [PubMed]
44. Kelsey, N.A.; Wilkins, H.M.; Linseman, D.A. Nutraceutical antioxidants as novel neuroprotective agents. *Molecules* **2010**, *15*, 7792–7814. [CrossRef] [PubMed]
45. Vauzour, D.; Buonfiglio, M.; Corona, G.; Chirafisi, J.; Vafeiadou, K.; Angeloni, C.; Hrelia, S.; Hrelia, P.; Spencer, J.P.E. Sulforaphane protects cortical neurons against 5-S-cysteinyl-dopamine-induced toxicity through the activation of ERK1/2, NrF-2 and the upregulation of detoxification enzymes. *Mol. Nutr. Food Res.* **2010**, *54*, 532–542. [CrossRef] [PubMed]
46. Tarozzi, A.; Angeloni, C.; Malaguti, M.; Morroni, F.; Hrelia, S.; Hrelia, P. Sulforaphane as a Potential protective phytochemical against neurodegenerative diseases. *Oxid. Med. Cell. Longev.* **2013**, *2013*, 415078. [CrossRef] [PubMed]
47. Newman, D.J.; Cragg, G.M. Natural Products as Sources of New Drugs from 1981 to 2014. *J. Nat. Prod.* **2016**, *79*, 629–661. [CrossRef]
48. Cheynier, V.; Comte, G.; Davies, K.M.; Lattanzio, V.; Martens, S. Plant phenolics: Recent advances on their biosynthesis, genetics, andecophysiology. *Plant Physiol. Biochem.* **2013**, *72*, 1–20. [CrossRef]
49. Spagnuolo, C.; Napolitano, M.; Tedesco, I.; Moccia, S.; Milito, A.; Russo, G.L. Neuroprotective role of natural polyphenols. *Curr.Top. Med. Chem.* **2016**, *16*, 1943–1950. [CrossRef]
50. Figueira, I.; Garcia, G.; Pimpão, R.C.; Terrasso, A.; Costa, I.; Almeida, A.; Tavares, L.; Pais, T.; Pinto, P.; Ventura, M. Polyphenols journey through blood-brain barrier towards neuronal protection. *Sci. Rep.* **2017**, *7*, 11456. [CrossRef]
51. Tsao, R. Chemistry and biochemistry of dietary polyphenols. *Nutrients* **2010**, *2*, 1231–1246. [CrossRef] [PubMed]
52. Eastwood, M.A. Interaction of dietary antioxidants in vivo: How fruit and vegetables prevent disease? *QJM* **1999**, *92*, 527–530. [CrossRef] [PubMed]
53. Hollman, P.C.H.; Katan, M.B. Health effects and bioavailability of dietary flavonols. *Free Radic. Res.* **1999**, *31*, 75–80. [CrossRef] [PubMed]
54. Prior, R.L.; Cao, G.; Martin, A.; Sofic, E.; McEwen, J.; O'Brien, C.; Lischner, N.; Ehlenfeldt, M.; Kalt, W.; Krewer, G.; et al. Antioxidant Capacity as Influenced by Total Phenolic and Anthocyanin Content, Maturity, and Variety of *Vaccinium* Species. *J. Agric. Food Chem.* **1998**, *46*, 2686–2693. [CrossRef]
55. Kim, H.K.; Jeong, T.-S.; Lee, M.-K.; Park, Y.B.; Choi, M.-S. Lipid-lowering efficacy of hesperetin metabolites in high-cholesterol fed rats. *Clin. Chim. Acta* **2003**, *327*, 129–137. [CrossRef] [PubMed]
56. Soobrattee, M.A.; Neergheen, V.S.; Luximon-Ramma, A.; Aruoma, O.I.; Bahorun, T. Phenolics as potential antioxidant therapeutic agents: Mechanism and actions. *Mutat. Res.* **2005**, *579*, 200–213. [CrossRef]
57. Wang, S.Y.; Lin, H.S. Antioxidant activity in fruits and leaves of blackberry, raspberry, and strawberry varies with cultivar and developmental stage. *J. Agric. Food Chem.* **2000**, *48*, 140–146. [CrossRef]
58. Eghorn, L.F.; Hoestgaard-Jensen, K.; Kongstad, K.T.; Bay, T.; Higgins, D.; Frølund, B.; Wellendorph, P. Positive allosteric modulation of the GHB high-affinity binding site by the GABAA receptor modulator monastrol and the flavonoid catechin. *Eur. J. Pharmacol.* **2014**, *740*, 570–577. [CrossRef]
59. Freyssin, A.; Page, G.; Fauconneau, B.; Bilan, A.R. Natural polyphenols effects on protein aggregates in Alzheimer's and Parkinson's prion-like diseases. *Neural Regen. Res.* **2018**, *13*, 955.
60. Gopinath, K.; Sudhandiran, G. Naringin modulates oxidative stress and inflammation in 3-nitropropionic acid-induced neurodegeneration through the activation of nuclear factor-erythroid 2-related factor-2 signalling pathway. *Neuroscience* **2012**, *227*, 134–143. [CrossRef]
61. Sandhir, R.; Mehrotra, A. Quercetin supplementation is effective in improving mitochondrial dysfunctions induced by 3-nitropropionic acid: Implications in Huntington's disease. *Biochim. Biophys. Acta Mol. Basis Dis.* **2013**, *1832*, 421–430. [CrossRef] [PubMed]

62. Lou, H.; Jing, X.; Wei, X.; Shi, H.; Ren, D.; Zhang, X. Naringenin protects against 6-OHDA-induced neurotoxicity via activation of the Nrf2/ARE signaling pathway. *Neuropharmacology* **2014**, *79*, 380–388. [CrossRef]
63. Katalinić, M.; Rusak, G.; Barović, J.D.; Šinko, G.; Jelić, D.; Antolović, R.; Kovarik, Z. Structural aspects of flavonoids as inhibitors of human butyrylcholinesterase. *Eur. J. Med. Chem.* **2010**, *45*, 186–192. [CrossRef] [PubMed]
64. Cho, N.; Choi, J.H.; Yang, H.; Jeong, E.J.; Lee, K.Y.; Kim, Y.C.; Sung, S.H. Neuroprotective and anti-inflammatory effects of flavonoids isolated from *Rhus verniciflua* in neuronal HT22 and microglial BV2 cell lines. *Food Chem. Toxicol.* **2012**, *50*, 1940–1945. [CrossRef] [PubMed]
65. Spencer, J.P.; Vafeiadou, K.; Williams, R.J.; Vauzour, D. Neuroinflammation: Modulation by flavonoids and mechanisms of action. *Mol. Asp. Med.* **2012**, *33*, 83–97. [CrossRef] [PubMed]
66. Wiciński, M.; Domanowska, A.; Wódkiewicz, E.; Malinowski, B. Neuroprotective Properties of Resveratrol and Its Derivatives—Influence on Potential Mechanisms Leading to the Development of Alzheimer's Disease. *Int. J. Mol. Sci.* **2020**, *21*, 2749. [CrossRef]
67. Pereira, L.R.; Fritzen, M.; Yunes, R.A.; Leal, P.C.; Creczynski-Pasa, T.B.; Pereira, A.F. Inhibitory effects of gallic acid ester derivatives on *Saccharomyces cerevisiae* multidrug resistance protein Pdr5p. *FEMS Yeast Res.* **2010**, *10*, 244–251. [CrossRef]
68. Iwaki, A.; Ohnuki, S.; Suga, Y.; Izawa, S.; Ohya, Y. Vanillin inhibits translation and induces messenger ribonucleoprotein (mRNP) granule formation in *Saccharomyces cerevisiae*: Application and validation of high-content, image-based profiling. *PLoS ONE* **2013**, *8*, e61748. [CrossRef]
69. Sunthonkun, P.; Palajai, R.; Somboon, P.; Suan, C.L.; Ungsurangsri, M.; Soontorngun, N. Life-span extension by pigmented rice bran in the model yeast *Saccharomyces cerevisiae*. *Sci. Rep.* **2019**, *9*, 18061. [CrossRef]
70. Costa, L.G.; Garrick, J.M.; Roquè, P.J.; Pellacani, C. Mechanisms of neuroprotection by quercetin: Counteracting oxidative stress and more. *Oxid. Med. Cell. Longev.* **2016**, *2016*, 2986796. [CrossRef]
71. Cui, X.; Lin, Q.; Liang, Y. Plant-derived antioxidants protect the nervous system from aging by inhibiting oxidative stress. *Front. aging Neurosci.* **2020**, *12*, 209. [CrossRef] [PubMed]
72. Scognamiglio, M.; Fiumano, V.; D'Abrosca, B.; Esposito, A.; Choi, Y.H.; Verpoorte, R.; Fiorentino, A. Chemical interactions between plants in Mediterranean vegetation: The influence of selected plant extracts on Aegilops geniculata metabolome. *Phytochemistry* **2014**, *106*, 69–85. [CrossRef] [PubMed]
73. Scognamiglio, M.; Graziani, V.; Tsafantakis, N.; Esposito, A.; Fiorentino, A.; D'Abrosca, B. NMR-based metabolomics and bioassays to study phytotoxic extracts and putative phytotoxins from Mediterranean plant species. *Phytochem. Anal.* **2019**, *30*, 512–523. [CrossRef] [PubMed]
74. Chengxu, W.; Mingxing, Z.; Xuhui, C.; Bo, Q. Review on allelopathy of exotic invasive plants. *Procedia Eng.* **2011**, *18*, 240–246. [CrossRef]
75. Chaves, N.; Alías, J.; Sosa, T. Phytotoxicity of *Cistus ladanifer* L.: Role of allelopathy. *Allelopath. J.* **2016**, *38*, 113–131. [CrossRef]
76. Rivas-Martínez, S. *Memoria y Mapas de la Series de Vegetación de España.1:400.000*; ICONA. Serie Técnica; MAPA: Madrid, Spain, 1987.
77. Plan Forestal de Extremadura. Análisis y Estudio del Paisaje Vegetal y su Dinámica en la región de Extremadura. Available online: http://extremambiente.juntaex.es/index.php?option=com_content&view=article&id=3609&Itemid=307 (accessed on 8 November 2023).
78. Chaves, N.; Ríos, J.J.; Gutierrez, C.; Escudero, J.C.; Olías, J.M. Analysis of secreted flavonoids of *Cistus ladanifer* L. by high-performance liquid chromatography–particle beam mass spectrometry. *J. Chromatogr. A* **1998**, *799*, 111–115. [CrossRef]
79. Chaves, N.; Sosa, T.; Alías, J.C.; Escudero, J.C. Identification and effects of interaction phytotoxic compounds from exudate of *Cistus ladanifer* leaves. *J. Chem. Ecol.* **2001**, *27*, 611–621. [CrossRef]
80. Einhellig, F.A.; Galindo, J.C.G.; Molinillo, J.M.G.; Cutler, H.G. Mode of allelochemical action of phenolic compounds. In *Allelopathy: Chemistry and Mode of Action of Allelochemicals*; CRC Press: Boca Raton, FL, USA, 2004; pp. 217–238.
81. Barrajón-Catalán, E.; Fernández-Arroyo, S.; Roldán, C.; Guillén, E.; Saura, D.; Segura-Carretero, A.; Micol, V. A systematic study of the polyphenolic composition of aqueous extracts deriving from several *Cistus* genus species: Evolutionary relationship. *Phytochem. Anal.* **2011**, *22*, 303–312. [CrossRef]
82. Barrajón-Catalán, E.; Fernández-Arroyo, S.; Saura, D.; Guillén, E.; Fernández-Gutiérrez, A.; Segura-Carretero, A.; Micol, V. Cistaceae aqueous extracts containing ellagitannins show antioxidant and antimicrobial capacity, and cytotoxic activity against human cancer cells. *Food Chem. Toxicol.* **2010**, *48*, 2273–2282. [CrossRef]
83. Viuda-Martos, M.; Sendra, E.; Alvarez, J.A.P.; Fernández-López, J.; Amensour, M.; Abrini, J. Identification of flavonoid content and chemical composition of the essential oils of moroccan herbs: Myrtle (*Myrtus communis* L.), rockrose (*Cistus ladanifer* L.) and montpellier cistus (*Cistus monspeliensis* L.). *J. Essent. Oil Res.* **2011**, *23*, 1–9. [CrossRef]
84. Barros, L.; Dueñas, M.; Alves, C.T.; Silva, S.; Henriques, M.; Santos-Buelga, C.; Ferreira, I.C.F.R. Antifungal activity and detailed chemical characterization of *Cistus ladanifer* phenolic extracts. *Ind. Crops Prod.* **2013**, *41*, 41–45. [CrossRef]
85. Gaweł-Bęben, K.; Kukula-Koch, W.; Hoian, U.; Czop, M.; Strzępek-Gomółka, M.; Antosiewicz, B. Characterization of *Cistus* × *incanus* L. and *Cistus ladanifer* L. extracts as potential multifunctional antioxidant ingredients for skin protecting cosmetics. *Antioxidants* **2020**, *9*, 202. [CrossRef] [PubMed]

86. Alves-Ferreira, J.; Miranda, I.; Duarte, L.C.; Roseiro, L.B.; Lourenço, A.; Quilhó, T.; Cardoso, S.; Fernandes, M.C.; Carvalheiro, F.; Pereira, H. Cistus ladanifer as a source of chemicals: Structural and chemical characterization. *Biomass Convers. Biorefinery* **2020**, *10*, 325–337. [CrossRef]
87. Carev, I.; Maravić, A.; Ilić, N.; Čulić, V.Č.; Politeo, O.; Zorić, Z.; Radan, M. UPLC-MS/MS phytochemical analysis of two Croatian *Cistus* species and their biological activity. *Life* **2020**, *10*, 112. [CrossRef] [PubMed]
88. Mastino, P.M.; Marchetti, M.; Costa, J.; Juliano, C.; Usai, M. Analytical Profiling of Phenolic Compounds in Extracts of Three *Cistus* Species from Sardinia and Their Potential Antimicrobial and Antioxidant Activity. *Chem. Biodivers.* **2021**, *18*, e2100053. [CrossRef] [PubMed]
89. Ben Jemia, M.; Kchouk, M.E.; Senatore, F.; Autore, G.; Marzocco, S.; De Feo, V.; Bruno, M. Antiproliferative activity of hexane extract from Tunisian *Cistus libanotis*, *Cistus monspeliensis* and *Cistus villosus*. *Chem. Cent. J.* **2013**, *7*, 47. [CrossRef]
90. Salomé-Abarca, L.F.; Mandrone, M.; Sanna, C.; Poli, F.; van der Hondel, C.A.M.J.J.; Klinkhamer, P.G.L.; Choi, Y.H. Metabolic variation in *Cistus monspeliensis* L. ecotypes correlated to their plant-fungal interactions. *Phytochemistry* **2020**, *176*, 112402. [CrossRef]
91. Tahiri, O.; Atmani-Kilani, D.; Sanchez-Fidalgo, S.; Aparicio-Soto, M.; Alarcón-de-la-Lastra, C.; Barrajón-Catalán, E.; Micol, V.; Atmani, D. The flavonol-enriched *Cistus albidus* chloroform extract possesses in vivo anti-inflammatory and anti-nociceptive activity. *J. Ethnopharmacol.* **2017**, *209*, 210–218. [CrossRef]
92. Luís, Â.; Domingues, F.; Duarte, A.P. Bioactive compounds, RP-HPLC analysis of phenolics, and antioxidant activity of some Portuguese shrub species extracts. *Nat. Prod. Commun.* **2011**, *6*, 1863–1872. [CrossRef]
93. Barros, L.; Dueñas, M.; Carvalho, A.M.; Ferreira, I.C.F.R.; Santos-Buelga, C. Characterization of phenolic compounds in flowers of wild medicinal plants from Northeastern Portugal. *Food Chem. Toxicol.* **2012**, *50*, 1576–1582. [CrossRef]
94. Pereira, O.R.; Silva, A.M.S.; Domingues, M.R.M.; Cardoso, S.M. Identification of phenolic constituents of *Cytisus multiflorus*. *Food Chem.* **2012**, *131*, 652–659. [CrossRef]
95. Pereira, O.R.; Macias, R.I.R.; Perez, M.J.; Marin, J.J.G.; Cardoso, S.M. Protective effects of phenolic constituents from *Cytisus multiflorus*, *Lamium album* L. and *Thymus citriodorus* on liver cells. *J. Funct. Foods* **2013**, *5*, 1170–1179. [CrossRef]
96. Garcia-Oliveira, P.; Carreira-Casais, A.; Pereira, E.; Dias, M.I.; Pereira, C.; Calhelha, R.C.; Stojković, D.; Sokovic, M.; Simal-Gandara, J.; Prieto, M.A.; et al. From Tradition to Health: Chemical and Bioactive Characterization of Five Traditional Plants. *Molecules* **2022**, *27*, 6495. [CrossRef] [PubMed]
97. González, N.; Ribeiro, D.; Fernandes, E.; Nogueira, D.R.; Conde, E.; Moure, A.; Vinardell, M.P.; Mitjans, M.; Domínguez, H. Potential use of *Cytisus scoparius* extracts in topical applications for skin protection against oxidative damage. *J. Photochem. Photobiol. B Biol.* **2013**, *125*, 83–89. [CrossRef] [PubMed]
98. Lores, M.; Pájaro, M.; Álvarez-Casas, M.; Domínguez, J.; García-Jares, C. Use of ethyl lactate to extract bioactive compounds from *Cytisus scoparius*: Comparison of pressurized liquid extraction and medium scale ambient temperature systems. *Talanta* **2015**, *140*, 134–142. [CrossRef] [PubMed]
99. González, N.; Otero, A.; Conde, E.; Falqué, E.; Moure, A.; Domínguez, H. Extraction of phenolics from broom branches using green technologies. *J. Chem. Technol. Biotechnol.* **2017**, *92*, 1345–1352. [CrossRef]
100. Abreu, A.C.; Coqueiro, A.; Sultan, A.R.; Lemmens, N.; Kim, H.K.; Verpoorte, R.; Van Wamel, W.J.; Simões, M.; Choi, Y.H. Looking to nature for a new concept in antimicrobial treatments: Isoflavonoids from *Cytisus striatus* as antibiotic adjuvants against MRSA. *Sci. Rep.* **2017**, *7*, 3777. [CrossRef]
101. Bekkai, D.; El Majdoub, Y.O.; Bekkai, H.; Cacciola, F.; Miceli, N.; Taviano, M.F.; Cavò, E.; Errabii, T.; Vinci, R.L.; Mondello, L. Determination of the phenolic profile by liquid chromatography, evaluation of antioxidant activity and toxicity of moroccan *Erica multiflora*, *Erica scoparia*, and *Calluna vulgaris* (Ericaceae). *Molecules* **2022**, *27*, 3979. [CrossRef]
102. Márquez-García, B.; Fernández, M.A.; Córdoba, F. Phenolics composition in *Erica* sp. differentially exposed to metal pollution in the Iberian Southwestern Pyritic Belt. *Bioresour. Technol.* **2009**, *100*, 446–451. [CrossRef]
103. Caleja, C.; Finimundy, T.C.; Pereira, C.; Barros, L.; Calhelha, R.C.; Sokovic, M.; Ivanov, M.; Carvalho, A.M.; Rosa, E.; Ferreira, I.C.F.R. Challenges of traditional herbal teas: Plant infusions and their mixtures with bioactive properties. *Food Funct.* **2019**, *10*, 5939–5951. [CrossRef]
104. Yangui, I.; Younsi, F.; Ghali, W.; Boussaid, M.; Messaoud, C. Phytochemicals, antioxidant and anti-proliferative activities of *Myrtus communis* L. genotypes from Tunisia. *S. Afr. J. Bot.* **2021**, *137*, 35–45. [CrossRef]
105. Amel, Z.; Nabila, B.B.; Nacéra, G.; Fethi, T.; Fawzia, A.B. Assessment of phytochemical composition and antioxidant properties of extracts from the leaf, stem, fruit and root of *Pistacia lentiscus* L. *Int. J. Pharmacogn. Phytochem. Res.* **2016**, *8*, 627–633.
106. Yemmen, M.; Landolsi, A.; Ben Hamida, J.; Mégraud, F.; Trabelsi Ayadi, M. Antioxidant activities, anticancer activity and polyphenolics profile, of leaf, fruit and stem extracts of *Pistacia lentiscus* from Tunisia. *Cell. Mol. Biol.* **2017**, *63*, 87–95. [CrossRef] [PubMed]
107. Sehaki, C.; Jullian, N.; Ayati, F.; Fernane, F.; Gontier, E. A Review of *Pistacia lentiscus* Polyphenols: Chemical Diversity and Pharmacological Activities. *Plants* **2023**, *12*, 279. [CrossRef] [PubMed]
108. Özcan, M.M.; Al Juhaimi, F.; Uslu, N.; Ahmed, I.A.M.; Babiker, E.E.; Osman, M.A.; Gassem, M.A.; Alqah, H.A.S.; Ghafoor, K. Effect of sonication process of terebinth (*Pistacia terebinthus* L.) fruits on antioxidant activity, phenolic compounds, fatty acids and tocopherol contents. *J. Food Sci. Technol.* **2020**, *57*, 2017–2025. [CrossRef]

109. Uysal, S.; Sinan, K.I.; Jekő, J.; Cziáky, Z.; Zengin, G. Chemical characterization, comprehensive antioxidant capacity, and enzyme inhibitory potential of leaves from *Pistacia terebinthus* L. (Anacardiaceae). *Food Biosci.* **2022**, *48*, 101820. [CrossRef]
110. Mena, P.; Cirlini, M.; Tassotti, M.; Herrlinger, K.A.; Dall'Asta, C.; Del Rio, D. Phytochemical Profiling of Flavonoids, Phenolic Acids, Terpenoids, and Volatile Fraction of a Rosemary (*Rosmarinus officinalis* L.) Extract. *Molecules* **2016**, *21*, 1576. [CrossRef]
111. Falade, A.O.; Omolaiye, G.I.; Adewole, K.E.; Agunloye, O.M.; Ishola, A.A.; Okaiyeto, K.; Oboh, G.; Oguntibeju, O.O. Aqueous Extracts of Bay Leaf (*Laurus nobilis*) and Rosemary (*Rosmarinus officinalis*) Inhibit Iron-Induced Lipid Peroxidation and Key-Enzymes Implicated in Alzheimer's Disease in Rat Brain-in Vitro. *Am. J. Biochem. Biotechnol.* **2022**, *18*, 9–22. [CrossRef]
112. Bellumori, M.; Innocenti, M.; Congiu, F.; Cencetti, G.; Raio, A.; Menicucci, F.; Mulinacci, N.; Michelozzi, M. Within-plant variation in *Rosmarinus officinalis* L. Terpenes and phenols and their antimicrobial activity against the rosemary phytopathogens *Alternaria alternata* and *Pseudomonas viridiflava*. *Molecules* **2021**, *26*, 3425. [CrossRef]
113. Chan, E.W.C.; Wong, S.K.; Chan, H.T. An overview of the chemistry and anticancer properties of rosemary extract and its diterpenes. *J. HerbMed Pharmacol.* **2022**, *11*, 10–19. [CrossRef]
114. Shaymaa, M.H.; Adnan, M.M.; Muthanna, J.M. The Effect of Extracts and Phenolic Compounds Isolation from *Rosmarinus officinalis* Plant Leaves on *Tribolium castaneum* Mortality. *Int. J. Drug Deliv. Technol.* **2022**, *12*, 814–819. [CrossRef]
115. Takayama, K.S.; Monteiro, M.C.; Saito, P.; Pinto, I.C.; Nakano, C.T.; Martinez, R.M.; Thomaz, D.V.; Verri, W.A.; Baracat, M.M.; Arakawa, N.S. *Rosmarinus officinalis* extract-loaded emulgel prevents UVB irradiation damage to the skin. *Anais Acad. Brasil. Ciências* **2022**, *94*, e20201058. [CrossRef] [PubMed]
116. Karioti, A.; Sokovic, M.; Ciric, A.; Koukoulitsa, C.; Bilia, A.R.; Skaltsa, H. Antimicrobial properties of *Quercus ilex* L. proanthocyanidin dimers and simple phenolics: Evaluation of their synergistic activity with conventional antimicrobials and prediction of their pharmacokinetic profile. *J. Agric. Food Chem.* **2011**, *59*, 6412–6422. [CrossRef] [PubMed]
117. Custódio, L.; Patarra, J.; Albericío, F.; Neng, N.R.; Nogueira, J.M.F.; Romano, A. Extracts from *Quercus* sp. acorns exhibit in vitro neuroprotective features through inhibition of cholinesterase and protection of the human dopaminergic cell line SH-SY5Y from hydrogen peroxide-induced cytotoxicity. *Ind. Crops Prod.* **2013**, *45*, 114–120. [CrossRef]
118. Hadidi, L.; Babou, L.; Zaidi, F.; Valentão, P.; Andrade, P.B.; Grosso, C. *Quercus ilex* L.: How season, Plant Organ and Extraction Procedure Can Influence Chemistry and Bioactivities. *Chem. Biodivers.* **2017**, *14*, e1600187. [CrossRef] [PubMed]
119. Pawlowska, A.M.; De Leo, M.; Braca, A. Phenolics of *Arbutus unedo* L.(Ericaceae) fruits: Identification of anthocyanins and gallic acid derivatives. *J. Agric. Food Chem.* **2006**, *54*, 10234–10238. [CrossRef] [PubMed]
120. Fiorentino, A.; Castaldi, S.; D'Abrosca, B.; Natale, A.; Carfora, A.; Messere, A.; Monaco, P. Polyphenols from the hydroalcoholic extract of *Arbutus unedo* living in a monospecific Mediterranean woodland. *Biochem. Syst. Ecol.* **2007**, *35*, 809. [CrossRef]
121. Pallauf, K.; Rivas-Gonzalo, J.C.; Del Castillo, M.; Cano, M.P.; de Pascual-Teresa, S. Characterization of the antioxidant composition of strawberry tree (*Arbutus unedo* L.) fruits. *J. Food Compos. Anal.* **2008**, *21*, 273–281. [CrossRef]
122. Guimarães, R.; Barros, L.; Dueñas, M.; Carvalho, A.M.; Queiroz, M.J.R.P.; Santos-Buelga, C.; Ferreira, I.C.F.R. Characterisation of phenolic compounds in wild fruits from Northeastern Portugal. *Food Chem.* **2013**, *141*, 3721–3730. [CrossRef]
123. Maleš, Ž.; Šarić, D.; Bojić, M. Quantitative determination of flavonoids and chlorogenic acid in the leaves of *Arbutus unedo* L. using thin layer chromatography. *J. Anal. Methods Chem.* **2013**, *2013*, 385473. [CrossRef]
124. Kachkoul, R.; Housseini, T.S.; Mohim, M.; El Habbani, R.; Miyah, Y.; Lahrichi, A. Chemical compounds as well as antioxidant and litholytic activities of *Arbutus unedo* L. leaves against calcium oxalate stones. *J. Integr. Med.* **2019**, *17*, 430–437. [CrossRef] [PubMed]
125. Maldini, M.; D'Urso, G.; Pagliuca, G.; Petretto, G.L.; Foddai, M.; Gallo, F.R.; Multari, G.; Caruso, D.; Montoro, P.; Pintore, G. HPTLC-PCA complementary to HRMS-PCA in the case study of *Arbutus unedo* antioxidant phenolic profiling. *Foods* **2019**, *8*, 294. [CrossRef] [PubMed]
126. Tenuta, M.C.; Deguin, B.; Loizzo, M.R.; Dugay, A.; Acquaviva, R.; Malfa, G.A.; Bonesi, M.; Bouzidi, C.; Tundis, R. Contribution of flavonoids and iridoids to the hypoglycaemic, antioxidant, and nitric oxide (NO) inhibitory activities of *Arbutus unedo* L. *Antioxidants* **2020**, *9*, 184. [CrossRef] [PubMed]
127. El Cadi, H.; El Cadi, A.; Kounnoun, A.; El Majdoub, Y.O.; Lovillo, M.P.; Brigui, J.; Dugo, P.; Mondello, L.; Cacciola, F. Wild strawberry (*Arbutus unedo*): Phytochemical screening and antioxidant properties of fruits collected in northern Morocco. *Arab. J. Chem.* **2020**, *13*, 6299–6311. [CrossRef]
128. Zitouni, H.; Hssaini, L.; Messaoudi, Z.; Ourradi, H.; Viuda-Martos, M.; Hernández, F.; Ercisli, S.; Hanine, H. Phytochemical components and bioactivity assessment among twelve strawberry (*Arbutus unedo* L.) genotypes growing in Morocco using chemometrics. *Foods* **2020**, *9*, 1345. [CrossRef] [PubMed]
129. Coimbra, A.T.; Luís, Â.F.; Batista, M.T.; Ferreira, S.M.; Duarte, A.P.C. Phytochemical characterization, bioactivities evaluation and synergistic effect of *Arbutus unedo* and *Crataegus monogyna* extracts with Amphotericin B. *Curr. Microbiol.* **2020**, *77*, 2143–2154. [CrossRef] [PubMed]
130. Macchioni, V.; Santarelli, V.; Carbone, K. Phytochemical profile, antiradical capacity and α-glucosidase inhibitory potential of wild *Arbutus unedo* L. Fruits from central italy: A chemometric approach. *Plants* **2020**, *9*, 1785. [CrossRef]
131. Izcara, S.; Morante-Zarcero, S.; Casado, N.; Sierra, I. Study of the Phenolic Compound Profile of *Arbutus unedo* L. Fruits at Different Ripening Stages by HPLC-TQ-MS/MS. *Appl. Sci.* **2021**, *11*, 11616. [CrossRef]
132. Martins, J.; Batista, T.; Pinto, G.; Canhoto, J. Seasonal variation of phenolic compounds in Strawberry tree (*Arbutus unedo* L.) leaves and inhibitory potential on *Phytophthora cinnamomi*. *Trees* **2021**, *35*, 1571–1586. [CrossRef]

133. Brčić Karačonji, I.; Jurica, K.; Gašić, U.; Dramićanin, A.; Tešić, Ž.; Milojković Opsenica, D. Comparative study on the phenolic fingerprint and antioxidant activity of strawberry tree (*Arbutus unedo* L.) leaves and fruits. *Plants* **2022**, *11*, 25. [CrossRef]
134. Contreras, M.D.M.; Algieri, F.; Rodriguez-Nogales, A.; Gálvez, J.; Segura-Carretero, A. Phytochemical profiling of anti-inflammatory *Lavandula* extracts via RP–HPLC–DAD–QTOF-MS and –MS/MS: Assessment of their qualitative and quantitative differences. *Electrophoresis* **2018**, *39*, 1284–1293. [CrossRef]
135. Karan, T. Metabolic profile and biological activities of *Lavandula stoechas* L. *Cell. Mol. Biol.* **2018**, *64*, 1–7. [CrossRef] [PubMed]
136. Dobros, N.; Zawada, K.D.; Paradowska, K. Phytochemical Profiling, Antioxidant and Anti-Inflammatory Activity of Plants Belonging to the *Lavandula* Genus. *Molecules* **2023**, *28*, 256. [CrossRef] [PubMed]
137. Sriti, J.; Fares, N.; Msaada, K.; Zarroug, Y.; Boulares, M.; Djebbi, S.; Selmi, S.; Limam, F. Phenological stage effect on phenolic composition, antioxidant, and antibacterial activity of *Lavandula stoechas* extract. *Riv. Ital. Sostanze Grasse* **2022**, *99*, 225–234.
138. Karabagias, I.K.; Karabagias, V.K.; Riganakos, K.A. Physico-Chemical Parameters, Phenolic Profile, In Vitro Antioxidant Activity and Volatile Compounds of Ladastacho (*Lavandula stoechas*) from the Region of Saidona. *Antioxidants* **2019**, *8*, 80. [CrossRef] [PubMed]
139. Domingues, J.; Delgado, F.; Gonçalves, J.C.; Zuzarte, M.; Duarte, A.P. Mediterranean Lavenders from Section Stoechas: An Undervalued Source of Secondary Metabolites with Pharmacological Potential. *Metabolites* **2023**, *13*, 337. [CrossRef]
140. Sánchez-Vioque, R.; Polissiou, M.; Astraka, K.; Mozos-Pascual, M.D.L.; Tarantilis, P.; Herraiz-Peñalver, D.; Santana-Méridas, O. Polyphenol composition and antioxidant and metal chelating activities of the solid residues from the essential oil industry. *Ind. Crops Prod.* **2013**, *49*, 150–159. [CrossRef]
141. Delgado, T.; Marinero, P.; Asensio-S.-Manzanera, M.C.; Asensio, C.; Herrero, B.; Pereira, J.A.; Ramalhosa, E. Antioxidant activity of twenty wild Spanish *Thymus mastichina* L. populations and its relation with their chemical composition. *LWT Food Sci. Technol.* **2014**, *57*, 412–418. [CrossRef]
142. Méndez-Tovar, I.; Sponza, S.; Asensio-S-Manzanera, M.C.; Novak, J. Contribution of the main polyphenols of *Thymus mastichina* subsp: Mastichina to its antioxidant properties. *Ind. Crops Prod.* **2015**, *66*, 291–298. [CrossRef]
143. Hossain, M.A.; Al-Raqmi, K.A.S.; Al-Mijizy, Z.H.; Weli, A.M.; Al-Riyami, Q. Study of total phenol, flavonoids contents and phytochemical screening of various leaves crude extracts of locally grown *Thymus vulgaris*. *Asian Pac. J. Trop. Biomed.* **2013**, *3*, 705–710. [CrossRef]
144. Vergara-Salinas, J.R.; Pérez-Jiménez, J.; Torres, J.L.; Agosin, E.; Pérez-Correa, J.R. Effects of temperature and time on polyphenolic content and antioxidant activity in the pressurized hot water extraction of deodorized thyme (*Thymus vulgaris*). *J. Agric. Food Chem.* **2012**, *60*, 10920–10929. [CrossRef] [PubMed]
145. Roby, M.H.H.; Sarhan, M.A.; Selim, K.A.H.; Khalel, K.I. Evaluation of antioxidant activity, total phenols and phenolic compounds in thyme (*Thymus vulgaris* L.), sage (*Salvia officinalis* L.), and marjoram (*Origanum majorana* L.) extracts. *Ind. Crops Prod.* **2013**, *43*, 827–831. [CrossRef]
146. Kaliora, A.C.; Kogiannou, D.A.A.; Kefalas, P.; Papassideri, I.S.; Kalogeropoulos, N. Phenolic profiles and antioxidant and anticarcinogenic activities of Greek herbal infusions; Balancing delight and chemoprevention? *Food Chem.* **2014**, *142*, 233–241. [CrossRef]
147. Pereira, E.; Barros, L.; Antonio, A.L.; Cabo Verde, S.; Santos-Buelga, C.; Ferreira, I.C.F.R. Infusions from *Thymus vulgaris* L. treated at different gamma radiation doses: Effects on antioxidant activity and phenolic composition. *LWT* **2016**, *74*, 34–39. [CrossRef]
148. Pereira, E.; Pimenta, A.I.; Barros, L.; Calhelha, R.C.; Antonio, A.L.; Cabo Verde, S.; Ferreira, I.C.F.R. Effects of gamma radiation on the bioactivity of medicinal and aromatic plants: *Mentha × piperita* L., *Thymus vulgaris* L. and *Aloysia citrodora Paláu* as case studies. *Food Funct.* **2018**, *9*, 5150–5161. [CrossRef] [PubMed]
149. Sonmezdag, A.S.; Kelebek, H.; Selli, S. Characterization of bioactive and volatile profiles of thyme (*Thymus vulgaris* L.) teas as affected by infusion times. *J. Food Meas. Charact.* **2018**, *12*, 2570–2580. [CrossRef]
150. Tlili, N.; Sarikurkcu, C. Bioactive compounds profile, enzyme inhibitory and antioxidant activities of water extracts from five selected medicinal plants. *Ind. Crops Prod.* **2020**, *151*, 112448. [CrossRef]
151. Patil, S.M.; Ramu, R.; Shirahatti, P.S.; Shivamallu, C.; Amachawadi, R.G. A systematic review on ethnopharmacology, phytochemistry and pharmacological aspects of *Thymus vulgaris* Linn. *Heliyon* **2021**, *7*, e07054. [CrossRef]
152. Mokhtari, R.; Kazemi Fard, M.; Rezaei, M.; Moftakharzadeh, S.A.; Mohseni, A. Antioxidant, Antimicrobial Activities, and Characterization of Phenolic Compounds of Thyme (*Thymus vulgaris*L.), Sage (*Salvia officinalis* L.), and Thyme–Sage Mixture Extracts. *J. Food Qual.* **2023**, 2602454. [CrossRef]
153. Martini, S.; D'Addario, C.; Colacevich, A.; Focardi, S.; Borghini, F.; Santucci, A.; Figura, N.; Rossi, C. Antimicrobial activity against *Helicobacter pylori* strains and antioxidant properties of blackberry leaves (*Rubus ulmifolius*) and isolated compounds. *Int. J. Antimicrob. Agents* **2009**, *34*, 50–59. [CrossRef]
154. Quave, C.L.; Estévez-Carmona, M.; Compadre, C.M.; Hobby, G.; Hendrickson, H.; Beenken, K.E.; Smeltzer, M.S. Ellagic acid derivatives from *Rubus ulmifolius* inhibit *Staphylococcus aureus* biofilm formation and improve response to antibiotics. *PLoS ONE* **2012**, *7*, e28737. [CrossRef] [PubMed]
155. Fazio, A.; Plastina, P.; Meijerink, J.; Witkamp, R.F.; Gabriele, B. Comparative analyses of seeds of wild fruits of *Rubus* and *Sambucus* species from Southern Italy: Fatty acid composition of the oil, total phenolic content, antioxidant and anti-inflammatory properties of the methanolic extracts. *Food Chem.* **2013**, *140*, 817–824. [CrossRef] [PubMed]

156. Ruiz-Rodríguez, B.M.; Sánchez-Moreno, C.; Ancos, B.D.; Sánchez-Mata, M.D.; Fernández-Ruíz, V.; Cámara, M.; Tardío, J. Wild *Arbutus unedo* L. and *Rubus ulmifolius* Schott fruits are underutilized sources of valuable bioactive compounds with antioxidant capacity. *Fruits* **2014**, *69*, 435–448. [CrossRef]
157. Martins, A.; Barros, L.; Carvalho, A.M.; Santos-Buelga, C.; Fernandes, I.P.; Barreiro, F.; Ferreira, I.C.F.R. Phenolic extracts of *Rubus ulmifolius* Schott flowers: Characterization, microencapsulation and incorporation into yogurts as nutraceutical sources. *Food Funct.* **2014**, *5*, 1091–1100. [CrossRef] [PubMed]
158. Tabarki, S.; Aouadhi, C.; Mechergui, K.; Hammi, K.M.; Ksouri, R.; Raies, A.; Toumi, L. Comparison of Phytochemical Composition and Biological Activities of *Rubus ulmifolius* Extracts Originating from Four Regions of Tunisia. *Chem. Biodivers.* **2017**, *14*, e1600168. [CrossRef] [PubMed]
159. Da Silva, L.P.; Pereira, E.; Pires, T.C.S.P.; Alves, M.J.; Pereira, O.R.; Barros, L.; Ferreira, I.C.F.R. *Rubus ulmifolius* Schott fruits: A detailed study of its nutritional, chemical and bioactive properties. *Food Res. Int.* **2019**, *119*, 34–43. [CrossRef] [PubMed]
160. Schulz, M.; Seraglio, S.K.T.; Della Betta, F.; Nehring, P.; Valese, A.C.; Daguer, H.; Gonzaga, L.V.; Costa, A.C.O.; Fett, R. Blackberry (*Rubus ulmifolius* Schott): Chemical composition, phenolic compounds and antioxidant capacity in two edible stages. *Food Res. Int.* **2019**, *122*, 627–634. [CrossRef]
161. Rodrigues, C.A.; Nicácio, A.E.; Boeing, J.S.; Garcia, F.P.; Nakamura, C.V.; Visentainer, J.V.; Maldaner, L. Rapid extraction method followed by a d-SPE clean-up step for determination of phenolic composition and antioxidant and antiproliferative activities from berry fruits. *Food Chem.* **2020**, *309*, 125694. [CrossRef]
162. Candela, R.G.; Lazzara, G.; Piacente, S.; Bruno, M.; Cavallaro, G.; Badalamenti, N. Conversion of organic dyes into pigments: Extraction of flavonoids from blackberries (*Rubus ulmifolius*) and stabilization. *Molecules* **2021**, *26*, 6878. [CrossRef]
163. Rice-Evans, C.A.; Miller, N.J.; Paganga, G. Structure-antioxidant activity relationships of flavonoids and phenolic acids. *Free Radic. Biol. Med.* **1996**, *20*, 933–956. [CrossRef]
164. Daglia, M.; Di Lorenzo, A.; F Nabavi, S.; S Talas, Z.; M Nabavi, S. Polyphenols: Well beyond the antioxidant capacity: Gallic acid and related compounds as neuroprotective agents: You are what you eat! *Curr. Pharm.Biotechnol.* **2014**, *15*, 362–372. [CrossRef] [PubMed]
165. Shabani, S.; Rabiei, Z.; Amini-Khoei, H. Exploring the multifaceted neuroprotective actions of gallic acid: A review. *Int. J. Food Prop.* **2020**, *23*, 736–752. [CrossRef]
166. Andrade, S.; Loureiro, J.A.; Pereira, M.C. Transferrin-functionalized liposomes for the delivery of gallic acid: A therapeutic approach for Alzheimer's disease. *Pharmaceutics* **2022**, *14*, 2163. [CrossRef] [PubMed]
167. Mansouri, M.T.; Farbood, Y.; Sameri, M.J.; Sarkaki, A.; Naghizadeh, B.; Rafeirad, M. Neuroprotective effects of oral gallic acid against oxidative stress induced by 6-hydroxydopamine in rats. *Food Chem.* **2013**, *138*, 1028–1033. [CrossRef] [PubMed]
168. Mirshekar, M.A.; Sarkaki, A.; Farbood, Y.; Gharib Naseri, M.K.; Badavi, M.; Mansouri, M.T.; Haghparast, A. Neuroprotective effects of gallic acid in a rat model of traumatic brain injury: Behavioral, electrophysiological, and molecular studies. *Iran. J. Basic Med. Sci.* **2018**, *21*, 1056–1063. [PubMed]
169. Maya, S.; Prakash, T.; Goli, D. Effect of wedelolactone and gallic acid on quinolinic acid-induced neurotoxicity and impaired motor function: Significance to sporadic amyotrophic lateral sclerosis. *NeuroToxicology* **2018**, *68*, 1–12. [CrossRef]
170. Zhu, J.-X.; Shan, J.-L.; Hu, W.-Q.; Zeng, J.-X.; Shu, J.-C. Gallic acid activates hippocampal BDNF-Akt-mTOR signaling in chronic mild stress. *Metab. Brain Dis.* **2019**, *34*, 93–101. [CrossRef]
171. Diaz, A.; Muñoz-Arenas, G.; Caporal-Hernandez, K.; Vázquez-Roque, R.; Lopez-Lopez, G.; Kozina, A.; Espinosa, B.; Flores, G.; Treviño, S.; Guevara, J. Gallic acid improves recognition memory and decreases oxidative-inflammatory damage in the rat hippocampus with metabolic syndrome. *Synapse* **2021**, *75*, e22186. [CrossRef]
172. Kim, M.-J.; Seong, A.-R.; Yoo, J.-Y.; Jin, C.-H.; Lee, Y.-H.; Kim, Y.J.; Lee, J.; Jun, W.J.; Yoon, H.-G. Gallic acid, a histone acetyltransferase inhibitor, suppresses β-amyloid neurotoxicity by inhibiting microglial-mediated neuroinflammation. *Mol. Nutr. Food Res.* **2011**, *55*, 1798–1808. [CrossRef]
173. Maya, S.; Prakash, T.; Goli, D. Evaluation of neuroprotective effects of wedelolactone and gallic acid on aluminium-induced neurodegeneration: Relevance to sporadic amyotrophic lateral sclerosis. *Eur. J. Pharmacol.* **2018**, *835*, 41–51. [CrossRef]
174. Ogunlade, B.; Adelakun, S.A.; Agie, J.A. Nutritional supplementation of gallic acid ameliorates Alzheimer-type hippocampal neurodegeneration and cognitive impairment induced by aluminum chloride exposure in adult Wistar rats. *Drug Chem. Toxicol.* **2022**, *45*, 651–662. [CrossRef] [PubMed]
175. Samad, N.; Jabeen, S.; Imran, I.; Zulfiqar, I.; Bilal, K. Protective effect of gallic acid against arsenic-induced anxiety−/depression-like behaviors and memory impairment in male rats. *Metab. Brain Dis.* **2019**, *34*, 1091–1102. [CrossRef] [PubMed]
176. Nabavi, S.F.; Tejada, S.; Setzer, W.N.; Gortzi, O.; Sureda, A.; Braidy, N.; Daglia, M.; Manayi, A.; Nabavi, S.M. Chlorogenic acid and mental diseases: From chemistry to medicine. *Curr. Neuropharmacol.* **2017**, *15*, 471–479. [CrossRef] [PubMed]
177. Shi, H.; Dong, L.; Jiang, J.; Zhao, J.; Zhao, G.; Dang, X.; Lu, X.; Jia, M. Chlorogenic acid reduces liver inflammation and fibrosis through inhibition of toll-like receptor 4 signaling pathway. *Toxicology* **2013**, *303*, 107–114. [CrossRef]
178. Rahimifard, M.; Maqbool, F.; Moeini-Nodeh, S.; Niaz, K.; Abdollahi, M.; Braidy, N.; Nabavi, S.M.; Nabavi, S.F. Targeting the TLR4 signaling pathway by polyphenols: A novel therapeutic strategy for neuroinflammation. *Ageing Res. Rev.* **2017**, *36*, 11–19. [CrossRef]
179. Kaur, S.; Dhiman, M.; Mantha, A.K. Ferulic Acid: A Natural Antioxidant with Application towards Neuroprotection against Alzheimer's Disease. In *Functional Food and Human Health*; Rani, V., Yadav, U.C.S., Eds.; Springer: Singapore, 2018; pp. 575–586.

180. Gulcin, İ. Antioxidants and antioxidant methods: An updated overview. *Arch. Toxicol.* **2020**, *94*, 651–715. [CrossRef]
181. Mancuso, C.; Santangelo, R. Ferulic acid: Pharmacological and toxicological aspects. *Food Chem. Toxicol.* **2014**, *65*, 185–195. [CrossRef]
182. Li, D.; Rui, Y.; Guo, S.-D.; Luan, F.; Liu, R.; Zeng, N. Ferulic acid: A review of its pharmacology, pharmacokinetics and derivatives. *Life Sci.* **2021**, *284*, 119921. [CrossRef]
183. Liu, Y.-M.; Shen, J.-D.; Xu, L.-P.; Li, H.-B.; Li, Y.-C.; Yi, L.-T. Ferulic acid inhibits neuro-inflammation in mice exposed to chronic unpredictable mild stress. *Int. Immunopharmacol.* **2017**, *45*, 128–134. [CrossRef]
184. Kikugawa, M.; Tsutsuki, H.; Ida, T.; Nakajima, H.; Ihara, H.; Sakamoto, T. Water-soluble ferulic acid derivatives improve amyloid-β-induced neuronal cell death and dysmnesia through inhibition of amyloid-β aggregation. *Biosci. Biotechnol. Biochem.* **2016**, *80*, 547–553. [CrossRef]
185. Wang, E.-J.; Wu, M.-Y.; Lu, J.-H. Ferulic Acid in Animal Models of Alzheimer's Disease: A Systematic Review of Preclinical Studies. *Cells* **2021**, *10*, 2653. [CrossRef] [PubMed]
186. Yan, J.-J.; Cho, J.-Y.; Kim, H.-S.; Kim, K.-L.; Jung, J.-S.; Huh, S.-O.; Suh, H.-W.; Kim, Y.-H.; Song, D.-K. Protection against β-amyloid peptide toxicity in vivo with long-term administration of ferulic acid. *Br. J. Pharmacol.* **2001**, *133*, 89–96. [CrossRef] [PubMed]
187. Cho, J.-Y.; Kim, H.-S.; Kim, D.-H.; Yan, J.-J.; Suh, H.-W.; Song, D.-K. Inhibitory effects of long-term administration of ferulic acid on astrocyte activation induced by intracerebroventricular injection of β-amyloid peptide (1–42) in mice. *Prog. Neuropsychopharmacol. Biol. Psychiatry* **2005**, *29*, 901–907. [CrossRef] [PubMed]
188. Wang, N.-Y.; Li, J.-N.; Liu, W.-L.; Huang, Q.; Li, W.-X.; Tan, Y.-H.; Liu, F.; Song, Z.-H.; Wang, M.-Y.; Xie, N.; et al. Ferulic Acid Ameliorates Alzheimer's Disease-like Pathology and Repairs Cognitive Decline by Preventing Capillary Hypofunction in APP/PS1 Mice. *Neurotherapeutics* **2021**, *18*, 1064–1080. [CrossRef] [PubMed]
189. AAlikhani, M.; Khalili, M.; Jahanshahi, M. The natural iron chelators' ferulic acid and caffeic acid rescue mice's brains from side effects of iron overload. *Front. Neurol.* **2022**, *13*, 951725. [CrossRef] [PubMed]
190. Jung, U.J.; Lee, M.K.; Park, Y.B.; Jeon, S.M.; Choi, M.S. Antihyperglycemic and antioxidant properties of caffeic acid in db/db mice. *J. Pharmacol. Exp. Ther.* **2006**, *318*, 476–483. [CrossRef] [PubMed]
191. Maass, A.; Düzel, S.; Brigadski, T.; Goerke, M.; Becke, A.; Sobieray, U.; Neumann, K.; Lövdén, M.; Lindenberger, U.; Bäckman, L.; et al. Relationships of peripheral IGF-1, VEGF and BDNF levels to exercise-related changes in memory, hippocampal perfusion and volumes in older adults. *NeuroImage* **2016**, *131*, 142–154. [CrossRef]
192. Xu, F.; Na, L.; Li, Y.; Chen, L. Roles of the PI3K/AKT/mTOR signalling pathways in neurodegenerative diseases and tumours. *Cell Biosci.* **2020**, *10*, 54. [CrossRef]
193. Ibrahim, A.M.; Chauhan, L.; Bhardwaj, A.; Sharma, A.; Fayaz, F.; Kumar, B.; Alhashmi, M.; AlHajri, N.; Alam, M.S.; Pottoo, F.H. Brain-Derived Neurotropic Factor in Neurodegenerative Disorders. *Biomedicines* **2022**, *10*, 1143. [CrossRef]
194. Chang, W.; Huang, D.; Lo, Y.M.; Tee, Q.; Kuo, P.; Wu, J.S.; Huang, W.; Shen, S. Protective effect of caffeic acid against Alzheimer's disease pathogenesis via modulating cerebral insulin signaling, β-amyloid accumulation, and synaptic plasticity in hyperinsulinemic rats. *J. Agric. Food Chem.* **2019**, *67*, 7684–7693. [CrossRef]
195. Siddiqui, S.; Kamal, A.; Khan, F.; Jamali, K.S.; Saify, Z.S. Gallic and vanillic acid suppress inflammation and promote myelination in an in vitro mouse model of neurodegeneration. *Mol. Biol. Rep.* **2019**, *46*, 997–1011. [CrossRef] [PubMed]
196. Venkatesan, R.; Ji, E.; Kim, S.Y. Phytochemicals that regulate neurodegenerative disease by targeting neurotrophins: A comprehensive review. *BioMed Res. Int.* **2015**, 814068. [CrossRef] [PubMed]
197. Sakamula, R.; Thong-asa, W. Neuroprotective effect of p-coumaric acid in mice with cerebral ischemia reperfusion injuries. *Metab. Brain Dis.* **2018**, *33*, 765–773. [CrossRef] [PubMed]
198. Yoon, J.-H.; Youn, K.; Ho, C.-T.; Karwe, M.V.; Jeong, W.-S.; Jun, M. p-Coumaric Acid and Ursolic Acid from Corni fructus Attenuated β-Amyloid25–35-Induced Toxicity through Regulation of the NF-κB Signaling Pathway in PC12 Cells. *J. Agric. Food Chem.* **2014**, *62*, 4911–4916. [CrossRef] [PubMed]
199. Oh, D.-R.; Kim, M.-J.; Choi, E.-J.; Kim, Y.; Lee, H.-S.; Bae, D.; Choi, C. Protective Effects of p-Coumaric Acid Isolated from *Vaccinium bracteatum* Thunb. Leaf Extract on Corticosterone-Induced Neurotoxicity in SH-SY5Y Cells and Primary Rat Cortical Neurons. *Processes* **2021**, *9*, 869. [CrossRef]
200. Daroi, P.A.; Dhage, S.N.; Juvekar, A.R. p-Coumaric acid mitigates lipopolysaccharide induced brain damage via alleviating oxidative stress, inflammation and apoptosis. *J. Pharm. Pharmacol.* **2021**, *74*, 556–564. [CrossRef]
201. Rashno, M.; Gholipour, P.; Salehi, I.; Komaki, A.; Rashidi, K.; Esmaeil Khoshnam, S.; Ghaderi, S. p-Coumaric acid mitigates passive avoidance memory and hippocampal synaptic plasticity impairments in aluminum chloride-induced Alzheimer's disease rat model. *J. Funct. Foods* **2022**, *94*, 105117. [CrossRef]
202. He, Y.; Chen, S.; Tsoi, B.; Qi, S.; Gu, B.; Wang, Z.; Peng, C.; Shen, J. *Alpinia oxyphylla* Miq. and Its Active Compound P-Coumaric Acid Promote Brain-Derived Neurotrophic Factor Signaling for Inducing Hippocampal Neurogenesis and Improving Post-cerebral Ischemic Spatial Cognitive Functions. *Front. Cell Develop. Biol.* **2021**, *8*, 577790. [CrossRef]
203. Mughal, E.U.; Sadiq, A.; Ashraf, J.; Zafar, M.N.; Sumrra, S.H.; Tariq, R.; Javed, C.O. Flavonols and 4-thioflavonols as potential acetylcholinesterase and butyrylcholinesterase inhibitors: Synthesis, structure-activity relationship and molecular docking studies. *Bioorg. Chem.* **2019**, *91*, 103124. [CrossRef]
204. Figueira, I.; Menezes, R.; Macedo, D.; Costa, I.; dos Santos, C.N. Polyphenols beyond barriers: A glimpse into the brain. *Curr. Neuropharmacol..* **2017**, *15*, 562–594. [CrossRef]

205. Manach, C.; Williamson, G.; Morand, C.; Scalbert, A.; Rémésy, C. Bioavailability and bioefficacy of polyphenols in humans. I. Review of 97 bioavailability studies. *Am. J. Clin. Nutr.* **2005**, *81*, 230–242. [CrossRef] [PubMed]
206. Renaud, J.; Martinoli, M.-G. Considerations for the use of polyphenols as therapies in neurodegenerative diseases. *Int. J. Mol. Sci.* **2019**, *20*, 1883. [CrossRef] [PubMed]
207. Ishisaka, A.; Ichikawa, S.; Sakakibara, H.; Piskula, M.K.; Nakamura, T.; Kato, Y.; Ito, M.; Miyamoto, K.-I.; Tsuji, A.; Kawai, Y. Accumulation of orally administered quercetin in brain tissue and its antioxidative effects in rats. *Free Rad. Biol. Med.* **2011**, *51*, 1329–1336. [CrossRef] [PubMed]
208. Dajas, F.; Abin-Carriquiry, J.A.; Arredondo, F.; Blasina, F.; Echeverry, C.; Martínez, M.; Rivera, F.; Vaamonde, L. Quercetin in brain diseases: Potential and limits. *Neurochem. Int.* **2015**, *89*, 140–148. [CrossRef] [PubMed]
209. Dajas, F. Life or death: Neuroprotective and anticancer effects of quercetin. *J. Ethnopharmacol.* **2012**, *143*, 383–396. [CrossRef] [PubMed]
210. Chen, W.; Zhuang, J.; Li, Y.; Shen, Y.; Zheng, X. Myricitrin protects against peroxynitrite-mediated DNA damage and cytotoxicity in astrocytes. *Food Chem.* **2013**, *141*, 927–933. [CrossRef] [PubMed]
211. Barreca, D.; Bellocco, E.; DOnofrio, G.; Fazel Nabavi, S.; Daglia, M.; Rastrelli, L.; Mohammad Nabavi, S. Neuroprotective effects of quercetin: From chemistry to medicine. *CNS Neurol. Disord. Drug Targets* **2016**, *15*, 964–975. [CrossRef]
212. Amanzadeh, E.; Esmaeili, A.; Rahgozar, S.; Nourbakhshnia, M. Application of quercetin in neurological disorders: From nutrition to nanomedicine. *Rev. Neurosci.* **2019**, *30*, 555–572. [CrossRef]
213. Azib, L.; Debbache-Benaida, N.; Costa, G.D.; Atmani-Kilani, D.; Saidene, N.; Ayouni, K.; Richard, T.; Atmani, D. *Pistacia lentiscus* L. leaves extract and its major phenolic compounds reverse aluminium-induced neurotoxicity in mice. *Ind. Crops Prod.* **2019**, *137*, 576–584. [CrossRef]
214. Moneim, A.E.A. Antioxidant activities of *Punica granatum* (pomegranate) peel extract on brain of rats. *J. Med. Plants Res.* **2012**, *6*, 195–199.
215. Martín, S.; González-Burgos, E.; Carretero, M.E.; Gómez-Serranillos, M.P. Neuroprotective properties of Spanish red wine and its isolated polyphenols on astrocytes. *Food Chem.* **2011**, *128*, 40–48. [CrossRef] [PubMed]
216. Sabogal-Guáqueta, A.M.; Munoz-Manco, J.I.; Ramírez-Pineda, J.R.; Lamprea-Rodriguez, M.; Osorio, E.; Cardona-Gómez, G.P. The flavonoid quercetin ameliorates Alzheimer's disease pathology and protects cognitive and emotional function in aged triple transgenic Alzheimer's disease model mice. *Neuropharmacol.* **2015**, *93*, 134–145. [CrossRef] [PubMed]
217. Abdalla, F.H.; Schmatz, R.; Cardoso, A.M.; Carvalho, F.B.; Baldissarelli, J.; de Oliveira, J.S.; Rosa, M.M.; Nunes, M.A.G.; Rubin, M.A.; da Cruz, I.B. Quercetin protects the impairment of memory and anxiogenic-like behavior in rats exposed to cadmium: Possible involvement of the acetylcholinesterase and Na^+, K^+-ATPase activities. *Physiol. Behav.* **2014**, *135*, 152–167. [CrossRef] [PubMed]
218. Khan, M.T.H.; Orhan, I.; Şenol, F.; Kartal, M.; Şener, B.; Dvorská, M.; Šmejkal, K.; Šlapetová, T. Cholinesterase inhibitory activities of some flavonoid derivatives and chosen xanthone and their molecular docking studies. *Chem. Biol. Interact.* **2009**, *181*, 383–389. [CrossRef] [PubMed]
219. Min, B.S.; Cuong, T.D.; Lee, J.-S.; Shin, B.-S.; Woo, M.H.; Hung, T.M. Cholinesterase inhibitors from *Cleistocalyx operculatus* buds. *Arch. Pharmacal Res.* **2010**, *33*, 1665–1670. [CrossRef]
220. Moeini, R.; Memariani, Z.; Asadi, F.; Bozorgi, M.; Gorji, N. Pistacia Genus as a Potential Source of Neuroprotective Natural Products. *Planta Med.* **2019**, *85*, 1326–1350. [CrossRef]
221. Zaplatic, E.; Bule, M.; Shah, S.Z.A.; Uddin, M.S.; Niaz, K. Molecular mechanisms underlying protective role of quercetin in attenuating Alzheimer's disease. *Life Sci.* **2019**, *224*, 109–119. [CrossRef]
222. Pervin, M.; Unno, K.; Ohishi, T.; Tanabe, H.; Miyoshi, N.; Nakamura, Y. Beneficial effects of green tea catechins on neurodegenerative diseases. *Molecules* **2018**, *23*, 1297. [CrossRef]
223. Ribeiro, G.A.C.; da Rocha, C.Q.; Veloso, W.B.; Fernandes, R.N.; da Silva, I.S.; Tanaka, A.A. Determination of the catechin contents of bioactive plant extracts using disposable screen-printed carbon electrodes in a batch injection analysis (BIA) system. *Microchem. J.* **2019**, *146*, 1249–1254. [CrossRef]
224. Farzaei, M.H.; Bahramsoltani, R.; Abbasabadi, Z.; Braidy, N.; Nabavi, S.M. Role of green tea catechins in prevention of age-related cognitive decline: Pharmacological targets and clinical perspective. *J. Cell. Physiol.* **2019**, *234*, 2447–2459. [CrossRef]
225. Farkhondeh, T.; Yazdi, H.S.; Samarghandian, S. The protective effects of green tea catechins in the management of neurodegenerative diseases: A review. *Curr. Drug Discov. Technol.* **2019**, *16*, 57–65. [CrossRef] [PubMed]
226. Cheruku, S.P.; Ramalingayya, G.V.; Chamallamudi, M.R.; Biswas, S.; Nandakumar, K.; Nampoothiri, M.; Gourishetti, K.; Kumar, N. Catechin ameliorates doxorubicin-induced neuronal cytotoxicity in in vitro and episodic memory deficit in in vivo in Wistar rats. *Cytotechnology* **2018**, *70*, 245–259. [CrossRef] [PubMed]
227. Ide, K.; Matsuoka, N.; Yamada, H.; Furushima, D.; Kawakami, K. Effects of tea catechins on Alzheimer's disease: Recent updates and perspectives. *Molecules* **2018**, *23*, 2357. [CrossRef] [PubMed]
228. Levites, Y.; Weinreb, O.; Maor, G.; Youdim, M.B.; Mandel, S. Green tea polyphenol (−)-epigallocatechin-3-gallate prevents N-methyl-4-phenyl-1, 2, 3, 6-tetrahydropyridine-induced dopaminergic neurodegeneration. *J. Neurochem.* **2001**, *78*, 1073–1082. [CrossRef] [PubMed]
229. Cuevas, E.; Limón, D.I.; Pérez-Severiano, F.; Díaz, A.; Ortega, L.; Zenteno, E.; Guevara, J. Antioxidant effects of epicatechin on the hippocampal toxicity caused by amyloid-beta 25-35 in rats. *Eur. J. Pharmacol.* **2009**, *616*, 122–127. [CrossRef]

230. Nan, S.; Wang, P.; Zhang, Y.; Fan, J. Epigallocatechin-3-Gallate Provides Protection Against Alzheimer's Disease-Induced Learning and Memory Impairments in Rats. *Drug Des. Devel. Ther.* **2021**, *13*, 2013–2024. [CrossRef]
231. Ali, A.A.; Abd El-Fattah, A.I.; Abu-Elfotuh, K.; Elariny, H.A. Natural antioxidants enhance the power of physical and mental activities versus risk factors inducing progression of Alzheimer's disease in rats. *Int. Immunopharmacol.* **2021**, *96*, 107729. [CrossRef]
232. Ez zoubi, Y.; Farah, A.; Zaroual, H.; El Ouali Lalami, A. Antimicrobial activity of *Lavandula stoechas* phenolic extracts against pathogenic bacteria isolated from a hospital in Morocco. *Vegetos* **2020**, *33*, 703–711. [CrossRef]
233. Sharma, D.R.; Wani, W.Y.; Sunkaria, A.; Kandimalla, R.J.; Verma, D.; Cameotra, S.S.; Gill, K.D. Quercetin protects against chronic aluminum-induced oxidative stress and ensuing biochemical, cholinergic, and neurobehavioral impairments in rats. *Neurotox. Res.* **2013**, *23*, 336–357. [CrossRef]
234. Bouyahya, A.; Bakri, Y.; Et-Touys, A.; Assemian, I.C.C.; Abrini, J.; Dakka, N. In vitro antiproliferative activity of selected medicinal plants from the North-West of Morocco on several cancer cell lines. *Eur. J. Integr. Med.* **2018**, *18*, 23–29. [CrossRef]
235. Bouyahya, A.; Dakka, N.; Talbaoui, A.; Moussaoui, N.E.; Abrini, J.; Bakri, Y. Phenolic contents and antiradical capacity of vegetable oil from *Pistacia lentiscus* (L). *J. Mater. Environ. Sci.* **2018**, *9*, 1518–1524.
236. Ghasemi Pirbalouti, A.; Emami Bistghani, Z.; Malekpoor, F. An overview on genus *Thymus*. *J. Med. Herb* **2015**, *6*, 93–100.

Disclaimer/Publisher's Note: The statements, opinions and data contained in all publications are solely those of the individual author(s) and contributor(s) and not of MDPI and/or the editor(s). MDPI and/or the editor(s) disclaim responsibility for any injury to people or property resulting from any ideas, methods, instructions or products referred to in the content.

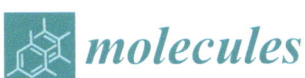 molecules

Review

Are There Lipid Membrane-Domain Subtypes in Neurons with Different Roles in Calcium Signaling?

Alejandro K. Samhan-Arias [1,2,*], Joana Poejo [3], Dorinda Marques-da-Silva [4,5,6], Oscar H. Martínez-Costa [1,2] and Carlos Gutierrez-Merino [3,*]

1. Departamento de Bioquímica, Universidad Autónoma de Madrid (UAM), C/Arturo Duperier 4, 28029 Madrid, Spain; oscar.martinez@uam.es
2. Instituto de Investigaciones Biomédicas 'Sols-Morreale' (CSIC-UAM), C/Arturo Duperier 4, 28029 Madrid, Spain
3. Instituto de Biomarcadores de Patologías Moleculares, Universidad de Extremadura, 06006 Badajoz, Spain; joanapoejo86@gmail.com
4. LSRE—Laboratory of Separation and Reaction Engineering and LCM—Laboratory of Catalysis and Materials, School of Management and Technology, Polytechnic Institute of Leiria, Morro do Lena-Alto do Vieiro, 2411-901 Leiria, Portugal; dorinda.silva@ipleiria.pt
5. ALiCE—Associate Laboratory in Chemical Engineering, Faculty of Engineering, University of Porto, Rua Dr. Roberto Frias, 4200-465 Porto, Portugal
6. School of Technology and Management, Polytechnic Institute of Leiria, Morro do Lena-Alto do Vieiro, 2411-901 Leiria, Portugal
* Correspondence: alejandro.samhan@uam.es (A.K.S.-A.); biocgm@gmail.com (C.G.-M.)

Abstract: Lipid membrane nanodomains or lipid rafts are 10–200 nm diameter size cholesterol- and sphingolipid-enriched domains of the plasma membrane, gathering many proteins with different roles. Isolation and characterization of plasma membrane proteins by differential centrifugation and proteomic studies have revealed a remarkable diversity of proteins in these domains. The limited size of the lipid membrane nanodomain challenges the simple possibility that all of them can coexist within the same lipid membrane domain. As caveolin-1, flotillin isoforms and gangliosides are currently used as neuronal lipid membrane nanodomain markers, we first analyzed the structural features of these components forming nanodomains at the plasma membrane since they are relevant for building supramolecular complexes constituted by these molecular signatures. Among the proteins associated with neuronal lipid membrane nanodomains, there are a large number of proteins that play major roles in calcium signaling, such as ionotropic and metabotropic receptors for neurotransmitters, calcium channels, and calcium pumps. This review highlights a large variation between the calcium signaling proteins that have been reported to be associated with isolated caveolin-1 and flotillin-lipid membrane nanodomains. Since these calcium signaling proteins are scattered in different locations of the neuronal plasma membrane, i.e., in presynapses, postsynapses, axonal or dendritic trees, or in the neuronal soma, our analysis suggests that different lipid membrane-domain subtypes should exist in neurons. Furthermore, we conclude that classification of lipid membrane domains by their content in calcium signaling proteins sheds light on the roles of these domains for neuronal activities that are dependent upon the intracellular calcium concentration. Some examples described in this review include the synaptic and metabolic activity, secretion of neurotransmitters and neuromodulators, neuronal excitability (long-term potentiation and long-term depression), axonal and dendritic growth but also neuronal cell survival and death.

Keywords: flotillin; caveolin; ganglioside; lipid rafts; lipid membrane domains; calcium channel; NMDA; PMCA; P2XR; membrane domains; neuron; brain

Citation: Samhan-Arias, A.K.; Poejo, J.; Marques-da-Silva, D.; Martínez-Costa, O.H.; Gutierrez-Merino, C. Are There Lipid Membrane-Domain Subtypes in Neurons with Different Roles in Calcium Signaling? *Molecules* **2023**, *28*, 7909. https://doi.org/10.3390/molecules28237909

Academic Editor: Angelina Angelova

Received: 20 October 2023
Revised: 24 November 2023
Accepted: 29 November 2023
Published: 2 December 2023

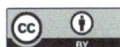

Copyright: © 2023 by the authors. Licensee MDPI, Basel, Switzerland. This article is an open access article distributed under the terms and conditions of the Creative Commons Attribution (CC BY) license (https://creativecommons.org/licenses/by/4.0/).

1. Lipid Membrane Nanodomains Organization in the Neuronal Plasma Membrane

The classical model of the plasma membrane, named the fluid mosaic model, described by Jonathan Singer and Garth Nicolson in 1972, is excessively reductionist for properly accounting for the well-organized plasma membrane domains. Lipid rafts are plasma membrane large areas of 10 and 200 nm diameter in size enriched in cholesterol and sphingolipids [1]. The existence lipid rafts was initially a subject of debate between physical chemists and histologists due to difficulties in visualizing them and their ill-defined molecular composition [1,2]. In the last two decades, a number of new techniques such as single-molecule spectroscopy, super-resolution microscopy, fluorescence recovery after photobleaching, stimulated emission depletion, Förster resonance energy transfer (FRET), total internal reflection fluorescence, and fluorescence correlation spectroscopy techniques allowed to estimate the lower limit of lipid rafts in <20 nm [3–6]. Plasma membrane domains of 26 ± 13 nm radius have been observed in living cells diffusing as one entity for minutes [7]. Further work using stimulated emission depletion (STED) far-field fluorescence nanoscopy revealed spots sized 70-fold below the diffraction barrier transiently trapped between 10 and 20 ms, in cholesterol-mediated molecular complexes dwelling within <20-nm diameter areas [3]. The diffraction limit of visible light impedes domains smaller than 1 µm to be directly visualized and indeed large micrometer-sized lipid rafts domains are readily observed in artificial membranes [3]. Also, associated proteins can mask the direct observation of lipid rafts in living cells. A tentative attempt to determine analogous domains in living cells has been made based on homo-FRET efficiencies obtained through the rate of fluorescence anisotropy loss and using GFP labeled glycosyl-phosphatidylinositol-anchored proteins which allow an estimation of the upper size limit of lipid rafts at ~5 nm [8,9]. Yethiraj and Weisshaar have suggested that the spatial heterogeneity in cell membranes limits the transferability of the conclusion drawn from artificial membranes to live cells, as integral membrane proteins attached to the cytoskeleton act as obstacles that limit the size of lipid domains [8]. For all these reasons, we introduce the concept of lipid membrane domains in this review, arising from the fact that some membrane proteins form oligomers and clusters in the membranes, which formation is favored by cholesterol and other lipid species.

Regarding the protein components associated with lipid membrane domains, widely named in the bibliography as lipid rafts, a proteomic study identified up to 36 integral membrane proteins associated with lipid membrane domain and flotillin, as a marker of these membrane domains where identified in the human brain [10]. In another study, 175 membrane-associated proteins were identified by proteomics, including L-type calcium channels and the plasma membrane calcium ATPase (PMCA), using caveolin-1 (Cav-1) and flotillin-1 (Flot-1), as biomarkers of lipid membrane domains isolated from brain neonatal mice [11]. Similarly, a proteomic assessment of proteins present in isolated lipid membrane domains of adult mouse brains identified 133 proteins, using Flot-1 as a marker of plasma membrane domains [12]. This study also highlighted the colocalization of this protein with several calcium channel subunits [12]. In cultured hippocampal neurons, sphingolipid-cholesterol-enriched microdomains have been localized flotillin 1, Thy-1 cell surface antigen or CD90, as specific lipid membrane-domain markers, associated with the ganglioside named monosialotetrahexosylganglioside (GM1) [13]. It is worth to mention at this point that although GM1 is not a definite lipid membrane-domain marker, its distribution into lipid membrane domains depends on the concentration. At elevated concentration, GM1 can form its own domains organizing in the plasma membrane in non-lipid membrane-domain areas located predominantly in the L_d phase [14]. Very recent discoveries regarding the molecular architecture of lipid membrane nanodomains support their organization in planar tightly packed nanodisks of Cav-1, with a 140Å external diameter size [15]. It is also probable that a similar size supramolecular complex based on flotillin might exist, based on the observed structural conformations of stomatin, prohibitin, flotillin, and the modulator for HflB protease specific for phage lambda cII repressor (HflK/C) domains (SPFH domain) [16]. Also, some studies have reported the isolation of up to 4 types of domains in the plasma membrane at physiological conditions [17]. Given the existence of these nanostructures, a question arises regarding how many of the reported protein molecules in the aforementioned proteomic and non-proteomic studies [10–13] could fit within a single of these nanostructures on one neuronal lipid membrane domain. The quantity of proteins reported in the neuronal lipid membrane domain contrasts with the number of proteins that could fit within or surrounding a 140Å diameter size nanodisk, if this type of structure stands alone as the main component of neuronal planar-lipid membrane domains in the plasma membrane. Neuronal lipid membrane domains are different from those of the invaginated *caveolae* in a variety of cell types, which require the presence of the protein named cavin and higher-order interactions with other proteins [18–20]. Cav-1–cavin interaction seems required to form mature *caveolae*, which have a polygonal shape to induce curvature in non-neuronal cells [21–24]. Cavin is absent or released when conforming planar-non-invaginated lipid membrane domains [20,25–27], like those described in neuronal lipid membrane domains.

In addition to these studies, more efforts are required to ascertain whether Cav-1 nanodisks independently exist in neuronal cells, either as discrete entities supporting non-invaginated areas on the plasma membrane or as components of supramolecular structures analogous to those observed in invaginated *caveolae* [20]. Since supramolecular structures with a similar protein composition to that of *caveolae* do not exist in neurons, the presence of a high number of proteins located in lipid membrane domains raises questions regarding the number of proteins that one Cav-1 nanodisk can hold due to steric hindrance. Methods for lipid membrane-domain isolation based on differential gradient centrifugation cannot discern the existence of lipid membrane nanodomain subtypes. Particularly, cytochemical and histochemical studies combined with physicochemical techniques based on quantitative fluorescence energy transfer (FRET) techniques, as those conducted by the research group led by Prof. Gutierrez-Merino, have provided insights into this matter by identification of proteins in clusters complexing with protein markers of lipid membrane domains (caveolin and flotillin isoforms) at a distance <100 nm in studies performed in neurons and brain tissue using the appropriate secondary fluorescent antibodies against the primary antibody of the selected lipid membrane-domain marker (Box 1) [28–36]. As discussed in these articles, this is a particular case of FRET from one donor to multiple acceptors, a situation in which the maximum range of FRET distance is significantly expanded, as analyzed in detail in former studies with purified biological membranes [23,37–39]. These research findings might support the existence of clusters that could stand alone as individual entities, such as Cav-1 nanodisks, with a diverse variety of calcium transporter elements. The well-recognized and wide distribution of these transporters in neurons, functioning as partners of lipid membrane-domain markers, strongly suggests the potential existence of multiple lipid membrane-domain subtypes within neurons. A neuronal lipid membrane-domain subtype is defined in this work as a plasma membrane, synaptic or extrasynaptic structure characterized by the presence of a protein biomarker of lipid membrane nanodomain and a specific calcium transport systems. The existence of these subdomains might correlate with the function of calcium gradients associated with cytosolic calcium microcompartments, near the plasma membrane [33,40], and such patterns may arise under certain conditions [41–44].

In this context, it is intriguing and controversial whether different types of lipid membrane domains might exist within a single cell or across different cell types based on the complex lipid and protein composition of these domains. This issue might be particularly notorious in tissues such as the brain, where recent findings using single-cell sequencing and methods to map the spatial location of gene expression have unraveled the extraordinary cellular diversity existing within this tissue [45]. Strategies for isolating lipid membrane domains, named rafts in these studies, that utilized membrane tension generate large observable membrane domains or lipid rafts, that are converted into small ones when the tension was relieved [17]. This result lends support to the hypothesis that a myriad of not well-described plasma membrane nanodomains might exist.

Box 1. FRET from one donor to multiple acceptors.

> Labeling of proteins with donor and acceptor secondary fluorescent antibodies forming a FRET pair is an approach that has been used to identify proteins clustered in lipid raft domains. This is a particular case of FRET from one donor to multiple acceptors because the density of labeling of commercial secondary fluorescent antibodies ranges between 2 and 10 dye molecules per antibody [46–49], and also because in theory, one primary IgG antibody can bind up to 2 secondary fluorescent IgG antibodies, one in each of the symmetrical domains of the primary antibody. Therefore, one dye molecule of the donor fluorescent antibody can form a FRET pair with 2–10 and 4–20 acceptor dyes bound to the acceptor secondary antibody for 1:1 and 1:2 stoichiometries of the primary/secondary antibody complex, respectively. The major advantage of a high density of labeling of the secondary fluorescent antibody is the amplification of the fluorescence intensity signal for fluorescence microscopy imaging of cells. In addition, it has another collateral advantage for FRET distance calculations, namely, that homotransfer between donors located in one fluorescent secondary antibody and time and space averaging of different orientations of donors and acceptors bound to different IgG molecules which should lead to a distribution close to a random orientation between donor and acceptors.
>
> The number of acceptor dyes available to a donor dye bound to a fluorescent antibody for FRET will be larger when the target protein units form clusters within lipid membrane-domains. In this case, FRET will extend to acceptor dyes of secondary antibodies bound to the primary antibodies that stain all neighbor protein targets present in the cluster within the area accessible to the IgG complex of primary/secondary antibodies plus the effective FRET distance between the selected donor and acceptor dyes. Each 1:1 complex of primary/secondary IgG antibodies will reach proteins located up to ≈30 nm from the target protein, taking into account the size of IgG molecules and their rotational mobility. Therefore, this implies that donor dyes bound to a primary/secondary IgG/ protein-1 complex can make contacts with acceptor dyes bound to the primary/secondary IgG complex attached to protein-2 separated up to ≈ 60 nm in the same lipid membrane-domain. If there is more than one unit of the target protein-2 stained with the secondary fluorescent antibody labeled with the acceptor dye, the number of acceptors/donor available for FRET will be proportionally increased.
>
> In addition, the overall rate (k_T) of FRET can be written for these cases as the sum of the rate of FRET between each one of the possible donor/acceptor pairs that can be formed in the system under study, i.e., $k_T = \Sigma\ k_i$, see for example [50,51]. Therefore, the overall FRET efficiency is the sum of the efficiency of energy transfer between all the possible donor/acceptor pairs that can be formed in the system [50–52]. This further increases the effective FRET distance using donor and acceptor secondary fluorescent antibodies. A simple calculation can serve to illustrate this point. For FRET from 1 donor to 10 acceptor molecules located at an equidistant distance, the apparent distance for 50% efficiency of FRET will be ~10 × R_0 from the target protein labeled with the donor secondary fluorescent antibody, where R_0 is the value of this distance for a single donor/acceptor pair, which ranges between 5 and 6 for the most frequently used FRET pairs in fluorescence microscopy. Let us remind here that the useful donor/acceptor distance range for a single donor/acceptor pair is approximately up to twice the distance for 50% efficiency of FRET [51,53]. Note that 10 acceptors per donor can be reached in any of the following cases: (i) 1:2 stoichiometry of the primary/secondary antibody complex and an average density of labeling of the acceptor fluorescent antibody of 5 dye molecules per antibody, and only one unit of the target proteins in the lipid membrane-domain; and (ii) 1:1 stoichiometry of the primary/secondary antibody complex and an average density of labeling of the acceptor fluorescent antibody of 5 dye molecules per antibody, with two protein units labeled with the acceptor fluorescent antibody within 60 nm in the same lipid membrane-domain. In summary, the effective FRET distance range extends to 80–200 nm when donor and acceptor dyes are bound to secondary fluorescent IgG antibodies directed against different target proteins present in lipid membrane-domains.
>
> Thus, FRET using donor and acceptor secondary fluorescent antibodies is a suitable approach to monitor the co-localization of proteins within lipid membrane-domains of 100–200 nm. Also, it follows from this analysis that when there is only one unit of one of the target proteins within each lipid membrane-domain, co-localization of proteins within smaller lipid membrane-domains of 40 or 20 nm can be studied with the use of fluorescent primary antibodies or antibody F_{ab} fragments, respectively, instead of using fluorescent secondary antibodies.

For cells, application of membrane tension resulted in several types of large domains; one class of domains was identified as a lipid raft, defined here as lipid membrane domain. Furthermore, the distribution of protein components of lipid domains [54–57] in planar non-invaginated regions of the neuronal plasma membrane [20,25–27], may be considered a robust evidence for the existence of not-so-transient, underlying structures that support several membrane nanodomains in neurons. This structural arrangement may differ from that observed in other cell types, where membrane invaginated areas forming *caveolae* have been described involved in membrane trafficking, with a transient formation and elimination of the protein content of these domains.

The objective of this review is to provide a comprehensive exploration and integrative analysis of information, suggesting the existence of lipid/protein-domain subtypes within neuronal cells. Several proteins that play major roles in neuronal calcium signaling have been described as components of lipid membrane domains [58], i.e., neurotransmitter receptors [59,60] and calcium transport systems [43,61], and they present a differential subcellular distribution within a single neuron and across different types of neurons, as shown in this review. The distribution pattern serves as a crucial tool for proposing the existence of diverse lipid membrane-domain subtypes in neurons.

2. Properties of Caveolin-, Flotillin- or Ganglioside-Containing Lipid Membrane Domains

Within neuronal lipid membrane domains, at least two classes of protein, named caveolin and flotillin, can scaffold cholesterol and have been used as biomarkers of these domains [62–68]. The differential spatial distribution of the caveolin-, flotillin- or some specific lipid-enriched domains of the neuronal plasma membrane suggests that various domains co-exist in one neuron. We will call them caveolin- and flotillin-enriched lipid membrane domains. Their differential association with plasma membrane receptors acting through calcium signaling, as well as with calcium channels and transport systems might be useful to classify lipid membrane nanodomains. Other lipids, such as gangliosides have been associated with both in certain contexts but not always [69–71]. This supports the idea that their presence might constitute a marker for additional lipid membrane nanodomain subtypes. The characterization and differentiation between these domains have been challenged by the limitations and insufficient resolution of the conventional methods for preparative isolation of lipid domains using a whole brain tissue or cells in culture (Figure 1). This is a major handicap for a proper classification of lipid membrane-domain subtypes. A potential dissection through immunohistochemical and immunocytochemical methods could offer insights of their precise intracellular and intercellular locations. Moreover, this dissection could contribute to a better comprehension of how key plasma membrane components in charge of calcium homeostasis are regulated in lipid membrane domains. The subsequent paragraphs of this review provide a brief account of the actual knowledge of these nanodomains in neurons.

2.1. Caveolin-Enriched Lipid Membrane Domains in Neurons

Cav-1 is the major component forming *caveolae* at the plasma membrane [27,72–75]. Several domains are recognized in the linear sequence of this protein related to its function and its interaction with lipids. Membrane binding, cholesterol recognition, and oligomerization functions have been attributed to the scaffolding domain (SD) of Cav-1 [76–78]. As part of the SD, a function for the intramembrane domain (IMD; residues 102−134) has been assigned, forming a unique α-helical hairpin that does not traverse the membrane [79–81]. Proteins associated with caveolin are characterized by the presence of an aromatic-rich caveolin binding motif (CBM) with the following compositions (ϕXϕXXXXϕ, ϕXXXXϕXXϕ or ϕXϕXXXXϕXXϕ, where ϕ is an aromatic and X an unspecified amino acid) [82–84]. Cav-1 also presents a cholesterol recognition/interaction amino acid consensus (CRAC) domain composed of the amino acid residues VTKYWFYR [85], which allows the interaction of this protein with cholesterol. It must be highlighted at this point that the presence of a CRAC domain in proteins is neither necessary nor sufficient for cholesterol binding [86,87]. In this sense, proteins including CRAC domains can be neutral with respect to cholesterol binding, and proteins lacking CRAC domain can bind cholesterol which is the case of transmembrane protein domains lacking a CRAC, a CARC or a tilted domain, as reviewed by Fantini and Barrantes [88]. For this reason, cholesterol interaction with caveolin might be beneficiated by additional interactions with the protein/membrane microenvironment.

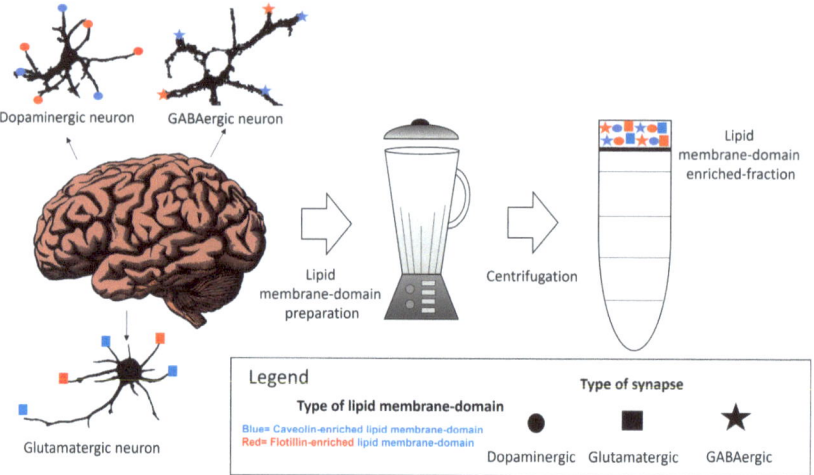

Figure 1. Some of the potential lipid membrane domains that can be isolated from brain tissue are associated with different neuronal types.

Cav-1 (Figure 2, panel a), which is one of the units required for *caveolae* formation, can hetero- or homo-oligomerize in complexes composed of 14–16 monomers (200–400 kDa) [89,90]. Recently, the typical supramolecular structure of this protein has been described by cryo-electron microscopy [15]. Cav-1 overexpression in *E. coli* formed 8S-like complexes and oligomerize, forming heterologous *caveolae* (*h-caveolae*) and sculpting membranes, which are two of the essential functions of mammalian cells *caveolae* [91,92]. Cav-1 can assemble in protomers organized into a tightly packed disc with a planar membrane-embedded surface [15]. Several Cav-1 protomers (11 protomers) can oligomerize to form an 8S complex, a type of complex with a proposed biological role essential for *caveolae* biogenesis since 8S complexes are known to concentrate in endoplasmic reticulum (ER) exit sites [93]. Also, they accumulate at the Golgi, where they lose their diffusional mobility and associate with cholesterol [94,95] and eventually assemble into 70S complexes [93]. The cholesterol-rich membranes containing 70S Cav1 complexes are then transported to the cell surface. The formation of the 8S complex occurs in a cooperative process mediated by its oligomerization domain (OD), which is aided by its SD and signature motif (SM). The crystallography study revealed that the 11 Cav-1 protomers can organize into a disc-shaped complex with a diameter of ~140 Å and a height of ~34 Å to form the 8S complex [15]. The nanodisk contains an outer "rim", a central β-barrel "hub", and 11 curved α-helical "spokes" with Cav-1 C-terminal ends oriented towards the hub and N-terminal ends towards the rim (Figure 2, panel b). This study supports that caveolin complexes may stabilize flat membrane surfaces of polyhedral structures rather than imposing continuous membrane curvature [15]. Although this structure is formed in an almost cholesterol-depleted environment, since cholesterol synthesis in *E. coli* is present in only freshly isolated strains [96,97], this study provides evidence of the structural dependence that *caveolae* might have on other proteins but also cholesterol in the membranes [98]. Interestingly, the location of the cholesterol interacting domain on the Cav-1 nanodisk surrounding this structure (Figure 2, panel c and d) is compatible with the "lipid belt" model proposed to mediate the interaction between some lipids and proteins, including ion channels, some of them described as Cav-1 protein partners in lipid membrane domains (Figure 2, panel e). This observation suggests that Cav-1 nanodisks may be a part of a lipid belt or a "shell" constituting the immediate perimeter of the protein channel [38,99–101], in those channels where no cholesterol interacting domain has been described, complexing and conforming a lipid-protein membrane domain (Figure 2, panel e).

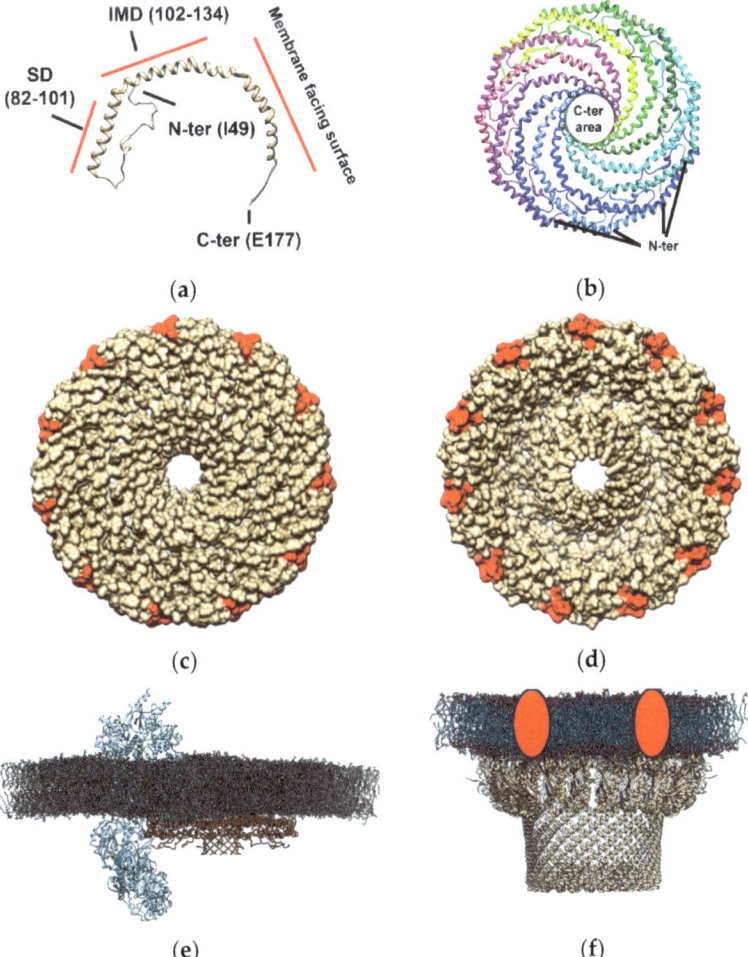

Figure 2. Molecular architecture of caveolin- and flotillin-enriched domains based on Cav-1 forming nanodisks based on the PDB model 7SC0 and as reported in the bibliography [15] and similar proteins to flotillin constituting SPFH domains. Cav-1 constitutes the singular unit for the formation of these structures. The amino and carboxyl end of the protein are labeled as N- and C-end (panel (a)). The scaffolding domains (SD, residues 82–101) and the intermembrane domain (IMD, residues 102–134) formed are shown in respect to the Cav-1 region that faces the membrane as shown in this panel. Nanodisks as formed by 11 Cav-1 protomers (individually labeled with different colors) which are tightly packed disks locating in planar membrane-embedded surfaces (panel (b)). The location of the C-ends oriented to form a central β-barrel "hub" (~28 Å wide), and N-terminal sides forming an outer "rim" (~23 Å wide) for generation of the nanodisks with a 140 Å diameter in size is shown in this panel. Representation of the membrane-oriented Cav-1 nanodisk surface in respect to cholesterol binding site (labeled in red is shown in panel (c). Representation of the cytoplasmic Cav-1 nanodisk surface in respect to cholesterol binding site (labeled in red is shown

in panel (**d**)). Location of the cholesterol binding site at the periphery of the nanodisk is compatible with the "lipid belt" proposed model for the interaction of some lipids with ion channels suggesting that cholesterol may be a part of a lipid belt or a "shell" constituting the immediate perimeter of the channel protein with could be mediated by complexation with Cav-1 nanodisks [38,99–101]. An artistic representation of a Cav-1 nanodisk (PDB: 7SC0, brown-colored backbone) interacting with voltage-dependent L-type calcium channel subunit α-1S (Cav1.1 subunit, PDB: 5GJW, blue-colored backbone) in a model membrane of dipalmitoyl phosphatidylcholine (colored in grey) is shown in panel (**e**). An artistic representation of the macromolecular structure of a flotillin-enriched domain based on that reported in the literature [102], (using 7VHP PDB model, light-brown-colored backbone) complexing with some proteases that might degrade misfolded/damaged membrane proteins or cytoplasmic proteins (red circles) at the membranes (panel (**f**)). Hydrophobic tails are represented in blue and polar heads in red, as described in bacterial membrane microdomains [102].

Regarding caveolin-enriched domains in neurons, certain studies have indicated that neuronal lipid membrane domains associated with caveolin are flat and do not have the invaginated appearance described for *caveolae* [103]. *Caveolae* curvature has been shown to be dependent upon cavin, and its release from lipid membrane domains has been associated with planar non-invaginated surfaces distinct from *caveolae* [20,25–27]. The crystallographic studies that provide evidence for the existence of macromolecular structures organized into Cav-1 nanodisks suggest that neuronal lipid membrane domains might at least be constituted by this structure, serving as fundamental units responsible for caveolin-enriched domains present in the plasma membrane of neurons.

Although the best-known endocytic route in cells is dependent upon clathrin and independent upon lipid membrane domains [104,105], alternative endocytic routes involving lipid membrane domains mediated by *caveolae* exist [106,107]. They rely on the protein named dynamin in some cases on Pacsin-2 and are dependent upon cholesterol, as shown by its sensitivity to cholesterol depletion [108–110]. They have been involved in the uptake of glycosylphosphatidylinositol (GPI)-anchored proteins (GPI-APs) and opportunistic ligands, including simian virus 40 and cholera toxin (CTx) [111]. Some authors have stated that distinct mechanisms of clathrin-independent endocytosis have unique sphingolipid requirements [112], but in many cases a role has been assigned to caveolin as an initiator of intracellular signaling via protein clustering, the segregation of proteins, and the protein trafficking to and from the membrane-associated with G proteins [113,114]. These processes can generally directly regulate channel permeability for calcium or modulate other components that regulate intracellular calcium concentration through the channel [82,115]. For example, secreted neurotrophins (including brain-derived neurotrophic factor (BDNF) and neurotrophic factors (NT): NT3, NT4, and NT5) can exert prolonged effects on presynaptic transmitter secretion or postsynaptic responses [116]. Neurotrophins binding to their receptors (tyrosine kinase (Trk)-A, Trk-B, Trk-C, etc.) occur in discontinuous regions of neuronal cell membranes associated with membrane lipid membrane domains [117].

Regarding the relevance of caveolin-enriched domains in brain neurons in *in vivo* studies, some of them have shown a correlation between Cav-1–knocking down (Cav-1–KD) and the disruption of Cav-1-enriched membrane domains found in neurodegenerative diseases, such Alzheimer's disease where an alteration of signaling processes associated with lipid membrane domains has been also described [118]. Caveolin has also been implicated in synaptic vesicle exocytosis impairment ascribed to changes in synaptic vesicle dynamics driven by Cav-1 palmitoylation using a Cav-1- knock-out animals (Cav-1-KO) [119]. Oppositely, an increase in caveolin expression was found to improve and preserve motor and cognitive function after brain trauma using animal models [120]. These experiments support that Cav-1 levels might enhance cellular survival and growth. Also, some researchers support its role as a candidate for its level modulation to repair the injured and neurodegenerative brain [121,122]. The opposite effect has been observed in some animal models of Huntington's disease, where a loss or reduction of Cav-1 expression rescues the phenotype in neurons and significantly delays the onset of motor decline and development of neurons. Therefore, aberrant interaction between Huntingtin and Cav-1 leading to altered cholesterol homeostasis in these diseases has been suggested [123].

2.2. Histological and Cytological Distribution of Caveolin-Enriched Lipid Membrane Domains in Neurons and Their Function in Calcium Signaling

Cav-1 has been identified as a component of lipid membrane domains localized within cell bodies and dendrites of primary culture of cerebellar granule neurons and Purkinje cells [33,119,124,125], soma and postsynapses of the anterior cingulate cortex neurons in tissue [126,127], cell body and *puncta* localized to areas of cellular outgrowth and synapses and dendritic spines of primary culture of hippocampal neurons [128–130].

A study has shown that Cav-1 partially colocalize with the N-methyl D-aspartate receptor subtype 2B (NR2B) subunit of the N-methyl-D-aspartic acid receptor (NMDAR), which is highly enriched in dendritic shafts and spines of rat cortical neurons at postsynaptic terminals [131,132]. NMDARs are glutamate-gated ion channels that mediate excitatory neurotransmission in the central nervous system (CNS) [133]. The presence of NMDARs at presynapses or postsynapses has a different function. In the case of presynapses, NMDA receptors have a function in neurotransmission and plasticity [134], and postsynaptic receptors are needed for spike-timing-dependent long-term depression (LTD) induction [135]. A study of Cav-1 overexpression in neurons showed that Cav-1 mediated expression of NMDAR subtypes promoting pathways dependent upon the membrane cholesterol associated with primary neuron arborization events [121]. Two regions on NR2B subunits ($W^{635}AFFAVIF^{642}$, and, $F^{1042}SFKSDRY^{1049}$) have been potentially suggested to interact with caveolin-binding motifs [84,132]. A disruption of the interaction between Cav-1 and NR2B has anti-nociceptive effects at the anterior cingulate cortex [126], which correlate with the observed effect of pain agonists promote a shift of the NR2B subunits of NMDA receptor subunit to non-lipid membrane-domain areas [132]. Also, an increased amount of caveolin promotes an enhanced surface level of NR2B in this brain area [126], which leads to an increase in cytosolic calcium concentration and activation of extracellular-signal-regulated kinase/cAMP response element (ERK/CREB) signaling pathways [136]. Thus, decreased caveolin expression in cells disrupts NMDAR signaling events, and reintroducing Cav-1 rescues proper NMDAR signaling. Since NR2B contains the binding site for glutamate [137], this suggests that caveolin is required for the signal transduction pathway activated by glutamate release from the presynaptic terminals [132]. It has been suggested that the regulation of the NR2B subunit by Cav-1 might be attributed to the modulation of proto-oncogene tyrosine-protein kinase (Src) activity since Cav-1 was observed to be essential for NMDA-mediated phosphorylation of Src and ERK1/2 activation [132], which is required for NMDA-mediated signaling (i.e.,: NMDA preconditioning stimuli) [121,132,138].

Src family tyrosine kinases (SFKs) serve as central regulators for the modulation of NMDAR signaling in normal and ischemic conditions and the induction of long-term potentiation (LTP) [139–141]. This modulation accounts for SFK-mediated tyrosine phosphorylation of NR2B, a subunit found highly phosphorylated in postsynaptic terminals [140,141]. Head and collaborators proposed that Cav-1, via its ability to scaffold key signaling components, mediates in the NMDAR localization to neuronal membrane domains, NMDAR/Src tyrosine kinase family/ERK signaling, and protection of neurons from ischemic injury and cell death [132]. Cav-1 promotes NR2B surface levels and has been shown to contribute to the modulation of chronic neuropathic pain in the anterior cingulate cortex [126]. Cellular stress events (i.e., superoxide anion radical, osmotic stress, and UV exposure) can increase SFK-mediated phosphorylation of caveolin [142]. In addition, some studies early reported the existence of a negative regulatory feedback loop in non-neuronal cells in which Y14 phosphorylated Cav-1, would bind and activates C-terminal Src kinase (Csk) and subsequently phosphorylates and inactivates Src [143–146]. In neurons, the regulatory role of Cav-1 phosphorylation/dephosphorylation by Src/Csk has been shown to mediate axonal outgrowth of motor neurons in Xenopus neuromuscular development [147]. Regarding the regulation of the system by oxidative stress, it should be noted that indeed it can activate both Src-kinases and their negative regulator Csk and induces phosphorylation of Cav-1 as a targeting protein for Csk [145]. These results suggest that caveolin could mediate in events mediated by NMDAR, such as those associated with neuronal plasticity and injury that might be associated with oxidative stress [132,148], by regulation of its level of phosphorylation.

Presynaptic NMDA receptors play pivotal roles in excitatory neurotransmission, contributing to synaptic plasticity and facilitating presynaptic neurotransmitter release, functions that are crucial for synaptic maturation and plasticity during formative periods of brain development [134,149,150]. It has been reported that presynaptic NMDA receptors might modulate superoxide anion production by NADPH oxidases (NOXs) [151]. In turn, NMDA receptors may be modulated by superoxide anion by a similar mechanism in postsynapses [142], and locations where NR2B subunits have been found at presynapses as the *cerebellum* [152] and neocortex [153]. In this case, modulation by superoxide anion might be associated with superoxide anion producing enzymes of very specific sources, also clustering within lipid membrane domains [32]. Flavoproteins, such as the enzyme cytochrome b_5 reductase (Cb_5R), have been established to form complexes within plasma membrane lipid membrane domains of cerebellar granule neurons, as those described by our laboratory [28]. Cb_5R is one of the major sources of superoxide anion in the plasma membrane lipid membrane domains of cerebellar granule neurons [29,31]. This protein holds the potential to facilitate certain superoxide anion-dependent adjustments of the NMDA receptor at the presynaptic terminals. The existence of these proteins associated with caveolin [33], might constitute an alternative form of caveolin-enriched lipid membrane-domain subtype in respect to those previously commented.

Both Cb_5R and neuronal nitric oxide synthases (nNOS), as alternative redox flavoproteins located within the neuronal plasma membrane lipid membrane domains, have been proposed to form complexes associated with caveolin-enriched domains [32,33]. These complexes have been postulated to function as redox nanotransducers, in charge of controlling calcium transporters such as the L-type calcium channels and NMDA receptors. These microchip-like structure have been proposed to tightly orchestrate coupling between calcium and nitric oxide signaling in presynapses of glutamatergic cerebellar granule neurons (CGNs) [32]. The co-localization of these components agrees with the suggested effect of glutamate on the activation of NMDA receptors in neuronal terminals containing nNOS, leading to nitric oxide (NO•) formation and amplifying neurotransmitter release, a mechanism early hypothesized by Snyder and Dawson [154]. These specialized domains can promote a localized and transient increase in calcium concentration up to 1 µM within a nearby microcompartments of 100 nm with low calcium buffering capacity [32]. nNOS is inactive at low calcium concentrations, but it active when calcium concentration is high enough to afford a significant saturation of calmodulin ($EC_{50} \approx 0.2$–0.4 µM). The mechanism by which nNOS is regulated by caveolin remains unknown. The modulation of nNOS activity by Cav-1 seems to be distinct from the one observed to regulate endothelial NOS [155].

In hippocampal and cortical neuron cultures, α-amino-3-hydroxy-5-methyl-4-isoxazolepropionic acid receptor (AMPAR) has been associated with caveolin-enriched lipid membrane domains [156]. The AMPAR present in lipid membrane domains is regulated by the activity of NMDAR and NO•-mediated pathways [129,156]. This regulation might be potentially interconnected with redox nanotransducers described above in adjacent domains observed in cerebellar granule neurons, particularly in presynaptic membranes [32]. NO• has a mimicking similar effect to that of NMDA, leading to the recruitment of AMPARs to the surface since lipid membrane domains are required for receptor insertion into the membrane [156]. Cholesterol depletion leads to instability of surface AMPAR, a gradual loss of synapses (both inhibitory and excitatory), and loss of dendritic spines [129].

Metabotropic glutamate receptors (mGluRs) are responsible for so-called slow synaptic transmission associated with the effects of peptide neurotransmitters and non-peptide neuromodulators [157,158]. Metabotropic receptors are G-protein-associated receptors enriched at excitatory synapses [159,160]. There are eight subtypes of mGluRs classified in presynapses as group I mGluRs (formed by mGluR1/mGluR5 subtypes) selectively activated by 3,5-dihydroxyphenylglycine and coupled to inositol phospholipid hydrolysis, group II mGluRs (formed by GluR2/mGluR3 subtypes) and group III mGluRs (formed by mGluR4/mGluR6/mGluR7/mGluR8 subtypes) [161–163]. Association of metabotropic mGluR with caveolin has been shown for group I and II [159,164,165], which might have a wide different location depending on the receptor type [166]. These group I of metabotropic glutamate receptors are modulated by Cav-1 [128] through the caveolin binding motif of the mGlu1 receptor (FVTLIFVLY-ϕXXXXϕXXϕ). Cav-1 interacts with mGluR1 through a motif contained within the last segment of the first transmembrane (TM) domain and the first intracellular loop of the receptor [159]. A second putative Cav-1 binding motif contained within i3 and the first segment of TM6 is also present in mGluR1/5 [159]. Localization of mGluR1/5 in lipid-protein membrane domains is promoted by Cav-1, which controls the rate of constitutive mGluR1 internalization and, therefore, regulates the expression of the receptor at the cell surface [128,159]. Indeed, the control of constitutive mGluR internalization rate and the surface level of mGlu1 has been shown to be dependent upon caveolar/lipid membrane-domain-dependent endocytosis associated with Cav-1 [159]. In addition, activation of other mGluR induced through complex to estrogen receptor subunits has been associated with different caveolin isoforms, including Cav-3 expression, in different brain areas: *striatum*, the estrogen receptor (ER) alpha (ERα)/Cav-1/mGLUR5/Gq GTPases (Gq) complex and the ERα or ERβ/Cav-3/mGLUR3/Gi/o proteins complex; *hippocampus*, ERα/Cav-1/mGLUR1a/Gq complex and the and the ERα or ERβ/Cav3/mGLUR2/Gi/o complex; the *arcuate nucleus*, ERα/Cav-1/mGLUR1a/Gq; astrocytes (*hypothalamus*) ERα/Cav-1/mGLUR1a/Gq; dorsal root ganglion neurons, ERα/Cav3/mGLUR2/Gi/o [167].

A G-protein-dependent intracellular calcium release by activation of phospholipase C (PLC), inositol-3-phosphate (IP3) pathway, and the transient receptor potential canonical channel (TRPC) are components associated with the group I of metabotropic receptors. These proteins are all present in lipid membrane domains [168–171]. Using dihydroxyphenylglycerol, an agonist of the group I mGluR, an increase in the mGluR1α clustering level to phosphorylated caveolin was found [172]. Other studies have shown that, the interaction between Cav-1 and group I mGluRs regulates mGluR-dependent phosphorylation/activation of MAPKs [159]. Lipid membrane-domain disruption with methyl-β-cyclodextrin induced a block in the agonist-dependent mGluR1α internalization, being the implication of caveolin suggested in synaptic plasticity in the *cerebellum* [173].

L-type calcium channels are known to regulate synaptic activity, contributing to the initiation of endosome recycling, which regulates the abundance of synaptic molecules such as AMPA-type glutamate receptors in neuronal dendrites [174]. This function might support the existence of L-type calcium channels associated with caveolin-enriched domain as a lipid membrane nanodomain subtype located at postsynaptic membranes [174]. Some subunits of the L-type calcium channel, such as A2δ-2 subunits, colocalize with proteins binding to gangliosides in alternative lipid membrane-domain structures to those described associated with caveolin [175]. Although non-invaginated caveolar structures have been suggested to exist in neurons, internalization of neurotrophins activated tyrosine kinases receptors (TrkA) [176] and TrkB [118], at growth cones might be dependent upon caveolin-associated endocytosis [177,178]. L-type calcium channels are also very sensitive to oxidative stress, as reported by the NMDA receptor, but in this case, by direct effect since these complexes present an allosteric thiol-containing "redox switch" that controls the activity of the L-type calcium channel [179].

Regulation of N-type calcium channel by Cav-1 has been observed in caveolin-enriched lipid membrane domains of neuroblastoma NG108-15 cell lines [180]. Downregulation of Cav-1 production in these cells induced a 79% reduction in the N-type current density without significant changes in the channel's activation and inactivation time course. The regulation of the channel by membrane cholesterol associated with caveolin was observed to be responsive to this effect rather than induced by direct modulation by caveolin [180]. A similar modulatory effect was observed for R-type voltage calcium channels and neurokinin receptors using kidney cell lines, where cholesterol was responsible for its modulation since intracellular diffusion of Cav-1 scaffolding peptide or overexpression of Cav-1 unaffected the channel function [180].

Localization of the PMCA has also been found at caveolin-enriched lipid membrane domains [33]. The cerebellar synaptosome isoform 4 of the PMCA was specifically localized in this domain with respect to other isoforms locating at non-lipid membrane domains [181]. Some studies show the stimulation of PMCA by acidic phospholipids such as phosphatidylserine [182]. This lipid is normally located at the inner leaflet of plasma membranes and enriched in caveolin-enriched domains in non-neuronal cells [183]. Phosphatidylserine externalization is typical of cell death processes associated with apoptosis [184], and this event might modulate PMCA activity and the interaction this lipid [185].

Purinergic receptors (P2X) have been associated with Cav-1-enriched lipid membrane domains [186–188]. Cooperatively, CaMKIIα and Cav-1 drive ATP-induced membrane delivery of the P2X3 receptor as reported in dorsal root ganglion neurons [187]. The NH_2-terminus of the P2X3 receptor was identified to interact with caveolin through the '$T^{12}KSVVVKSWTI^{22}$' motif and the extended motif '$F^6FTYETTKSVVVKSWTI^{22}$' was engaged to CaMKIIα binding [187]. P2X3 receptors are associated with calcium influxes, which further activate the calcium/calmodulin-dependent protein kinase IIa (CaMKIIa), and are primarily expressed in primary sensory neurons located in dorsal root ganglion (DRG) responsible for pain [189,190]. Upon receptor phosphorylation, an increase in P2X3 interaction with Cav-1 has been observed, providing a mechanism for P2X3 receptor sensitization in pain development [187]. It is particularly noteworthy that immunoreactivity of P2X3 in the plasma membrane was not decreased by the cholesterol depletion with methyl-β-cyclodextrin and cholesterol sequestering had no effect on P2X3- or P2X2/3-mediated inward currents [191]. This result support that the P2X3 receptor may be diffusely distributed in lipid membrane domains and in non-lipid membrane domains in primary sensory neurons [191].

2.3. Flotillin and Neuronal Lipid Membrane Domains

Domains formed by flotillin in the plasma membrane differ from those in which Cav-1 is present. Furthermore, they are dynamic and bud into the cell [192]. The main protein components of these domains are the flotillin isoforms, Flot-1 and Flot-2, which share 50% sequence identity [193]. They are in charge of membrane curvature induction in non-neuronal cells, the formation of plasma-membrane invaginations morphologically similar to *caveolae*, and the accumulation of intracellular vesicles [192]. Early studies suggested flotillin proteins organization into stable tetramers in membrane microdomains [194]. Some studies suggested the possible role of flotillin as a new marker of *caveolae* [194], and subsequent studies have shown that flotillin and caveolin do not always co-localize [56]. Nevertheless, it cannot be discarded that a certain amount of flotillin could be enriched at *caveolae* [195]. An estimation of the size dimension of flotillin-enriched lipid membrane domains by immunolabelling suggests the formation of patches ranging 40–200 nm in neurons [196]. These studies correlate with a description of flotillin protein complexes as part of a family of proteins named SPFH (stomatin, prohibitin, flotillin, and HflK/C) forming an operon with NfeD proteins [197]. The ancient origin of SPFH-domain proteins and the Nodulation efficiency protein D (NfeD) protein and the stomatin operon partner protein (STOPP) can be traced back to the ancient living cells that diverged and evolved to *Archaea* and *Bacteria* to constitute the main binding region of apolar polyisoprenoids as well as cholesterol, contributing to lipid membrane-domain formation [197].

SPFH are proteins enriched in the plasma membranes and also in other subcellular membranes, of prokaryotic and eukaryotic cells [111,198]. Electron microscopy studies have shown a wide distribution of Flot-1 in cells localizing at the cytoplasmic side of the plasma membrane, the cytoplasmic side of primary and secondary lysosome membrane, lipofuscin, multivesicular bodies, Golgi saccules, the cytoplasmic leaflet of the vesicles associated with Golgi apparatus and the lumen side of ER of neuronal cells of rat brain [196]. They have an SPFH domain in common in their structure formed by an N-terminal hydrophobic region that associates proteins to the membrane [111,198]. Flotillin isoforms contain a conserved domain C-terminal to the SPFH domain, called the 'flotillin domain', although is not present in the other SPFH domain-containing proteins [193]. SPFHs can form high ordered structures complexes organized as circular structures comprising homo- or hetero-oligomers [102,199,200]. Several structural membrane microdomain organizations by SPFH family proteins have been proposed [102] (Figure 2, panel f). In flotillin structure, two domains with unclear functions have been shown to be present. The first SPFH domain contains sites for acylation [201,202]. In contrast, the C-terminal domain mediates the oligomerization and contains Ala-Glu repeats and phosphorable Tyr residues [203–205], which are important for flotillin function.

In brain, anatomical and physiological studies have shown that Flot-1 enhances the formation of glutamatergic synapses but not GABAergic synapses, and it has been suggested that this protein might have a role in neurodevelopmental disorders and axon regeneration and growth [206]. Flotillin is recognized as essential for growth cone elongation and regeneration in retinal ganglion cells and mouse hippocampal neurons [207,208]. Notably, when flotillin isoforms are downregulated, and the signaling pathways that govern actin dynamics are disrupted, axon formation fails to occur [209].

Some studies have demonstrated that flotillin directly regulates the formation of cadherin complexes [210,211]. Flotillin-enriched domains have been observed to be required for the dynamic association, stabilization of cadherins at cell–cell junctions [212], transducing extracellular signals into intracellular signaling events, and modulating alterations in the cytoskeleton in response to various external stimuli [213], signal transduction of Trk receptors, and participates in cellular trafficking pathways [214]. However, the molecular mechanism of action of this protein in these processes is not well understood [215].

It is known that Flot-1 acylation determines this protein traffic from the endoplasmic reticulum toward the plasma membrane [210]. Palmitoylated Flot-1 efflux from the endoplasmic reticulum also mediates Cav-1 traffic to the plasma membrane, avoiding the endoplasmic reticulum stress by inhibiting the synthesis of Cav-1 [210]. Once Flot-1 reaches the plasma membrane, it hetero-oligomerizes with Flot-2 and undergoes depalmitoylation/repalmitoylation, which evokes prolonged insulin-like growth factor-1 (IGF-1) signaling [210]. Recently, a role of Flot-1 in mediating the membrane expression and cellular responses of the transient receptor potential vanilloid type 2 (TRPV2) has been described in primary neuronal culture of dorsal root ganglion [216]. This suggests a crosstalk between TRPV2 and lipid membrane-domain components may influence the cellular morphology and play critical roles in nociception and pain [216]. Also, flotillin depalmitoylation has been linked to receptor cycling between the plasma membrane and endosomes alone or with Flot-2 [210].

Although palmitoylation/palmitoylation of flotillins regulate this protein location into lipid membrane domains, the regulatory role of palmitoylation is not exclusive for this protein. Cav-1 can be palmitoylated on multiple cysteine residues although palmitoylation is not necessary for localization of caveolin to *caveolae* [217]. Palmitoylated Cav-1 has been involved in signaling molecules assembly in plasma membrane *caveolae* and in intracellular cholesterol transport [218]. Also, cav-1 palmiltoylation for example, can regulate synaptic vesicle dynamics events [119], which are processes associated with SNARE machinery [219] linked with different plasma membrane domains [220]. Some of the proteins constituting the SNARE complexes might eventually be associated with lipid membrane domains [221,222]. Therefore, this process should not be directly associated with lipid membrane domains [223].

Glebov and collaborators have suggested flotillin participation in a third endocytosis pathway different from those described for clathrin and caveolin [224]. Flot-1 can colocalize in endosomes with the fluid-phase marker dextran, the glycosylphosphatidylinositol-anchored CD59 (GPI-AP CD59), and CTx and is required for a dynamin-independent endocytic pathway that mediates receptor-independent fluid-phase endocytosis and these markers [224]. This supports that gangliosides colocalization might be used to track endocytosis processes, as also suggested for caveolin-enriched lipid membrane domains. In neurons, flotillin was initially discovered in caveolin-independent cholesterol- and glycosphingolipid-enriched membrane microdomains expressed during axon regeneration [212].

2.4. Histological Cytological Distribution of Flotillin-Enriched Lipid Membrane Domains in Neurons and Function Calcium Signaling

Flotillin isoforms have been widely used as a lipid membrane-domain biomarker. Flotillin isoforms have been observed to colocalize with calcium channel $\alpha 1$ subunit CaV2.1, which are subunits of P/Q type calcium channels located presynaptic areas of the brain [175,225], GPI-enriched areas [226] and small uniform *puncta* of pre and postsynapse of hippocampal neurons [206,227], soma and postsynapses of rat cerebral cortex [127]. Flotillin-enriched lipid membrane domains are abundant in the axonal plasma membrane and are found in less amount in somatodendritic membranes [228]. This correlated with electrophysiological results using whole-cell patch clamp, showing that Flot-1 increases in the frequency of miniature excitatory postsynaptic currents but not miniature inhibitory postsynaptic currents. In contrast, amplitude and decay kinetics of either type of synaptic current were unaffected, linking these domains with calcium homeostasis [206].

One-third of the NMDAR clusters with flotillin in cultured hippocampal neurons [227]. In hippocampal neurons, both NR2A and NR2B subunits of NMDARs interact with Flot-1 [227]. Flot-1 has been associated with the NR1 subunit preferentially at synaptic areas rather than non-synaptic NR1-enriched areas of hippocampal neurons [206]. It has been suggested that NMDAR interaction with flotillin is involved in recruiting NMDARs into lipid membrane domains to initiate second messenger signaling cascades linked with receptor depletion for neuronal protection during NMDAR-induced excitotoxicity [229]. Indeed, some lipoprotein receptor involved in cholesterol traffic from astrocytes to neurons, such as low-density lipoprotein receptor-related protein 1 (LRP1) [230–232], has been suggested to influence the composition of postsynaptic protein complexes through NMDA-induced degradation of the postsynaptic density protein 95 (PSD-95) [233], which might link this process with cholesterol homeostasis and regulation of lipid membrane domains enriched on PSD-95. NMDARs can associate with scaffold protein PSD-95 and form signaling complexes that differ in composition depending on whether they are found in the postsynaptic density or the presynaptic lipid membrane domains. Recently, enhancement in the formation of glutamatergic synapses but not gamma-aminobutyric acid-dependent (GABAergic) synapses has been observed by modulation of Flot-1 level, which suggests further exploration of Flot-1 effect in neurodevelopmental disorders [206]. The authors have postulated that flotillin might have a role in the endocytic internalization of the NMDA receptors after high neuronal stimulation, thereby implicating a subtype of flotillin-enriched domain in the modulation of this process [227]. Flot-1 acylation determines this protein traffic from the endoplasmic reticulum toward the plasma membrane and supports the idea that these domains might be involved with the trafficking of these receptors toward the membrane [168].

Flot-1 and Flot-2 are associated with Ras-binding family of small GTPase 11A (Rab11A) and sorting nexin 4 (SNX4) binding proteins that participates in the recycling and co-transportation of PSD-95, N-cadherin, the glutamate receptors GluA1 and GluN1 to be delivered to the postsynaptic membrane in spines of hippocampal neurons [234]. The mechanism of action remains to be determined [234].

The Cav 2.1 subunit (also known as α (1A) subunit) is a component of the P- and Q-type calcium channels [235], which have different locations and properties than the L-type calcium channels associated with caveolin domains. The $\alpha 2\delta$-2 subunit of P- and

Q-type calcium channels [236–238], partitions with Cav2.1 subunit into flotillin-enriched lipid domains isolated from the *cerebellum* [175].

PMCA has also been found in isolated flotillin-enriched lipid membrane domains from dissociated cortical and hippocampal primary neurons in culture, and its activity has been affected by cholesterol depletion [181,239]. The PMCA activity in these domains has been described to be higher than the PMCA activity excluded from these microdomains [240]. The activity decreased when cholesterol was depleted from these domains [240].

2.5. Gangliosides as a Lipid Membrane-Domain Biomarkers for Some Caveolin- and Flotillin-Enriched Lipid Membrane Domains

The presence of gangliosides has been observed in both caveolin- and flotillin-enriched lipid membrane domains [241–243], although they are not specifically localized at the plasma membrane and their properties are not exclusively dependent on their polar head group [244]. This type of lipid is strongly abundant in the brain, i.e., in cerebellar granule neurons, they are 5% of total amphipathic lipids [245]. The resulting ganglioside-driven membrane organization are reliant on its production pattern, which is tightly regulated [244]. Not all gangliosides colocalize at the same type of plasma membrane domains [246]. Some authors have concluded that proteins binding to plasma membrane gangliosides can be divided into host plasma membrane proteins and extracellular proteins [247]. Some gangliosides such as GM1 are known to be particularly enriched in the outer leaflet of neuronal lipid membrane domains and exhibit a nearly exclusive presence within these domains compared to non-lipid membrane domains regions. The lipid membrane domain/non-lipid membrane domain ratio values range from 10 to 1000 [248]. Recent molecular dynamics simulation data have shown that three different subpopulations of gangliosides such as GM1 can be characterized in the same lipid membrane domain [14,249], distributed into the central, peripheric and edge areas, which defines their mobility from less to high [247]. Gangliosides at the edge adopt the typical chalice or butterfly-like (open wings) dimeric conformation [250], although conformational possibilities might be further extended by the biochemical diversity of gangliosides. Ganglioside concentration in the same lipid membrane domain creates a large negative electrostatic surface potential, which is one of the essential properties of lipid membrane domains for protein, toxin, or pathogenic agents easily binding due to the electropositive potential [247].

Two types of gangliosides binding domains (GBD) have been described in proteins present in lipid membrane domains:

- Type 1 GBD, or GBD-1, comprises any membrane protein ganglioside-binding domain able to form a stoichiometric (1:1, mol:mol) complex with a single ganglioside molecule [247]. GBD-1 is generally present at the flexible juxta membrane region interacting with transmembrane glycoproteins [113]. The serotonin 5-HT1A receptor, the tumor stem cell marker CD133 are candidates the EGF and PDGF receptors and ion transporters [247]. These membrane proteins are expected to reside at the edge of a lipid raft.
- Type 2 GBD, or GBD-2 are represented by protein dimeric structures resembling a flower chalice or the open wings of a butterfly [250,251]. The typical protein insertion processes have been associated with these domains in which proteins with a hairpin loop interact with the ganglioside, leading to a conformational change that implicates a deep interaction with the ganglioside [251]. This type of ganglioside-dependent insertion process accounts at the edge of a lipid raft or at the periphery since they need to have sufficient conformational flexibility to accommodate the loop [251]. Chalice-shaped ganglioside dimers are required for HIV fusion with host cell membranes [247,252] and the formation of oligomeric calcium permeable amyloid pores [247,253].

In this organization, it is unclear which proteins present in flotillin and caveolin-enriched domains, and more specifically in the brain, might contain GBDs. Cav-1 and Flot 1 have been shown to colocalize with 5-hydroxytryptamine receptor (5-HT1A) [254], and CD133 colocalize with Cav-1-enriched lipid membrane domains [255], which present GBD-1. Caveolin, but no flotillin [256], has been associated with HIV infection and latency [257,258], and this might correlate with the presence of HIV proteins associated with GBD-2 domain. Increased GM1 concentrations have been found in cerebrospinal fluid ganglioside, indicating neuronal involvement in all stages of HIV-1 infection [259].

2.6. Histological Cytological Distribution of Gangliosides-Enriched Lipid Membrane Domains in Neurons and Function Calcium Signaling

Regarding calcium transport systems, gangliosides are well-known modulators of calcium homeostasis [260]. PMCA2 and 3 are known to be regulated by endogenous ganglioside content, such as the asialoGM1 that promotes a decrease in pump activity [261,262]. This correlates with the identification of PMCA location in caveolin-enriched lipid membrane domains in cerebellar granule neurons by Marques-da-Silva and Gutiérrez-Merino [33]. The highest PMCA activity is present in the lipid membrane domains enriched in cholesterol and gangliosides [263], which correlates with a report showing that neuraminidase treatment and D-threo-1-phenyl-2-decanoylamino-3-morpholino-1-propanol (d-PDMP), a used inhibitor of glycosphingolipid biosynthesis, induce a decrease in PMCA activity [261]. However, the mechanism of PMCA inhibition by GM1 is still under discussion. Some researchers have suggested that GM1 affects the PMCA interaction via calmodulin modulation of calcium pump affinity and the V_{max} [262]. This contrasts with the suggestion of modulation based on the interaction with the calmodulin-binding domain stimulating the phosphatase activity of PMCA by stabilizing E(2) conformer [264,265]. Total lipid membrane domains associated PMCA activity is higher than the PMCA activity excluded from lipid membrane-microdomains [240]. Depletion of cellular cholesterol dramatically inhibited the activity of the lipid membrane-domain-associated PMCA with no effect on the activity of the non-lipid membrane-domain pool [240]. This modulatory function of gangliosides contrasts with that inducing activation of L-type calcium channels, as shown in N18 neuroblastoma cells by the same gangliosides [266].

An almost complete colocalization of NMDARs with the lipid membrane-domain marker ganglioside GM1 has been found in postsynaptic densities close to GM1 [267]. GM1 has been shown to reduce the neurotoxicity of NMDAR, which suggests that receptors located at this location might differentially response to glutamate in this location. However, GM1 does not suppress the function of the NMDAR channel directly [268–270]. This protection might be associated with endocytic internalization of the NMDA receptors associated with flotillin-enriched lipid membrane domains, as indicate above [227].

By electron microscopy, a subpopulation of synaptic membrane fractions has been found to be enriched in GM1, and 46 percent of the labeled vesicles are also labeled the GluR2 subunit of the AMPAR [271]. SFKs has been associated with gangliosides and caveolin-enriched lipid membrane domains [272]. They are important since they also mediate the phosphorylation of the AMPARs [273], and they can mediate GluA2-binding protein exchange through endocytosis of GluA2-containing synaptic AMPARs [60]. This might constitute an additional subtype of lipid membrane domains enriched in gangliosides and implicated in endocytic processes or the same associated with Src and NMDA receptors at excitatory synapses. Location studies suggest that AMPAR within PSD are segregated from NMDA receptor clusters [274,275]. In addition, a study has shown that GM1-bound to GluR2-containing AMPARs are functionally segregated from the AMPAR-trafficking complexes (ATCs) containing Thorase, n-ethylmaleimide-sensitive factor attachment protein gamma (γ-SNAP), N-ethylmaleimide sensitive fusion protein (NSF), and nicalin bind selectively to trisialoganglioside gt1b (GT1b) [276], which could define alternative AMPAR domains at the plasma membrane.

GM1 modulation of calcium channels was first described in neurons using N18 neuroblastoma cells [266,277,278] and primary neurons [279,280]. Studies with N18 cells showed that GM1 blocked the intracellular calcium increase sensitive to dihydropyridine blockers at a concentration of 5 mM [266], proposing GM1 function as a constitutive inhibitor of L-type calcium channels [260]. GM1 functions as neuritogenic molecules in neuronal differentiation phases [278]. Upregulation of this lipid has been found in the plasma and nuclear membranes during axonogenesis [278]. In the presence of neuraminidase (N'ase), an enzyme that increases the cell surface content of GM1, a prolific outgrowth of neurites has been found in Neuro-2a and NG108-15 cells [278]. This effect can be blocked by the cholera toxin B, a biochemical tool extensively used for labeling lipid membrane domains using fluorescent conjugates, which potentiated the effect of N'ase in NG108-15 cells [278].

Although cholera toxin binding to ganglioside GM1 supports that this regulation is mediated by lowering free GM1 concentration in the plasma membrane, it remains to be known whether cholera toxin can be sequestered the GM1 localizing in lipid membrane domains, which might modulate the L-type calcium channels associated with these domains. Neurite outgrowth correlated with the influx of extracellular calcium, which correlates with the reported modulation of calcium channels by gangliosides [260].

Using synaptosomes, the N-type calcium channels has also been found to be activated by GM1 ganglioside, followed by the P-type, and very weakly influencing other channels in cerebrocortical synapses [281]. Based on previous indications showing gangliosides with association with caveolin- and flotillin-enriched lipid membrane domains, it is not clear if calcium transporter elements modulated by this lipid might constitute a population implicated in the endocytic process or just be simply subjected to endocytosis.

3. The Summary of the Distribution Map

A wide range of possible complexes enriched in lipid membrane nanodomain subtypes in the same or different glutamatergic neurons has been described. The organization of NMDAR, L-P/Q calcium channels, some metabotropic receptors, and PMCA located in the synapses of glutamatergic neurons are shown in Figure 3.

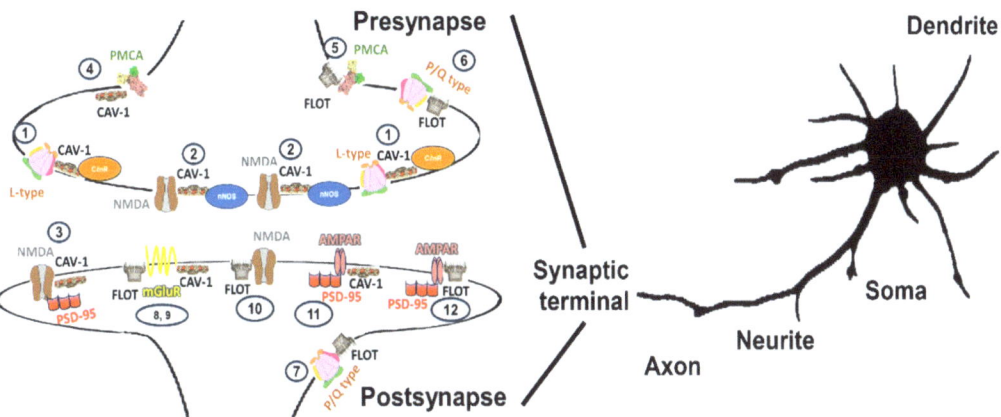

Figure 3. Illustration of a variety of caveolin- and flotillin-enriched lipid membrane domains location complexing with calcium transporter elements (NMDAR, L-P/Q calcium channels, some metabotropic receptors, and PMCA) in synaptic terminals described to exist in glutamatergic neuronal cells. Calcium transporter elements have been differentially described to be present in many neuronal locations, including somas, neurites, axons, dendrites, spines, and synaptic terminals. In synaptic terminals a variability of subunits may yield specific calcium transporters for that location (i.e.,: presynaptic and postsynaptic NMDAR might be differentiated by the type of subunits that configure them in hippocampal neurons [282]) that might differ in configuration from those distributed in other neuronal locations and vary in respect to the neuronal cell type [135]. In this figure, we are focusing on calcium-transporting elements associated with caveolin- and flotillin-enriched lipid membrane domains, that should be added to those elements that are not located in lipid membrane-domain areas (not shown in this figure) and omitted in synaptic terminals

that comprise areas of 0.5 to 2 μm size [283]. Lipid membrane domains associated with gangliosides are suggested to be involved in endocytic processes in some membranes and have been omitted from this figure for the sake of clarity. NMDA (1) and L-type calcium channels (2) located in caveolin-enriched domains might function as redox nanotransducers in charge of the control of these calcium transporters working as a microchip-like structure for a tighter functional coupling between calcium, nitric oxide and superoxide anion signaling in presynapses [32,154,155] and postsynapses (3) also sensitive to superoxide anion [132,142], in glutamatergic CGNs. Also, in associated caveolin-enriched domains at presynapses, we can allocate PMCA (4), which are susceptible of inhibition by GM1 contained in these subdomains [33,261,262]. PMCA has also been described to be present in flotillin-enriched lipid membrane domains (5), which are very sensitive to cholesterol content. The activity in these domains is higher than the one not present in lipid membrane domains [240]. The differential response to endogenous cholesterol and gangliosides seems to support that caveolin and flotillin-enriches domains constitute different lipid membrane nanodomain subtypes in presynaptic terminals. We can also find P/Q-type calcium channels at presynaptic terminals (6) associated with flotillin-enriched domains and GPI-enriched areas [175,225,226]. This type of cluster can also be found in postsynaptic terminals (7) [206], and the physiological behavior has been characterized by the presence of Flot-1 and has been related to and increases in the frequency of miniature excitatory postsynaptic currents. Several subunits of metabotropic receptors have been described to colocalize in caveolin- and flotillin-enriched domains (8) and (9). Subunit interaction with caveolin has been better described than for flotillin. Several motifs of mGlu subunits have been described to interact with cav-1 [128,159], which controls the rate of receptor internalization and location at the surface [128,159]. A function of recruitment of NMDARs into lipid membrane domains at postsynapses to initiate second messenger signaling cascades linked with receptor depletion for neuronal protection in NMDAR-induced excitotoxicity has been suggested for NMDAR located at flotillin-enriched domains (10) [212]. As previously indicated, NMDARs can associate with scaffold protein PSD-95 and form signaling complexes that differ in their composition. Some subunits of the AMPAR have also been located in caveolin- (11) and flotillin-enriched domains (12) at post synaptic terminals associated with PSD-95. NO• has a similar effect mimicking that of NMDA, recruiting AMPARs to lipid membrane-domain surface which suggest a counterplay with lipid membrane domains associated with postsynaptic domains (3) or presynaptic (1) and (2) domains since NO• can reach this location by diffusion from presynaptic sources.

A summary of the components implicated in calcium signaling in neurons and their association and function with each lipid membrane-domain subtype can be found in the Table 1.

Table 1. Calcium signaling components and distribution map in lipid raft-domain subtypes.

Type	Subunit	Neuronal Type	Associated with Raft Component	Main Distribution in Brain and Subcellular Location	Function
L-type	Cav1.2	Primary culture of cerebellar granule neurons and Purkinje cells [30,279]	Cav-1 and GM1 [30], GM1 [279]		Neuronal calcium transients in cell bodies and dendrites, regulation of enzyme activity, regulation of transcription [125]
P/Q-type	Cav2.1	Cerebellar Purkinje neurons (tissue [175]; primary culture [284]; brain synaptosomal fraction [225])	Flot-1 [175], GM1 [225,284]	Hippocampus [285], dorsal root ganglion neurons [286], presynaptic areas [225,286]	Neurotransmitter release, dendritic calcium transients [125]
L/P/Q/N-type	α2δ-2, α2δ-3 [226]	Hippocampal neurons (raft isolation and microscopy) [226]	Flot-1 [226]	GPI-enriched areas [226]	
NMDA	NR1	Primary cultures of hippocampal neurons [206]; ganglion cells in rat retina (tissue) [287,288]; ventral part of lamina III and in laminae III and IV [289]	Flot-1 [206]; GM1 [287–289]	Small uniform puncta throughout the neuron, pre and postsynapses [206,289]; ganglion cell dendrites [287], extrasynaptic plasma membrane [288]	Signaling complexes in the postsynaptic density [290], glutamatergic signaling, synaptic plasticity, excitotoxicity, and memory [132], neurite outgrowth and axonal growth cone motility [291,292]
	NR2B	Anterior cingulate cortex neurons in tissue and cultured (microscopy and immunoprecipitation) [126]; neurons from normal rat cerebral cortex (raft isolation, microscopy and immunoprecipitation) [127]; primary culture of cortical neurons (microscopy and raft isolation) [132]; ganglion cells in rat retina (tissue) [287,288]	Cav-1 [126,127], Flot-1 [127]; GM1 [287,288]	Soma and postsynapses [126,127]; ganglion cell dendrites extrasynapses peri-synapses [287,288]	
	NR2A [227]	Cultured hippocampal neurons (microscopy and raft isolation) [227]	Flot-1 and -2 [227]	Small uniform puncta throughout the neuron [227]	

Table 1. Cont.

Type	Subunit	Neuronal Type	Associated with Raft Component	Main Distribution in Brain and Subcellular Location	Function
AMPAR	GluA2 [130]	Primary culture of hippocampal neurons (microscopy, immunoprecipitation and raft preparation) [130]	Cav-1 [130]	Cell body and as puncta localized to areas of cellular outgrowth [130]	Postsynaptic currents mediated by the AMPA subtype of glutamate receptors in LTP [293]; long-term potentiation (LTP) induced GluA1 surface exposure [294]
	GluA1 [156,234]	Primary culture of hippocampal neurons (microscopy and raft isolation) [156,234]	Flot-1 and -2 [234], Cav-1 [129], GM1 [156]	Postsynapses [156], synapses and dendritic Spines [129]	
	GluR2/3 [129]	Primary culture of hippocampal neurons (microscopy) [129], synaptosomes [271]; ganglion cells in rat retina (tissue) [287]	Cav-1 [129], GM1 [271,287]	Synapses and dendritic spines [129]; dendrites and somata [287]	
	GluR4	Ganglion cells in rat retina (tissue) [287]	GM1 [287]	Dendrites and somata [287]	
mGluR	mGluR1/5	Primary hippocampal neurons (microscopy and immunoprecipitation) [128]	Cav-1 [128]	Soma and dendrites [128]; postsynaptic density late in development [295]	Synapse formation and plasticity [159]
	mGluR1a	Hippocampus, *arcuate nucleus, hypothalamus* [167]	Cav-1 [167]		Caveolin proteins act to functionally isolate distinct estrogen receptors and mGluRs, leading to activation of specific second messenger signaling cascades [167]
	mGluR1α	Synaptosomes from pig *cerebellum*	Cav-1 and Flot [173,248]		By application of MβCD, interaction of phosphorylated caveolin with the receptor decreased, and finally, internalization of the receptor was blocked [173]

Table 1. *Cont.*

Type	Subunit	Neuronal Type	Associated with Raft Component	Main Distribution in Brain and Subcellular Location	Function
Pumps	PMCA isoform 4	Synaptosomes from pig *cerebellum* (Brij96 extracts) [181]	ganglioside GM1 [181]		Discrete functional positions on the synaptic nerve terminals [181]
Purinergic receptors	P2X3	Rat brain, cerebellar granule neurons in culture (microscopy, immunoprecipitation and raft preparation), dorsal root ganglion neurons in culture	Flot-2, Cav-1	P2X3 subunit is expressed in cell bodies as well as in peripheral and central terminals of sensory neurons in dorsal root ganglia (DRG) [296,297]	Well-defined role in pain perception [298,299]. Cav-1 is required for basal and ligand-induced membrane delivery of the P2X3 receptor [187]

Note: The reason for no data regarding some of the calcium components and the main distribution in brain and subcellular location is the description of these calcium components in experiments performed *in vitro* in culture. Although some of these cultures were prepared from tissue, we thought this should be differentiated from histochemical studies reporting calcium transported elements in rafts directly visualized on tissue slices or directly prepared or isolated from those tissues.

4. Conclusions

Future work should further elucidate the relationship between caveolin- and flotillin-enriched domains and the proteins and lipid partners present in each type of platform that, as shown in this review, may form different lipid membrane-domain subtypes. This includes the effect of cholesterol in calcium signaling and the potential modulation of elements in charge, including calcium channels, that might differentially interact with this lipid in neurons, concerning the same population of protein that might present in non- lipid membrane-domain areas. The cumulative experimental evidence analyzed in this review suggest that lipid membrane-domain subtypes are likely to exist in neurons, largely based on the well-known location and distribution of calcium transporter elements differentially interacting with caveolin- and flotillin-enriched domains.

There is a need for a better characterization of the molecular components of different lipid membrane-domain subtypes in different types of neurons, and of the role of protein-protein and protein-lipid interactions in the functional modulation of the components of these domains. One of the open questions to be answered is associated with the role of cholesterol and its effects, induced by direct interaction with proteins or by changes in the physical-chemical properties of the membranes. Cholesterol enantiomers are potential tools that might help to answer this question since they have identical physical properties to cholesterol but opposite three-dimensional configurations compared to cholesterol [300]. An additional question that needs to be addressed in the future concerns the presence of proteins such as cavin that are present in *caveolae* of non-neuronal cells and seem to be required for the plasma membrane curvature. Neuronal plasma membranes are non-invaginated, suggesting that cavin is not present in these structures, but it should not be discarded the presence of other Cav-1 homologous partners at the neuronal lipid membrane domains that have been determined to be present in non-neuronal cells such as caveolin-2 (Cav-2). Cav-2 is a protein that has also been located at neuronal plasma membrane lipid membrane domains. Indeed, antibodies against this protein have been shown to be helpful in inhibiting some of the protein activities associated with plasma membrane lipid membrane nanodomains of synaptosomes, such as Cb_5R activity [29,31]. Although an antagonist role has been described for Cav-2 with respect to Cav-1 due to the ability of Cav-2 to bind cholesterol [301], it cannot be discarded the presence of Cav-2 in the same domains or its role as a major component of some lipid membrane nanodomain subtype. Besides calcium transport channels, the majority of the proteins associated with lipid membrane domains are lipid-anchored proteins [302,303]. Cholesterol might also modulate the dynamics of bulk phases in membranes, altering membrane proteins' folding and stability, and impacting energetics for protein oligomerization [304]. The hypothetical role of recently discovered molecular architectures enriched in caveolin-forming nanodisks [15], in buffering, distributing, or controlling cholesterol availability for neuronal plasma membrane proteins deserves to be studied in future studies.

Author Contributions: Conceptualization, A.K.S.-A. and C.G.-M.; writing—original draft preparation, A.K.S.-A.; writing—review and editing, A.K.S.-A., J.P., D.M.-d.-S., O.H.M.-C. and C.G.-M.; visualization, A.K.S.-A.; supervision, C.G.-M. All authors have read and agreed to the published version of the manuscript.

Funding: This research received no external funding.

Acknowledgments: We would like to thank *Molecules* and MDPI for the support and organization of the Special Issue dedicated to Carlos Gutiérrez-Merino: "Themed Issue in Honor of Carlos Gutiérrez Merino: Forty Years of Research Excellence in the Field of Membrane Proteins and Bioenergetics.".

Conflicts of Interest: The authors declare no conflict of interest.

Abbreviations

5-hydroxytryptamine receptor (5-HT1A); NSF attachment protein (γ-SNAP); α-amino-3-hydroxy-5-methyl-4-isoxazolepropionic acid receptor (AMPAR); AMPAR-trafficking complexes (ATCs); brain-derived neurotrophic factor (BDNF); calcium/calmodulin-dependent protein kinase IIa (CaMKIIa); caveolin-1 (Cav-1); Cav-1–knocking down (Cav-1–KD); caveolin-2 (Cav-2); cytochrome b_5 reductase (Cb_5R); cerebellar granule neurons (CGN); caveolin binding motif (CMB); central nervous system (CNS); Cholesterol Recognition/Interaction Amino Acid Consensus (CRAC); C-terminal Src kinase (CsK); cholera toxin (CTx); dorsal root ganglion (DRG); estrogen receptor (ER); fluorescence energy transfer (FRET); ganglioside binding domains (GBD); monosialotetrahexosylganglioside (GM1); glycosylphosphatidylinositol (GPI); trisialoganglioside gt1b (GT1b); insulin-like growth factor-1 (IGF-1); intermembrane domain (IMD); inositol-3-phosphate (IP3); long-term depression (LTD); low-density lipoprotein receptor-related protein 1 (LRP1); metabotropic glutamate receptors (mGluRs); neuraminidase (N'ase); modulation efficiency protein D (NfeD); N-methyl-D-aspartate receptor (NMDAr); neuronal nitric oxide synthase (nNOS); NADPH oxidases (NOXs); N-ethylmaleimide sensitive fusion protein (NSF); NMDAr subtype 2B subunit (NR2B); oligomerization domain (OD); purinergic P2X receptor (P2XR); protein data bank (PBD); phospholipase C (PLC); plasma membrane calcium ATPase (PMCA); postsynaptic density protein 95 (PSD-95); scaffolding domain (SD); Src tyrosine kinase family (SFK); signature motif (SM); stomatin, prohibitin, flotillin, and HflK/C domains (SPFH); stomatin operon partner protein (STOPP); transmembrane (TM); tyrosine kinase receptors (Trk); transient receptor potential canonical channel (TRPC); transient receptor potential vanilloid type 2 (TRPV2).

References

1. Pike, L.J. Rafts Defined: A Report on the Keystone Symposium on Lipid Rafts and Cell Function. *J. Lipid Res.* **2006**, *47*, 1597–1598. [CrossRef] [PubMed]
2. Goñi, F.M. "Rafts": A Nickname for Putative Transient Nanodomains. *Chem. Phys. Lipids* **2019**, *218*, 34–39. [CrossRef]
3. Eggeling, C.; Ringemann, C.; Medda, R.; Schwarzmann, G.; Sandhoff, K.; Polyakova, S.; Belov, V.N.; Hein, B.; von Middendorff, C.; Schönle, A.; et al. Direct Observation of the Nanoscale Dynamics of Membrane Lipids in a Living Cell. *Nature* **2009**, *457*, 1159–1162. [CrossRef] [PubMed]
4. Klotzsch, E.; Schütz, G.J. A Critical Survey of Methods to Detect Plasma Membrane Rafts. *Philos. Trans. R. Soc. B Biol. Sci.* **2013**, *368*, 20120033. [CrossRef]
5. Kusumi, A.; Fujiwara, T.K.; Tsunoyama, T.A.; Kasai, R.S.; Liu, A.-A.; Hirosawa, K.M.; Kinoshita, M.; Matsumori, N.; Komura, N.; Ando, H.; et al. Defining Raft Domains in the Plasma Membrane. *Traffic* **2020**, *21*, 106–137. [CrossRef] [PubMed]
6. Hernández-Adame, P.L.; Meza, U.; Rodríguez-Menchaca, A.A.; Sánchez-Armass, S.; Ruiz-García, J.; Gomez, E. Determination of the Size of Lipid Rafts Studied through Single-Molecule FRET Simulations. *Biophys. J.* **2021**, *120*, 2287–2295. [CrossRef] [PubMed]
7. Pralle, A.; Keller, P.; Florin, E.L.; Simons, K.; Hörber, J.K. Sphingolipid-Cholesterol Rafts Diffuse as Small Entities in the Plasma Membrane of Mammalian Cells. *J. Cell Biol.* **2000**, *148*, 997–1008. [CrossRef]
8. Yethiraj, A.; Weisshaar, J.C. Why Are Lipid Rafts Not Observed In Vivo? *Biophys. J.* **2007**, *93*, 3113–3119. [CrossRef]
9. Sharma, P.; Varma, R.; Sarasij, R.C.; Ira; Gousset, K.; Krishnamoorthy, G.; Rao, M.; Mayor, S. Nanoscale Organization of Multiple GPI-Anchored Proteins in Living Cell Membranes. *Cell* **2004**, *116*, 577–589. [CrossRef]
10. Martosella, J.; Zolotarjova, N.; Liu, H.; Moyer, S.C.; Perkins, P.D.; Boyes, B.E. High Recovery HPLC Separation of Lipid Rafts for Membrane Proteome Analysis. *J. Proteome Res.* **2006**, *5*, 1301–1312. [CrossRef]
11. Yu, H.; Wakim, B.; Li, M.; Halligan, B.; Tint, G.S.; Patel, S.B. Quantifying Raft Proteins in Neonatal Mouse Brain by "tube-Gel" Protein Digestion Label-Free Shotgun Proteomics. *Proteome Sci.* **2007**, *5*, 17. [CrossRef] [PubMed]
12. Kalinowska, M.; Castillo, C.; Francesconi, A. Quantitative Profiling of Brain Lipid Raft Proteome in a Mouse Model of Fragile X Syndrome. *PLoS ONE* **2015**, *10*, e0121464. [CrossRef]
13. Ledesma, M.D.; Da Silva, J.S.; Schevchenko, A.; Wilm, M.; Dotti, C.G. Proteomic Characterisation of Neuronal Sphingolipid-Cholesterol Microdomains: Role in Plasminogen Activation. *Brain Res.* **2003**, *987*, 107–116. [CrossRef]
14. Galimzyanov, T.R.; Lyushnyak, A.S.; Aleksandrova, V.V.; Shilova, L.A.; Mikhalyov, I.I.; Molotkovskaya, I.M.; Akimov, S.A.; Batishchev, O.V. Line Activity of Ganglioside GM1 Regulates the Raft Size Distribution in a Cholesterol-Dependent Manner. *Langmuir* **2017**, *33*, 3517–3524. [CrossRef]
15. Porta, J.C.; Han, B.; Gulsevin, A.; Chung, J.M.; Peskova, Y.; Connolly, S.; Mchaourab, H.S.; Meiler, J.; Karakas, E.; Kenworthy, A.K.; et al. Molecular Architecture of the Human Caveolin-1 Complex. *Sci. Adv.* **2022**, *8*, eabn7232. [CrossRef] [PubMed]
16. Yokoyama, H.; Matsui, I. Higher-Order Structure Formation Using Refined Monomer Structures of Lipid Raft Markers, Stomatin, Prohibitin, Flotillin, and HflK/C-Related Proteins. *FEBS Open Bio* **2023**, *13*, 926–937. [CrossRef]

17. Ayuyan, A.G.; Cohen, F.S. Raft Composition at Physiological Temperature and pH in the Absence of Detergents. *Biophys. J.* **2008**, *94*, 2654–2666. [CrossRef]
18. Lamaze, C.; Tardif, N.; Dewulf, M.; Vassilopoulos, S.; Blouin, C.M. The Caveolae Dress Code: Structure and Signaling. *Curr. Opin. Cell Biol.* **2017**, *47*, 117–125. [CrossRef]
19. Stoeber, M.; Schellenberger, P.; Siebert, C.A.; Leyrat, C.; Helenius, A.; Grünewald, K. Model for the Architecture of Caveolae Based on a Flexible, Net-like Assembly of Cavin1 and Caveolin Discs. *Proc. Natl. Acad. Sci. USA* **2016**, *113*, E8069–E8078. [CrossRef]
20. Matthaeus, C.; Sochacki, K.A.; Dickey, A.M.; Puchkov, D.; Haucke, V.; Lehmann, M.; Taraska, J.W. The Molecular Organization of Differentially Curved Caveolae Indicates Bendable Structural Units at the Plasma Membrane. *Nat. Commun.* **2022**, *13*, 7234. [CrossRef]
21. Lee, J.; Glover, K.J. The Transmembrane Domain of Caveolin-1 Exhibits a Helix-Break-Helix Structure. *Biochim. Biophys. Acta* **2012**, *1818*, 1158–1164. [CrossRef] [PubMed]
22. Parton, R.G.; Tillu, V.; McMahon, K.-A.; Collins, B.M. Key Phases in the Formation of Caveolae. *Curr. Opin. Cell Biol.* **2021**, *71*, 7–14. [CrossRef] [PubMed]
23. Jarsch, I.K.; Daste, F.; Gallop, J.L. Membrane Curvature in Cell Biology: An Integration of Molecular Mechanisms. *J. Cell Biol.* **2016**, *214*, 375–387. [CrossRef] [PubMed]
24. Has, C.; Das, S.L. Recent Developments in Membrane Curvature Sensing and Induction by Proteins. *Biochim. Biophys. Acta Gen. Subj.* **2021**, *1865*, 129971. [CrossRef] [PubMed]
25. Gambin, Y.; Ariotti, N.; McMahon, K.-A.; Bastiani, M.; Sierecki, E.; Kovtun, O.; Polinkovsky, M.E.; Magenau, A.; Jung, W.; Okano, S.; et al. Single-Molecule Analysis Reveals Self Assembly and Nanoscale Segregation of Two Distinct Cavin Subcomplexes on Caveolae. *Elife* **2013**, *3*, e01434. [CrossRef] [PubMed]
26. Sinha, B.; Köster, D.; Ruez, R.; Gonnord, P.; Bastiani, M.; Abankwa, D.; Stan, R.V.; Butler-Browne, G.; Vedie, B.; Johannes, L.; et al. Cells Respond to Mechanical Stress by Rapid Disassembly of Caveolae. *Cell* **2011**, *144*, 402–413. [CrossRef] [PubMed]
27. Parton, R.G.; McMahon, K.-A.; Wu, Y. Caveolae: Formation, Dynamics, and Function. *Curr. Opin. Cell Biol.* **2020**, *65*, 8–16. [CrossRef]
28. Samhan-Arias, A.K.; García-Bereguiaín, M.A.; Martín-Romero, F.J.; Gutiérrez-Merino, C. Regionalization of Plasma Membrane-Bound Flavoproteins of Cerebellar Granule Neurons in Culture by Fluorescence Energy Transfer Imaging. *J. Fluoresc.* **2006**, *16*, 393–401. [CrossRef]
29. Samhan-Arias, A.K.; Garcia-Bereguiain, M.A.; Martin-Romero, F.J.; Gutierrez-Merino, C. Clustering of Plasma Membrane-Bound Cytochrome B5 Reductase within "lipid Raft" Microdomains of the Neuronal Plasma Membrane. *Mol. Cell Neurosci.* **2009**, *40*, 14–26. [CrossRef]
30. Marques-da-Silva, D.; Samhan-Arias, A.K.; Tiago, T.; Gutierrez-Merino, C. L-Type Calcium Channels and Cytochrome B5 Reductase Are Components of Protein Complexes Tightly Associated with Lipid Rafts Microdomains of the Neuronal Plasma Membrane. *J. Proteom.* **2010**, *73*, 1502–1510. [CrossRef]
31. Samhan-Arias, A.K.; Marques-da-Silva, D.; Yanamala, N.; Gutierrez-Merino, C. Stimulation and Clustering of Cytochrome B5 Reductase in Caveolin-Rich Lipid Microdomains Is an Early Event in Oxidative Stress-Mediated Apoptosis of Cerebellar Granule Neurons. *J. Proteom.* **2012**, *75*, 2934–2949. [CrossRef]
32. Marques-da-Silva, D.; Gutierrez-Merino, C. L-Type Voltage-Operated Calcium Channels, N-Methyl-d-Aspartate Receptors and Neuronal Nitric-Oxide Synthase Form a Calcium/Redox Nano-Transducer within Lipid Rafts. *Biochem. Biophys. Res. Commun.* **2012**, *420*, 257–262. [CrossRef]
33. Marques-da-Silva, D.; Gutierrez-Merino, C. Caveolin-Rich Lipid Rafts of the Plasma Membrane of Mature Cerebellar Granule Neurons Are Microcompartments for Calcium/Reactive Oxygen and Nitrogen Species Cross-Talk Signaling. *Cell Calcium* **2014**, *56*, 108–123. [CrossRef]
34. Samhan-Arias, A.K.; López-Sánchez, C.; Marques-da-Silva, D.; Lagoa, R.; Garcia-Lopez, V.; García-Martínez, V.; Gutierrez-Merino, C. High Expression of Cytochrome B5 Reductase Isoform 3/Cytochrome B5 System in the Cerebellum and Pyramidal Neurons of Adult Rat Brain. *Brain Struct. Funct.* **2016**, *221*, 2147–2162. [CrossRef]
35. Poejo, J.; Salazar, J.; Mata, A.M.; Gutierrez-Merino, C. Binding of Amyloid β(1-42)-Calmodulin Complexes to Plasma Membrane Lipid Rafts in Cerebellar Granule Neurons Alters Resting Cytosolic Calcium Homeostasis. *Int. J. Mol. Sci.* **2021**, *22*, 1984. [CrossRef]
36. Poejo, J.; Orantos-Aguilera, Y.; Martin-Romero, F.J.; Mata, A.M.; Gutierrez-Merino, C. Internalized Amyloid-β (1–42) Peptide Inhibits the Store-Operated Calcium Entry in HT-22 Cells. *Int. J. Mol. Sci.* **2022**, *23*, 12678. [CrossRef]
37. Bonini, I.C.; Antollini, S.S.; Gutiérrez-Merino, C.; Barrantes, F.J. Sphingomyelin Composition and Physical Asymmetries in Native Acetylcholine Receptor-Rich Membranes. *Eur. Biophys. J.* **2002**, *31*, 417–427. [CrossRef]
38. Antollini, S.S.; Soto, M.A.; Bonini de Romanelli, I.; Gutiérrez-Merino, C.; Sotomayor, P.; Barrantes, F.J. Physical State of Bulk and Protein-Associated Lipid in Nicotinic Acetylcholine Receptor-Rich Membrane Studied by Laurdan Generalized Polarization and Fluorescence Energy Transfer. *Biophys. J.* **1996**, *70*, 1275–1284. [CrossRef]
39. Gutiérrez-Merino, C.; Bonini de Romanelli, I.C.; Pietrasanta, L.I.; Barrantes, F.J. Preferential Distribution of the Fluorescent Phospholipid Probes NBD-Phosphatidylcholine and Rhodamine-Phosphatidylethanolamine in the Exofacial Leaflet of Acetylcholine Receptor-Rich Membranes from Torpedo Marmorata. *Biochemistry* **1995**, *34*, 4846–4855. [CrossRef]

40. Parekh, A.B. Ca^{2+} Microdomains near Plasma Membrane Ca^{2+} Channels: Impact on Cell Function. *J. Physiol.* **2008**, *586*, 3043–3054. [CrossRef]
41. Mironov, S.L. Rethinking Calcium Profiles around Single Channels: The Exponential and Periodic Calcium Nanodomains. *Sci. Rep.* **2019**, *9*, 17196. [CrossRef] [PubMed]
42. Wu, Y.-L.; Tschanz, A.; Krupnik, L.; Ries, J. Quantitative Data Analysis in Single-Molecule Localization Microscopy. *Trends Cell Biol.* **2020**, *30*, 837–851. [CrossRef]
43. Wang, L.-Y.; Augustine, G.J. Presynaptic Nanodomains: A Tale of Two Synapses. *Front. Cell. Neurosci.* **2015**, *8*, 455. [CrossRef]
44. Chen, Y.; Matveev, V. Stationary Ca2+ Nanodomains in the Presence of Buffers with Two Binding Sites. *Biophys. J.* **2021**, *120*, 1942–1956. [CrossRef]
45. Kwon, D. The Quest to Map the Mouse Brain. *Nature* **2023**, *620*, 685–687. [CrossRef]
46. Holmes, K.L.; Lantz, L.M.; Russ, W. Conjugation of Fluorochromes to Monoclonal Antibodies. In *Current Protocols in Cytometry*; Chapter 4, Unit 4.2; Wiley Periodicals LLC.: Hoboken, NJ, USA, 2001. [CrossRef]
47. Haugland, R.P. Antibody Conjugates for Cell Biology. In *Current Protocols in Molecular Biology*; Chapter 16, Unit 16.5; Wiley Periodicals LLC.: Hoboken, NJ, USA, 2001. [CrossRef]
48. Haugland, R.P. Coupling of Monoclonal Antibodies with Fluorophores. *Methods Mol. Biol.* **1995**, *45*, 205–221. [CrossRef]
49. Vira, S.; Mekhedov, E.; Humphrey, G.; Blank, P.S. Fluorescent-Labeled Antibodies: Balancing Functionality and Degree of Labeling. *Anal. Biochem.* **2010**, *402*, 146–150. [CrossRef]
50. Gutierrez-Merino, C. Quantitation of the Förster Energy Transfer for Two-Dimensional Systems. II. Protein Distribution and Aggregation State in Biological Membranes. *Biophys. Chem.* **1981**, *14*, 259–266. [CrossRef]
51. Gutierrez-Merino, C.; Centeno, F.; Garcia-Martin, E.; Merino, J.M. Fluorescence Resonance Energy Transfer as a Tool to Locate Functional Sites in Membrane Proteins. *Biochem. Soc. Trans.* **1994**, *22*, 784–788. [CrossRef] [PubMed]
52. Dewey, T.G.; Hammes, G.G. Calculation on Fluorescence Resonance Energy Transfer on Surfaces. *Biophys. J.* **1980**, *32*, 1023–1035. [CrossRef]
53. Stryer, L. Fluorescence Energy Transfer as a Spectroscopic Ruler. *Annu. Rev. Biochem.* **1978**, *47*, 819–846. [CrossRef]
54. Pol, A.; Morales-Paytuví, F.; Bosch, M.; Parton, R.G. Non-Caveolar Caveolins—Duties Outside the Caves. *J. Cell Sci.* **2020**, *133*, jcs241562. [CrossRef]
55. Simons, K.; Toomre, D. Lipid Rafts and Signal Transduction. *Nat. Rev. Mol. Cell Biol.* **2000**, *1*, 31–39. [CrossRef]
56. Lang, D.M.; Lommel, S.; Jung, M.; Ankerhold, R.; Petrausch, B.; Laessing, U.; Wiechers, M.F.; Plattner, H.; Stuermer, C.A. Identification of Reggie-1 and Reggie-2 as Plasmamembrane-Associated Proteins Which Cocluster with Activated GPI-Anchored Cell Adhesion Molecules in Non-Caveolar Micropatches in Neurons. *J. Neurobiol.* **1998**, *37*, 502–523. [CrossRef]
57. Lipid Raft Microdomains and Neurotransmitter Signalling | Nature Reviews Neuroscience. Available online: https://www.nature.com/articles/nrn2059 (accessed on 26 August 2023).
58. Muallem, S.; Chung, W.Y.; Jha, A.; Ahuja, M. Lipids at Membrane Contact Sites: Cell Signaling and Ion Transport. *EMBO Rep.* **2017**, *18*, 1893–1904. [CrossRef]
59. Grassi, S.; Giussani, P.; Mauri, L.; Prioni, S.; Sonnino, S.; Prinetti, A. Lipid Rafts and Neurodegeneration: Structural and Functional Roles in Physiologic Aging and Neurodegenerative Diseases. *J. Lipid Res.* **2020**, *61*, 636–654. [CrossRef]
60. Hayashi, T. Membrane Lipid Rafts Are Required for AMPA Receptor Tyrosine Phosphorylation. *Front. Synaptic Neurosci.* **2022**, *14*, 921772. [CrossRef]
61. Chen, J.; Sitsel, A.; Benoy, V.; Sepúlveda, M.R.; Vangheluwe, P. Primary Active Ca^{2+} Transport Systems in Health and Disease. *Cold Spring Harb. Perspect. Biol.* **2020**, *12*, a035113. [CrossRef] [PubMed]
62. Ge, L.; Qi, W.; Wang, L.-J.; Miao, H.-H.; Qu, Y.-X.; Li, B.-L.; Song, B.-L. Flotillins Play an Essential Role in Niemann-Pick C1-like 1-Mediated Cholesterol Uptake. *Proc. Natl. Acad. Sci. USA* **2011**, *108*, 551–556. [CrossRef] [PubMed]
63. Roitbak, T.; Surviladze, Z.; Tikkanen, R.; Wandinger-Ness, A. A Polycystin Multiprotein Complex Constitutes a Cholesterol-Containing Signalling Microdomain in Human Kidney Epithelia. *Biochem. J.* **2005**, *392*, 29–38. [CrossRef] [PubMed]
64. Volonte, D.; Galbiati, F.; Li, S.; Nishiyama, K.; Okamoto, T.; Lisanti, M.P. Flotillins/Cavatellins Are Differentially Expressed in Cells and Tissues and Form a Hetero-Oligomeric Complex with Caveolins in Vivo. Characterization and Epitope-Mapping of a Novel Flotillin-1 Monoclonal Antibody Probe. *J. Biol. Chem.* **1999**, *274*, 12702–12709. [CrossRef]
65. Yang, G.; Xu, H.; Li, Z.; Li, F. Interactions of Caveolin-1 Scaffolding and Intramembrane Regions Containing a CRAC Motif with Cholesterol in Lipid Bilayers. *Biochim. Biophys. Acta* **2014**, *1838*, 2588–2599. [CrossRef]
66. Hanafusa, K.; Hayashi, N. The Flot2 Component of the Lipid Raft Changes Localization during Neural Differentiation of P19C6 Cells. *BMC Mol. Cell Biol.* **2019**, *20*, 38. [CrossRef]
67. Wåhlén, E.; Olsson, F.; Söderberg, O.; Lennartsson, J.; Heldin, J. Differential Impact of Lipid Raft Depletion on Platelet-Derived Growth Factor (PDGF)-Induced ERK1/2 MAP-Kinase, SRC and AKT Signaling. *Cell. Signal.* **2022**, *96*, 110356. [CrossRef]
68. Ouweneel, A.B.; Thomas, M.J.; Sorci-Thomas, M.G. The Ins and Outs of Lipid Rafts: Functions in Intracellular Cholesterol Homeostasis, Microparticles, and Cell Membranes. *J. Lipid Res.* **2020**, *61*, 676–686. [CrossRef]
69. Davidović, D.; Kukulka, M.; Sarmento, M.J.; Mikhalyov, I.; Gretskaya, N.; Chmelová, B.; Ricardo, J.C.; Hof, M.; Cwiklik, L.; Šachl, R. Which Moiety Drives Gangliosides to Form Nanodomains? *J. Phys. Chem. Lett.* **2023**, *14*, 5791–5797. [CrossRef]
70. Matsubara, T.; Iljima, K.; Kojima, T.; Hirai, M.; Miyamoto, E.; Sato, T. Heterogeneous Ganglioside-Enriched Nanoclusters with Different Densities in Membrane Rafts Detected by a Peptidyl Molecular Probe. *Langmuir* **2021**, *37*, 646–654. [CrossRef]

71. Sipione, S.; Monyror, J.; Galleguillos, D.; Steinberg, N.; Kadam, V. Gangliosides in the Brain: Physiology, Pathophysiology and Therapeutic Applications. *Front. Neurosci.* **2020**, *14*, 572965. [CrossRef] [PubMed]
72. Huang, Q.; Zhong, W.; Hu, Z.; Tang, X. A Review of the Role of Cav-1 in Neuropathology and Neural Recovery after Ischemic Stroke. *J. Neuroinflammation* **2018**, *15*, 348. [CrossRef] [PubMed]
73. Simón, L.; Campos, A.; Leyton, L.; Quest, A.F.G. Caveolin-1 Function at the Plasma Membrane and in Intracellular Compartments in Cancer. *Cancer Metastasis Rev.* **2020**, *39*, 435–453. [CrossRef] [PubMed]
74. Luo, S.; Yang, M.; Zhao, H.; Han, Y.; Jiang, N.; Yang, J.; Chen, W.; Li, C.; Liu, Y.; Zhao, C.; et al. Caveolin-1 Regulates Cellular Metabolism: A Potential Therapeutic Target in Kidney Disease. *Front. Pharmacol.* **2021**, *12*, 768100. [CrossRef]
75. Razani, B.; Engelman, J.A.; Wang, X.B.; Schubert, W.; Zhang, X.L.; Marks, C.B.; Macaluso, F.; Russell, R.G.; Li, M.; Pestell, R.G.; et al. Caveolin-1 Null Mice Are Viable but Show Evidence of Hyperproliferative and Vascular Abnormalities. *J. Biol. Chem.* **2001**, *276*, 38121–38138. [CrossRef]
76. Schlegel, A.; Schwab, R.B.; Scherer, P.E.; Lisanti, M.P. A Role for the Caveolin Scaffolding Domain in Mediating the Membrane Attachment of Caveolin-1. The Caveolin Scaffolding Domain Is Both Necessary and Sufficient for Membrane Binding in Vitro. *J. Biol. Chem.* **1999**, *274*, 22660–22667. [CrossRef]
77. Wong, T.H.; Khater, I.M.; Joshi, B.; Shahsavari, M.; Hamarneh, G.; Nabi, I.R. Single Molecule Network Analysis Identifies Structural Changes to Caveolae and Scaffolds Due to Mutation of the Caveolin-1 Scaffolding Domain. *Sci. Rep.* **2021**, *11*, 7810. [CrossRef]
78. Reese, C.F.; Chinnakkannu, P.; Tourkina, E.; Hoffman, S.; Kuppuswamy, D. Multiple Subregions within the Caveolin-1 Scaffolding Domain Inhibit Fibrosis, Microvascular Leakage, and Monocyte Migration. *PLoS ONE* **2022**, *17*, e0264413. [CrossRef]
79. Aoki, S.; Thomas, A.; Decaffmeyer, M.; Brasseur, R.; Epand, R.M. The Role of Proline in the Membrane Re-Entrant Helix of Caveolin-1. *J. Biol. Chem.* **2010**, *285*, 33371–33380. [CrossRef]
80. Root, K.T.; Julien, J.A.; Glover, K.J. Secondary Structure of Caveolins: A Mini Review. *Biochem. Soc. Trans.* **2019**, *47*, 1489–1498. [CrossRef]
81. Yang, G.; Dong, Z.; Xu, H.; Wang, C.; Li, H.; Li, Z.; Li, F. Structural Study of Caveolin-1 Intramembrane Domain by Circular Dichroism and Nuclear Magnetic Resonance. *Pept. Sci.* **2015**, *104*, 11–20. [CrossRef]
82. Fielding, C.J.; Fielding, P.E. Role of Cholesterol in Signal Transduction from Caveolae. In *Lipid Rafts and Caveolae*; John Wiley & Sons, Ltd.: Hoboken, NJ, USA, 2006; pp. 91–113, ISBN 978-3-527-60807-2.
83. Kenworthy, A.K. The Building Blocks of Caveolae Revealed: Caveolins Finally Take Center Stage. *Biochem. Soc. Trans.* **2023**, *51*, 855–869. [CrossRef]
84. Couet, J.; Li, S.; Okamoto, T.; Ikezu, T.; Lisanti, M.P. Identification of Peptide and Protein Ligands for the Caveolin-Scaffolding Domain. Implications for the Interaction of Caveolin with Caveolae-Associated Proteins. *J. Biol. Chem.* **1997**, *272*, 6525–6533. [CrossRef] [PubMed]
85. Li, H.; Yao, Z.; Degenhardt, B.; Teper, G.; Papadopoulos, V. Cholesterol Binding at the Cholesterol Recognition/ Interaction Amino Acid Consensus (CRAC) of the Peripheral-Type Benzodiazepine Receptor and Inhibition of Steroidogenesis by an HIV TAT-CRAC Peptide. *Proc. Natl. Acad. Sci. USA* **2001**, *98*, 1267–1272. [CrossRef]
86. Sheng, R.; Chen, Y.; Yung Gee, H.; Stec, E.; Melowic, H.R.; Blatner, N.R.; Tun, M.P.; Kim, Y.; Källberg, M.; Fujiwara, T.K.; et al. Cholesterol Modulates Cell Signaling and Protein Networking by Specifically Interacting with PDZ Domain-Containing Scaffold Proteins. *Nat. Commun.* **2012**, *3*, 1249. [CrossRef]
87. Epand, R.M. Proteins and Cholesterol-Rich Domains. *Biochim. Biophys. Acta (BBA)-Biomembr.* **2008**, *1778*, 1576–1582. [CrossRef]
88. Fantini, J.; Barrantes, F.J. How Cholesterol Interacts with Membrane Proteins: An Exploration of Cholesterol-Binding Sites Including CRAC, CARC, and Tilted Domains. *Front. Physiol.* **2013**, *4*, 31. [CrossRef]
89. Monier, S.; Parton, R.G.; Vogel, F.; Behlke, J.; Henske, A.; Kurzchalia, T.V. VIP21-Caveolin, a Membrane Protein Constituent of the Caveolar Coat, Oligomerizes in Vivo and in Vitro. *Mol. Biol. Cell* **1995**, *6*, 911–927. [CrossRef]
90. Sargiacomo, M.; Scherer, P.E.; Tang, Z.; Kübler, E.; Song, K.S.; Sanders, M.C.; Lisanti, M.P. Oligomeric Structure of Caveolin: Implications for Caveolae Membrane Organization. *Proc. Natl. Acad. Sci. USA* **1995**, *92*, 9407–9411. [CrossRef]
91. Ariotti, N.; Rae, J.; Leneva, N.; Ferguson, C.; Loo, D.; Okano, S.; Hill, M.M.; Walser, P.; Collins, B.M.; Parton, R.G. Molecular Characterization of Caveolin-Induced Membrane Curvature. *J. Biol. Chem.* **2015**, *290*, 24875–24890. [CrossRef] [PubMed]
92. Walser, P.J.; Ariotti, N.; Howes, M.; Ferguson, C.; Webb, R.; Schwudke, D.; Leneva, N.; Cho, K.-J.; Cooper, L.; Rae, J.; et al. Constitutive Formation of Caveolae in a Bacterium. *Cell* **2012**, *150*, 752–763. [CrossRef] [PubMed]
93. Hayer, A.; Stoeber, M.; Bissig, C.; Helenius, A. Biogenesis of Caveolae: Stepwise Assembly of Large Caveolin and Cavin Complexes. *Traffic* **2010**, *11*, 361–382. [CrossRef] [PubMed]
94. Hayer, A.; Stoeber, M.; Ritz, D.; Engel, S.; Meyer, H.H.; Helenius, A. Caveolin-1 Is Ubiquitinated and Targeted to Intralumenal Vesicles in Endolysosomes for Degradation. *J. Cell Biol.* **2010**, *191*, 615–629. [CrossRef] [PubMed]
95. Han, B.; Copeland, C.A.; Tiwari, A.; Kenworthy, A.K. Assembly and Turnover of Caveolae: What Do We Really Know? *Front. Cell Dev. Biol.* **2016**, *4*, 68. [CrossRef] [PubMed]
96. Panchishina, M.V. [Cholesterol synthesis by several strains of Escherichia]. *Zhurnal Mikrobiol. Epidemiol. Immunobiol.* **1979**, *9*, 65–68.
97. Santoscoy, M.C.; Jarboe, L.R. Production of Cholesterol-like Molecules Impacts Escherichia Coli Robustness, Production Capacity, and Vesicle Trafficking. *Metab. Eng.* **2022**, *73*, 134–143. [CrossRef]

98. Alberts, B.; Johnson, A.; Lewis, J.; Raff, M.; Roberts, K.; Walter, P. *Molecular Biology of the Cell*, 4th ed.; Garland Science: New York, NY, USA, 2002; ISBN 978-0-8153-3218-3.
99. Barrantes, F.J. Structural Basis for Lipid Modulation of Nicotinic Acetylcholine Receptor Function. *Brain Res. Brain Res. Rev.* **2004**, *47*, 71–95. [CrossRef]
100. Criado, M.; Eibl, H.; Barrantes, F.J. Effects of Lipids on Acetylcholine Receptor. Essential Need of Cholesterol for Maintenance of Agonist-Induced State Transitions in Lipid Vesicles. *Biochemistry* **1982**, *21*, 3622–3629. [CrossRef]
101. Marsh, D.; Barrantes, F.J. Immobilized Lipid in Acetylcholine Receptor-Rich Membranes from Torpedo Marmorata. *Proc. Natl. Acad. Sci. USA* **1978**, *75*, 4329–4333. [CrossRef] [PubMed]
102. Ma, C.; Wang, C.; Luo, D.; Yan, L.; Yang, W.; Li, N.; Gao, N. Structural Insights into the Membrane Microdomain Organization by SPFH Family Proteins. *Cell Res.* **2022**, *32*, 176–189. [CrossRef]
103. Head, B.P.; Insel, P.A. Do Caveolins Regulate Cells by Actions Outside of Caveolae? *Trends Cell Biol.* **2007**, *17*, 51–57. [CrossRef]
104. Kaksonen, M.; Roux, A. Mechanisms of Clathrin-Mediated Endocytosis. *Nat. Rev. Mol. Cell Biol.* **2018**, *19*, 313–326. [CrossRef]
105. Smith, S.M.; Smith, C.J. Capturing the Mechanics of Clathrin-Mediated Endocytosis. *Curr. Opin. Struct. Biol.* **2022**, *75*, 102427. [CrossRef]
106. Mayor, S.; Parton, R.G.; Donaldson, J.G. Clathrin-Independent Pathways of Endocytosis. *Cold Spring Harb. Perspect. Biol.* **2014**, *6*, a016758. [CrossRef] [PubMed]
107. Ripa, I.; Andreu, S.; López-Guerrero, J.A.; Bello-Morales, R. Membrane Rafts: Portals for Viral Entry. *Front. Microbiol.* **2021**, *12*, 631274. [CrossRef] [PubMed]
108. Gusmira, A.; Takemura, K.; Lee, S.Y.; Inaba, T.; Hanawa-Suetsugu, K.; Oono-Yakura, K.; Yasuhara, K.; Kitao, A.; Suetsugu, S. Regulation of Caveolae through Cholesterol-Depletion-Dependent Tubulation Mediated by PACSIN2. *J. Cell Sci.* **2020**, *133*, jcs246785. [CrossRef] [PubMed]
109. Nabi, I.R.; Le, P.U. Caveolae/Raft-Dependent Endocytosis. *J. Cell Biol.* **2003**, *161*, 673–677. [CrossRef] [PubMed]
110. Rennick, J.J.; Johnston, A.P.R.; Parton, R.G. Key Principles and Methods for Studying the Endocytosis of Biological and Nanoparticle Therapeutics. *Nat. Nanotechnol.* **2021**, *16*, 266–276. [CrossRef] [PubMed]
111. Browman, D.T.; Hoegg, M.B.; Robbins, S.M. The SPFH Domain-Containing Proteins: More than Lipid Raft Markers. *Trends Cell Biol.* **2007**, *17*, 394–402. [CrossRef] [PubMed]
112. Cheng, Z.-J.; Singh, R.D.; Sharma, D.K.; Holicky, E.L.; Hanada, K.; Marks, D.L.; Pagano, R.E. Distinct Mechanisms of Clathrin-Independent Endocytosis Have Unique Sphingolipid Requirements. *Mol. Biol. Cell* **2006**, *17*, 3197–3210. [CrossRef]
113. Stern, C.M.; Mermelstein, P.G. Caveolin Regulation of Neuronal Intracellular Signaling. *Cell Mol. Life Sci.* **2010**, *67*, 3785–3795. [CrossRef]
114. Monier, S.; Dietzen, D.J.; Hastings, W.R.; Lublin, D.M.; Kurzchalia, T.V. Oligomerization of VIP21-Caveolin in Vitro Is Stabilized by Long Chain Fatty Acylation or Cholesterol. *FEBS Lett.* **1996**, *388*, 143–149. [CrossRef]
115. Boulware, M.I.; Kordasiewicz, H.; Mermelstein, P.G. Caveolin Proteins Are Essential for Distinct Effects of Membrane Estrogen Receptors in Neurons. *J. Neurosci.* **2007**, *27*, 9941–9950. [CrossRef]
116. Poo, M.M. Neurotrophins as Synaptic Modulators. *Nat. Rev. Neurosci.* **2001**, *2*, 24–32. [CrossRef]
117. Zhong, W.; Huang, Q.; Zeng, L.; Hu, Z.; Tang, X. Caveolin-1 and MLRs: A Potential Target for Neuronal Growth and Neuroplasticity after Ischemic Stroke. *Int. J. Med. Sci.* **2019**, *16*, 1492–1503. [CrossRef]
118. Head, B.P.; Peart, J.N.; Panneerselvam, M.; Yokoyama, T.; Pearn, M.L.; Niesman, I.R.; Bonds, J.A.; Schilling, J.M.; Miyanohara, A.; Headrick, J.; et al. Loss of Caveolin-1 Accelerates Neurodegeneration and Aging. *PLoS ONE* **2010**, *5*, e15697. [CrossRef]
119. Koh, S.; Lee, W.; Park, S.M.; Kim, S.H. Caveolin-1 Deficiency Impairs Synaptic Transmission in Hippocampal Neurons. *Mol. Brain* **2021**, *14*, 53. [CrossRef]
120. Egawa, J.; Schilling, J.M.; Cui, W.; Posadas, E.; Sawada, A.; Alas, B.; Zemljic-Harpf, A.E.; Fannon-Pavlich, M.J.; Mandyam, C.D.; Roth, D.M.; et al. Neuron-Specific Caveolin-1 Overexpression Improves Motor Function and Preserves Memory in Mice Subjected to Brain Trauma. *FASEB J.* **2017**, *31*, 3403–3411. [CrossRef] [PubMed]
121. Head, B.P.; Hu, Y.; Finley, J.C.; Saldana, M.D.; Bonds, J.A.; Miyanohara, A.; Niesman, I.R.; Ali, S.S.; Murray, F.; Insel, P.A.; et al. Neuron-Targeted Caveolin-1 Protein Enhances Signaling and Promotes Arborization of Primary Neurons. *J. Biol. Chem.* **2011**, *286*, 33310–33321. [CrossRef] [PubMed]
122. Wang, S.; Head, B.P. Caveolin-1 in Stroke Neuropathology and Neuroprotection: A Novel Molecular Therapeutic Target for Ischemic-Related Injury. *Curr. Vasc. Pharmacol.* **2019**, *17*, 41–49. [CrossRef] [PubMed]
123. Trushina, E.; Canaria, C.A.; Lee, D.Y.; McMurray, C.T. Loss of Caveolin-1 Expression in Knock-in Mouse Model of Huntington's Disease Suppresses Pathophysiology In Vivo. *Hum. Mol. Genet.* **2014**, *23*, 129–144. Available online: https://www.ncbi.nlm.nih.gov/pmc/articles/PMC3857950/ (accessed on 11 May 2023). [CrossRef]
124. Fortalezas, S.; Marques-da-Silva, D.; Gutierrez-Merino, C. Methyl-β-Cyclodextrin Impairs the Phosphorylation of the B_2 Subunit of L-Type Calcium Channels and Cytosolic Calcium Homeostasis in Mature Cerebellar Granule Neurons. *Int. J. Mol. Sci.* **2018**, *19*, 3667. [CrossRef] [PubMed]
125. Atlas, D. Voltage-Gated Calcium Channels Function as Ca2+-Activated Signaling Receptors. *Trends Biochem. Sci.* **2014**, *39*, 45–52. [CrossRef] [PubMed]

126. Yang, J.-X.; Hua, L.; Li, Y.-Q.; Jiang, Y.-Y.; Han, D.; Liu, H.; Tang, Q.-Q.; Yang, X.-N.; Yin, C.; Hao, L.-Y.; et al. Caveolin-1 in the Anterior Cingulate Cortex Modulates Chronic Neuropathic Pain via Regulation of NMDA Receptor 2B Subunit. *J. Neurosci.* **2015**, *35*, 36–52. [CrossRef] [PubMed]
127. Bigford, G.E.; Alonso, O.F.; Dietrich, W.D.; Keane, R.W. A Novel Protein Complex in Membrane Rafts Linking the NR2B Glutamate Receptor and Autophagy Is Disrupted Following Traumatic Brain Injury. *J. Neurotrauma* **2009**, *26*, 703–720. [CrossRef] [PubMed]
128. Roh, S.-E.; Hong, Y.H.; Jang, D.C.; Kim, J.; Kim, S.J. Lipid Rafts Serve as Signaling Platforms for mGlu1 Receptor-Mediated Calcium Signaling in Association with Caveolin. *Mol. Brain* **2014**, *7*, 9. [CrossRef] [PubMed]
129. Hering, H.; Lin, C.-C.; Sheng, M. Lipid Rafts in the Maintenance of Synapses, Dendritic Spines, and Surface AMPA Receptor Stability. *J. Neurosci.* **2003**, *23*, 3262–3271. [CrossRef] [PubMed]
130. Gaudreault, S.B.; Chabot, C.; Gratton, J.-P.; Poirier, J. The Caveolin Scaffolding Domain Modifies 2-Amino-3-Hydroxy-5-Methyl-4-Isoxazole Propionate Receptor Binding Properties by Inhibiting Phospholipase A2 Activity. *J. Biol. Chem.* **2004**, *279*, 356–362. [CrossRef]
131. Li, X.-H.; Miao, H.-H.; Zhuo, M. NMDA Receptor Dependent Long-Term Potentiation in Chronic Pain. *Neurochem. Res.* **2019**, *44*, 531–538. [CrossRef]
132. Head, B.P.; Patel, H.H.; Tsutsumi, Y.M.; Hu, Y.; Mejia, T.; Mora, R.C.; Insel, P.A.; Roth, D.M.; Drummond, J.C.; Patel, P.M. Caveolin-1 Expression Is Essential for N-Methyl-D-Aspartate Receptor-Mediated Src and Extracellular Signal-Regulated Kinase 1/2 Activation and Protection of Primary Neurons from Ischemic Cell Death. *FASEB J.* **2008**, *22*, 828–840. [CrossRef]
133. Hansen, K.B.; Yi, F.; Perszyk, R.E.; Furukawa, H.; Wollmuth, L.P.; Gibb, A.J.; Traynelis, S.F. Structure, Function, and Allosteric Modulation of NMDA Receptors. *J. Gen. Physiol.* **2018**, *150*, 1081–1105. [CrossRef]
134. Banerjee, A.; Larsen, R.S.; Philpot, B.D.; Paulsen, O. Roles of Presynaptic NMDA Receptors in Neurotransmission and Plasticity. *Trends Neurosci.* **2016**, *39*, 26–39. [CrossRef]
135. Carter, B.C.; Jahr, C.E. Postsynaptic, Not Presynaptic NMDA Receptors Are Required for Spike-Timing-Dependent LTD Induction. *Nat. Neurosci.* **2016**, *19*, 1218–1224. [CrossRef]
136. Paul, S.; Connor, J.A. NR2B-NMDA Receptor Mediated Increases in Intracellular Ca^{2+} Concentration Regulate the Tyrosine Phosphatase, STEP, and ERK MAP Kinase Signaling. *J. Neurochem.* **2010**, *114*, 1107–1118. [CrossRef]
137. Laube, B.; Hirai, H.; Sturgess, M.; Betz, H.; Kuhse, J. Molecular Determinants of Agonist Discrimination by NMDA Receptor Subunits: Analysis of the Glutamate Binding Site on the NR2B Subunit. *Neuron* **1997**, *18*, 493–503. [CrossRef] [PubMed]
138. Stary, C.; Tsutsumi, Y.; Patel, P.; Head, B.; Patel, H.; Roth, D. Caveolins: Targeting pro-Survival Signaling in the Heart and Brain. *Front. Physiol.* **2012**, *3*, 393. [CrossRef] [PubMed]
139. Lu, Y.M.; Roder, J.C.; Davidow, J.; Salter, M.W. Src Activation in the Induction of Long-Term Potentiation in CA1 Hippocampal Neurons. *Science* **1998**, *279*, 1363–1367. [CrossRef]
140. Rostas, J.A.; Brent, V.A.; Voss, K.; Errington, M.L.; Bliss, T.V.; Gurd, J.W. Enhanced Tyrosine Phosphorylation of the 2B Subunit of the N-Methyl-D-Aspartate Receptor in Long-Term Potentiation. *Proc. Natl. Acad. Sci. USA* **1996**, *93*, 10452–10456. [CrossRef] [PubMed]
141. Nakazawa, T.; Komai, S.; Tezuka, T.; Hisatsune, C.; Umemori, H.; Semba, K.; Mishina, M.; Manabe, T.; Yamamoto, T. Characterization of Fyn-Mediated Tyrosine Phosphorylation Sites on GluR Epsilon 2 (NR2B) Subunit of the N-Methyl-D-Aspartate Receptor. *J. Biol. Chem.* **2001**, *276*, 693–699. [CrossRef] [PubMed]
142. Volonté, D.; Galbiati, F.; Pestell, R.G.; Lisanti, M.P. Cellular Stress Induces the Tyrosine Phosphorylation of Caveolin-1 (Tyr(14)) via Activation of P38 Mitogen-Activated Protein Kinase and c-Src Kinase. Evidence for Caveolae, the Actin Cytoskeleton, and Focal Adhesions as Mechanical Sensors of Osmotic Stress. *J. Biol. Chem.* **2001**, *276*, 8094–8103. [CrossRef]
143. Grande-García, A.; Echarri, A.; de Rooij, J.; Alderson, N.B.; Waterman-Storer, C.M.; Valdivielso, J.M.; del Pozo, M.A. Caveolin-1 Regulates Cell Polarization and Directional Migration through Src Kinase and Rho GTPases. *J. Cell Biol.* **2007**, *177*, 683–694. [CrossRef]
144. Radel, C.; Rizzo, V. Integrin Mechanotransduction Stimulates Caveolin-1 Phosphorylation and Recruitment of Csk to Mediate Actin Reorganization. *Am. J. Physiol.-Heart Circ. Physiol.* **2005**, *288*, H936–H945. [CrossRef]
145. Cao, H.; Sanguinetti, A.R.; Mastick, C.C. Oxidative Stress Activates Both Src-Kinases and Their Negative Regulator Csk and Induces Phosphorylation of Two Targeting Proteins for Csk: Caveolin-1 and Paxillin. *Exp. Cell Res.* **2004**, *294*, 159–171. [CrossRef]
146. Okada, M. Regulation of the Src Family Kinases by Csk. *Int. J. Biol. Sci.* **2012**, *8*, 1385–1397. [CrossRef] [PubMed]
147. Breuer, M.; Berger, H.; Borchers, A. Caveolin 1 Is Required for Axonal Outgrowth of Motor Neurons and Affects Xenopus Neuromuscular Development. *Sci. Rep.* **2020**, *10*, 16546. [CrossRef] [PubMed]
148. Gaudreault, S.B.; Blain, J.-F.; Gratton, J.-P.; Poirier, J. A Role for Caveolin-1 in Post-Injury Reactive Neuronal Plasticity. *J. Neurochem.* **2005**, *92*, 831–839. [CrossRef] [PubMed]
149. Lituma, P.J.; Kwon, H.-B.; Alviña, K.; Luján, R.; Castillo, P.E. Presynaptic NMDA Receptors Facilitate Short-Term Plasticity and BDNF Release at Hippocampal Mossy Fiber Synapses. *eLife* **2021**, *10*, e66612. [CrossRef] [PubMed]
150. Neubauer, F.B.; Min, R.; Nevian, T. Presynaptic NMDA Receptors Influence Ca^{2+} Dynamics by Interacting with Voltage-Dependent Calcium Channels during the Induction of Long-Term Depression. *Neural Plast.* **2022**, *2022*, e2900875. [CrossRef] [PubMed]
151. Brennan, A.M.; Suh, S.W.; Won, S.J.; Narasimhan, P.; Kauppinen, T.M.; Lee, H.; Edling, Y.; Chan, P.H.; Swanson, R.A. NADPH Oxidase Is the Primary Source of Superoxide Induced by NMDA Receptor Activation. *Nat. Neurosci.* **2009**, *12*, 857–863. [CrossRef] [PubMed]

152. Casado, M.; Isope, P.; Ascher, P. Involvement of Presynaptic N-Methyl-D-Aspartate Receptors in Cerebellar Long-Term Depression. *Neuron* **2002**, *33*, 123–130. [CrossRef]
153. Sjöström, P.J.; Turrigiano, G.G.; Nelson, S.B. Neocortical LTD via Coincident Activation of Presynaptic NMDA and Cannabinoid Receptors. *Neuron* **2003**, *39*, 641–654. [CrossRef]
154. Dawson, T.M.; Snyder, S.H. Gases as Biological Messengers: Nitric Oxide and Carbon Monoxide in the Brain. *J. Neurosci.* **1994**, *14*, 5147–5159. [CrossRef]
155. Sato, Y.; Sagami, I.; Shimizu, T. Identification of Caveolin-1-Interacting Sites in Neuronal Nitric-Oxide Synthase: Molecular Mechanism for Inhibition of No Formation. *J. Biol. Chem.* **2004**, *279*, 8827–8836. [CrossRef]
156. Hou, Q.; Huang, Y.; Amato, S.; Snyder, S.H.; Huganir, R.L.; Man, H.-Y. Regulation of AMPA Receptor Localization in Lipid Rafts. *Mol. Cell Neurosci.* **2008**, *38*, 213–223. [CrossRef] [PubMed]
157. Roth, B.L. Molecular Pharmacology of Metabotropic Receptors Targeted by Neuropsychiatric Drugs. *Nat. Struct. Mol. Biol.* **2019**, *26*, 535–544. [CrossRef] [PubMed]
158. Pereira, V.; Goudet, C. Emerging Trends in Pain Modulation by Metabotropic Glutamate Receptors. *Front. Mol. Neurosci.* **2019**, *11*, 464. [CrossRef] [PubMed]
159. Francesconi, A.; Kumari, R.; Zukin, R.S. Regulation of Group I Metabotropic Glutamate Receptor Trafficking and Signaling by the Caveolar/Lipid Raft Pathway. *J. Neurosci.* **2009**, *29*, 3590–3602. [CrossRef] [PubMed]
160. Reiner, A.; Levitz, J. Glutamatergic Signaling in the Central Nervous System: Ionotropic and Metabotropic Receptors in Concert. *Neuron* **2018**, *98*, 1080–1098. [CrossRef] [PubMed]
161. Nakanishi, S. Molecular Diversity of Glutamate Receptors and Implications for Brain Function. *Science* **1992**, *258*, 597–603. [CrossRef]
162. Nakanishi, S.; Masu, M. Molecular Diversity and Functions of Glutamate Receptors. *Annu. Rev. Biophys. Biomol. Struct.* **1994**, *23*, 319–348. [CrossRef]
163. Huh, E.; Agosto, M.A.; Wensel, T.G.; Lichtarge, O. Coevolutionary Signals in Metabotropic Glutamate Receptors Capture Residue Contacts and Long-Range Functional Interactions. *J. Biol. Chem.* **2023**, *299*, 103030. [CrossRef]
164. Gandasi, N.R.; Arapi, V.; Mickael, M.E.; Belekar, P.A.; Granlund, L.; Kothegala, L.; Fredriksson, R.; Bagchi, S. Glutamine Uptake via SNAT6 and Caveolin Regulates Glutamine–Glutamate Cycle. *Int. J. Mol. Sci.* **2021**, *22*, 1167. [CrossRef]
165. Mango, D.; Ledonne, A. Updates on the Physiopathology of Group I Metabotropic Glutamate Receptors (mGluRI)-Dependent Long-Term Depression. *Cells* **2023**, *12*, 1588. [CrossRef]
166. Shigemoto, R.; Kinoshita, A.; Wada, E.; Nomura, S.; Ohishi, H.; Takada, M.; Flor, P.J.; Neki, A.; Abe, T.; Nakanishi, S.; et al. Differential Presynaptic Localization of Metabotropic Glutamate Receptor Subtypes in the Rat Hippocampus. *J. Neurosci.* **1997**, *17*, 7503–7522. [CrossRef] [PubMed]
167. Grove-Strawser, D.; Boulware, M.I.; Mermelstein, P.G. Membrane Estrogen Receptors Activate the Metabotropic Glutamate Receptors mGluR5 and mGluR3 to Bidirectionally Regulate CREB Phosphorylation in Female Rat Striatal Neurons. *Neuroscience* **2010**, *170*, 1045–1055. [CrossRef] [PubMed]
168. Fujimoto, T.; Nakade, S.; Miyawaki, A.; Mikoshiba, K.; Ogawa, K. Localization of Inositol 1,4,5-Trisphosphate Receptor-like Protein in Plasmalemmal Caveolae. *J. Cell Biol.* **1992**, *119*, 1507–1513. [CrossRef] [PubMed]
169. Fujimoto, T.; Miyawaki, A.; Mikoshiba, K. Inositol 1,4,5-Trisphosphate Receptor-like Protein in Plasmalemmal Caveolae Is Linked to Actin Filaments. *J. Cell Sci.* **1995**, *108*, 7–15. [CrossRef] [PubMed]
170. Lockwich, T.P.; Liu, X.; Singh, B.B.; Jadlowiec, J.; Weiland, S.; Ambudkar, I.S. Assembly of Trp1 in a Signaling Complex Associated with Caveolin-Scaffolding Lipid Raft Domains. *J. Biol. Chem.* **2000**, *275*, 11934–11942. [CrossRef] [PubMed]
171. Dunphy, J.T.; Greentree, W.K.; Linder, M.E. Enrichment of G-Protein Palmitoyltransferase Activity in Low Density Membranes: In Vitro Reconstitution of Gαi to These Domains Requires Palmitoyltransferase Activity. *J. Biol. Chem.* **2001**, *276*, 43300–43304. [CrossRef] [PubMed]
172. Kumari, R.; Castillo, C.; Francesconi, A. Agonist-Dependent Signaling by Group I Metabotropic Glutamate Receptors Is Regulated by Association with Lipid Domains. *J. Biol. Chem.* **2013**, *288*, 32004–32019. [CrossRef]
173. Hong, Y.H.; Kim, J.Y.; Lee, J.H.; Chae, H.G.; Jang, S.S.; Jeon, J.H.; Kim, C.H.; Kim, J.; Kim, S.J. Agonist-Induced Internalization of mGluR1α Is Mediated by Caveolin. *J. Neurochem.* **2009**, *111*, 61–71. [CrossRef]
174. Hiester, B.G.; Bourke, A.M.; Sinnen, B.L.; Cook, S.G.; Gibson, E.S.; Smith, K.R.; Kennedy, M.J. L-Type Voltage-Gated Ca2+ Channels Regulate Synaptic-Activity-Triggered Recycling Endosome Fusion in Neuronal Dendrites. *Cell Rep.* **2017**, *21*, 2134–2146. [CrossRef]
175. Davies, A.; Douglas, L.; Hendrich, J.; Wratten, J.; Tran Van Minh, A.; Foucault, I.; Koch, D.; Pratt, W.S.; Saibil, H.R.; Dolphin, A.C. The Calcium Channel A2δ-2 Subunit Partitions with CaV2.1 into Lipid Rafts in Cerebellum: Implications for Localization and Function. *J. Neurosci.* **2006**, *26*, 8748–8757. [CrossRef]
176. Spencer, A.; Yu, L.; Guili, V.; Reynaud, F.; Ding, Y.; Ma, J.; Jullien, J.; Koubi, D.; Gauthier, E.; Cluet, D.; et al. Nerve Growth Factor Signaling from Membrane Microdomains to the Nucleus: Differential Regulation by Caveolins. *Int. J. Mol. Sci.* **2017**, *18*, 693. [CrossRef] [PubMed]
177. Bilderback, T.R.; Gazula, V.R.; Lisanti, M.P.; Dobrowsky, R.T. Caveolin Interacts with Trk A and P75(NTR) and Regulates Neurotrophin Signaling Pathways. *J. Biol. Chem.* **1999**, *274*, 257–263. [CrossRef] [PubMed]

178. Huang, C.S.; Zhou, J.; Feng, A.K.; Lynch, C.C.; Klumperman, J.; DeArmond, S.J.; Mobley, W.C. Nerve Growth Factor Signaling in Caveolae-like Domains at the Plasma Membrane. *J. Biol. Chem.* **1999**, *274*, 36707–36714. [CrossRef] [PubMed]
179. Campbell, D.L.; Stamler, J.S.; Strauss, H.C. Redox Modulation of L-Type Calcium Channels in Ferret Ventricular Myocytes. Dual Mechanism Regulation by Nitric Oxide and S-Nitrosothiols. *J. Gen. Physiol.* **1996**, *108*, 277–293. [CrossRef]
180. Toselli, M.; Biella, G.; Taglietti, V.; Cazzaniga, E.; Parenti, M. Caveolin-1 Expression and Membrane Cholesterol Content Modulate N-Type Calcium Channel Activity in NG108-15 Cells. *Biophys. J.* **2005**, *89*, 2443–2457. [CrossRef]
181. Sepúlveda, M.R.; Berrocal-Carrillo, M.; Gasset, M.; Mata, A.M. The Plasma Membrane Ca2+-ATPase Isoform 4 Is Localized in Lipid Rafts of Cerebellum Synaptic Plasma Membranes. *J. Biol. Chem.* **2006**, *281*, 447–453. [CrossRef]
182. Lopreiato, R.; Giacomello, M.; Carafoli, E. The Plasma Membrane Calcium Pump: New Ways to Look at an Old Enzyme. *J. Biol. Chem.* **2014**, *289*, 10261–10268. [CrossRef]
183. Hirama, T.; Das, R.; Yang, Y.; Ferguson, C.; Won, A.; Yip, C.M.; Kay, J.G.; Grinstein, S.; Parton, R.G.; Fairn, G.D. Phosphatidylserine Dictates the Assembly and Dynamics of Caveolae in the Plasma Membrane. *J. Biol. Chem.* **2017**, *292*, 14292–14307. [CrossRef]
184. Kagan, V.E.; Fabisiak, J.P.; Shvedova, A.A.; Tyurina, Y.Y.; Tyurin, V.A.; Schor, N.F.; Kawai, K. Oxidative Signaling Pathway for Externalization of Plasma Membrane Phosphatidylserine during Apoptosis. *FEBS Lett.* **2000**, *477*, 1–7. [CrossRef]
185. Zhang, J.; Xiao, P.; Zhang, X. Phosphatidylserine Externalization in Caveolae Inhibits Ca2+ Efflux through Plasma Membrane Ca2+-ATPase in ECV304. *Cell Calcium* **2009**, *45*, 177–184. [CrossRef]
186. Vacca, F.; Amadio, S.; Sancesario, G.; Bernardi, G.; Volonté, C. P2X3 Receptor Localizes into Lipid Rafts in Neuronal Cells. *J. Neurosci. Res.* **2004**, *76*, 653–661. [CrossRef] [PubMed]
187. Chen, X.-Q.; Zhu, J.-X.; Wang, Y.; Zhang, X.; Bao, L. CaMKIIα and Caveolin-1 Cooperate to Drive ATP-Induced Membrane Delivery of the P2X3 Receptor. *J. Mol. Cell Biol.* **2014**, *6*, 140–153. [CrossRef] [PubMed]
188. Mojsilovic-Petrovic, J.; Jeong, G.-B.; Crocker, A.; Arneja, A.; David, S.; Russell, D.S.; Kalb, R.G. Protecting Motor Neurons from Toxic Insult by Antagonism of Adenosine A2a and Trk Receptors. *J. Neurosci.* **2006**, *26*, 9250–9263. [CrossRef]
189. North, R.A. P2X3 Receptors and Peripheral Pain Mechanisms. *J. Physiol.* **2004**, *554*, 301–308. [CrossRef] [PubMed]
190. Wirkner, K.; Sperlagh, B.; Illes, P. P2X3 Receptor Involvement in Pain States. *Mol. Neurobiol.* **2007**, *36*, 165–183. [CrossRef]
191. Liu, M.; Huang, W.; Wu, D.; Priestley, J.V. TRPV1, but Not P2X3, Requires Cholesterol for Its Function and Membrane Expression in Rat Nociceptors. *Eur. J. Neurosci.* **2006**, *24*, 1–6. [CrossRef]
192. Frick, M.; Bright, N.A.; Riento, K.; Bray, A.; Merrifield, C.; Nichols, B.J. Coassembly of Flotillins Induces Formation of Membrane Microdomains, Membrane Curvature, and Vesicle Budding. *Curr. Biol.* **2007**, *17*, 1151–1156. [CrossRef]
193. Rivera-Milla, E.; Stuermer, C.A.O.; Málaga-Trillo, E. Ancient Origin of Reggie (Flotillin), Reggie-like, and Other Lipid-Raft Proteins: Convergent Evolution of the SPFH Domain. *Cell Mol. Life Sci.* **2006**, *63*, 343–357. [CrossRef]
194. Bickel, P.E.; Scherer, P.E.; Schnitzer, J.E.; Oh, P.; Lisanti, M.P.; Lodish, H.F. Flotillin and Epidermal Surface Antigen Define a New Family of Caveolae-Associated Integral Membrane Proteins. *J. Biol. Chem.* **1997**, *272*, 13793–13802. [CrossRef]
195. Morrow, I.C.; Rea, S.; Martin, S.; Prior, I.A.; Prohaska, R.; Hancock, J.F.; James, D.E.; Parton, R.G. Flotillin-1/Reggie-2 Traffics to Surface Raft Domains via a Novel Golgi-Independent Pathway. Identification of a Novel Membrane Targeting Domain and a Role for Palmitoylation. *J. Biol. Chem.* **2002**, *277*, 48834–48841. [CrossRef]
196. Kokubo, H.; Helms, J.B.; Ohno-Iwashita, Y.; Shimada, Y.; Horikoshi, Y.; Yamaguchi, H. Ultrastructural Localization of Flotillin-1 to Cholesterol-Rich Membrane Microdomains, Rafts, in Rat Brain Tissue. *Brain Res.* **2003**, *965*, 83–90. [CrossRef] [PubMed]
197. Yokoyama, H.; Matsui, I. The Lipid Raft Markers Stomatin, Prohibitin, Flotillin, and HflK/C (SPFH)-Domain Proteins Form an Operon with NfeD Proteins and Function with Apolar Polyisoprenoid Lipids. *Crit. Rev. Microbiol.* **2020**, *46*, 38–48. [CrossRef] [PubMed]
198. Lapatsina, L.; Brand, J.; Poole, K.; Daumke, O.; Lewin, G.R. Stomatin-Domain Proteins. *Eur. J. Cell Biol.* **2012**, *91*, 240–245. [CrossRef] [PubMed]
199. Tatsuta, T.; Model, K.; Langer, T. Formation of Membrane-Bound Ring Complexes by Prohibitins in Mitochondria. *Mol. Biol. Cell* **2005**, *16*, 248–259. [CrossRef] [PubMed]
200. Daumke, O.; Lewin, G.R. SPFH Protein Cage—One Ring to Rule Them All. *Cell Res.* **2022**, *32*, 117–118. [CrossRef]
201. Li, Y.; Martin, B.R.; Cravatt, B.F.; Hofmann, S.L. DHHC5 Protein Palmitoylates Flotillin-2 and Is Rapidly Degraded on Induction of Neuronal Differentiation in Cultured Cells. *J. Biol. Chem.* **2012**, *287*, 523–530. [CrossRef] [PubMed]
202. Strauss, K.; Goebel, C.; Runz, H.; Möbius, W.; Weiss, S.; Feussner, I.; Simons, M.; Schneider, A. Exosome Secretion Ameliorates Lysosomal Storage of Cholesterol in Niemann-Pick Type C Disease. *J. Biol. Chem.* **2010**, *285*, 26279–26288. [CrossRef]
203. Solis, G.P.; Hoegg, M.; Munderloh, C.; Schrock, Y.; Malaga-Trillo, E.; Rivera-Milla, E.; Stuermer, C.A.O. Reggie/Flotillin Proteins Are Organized into Stable Tetramers in Membrane Microdomains. *Biochem. J.* **2007**, *403*, 313–322. [CrossRef]
204. Riento, K.; Frick, M.; Schafer, I.; Nichols, B.J. Endocytosis of Flotillin-1 and Flotillin-2 Is Regulated by Fyn Kinase. *J. Cell Sci.* **2009**, *122*, 912–918. [CrossRef]
205. Neumann-Giesen, C.; Fernow, I.; Amaddii, M.; Tikkanen, R. Role of EGF-Induced Tyrosine Phosphorylation of Reggie-1/Flotillin-2 in Cell Spreading and Signaling to the Actin Cytoskeleton. *J. Cell Sci.* **2007**, *120*, 395–406. [CrossRef]
206. Swanwick, C.C.; Shapiro, M.E.; Vicini, S.; Wenthold, R.J. Flotillin-1 Promotes Formation of Glutamatergic Synapses in Hippocampal Neurons. *Dev. Neurobiol.* **2010**, *70*, 875–883. [CrossRef]

207. Munderloh, C.; Solis, G.P.; Bodrikov, V.; Jaeger, F.A.; Wiechers, M.; Málaga-Trillo, E.; Stuermer, C.A.O. Reggies/Flotillins Regulate Retinal Axon Regeneration in the Zebrafish Optic Nerve and Differentiation of Hippocampal and N2a Neurons. *J. Neurosci.* **2009**, *29*, 6607–6615. [CrossRef] [PubMed]
208. Koch, J.C.; Solis, G.P.; Bodrikov, V.; Michel, U.; Haralampieva, D.; Shypitsyna, A.; Tönges, L.; Bähr, M.; Lingor, P.; Stuermer, C.A.O. Upregulation of Reggie-1/Flotillin-2 Promotes Axon Regeneration in the Rat Optic Nerve in Vivo and Neurite Growth in Vitro. *Neurobiol. Dis.* **2013**, *51*, 168–176. [CrossRef] [PubMed]
209. Stuermer, C.A.O. The Reggie/Flotillin Connection to Growth. *Trends Cell Biol.* **2010**, *20*, 6–13. [CrossRef]
210. Kwiatkowska, K.; Matveichuk, O.V.; Fronk, J.; Ciesielska, A. Flotillins: At the Intersection of Protein S-Palmitoylation and Lipid-Mediated Signaling. *Int. J. Mol. Sci.* **2020**, *21*, 2283. [CrossRef] [PubMed]
211. Guillaume, E.; Comunale, F.; Do Khoa, N.; Planchon, D.; Bodin, S.; Gauthier-Rouvière, C. Flotillin Microdomains Stabilize Cadherins at Cell-Cell Junctions. *J. Cell Sci.* **2013**, *126*, 5293–5304. [CrossRef]
212. Bodin, S.; Planchon, D.; Rios Morris, E.; Comunale, F.; Gauthier-Rouvière, C. Flotillins in Intercellular Adhesion-from Cellular Physiology to Human Diseases. *J. Cell Sci.* **2014**, *127*, 5139–5147. [CrossRef]
213. Seong, E.; Yuan, L.; Arikkath, J. Cadherins and Catenins in Dendrite and Synapse Morphogenesis. *Cell Adhes. Migr.* **2015**, *9*, 202–213. [CrossRef]
214. Meister, M.; Tikkanen, R. Endocytic Trafficking of Membrane-Bound Cargo: A Flotillin Point of View. *Membranes* **2014**, *4*, 356–371. [CrossRef]
215. Otto, G.P.; Nichols, B.J. The Roles of Flotillin Microdomains--Endocytosis and Beyond. *J. Cell Sci.* **2011**, *124*, 3933–3940. [CrossRef]
216. Hu, J.; Gao, Y.; Huang, Q.; Wang, Y.; Mo, X.; Wang, P.; Zhang, Y.; Xie, C.; Li, D.; Yao, J. Flotillin-1 Interacts With and Sustains the Surface Levels of TRPV2 Channel. *Front. Cell Dev. Biol.* **2021**, *9*, 634160. [CrossRef]
217. Dietzen, D.J.; Hastings, W.R.; Lublin, D.M. Caveolin Is Palmitoylated on Multiple Cysteine Residues: Palmitoylation IS Not Necessary for Localization of Caveolin to Caveolae. *J. Biol. Chem.* **1995**, *270*, 6838–6842. [CrossRef]
218. Parat, M.-O.; Fox, P.L. Palmitoylation of Caveolin-1 in Endothelial Cells Is Post-Translational but Irreversible. *J. Biol. Chem.* **2001**, *276*, 15776–15782. [CrossRef] [PubMed]
219. Südhof, T.C.; Rizo, J. Synaptic Vesicle Exocytosis. *Cold Spring Harb. Perspect. Biol.* **2011**, *3*, a005637. [CrossRef] [PubMed]
220. Ogunmowo, T.H.; Jing, H.; Raychaudhuri, S.; Kusick, G.F.; Imoto, Y.; Li, S.; Itoh, K.; Ma, Y.; Jafri, H.; Dalva, M.B.; et al. Membrane Compression by Synaptic Vesicle Exocytosis Triggers Ultrafast Endocytosis. *Nat. Commun.* **2023**, *14*, 2888. [CrossRef]
221. Braun, J.E.A.; Madison, D.V. A Novel SNAP25–Caveolin Complex Correlates with the Onset of Persistent Synaptic Potentiation. *J. Neurosci.* **2000**, *20*, 5997–6006. [CrossRef] [PubMed]
222. Pombo, I.; Rivera, J.; Blank, U. Munc18-2/Syntaxin3 Complexes Are Spatially Separated from Syntaxin3-Containing SNARE Complexes. *FEBS Lett.* **2003**, *550*, 144–148. [CrossRef] [PubMed]
223. Wang, C.; Tu, J.; Zhang, S.; Cai, B.; Liu, Z.; Hou, S.; Zhong, Q.; Hu, X.; Liu, W.; Li, G.; et al. Different Regions of Synaptic Vesicle Membrane Regulate VAMP2 Conformation for the SNARE Assembly. *Nat. Commun.* **2020**, *11*, 1531. [CrossRef]
224. Glebov, O.O.; Bright, N.A.; Nichols, B.J. Flotillin-1 Defines a Clathrin-Independent Endocytic Pathway in Mammalian Cells. *Nat. Cell Biol.* **2006**, *8*, 46–54. [CrossRef]
225. Taverna, E.; Saba, E.; Rowe, J.; Francolini, M.; Clementi, F.; Rosa, P. Role of Lipid Microdomains in P/Q-Type Calcium Channel (Cav2.1) Clustering and Function in Presynaptic Membranes. *J. Biol. Chem.* **2004**, *279*, 5127–5134. [CrossRef]
226. Davies, A.; Kadurin, I.; Alvarez-Laviada, A.; Douglas, L.; Nieto-Rostro, M.; Bauer, C.S.; Pratt, W.S.; Dolphin, A.C. The A2δ Subunits of Voltage-Gated Calcium Channels Form GPI-Anchored Proteins, a Posttranslational Modification Essential for Function. *Proc. Natl. Acad. Sci. USA* **2010**, *107*, 1654–1659. [CrossRef]
227. Swanwick, C.C.; Shapiro, M.E.; Yi, Z.; Chang, K.; Wenthold, R.J. NMDA Receptors Interact with Flotillin-1 and -2, Lipid Raft-Associated Proteins. *FEBS Lett.* **2009**, *583*, 1226–1230. [CrossRef]
228. Simons, K.; Ikonen, E. Functional Rafts in Cell Membranes. *Nature* **1997**, *387*, 569–572. [CrossRef] [PubMed]
229. Abulrob, A.; Tauskela, J.S.; Mealing, G.; Brunette, E.; Faid, K.; Stanimirovic, D. Protection by Cholesterol-Extracting Cyclodextrins: A Role for N-Methyl-d-Aspartate Receptor Redistribution. *J. Neurochem.* **2005**, *92*, 1477–1486. [CrossRef] [PubMed]
230. Arenas, F.; Garcia-Ruiz, C.; Fernandez-Checa, J.C. Intracellular Cholesterol Trafficking and Impact in Neurodegeneration. *Front. Mol. Neurosci.* **2017**, *10*, 382. [CrossRef] [PubMed]
231. Ramanathan, A.; Nelson, A.R.; Sagare, A.P.; Zlokovic, B.V. Impaired Vascular-Mediated Clearance of Brain Amyloid Beta in Alzheimer's Disease: The Role, Regulation and Restoration of LRP1. *Front. Aging Neurosci.* **2015**, *7*, 136. [CrossRef]
232. Beffert, U.; Stolt, P.C.; Herz, J. Functions of Lipoprotein Receptors in Neurons. *J. Lipid Res.* **2004**, *45*, 403–409. [CrossRef] [PubMed]
233. Nakajima, C.; Kulik, A.; Frotscher, M.; Herz, J.; Schäfer, M.; Bock, H.H.; May, P. Low Density Lipoprotein Receptor-Related Protein 1 (LRP1) Modulates N-Methyl-D-Aspartate (NMDA) Receptor-Dependent Intracellular Signaling and NMDA-Induced Regulation of Postsynaptic Protein Complexes. *J. Biol. Chem.* **2013**, *288*, 21909–21923. [CrossRef]
234. Bodrikov, V.; Pauschert, A.; Kochlamazashvili, G.; Stuermer, C.A.O. Reggie-1 and Reggie-2 (Flotillins) Participate in Rab11a-Dependent Cargo Trafficking, Spine Synapse Formation and LTP-Related AMPA Receptor (GluA1) Surface Exposure in Mouse Hippocampal Neurons. *Exp. Neurol.* **2017**, *289*, 31–45. [CrossRef]
235. Rajakulendran, S.; Hanna, M.G. The Role of Calcium Channels in Epilepsy. *Cold Spring Harb. Perspect. Med.* **2016**, *6*, a022723. [CrossRef]

236. Arikkath, J.; Campbell, K.P. Auxiliary Subunits: Essential Components of the Voltage-Gated Calcium Channel Complex. *Curr. Opin. Neurobiol.* **2003**, *13*, 298–307. [CrossRef]
237. Schlick, B.; Flucher, B.E.; Obermair, G.J. Voltage-Activated Calcium Channel Expression Profiles in Mouse Brain and Cultured Hippocampal Neurons. *Neuroscience* **2010**, *167*, 786–798. [CrossRef]
238. Catterall, W.A. Voltage-Gated Calcium Channels. *Cold Spring Harb. Perspect. Biol.* **2011**, *3*, a003947. [CrossRef]
239. Ilic, K.; Lin, X.; Malci, A.; Stojanović, M.; Puljko, B.; Rožman, M.; Vukelić, Ž.; Heffer, M.; Montag, D.; Schnaar, R.L.; et al. Plasma Membrane Calcium ATPase-Neuroplastin Complexes Are Selectively Stabilized in GM1-Containing Lipid Rafts. *Int. J. Mol. Sci.* **2021**, *22*, 13590. [CrossRef]
240. Jiang, L.; Fernandes, D.; Mehta, N.; Bean, J.L.; Michaelis, M.L.; Zaidi, A. Partitioning of the Plasma Membrane Ca^{2+}-ATPase into Lipid Rafts in Primary Neurons: Effects of Cholesterol Depletion. *J. Neurochem.* **2007**, *102*, 378–388. [CrossRef]
241. Stuermer, C.A.; Lang, D.M.; Kirsch, F.; Wiechers, M.; Deininger, S.O.; Plattner, H. Glycosylphosphatidyl Inositol-Anchored Proteins and Fyn Kinase Assemble in Noncaveolar Plasma Membrane Microdomains Defined by Reggie-1 and -2. *Mol. Biol. Cell* **2001**, *12*, 3031–3045. [CrossRef] [PubMed]
242. Arvanitis, D.N.; Min, W.; Gong, Y.; Heng, Y.M.; Boggs, J.M. Two Types of Detergent-Insoluble, Glycosphingolipid/Cholesterol-Rich Membrane Domains from Isolated Myelin. *J. Neurochem.* **2005**, *94*, 1696–1710. [CrossRef] [PubMed]
243. del Toro, D.; Xifró, X.; Pol, A.; Humbert, S.; Saudou, F.; Canals, J.M.; Alberch, J. Altered Cholesterol Homeostasis Contributes to Enhanced Excitotoxicity in Huntington's Disease. *J. Neurochem.* **2010**, *115*, 153–167. [CrossRef] [PubMed]
244. Sonnino, S.; Chiricozzi, E.; Grassi, S.; Mauri, L.; Prioni, S.; Prinetti, A. Chapter Three-Gangliosides in Membrane Organization. In *Progress in Molecular Biology and Translational Science*; Schnaar, R.L., Lopez, P.H.H., Eds.; Gangliosides in Health and Disease; Academic Press: Cambridge, MA, USA, 2018; Volume 156, pp. 83–120.
245. Prinetti, A.; Chigorno, V.; Tettamanti, G.; Sonnino, S. Sphingolipid-Enriched Membrane Domains from Rat Cerebellar Granule Cells Differentiated in Culture: A Compositional Study. *J. Biol. Chem.* **2000**, *275*, 11658–11665. [CrossRef] [PubMed]
246. Vyas, K.A.; Patel, H.V.; Vyas, A.A.; Schnaar, R.L. Segregation of Gangliosides GM1 and GD3 on Cell Membranes, Isolated Membrane Rafts, and Defined Supported Lipid Monolayers. *Biol. Chem.* **2001**, *382*, 241–250. [CrossRef] [PubMed]
247. Fantini, J. Lipid Rafts and Human Diseases: Why We Need to Target Gangliosides. *FEBS Open Bio* **2023**, *13*, 1636–1650. [CrossRef]
248. Díaz, M.; de Pablo, D.P.; Valdés-Baizabal, C.; Santos, G.; Marin, R. Molecular and Biophysical Features of Hippocampal "Lipid Rafts Aging" Are Modified by Dietary N-3 Long-chain Polyunsaturated Fatty Acids. *Aging Cell* **2023**, *22*, e13867. [CrossRef] [PubMed]
249. Azzaz, F.; Chahinian, H.; Yahi, N.; Fantini, J.; Di Scala, C. AmyP53 Prevents the Formation of Neurotoxic β-Amyloid Oligomers through an Unprecedent Mechanism of Interaction with Gangliosides: Insights for Alzheimer's Disease Therapy. *Int. J. Mol. Sci.* **2023**, *24*, 1760. [CrossRef] [PubMed]
250. Yahi, N.; Fantini, J. Deciphering the Glycolipid Code of Alzheimer's and Parkinson's Amyloid Proteins Allowed the Creation of a Universal Ganglioside-Binding Peptide. *PLoS ONE* **2014**, *9*, e104751. [CrossRef] [PubMed]
251. Fantini, J.; Yahi, N. The Driving Force of Alpha-Synuclein Insertion and Amyloid Channel Formation in the Plasma Membrane of Neural Cells: Key Role of Ganglioside- and Cholesterol-Binding Domains. *Adv. Exp. Med. Biol.* **2013**, *991*, 15–26. [CrossRef] [PubMed]
252. Mahfoud, R.; Garmy, N.; Maresca, M.; Yahi, N.; Puigserver, A.; Fantini, J. Identification of a Common Sphingolipid-Binding Domain in Alzheimer, Prion, and HIV-1 Proteins. *J. Biol. Chem.* **2002**, *277*, 11292–11296. [CrossRef]
253. Di Scala, C.; Yahi, N.; Boutemeur, S.; Flores, A.; Rodriguez, L.; Chahinian, H.; Fantini, J. Common Molecular Mechanism of Amyloid Pore Formation by Alzheimer's β-Amyloid Peptide and α-Synuclein. *Sci. Rep.* **2016**, *6*, 28781. [CrossRef]
254. Sahu, S.K.; Saxena, R.; Chattopadhyay, A. Cholesterol Depletion Modulates Detergent Resistant Fraction of Human serotonin1A Receptors. *Mol. Membr. Biol.* **2012**, *29*, 290–298. [CrossRef]
255. Gupta, V.K.; Sharma, N.S.; Kesh, K.; Dauer, P.; Nomura, A.; Giri, B.; Dudeja, V.; Banerjee, S.; Bhattacharya, S.; Saluja, A.; et al. Metastasis and Chemoresistance in CD133 Expressing Pancreatic Cancer Cells Are Dependent on Their Lipid Raft Integrity. *Cancer Lett.* **2018**, *439*, 101–112. [CrossRef]
256. Brügger, B.; Glass, B.; Haberkant, P.; Leibrecht, I.; Wieland, F.T.; Kräusslich, H.-G. The HIV Lipidome: A Raft with an Unusual Composition. *Proc. Natl. Acad. Sci. USA* **2006**, *103*, 2641–2646. [CrossRef]
257. Mergia, A. The Role of Caveolin 1 in HIV Infection and Pathogenesis. *Viruses* **2017**, *9*, 129. [CrossRef]
258. Sahay, B.; Mergia, A. The Potential Contribution of Caveolin 1 to HIV Latent Infection. *Pathogens* **2020**, *9*, 896. Available online: https://www.mdpi.com/2076-0817/9/11/896 (accessed on 26 July 2023). [CrossRef]
259. Gisslén, M.; Hagberg, L.; Norkrans, G.; Lekman, A.; Fredman, P. Increased Cerebrospinal Fluid Ganglioside GM1 Concentrations Indicating Neuronal Involvement in All Stages of HIV-1 Infection. *J. Neurovirol* **1997**, *3*, 148–152. [CrossRef]
260. Ledeen, R.W.; Wu, G. Ganglioside Function in Calcium Homeostasis and Signaling. *Neurochem. Res.* **2002**, *27*, 637–647. [CrossRef]
261. Jiang, L.; Bechtel, M.D.; Bean, J.L.; Winefield, R.; Williams, T.D.; Zaidi, A.; Michaelis, E.K.; Michaelis, M.L. Effects of Gangliosides on the Activity of the Plasma Membrane Ca2+-ATPase. *Biochim. Biophys. Acta* **2014**, *1838*, 1255–1265. [CrossRef]
262. Zhao, Y.; Fan, X.; Yang, F.; Zhang, X. Gangliosides Modulate the Activity of the Plasma Membrane Ca^{2+}-ATPase from Porcine Brain Synaptosomes. *Arch. Biochem. Biophys.* **2004**, *427*, 204–212. [CrossRef] [PubMed]
263. Jiang, L.; Bechtel, M.D.; Galeva, N.A.; Williams, T.D.; Michaelis, E.K.; Michaelis, M.L. Decreases in Plasma Membrane Ca2+-ATPase in Brain Synaptic Membrane Rafts from Aged Rats. *J. Neurochem.* **2012**, *123*, 689–699. [CrossRef] [PubMed]

264. Colina, C.; Cervino, V.; Benaim, G. Ceramide and Sphingosine Have an Antagonistic Effect on the Plasma-Membrane Ca2+-ATPase from Human Erythrocytes. *Biochem. J.* **2002**, *362*, 247–251. [CrossRef] [PubMed]
265. Zhang, J.; Zhao, Y.; Duan, J.; Yang, F.; Zhang, X. Gangliosides Activate the Phosphatase Activity of the Erythrocyte Plasma Membrane Ca2+-ATPase. *Arch. Biochem. Biophys.* **2005**, *444*, 1–6. [CrossRef] [PubMed]
266. Carlson, R.O.; Masco, D.; Brooker, G.; Spiegel, S. Endogenous Ganglioside GM1 Modulates L-Type Calcium Channel Activity in N18 Neuroblastoma Cells. *J. Neurosci.* **1994**, *14*, 2272–2281. [CrossRef]
267. Frank, C.; Giammarioli, A.M.; Pepponi, R.; Fiorentini, C.; Rufini, S. Cholesterol Perturbing Agents Inhibit NMDA-Dependent Calcium Influx in Rat Hippocampal Primary Culture. *FEBS Lett.* **2004**, *566*, 25–29. [CrossRef]
268. de Erausquin, G.A.; Manev, H.; Guidotti, A.; Costa, E.; Brooker, G. Gangliosides Normalize Distorted Single-Cell Intracellular Free Ca2+ Dynamics after Toxic Doses of Glutamate in Cerebellar Granule Cells. *Proc. Natl. Acad. Sci. USA* **1990**, *87*, 8017–8021. [CrossRef] [PubMed]
269. Manev, H.; Favaron, M.; Vicini, S.; Guidotti, A.; Costa, E. Glutamate-Induced Neuronal Death in Primary Cultures of Cerebellar Granule Cells: Protection by Synthetic Derivatives of Endogenous Sphingolipids. *J. Pharmacol. Exp. Ther.* **1990**, *252*, 419–427. [PubMed]
270. Costa, E.; Armstrong, D.M.; Guidotti, A.; Kharlamov, A.; Kiedrowski, L.; Manev, H.; Polo, A.; Wroblewski, J.T. Gangliosides in the Protection against Glutamate Excitotoxicity. *Prog. Brain Res.* **1994**, *101*, 357–373. [CrossRef] [PubMed]
271. Cole, A.A.; Dosemeci, A.; Reese, T.S. Co-Segregation of AMPA Receptors with GM1 Ganglioside in Synaptosomal Membrane Sub-Fractions. *Biochem. J.* **2010**, *427*, 535–540. [CrossRef]
272. Kasahara, K.; Watanabe, Y.; Yamamoto, T.; Sanai, Y. Association of Src Family Tyrosine Kinase Lyn with Ganglioside GD3 in Rat Brain. Possible Regulation of Lyn by Glycosphingolipid in Caveolae-like Domains. *J. Biol. Chem.* **1997**, *272*, 29947–29953. [CrossRef]
273. Hayashi, T.; Huganir, R.L. Tyrosine Phosphorylation and Regulation of the AMPA Receptor by SRC Family Tyrosine Kinases. *J. Neurosci.* **2004**, *24*, 6152–6160. [CrossRef]
274. Goncalves, J.; Bartol, T.M.; Camus, C.; Levet, F.; Menegolla, A.P.; Sejnowski, T.J.; Sibarita, J.-B.; Vivaudou, M.; Choquet, D.; Hosy, E. Nanoscale Co-Organization and Coactivation of AMPAR, NMDAR, and mGluR at Excitatory Synapses. *Proc. Natl. Acad. Sci. USA* **2020**, *117*, 14503–14511. [CrossRef]
275. Li, S.; Raychaudhuri, S.; Lee, S.A.; Brockmann, M.M.; Wang, J.; Kusick, G.; Prater, C.; Syed, S.; Falahati, H.; Ramos, R.; et al. Asynchronous Release Sites Align with NMDA Receptors in Mouse Hippocampal Synapses. *Nat. Commun.* **2021**, *12*, 677. [CrossRef]
276. Prendergast, J.; Umanah, G.K.E.; Yoo, S.-W.; Lagerlöf, O.; Motari, M.G.; Cole, R.N.; Huganir, R.L.; Dawson, T.M.; Dawson, V.L.; Schnaar, R.L. Ganglioside Regulation of AMPA Receptor Trafficking. *J. Neurosci.* **2014**, *34*, 13246–13258. [CrossRef]
277. Wu, G.; Ledeen, R.W. Gangliosides as Modulators of Neuronal Calcium. *Prog. Brain Res.* **1994**, *101*, 101–112. [CrossRef]
278. Fang, Y.; Wu, G.; Xie, X.; Lu, Z.H.; Ledeen, R.W. Endogenous GM1 Ganglioside of the Plasma Membrane Promotes Neuritogenesis by Two Mechanisms. *Neurochem. Res.* **2000**, *25*, 931–940. [CrossRef]
279. Wu, G.; Lu, Z.-H.; Nakamura, K.; Spray, D.C.; Ledeen, R.W. Trophic Effect of Cholera Toxin B Subunit in Cultured Cerebellar Granule Neurons: Modulation of Intracellular Calcium by GM1 Ganglioside. *J. Neurosci. Res.* **1996**, *44*, 243–254. [CrossRef]
280. Milani, D.; Minozzi, M.C.; Petrelli, L.; Guidolin, D.; Skaper, S.D.; Spoerri, P.E. Interaction of Ganglioside GM1 with the B Subunit of Cholera Toxin Modulates Intracellular Free Calcium in Sensory Neurons. *J. Neurosci. Res.* **1992**, *33*, 466–475. [CrossRef]
281. Ando, S.; Tanaka, Y.; Waki, H.; Kon, K.; Iwamoto, M.; Fukui, F. Gangliosides and Sialylcholesterol as Modulators of Synaptic Functionsa. *Ann. N. Y. Acad. Sci.* **1998**, *845*, 232–239. [CrossRef]
282. Berg, L.K.; Larsson, M.; Morland, C.; Gundersen, V. Pre- and Postsynaptic Localization of NMDA Receptor Subunits at Hippocampal Mossy Fibre Synapses. *Neuroscience* **2013**, *230*, 139–150. [CrossRef]
283. Nosov, G.; Kahms, M.; Klingauf, J. The Decade of Super-Resolution Microscopy of the Presynapse. *Front. Synaptic Neurosci.* **2020**, *12*, 32. [CrossRef]
284. Nakatani, Y.; Hotta, S.; Utsunomiya, I.; Tanaka, K.; Hoshi, K.; Ariga, T.; Yu, R.K.; Miyatake, T.; Taguchi, K. Cav2.1 Voltage-Dependent Ca2+ Channel Current Is Inhibited by Serum from Select Patients with Guillain-Barré Syndrome. *Neurochem. Res.* **2009**, *34*, 149–157. [CrossRef]
285. Taylor, C.P.; Garrido, R. Immunostaining of Rat Brain, Spinal Cord, Sensory Neurons and Skeletal Muscle for Calcium Channel Alpha2-Delta (Alpha2-Delta) Type 1 Protein. *Neuroscience* **2008**, *155*, 510–521. [CrossRef]
286. Bauer, C.S.; Nieto-Rostro, M.; Rahman, W.; Tran-Van-Minh, A.; Ferron, L.; Douglas, L.; Kadurin, I.; Sri Ranjan, Y.; Fernandez-Alacid, L.; Millar, N.S.; et al. The Increased Trafficking of the Calcium Channel Subunit Alpha2delta-1 to Presynaptic Terminals in Neuropathic Pain Is Inhibited by the Alpha2delta Ligand Pregabalin. *J. Neurosci.* **2009**, *29*, 4076–4088. [CrossRef]
287. Zhang, J.; Diamond, J.S. Distinct Perisynaptic and Synaptic Localization of NMDA and AMPA Receptors on Ganglion Cells in Rat Retina. *J. Comp. Neurol.* **2006**, *498*, 810–820. [CrossRef]
288. Zhang, J.; Diamond, J.S. Subunit- and Pathway-Specific Localization of NMDA Receptors and Scaffolding Proteins at Ganglion Cell Synapses in Rat Retina. *J. Neurosci.* **2009**, *29*, 4274–4286. [CrossRef]
289. Lu, C.-R.; Hwang, S.J.; Phend, K.D.; Rustioni, A.; Valtschanoff, J.G. Primary Afferent Terminals That Express Presynaptic NR1 in Rats Are Mainly from Myelinated, Mechanosensitive Fibers. *J. Comp. Neurol.* **2003**, *460*, 191–202. [CrossRef]

290. Grant, S.G.N. Synapse Signalling Complexes and Networks: Machines Underlying Cognition. *Bioessays* **2003**, *25*, 1229–1235. [CrossRef]
291. Henley, J.; Poo, M. Guiding Neuronal Growth Cones Using Ca2+ Signals. *Trends Cell Biol.* **2004**, *14*, 320–330. [CrossRef] [PubMed]
292. Zheng, J.Q.; Poo, M.-M. Calcium Signaling in Neuronal Motility. *Annu. Rev. Cell Dev. Biol.* **2007**, *23*, 375–404. [CrossRef]
293. Davies, S.N.; Lester, R.A.; Reymann, K.G.; Collingridge, G.L. Temporally Distinct Pre- and Post-Synaptic Mechanisms Maintain Long-Term Potentiation. *Nature* **1989**, *338*, 500–503. [CrossRef]
294. Brown, T.C.; Correia, S.S.; Petrok, C.N.; Esteban, J.A. Functional Compartmentalization of Endosomal Trafficking for the Synaptic Delivery of AMPA Receptors during Long-Term Potentiation. *J. Neurosci.* **2007**, *27*, 13311–13315. [CrossRef]
295. Petralia, R.S.; Wang, Y.-X.; Wenthold, R.J. Internalization at Glutamatergic Synapses during Development. *Eur. J. Neurosci.* **2003**, *18*, 3207–3217. [CrossRef]
296. Vulchanova, L.; Riedl, M.S.; Shuster, S.J.; Buell, G.; Surprenant, A.; North, R.A.; Elde, R. Immunohistochemical Study of the P2X2 and P2X3 Receptor Subunits in Rat and Monkey Sensory Neurons and Their Central Terminals. *Neuropharmacology* **1997**, *36*, 1229–1242. [CrossRef]
297. Llewellyn-Smith, I.J.; Burnstock, G. Ultrastructural Localization of P2X3 Receptors in Rat Sensory Neurons. *Neuroreport* **1998**, *9*, 2545–2550. [CrossRef]
298. Cook, S.P.; Vulchanova, L.; Hargreaves, K.M.; Elde, R.; McCleskey, E.W. Distinct ATP Receptors on Pain-Sensing and Stretch-Sensing Neurons. *Nature* **1997**, *387*, 505–508. [CrossRef]
299. Souslova, V.; Cesare, P.; Ding, Y.; Akopian, A.N.; Stanfa, L.; Suzuki, R.; Carpenter, K.; Dickenson, A.; Boyce, S.; Hill, R.; et al. Warm-Coding Deficits and Aberrant Inflammatory Pain in Mice Lacking P2X3 Receptors. *Nature* **2000**, *407*, 1015–1017. [CrossRef] [PubMed]
300. Westover, E.J.; Covey, D.F. The Enantiomer of Cholesterol. *J. Membr. Biol.* **2004**, *202*, 61–72. [CrossRef] [PubMed]
301. Gorospe, B.; Moura, J.J.G.; Gutierrez-Merino, C.; Samhan-Arias, A.K. Biochemical and Biophysical Characterization of the Caveolin-2 Interaction with Membranes and Analysis of the Protein Structural Alteration by the Presence of Cholesterol. *Int. J. Mol. Sci.* **2022**, *23*, 15203. [CrossRef] [PubMed]
302. Levental, I.; Grzybek, M.; Simons, K. Greasing Their Way: Lipid Modifications Determine Protein Association with Membrane Rafts. *Biochemistry* **2010**, *49*, 6305–6316. [CrossRef]
303. Levental, I.; Lingwood, D.; Grzybek, M.; Coskun, U.; Simons, K. Palmitoylation Regulates Raft Affinity for the Majority of Integral Raft Proteins. *Proc. Natl. Acad. Sci. USA* **2010**, *107*, 22050–22054. [CrossRef]
304. Song, Y.; Kenworthy, A.K.; Sanders, C.R. Cholesterol as a Co-Solvent and a Ligand for Membrane Proteins. *Protein Sci.* **2014**, *23*, 1–22. [CrossRef]

Disclaimer/Publisher's Note: The statements, opinions and data contained in all publications are solely those of the individual author(s) and contributor(s) and not of MDPI and/or the editor(s). MDPI and/or the editor(s) disclaim responsibility for any injury to people or property resulting from any ideas, methods, instructions or products referred to in the content.

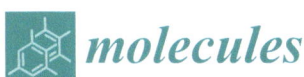

Review

Rafting on the Evidence for Lipid Raft-like Domains as Hubs Triggering Environmental Toxicants' Cellular Effects

Dorinda Marques-da-Silva [1,2,3,*] and Ricardo Lagoa [1,2,3]

1. LSRE—Laboratory of Separation and Reaction Engineering and LCM—Laboratory of Catalysis and Materials, School of Management and Technology, Polytechnic Institute of Leiria, Morro do Lena-Alto do Vieiro, 2411-901 Leiria, Portugal; ricardo.lagoa@ipleiria.pt
2. ALiCE—Associate Laboratory in Chemical Engineering, Faculty of Engineering, University of Porto, Rua Dr. Roberto Frias, 4200-465 Porto, Portugal
3. School of Technology and Management, Polytechnic Institute of Leiria, Morro do Lena-Alto do Vieiro, 2411-901 Leiria, Portugal
* Correspondence: dorinda.silva@ipleiria.pt

Abstract: The plasma membrane lipid rafts are cholesterol- and sphingolipid-enriched domains that allow regularly distributed, sub-micro-sized structures englobing proteins to compartmentalize cellular processes. These membrane domains can be highly heterogeneous and dynamic, functioning as signal transduction platforms that amplify the local concentrations and signaling of individual components. Moreover, they participate in cell signaling routes that are known to be important targets of environmental toxicants affecting cell redox status and calcium homeostasis, immune regulation, and hormonal functions. In this work, the evidence that plasma membrane raft-like domains operate as hubs for toxicants' cellular actions is discussed, and suggestions for future research are provided. Several studies address the insertion of pesticides and other organic pollutants into membranes, their accumulation in lipid rafts, or lipid rafts' disruption by polychlorinated biphenyls (PCBs), benzo[a]pyrene (B[a]P), and even metals/metalloids. In hepatocytes, macrophages, or neurons, B[a]P, airborne particulate matter, and other toxicants caused rafts' protein and lipid remodeling, oxidative changes, or amyloidogenesis. Different studies investigated the role of the invaginated lipid rafts present in endothelial cells in mediating the vascular inflammatory effects of PCBs. Furthermore, in vitro and in vivo data strongly implicate raft-localized NADPH oxidases, the aryl hydrocarbon receptor, caveolin-1, and protein kinases in the toxic mechanisms of occupational and environmental chemicals.

Keywords: caveolae; cholesterol; endocrine disruptors; environmental toxicology; inflammatory signaling; lipophilic agents; membrane rafts; pollutants; polycyclic aromatic hydrocarbons; toxic agents

1. Introduction

Lipid rafts and plasma membrane domains abundant in cholesterol and sphingolipids have been reported to participate in important cellular processes, namely, in terms of the space-time dimension of signal transduction and cell signaling [1–3], and so act as molecular signaling hubs.

Environmental and occupational toxicants can bring about a great diversity of cellular and systemic alterations implicated in the short-term and long-term outcomes of toxic exposures [4–9]. The cellular effects of common pollutants (or their metabolites) can affect redox status, calcium homeostasis, metabolic and epigenetic programs, among other disturbances, but the key molecular targets and mechanisms of action of specific compounds remain unresolved [4,10–14].

Many environmental chemicals are lipophilic, which allows them to accumulate in the plasma membrane, but the potential role of membrane raft-like domains unleashing their cellular effects is debatable. As it will be discussed in the following sections, experimental evidence exists for the targeting of lipid rafts—on cells in vitro—by some toxicants, such as polychlorinated biphenyls (PCBs) and air pollutants [15–17]. In addition, environmental or occupational exposures have been demonstrated to alter the levels of raft-related lipids [18–20], and to disturb signaling events associated with these membrane domains [6,15,21–23].

Therefore, it is plausible that raft-like domains at the plasma membrane play a role as hubs/platforms for environmental and occupational toxicants to trigger or amplify their toxic actions in cells. The present work aimed to collect and discuss the existing evidence supporting this hypothesis and to identify gaps to be addressed in future research.

2. Lipid Rafts—Structure and Composition

2.1. Plasma Membrane Domains

The lipid rafts concept marked a change in the understanding of the plasma membrane organization and function. Before it, the plasma membrane was understood by Singer and Nicholson's classical membrane fluid mosaic model. Nevertheless, the new concept amplified the understanding related to the structure and function of the plasma membrane [24,25] into a more complex structure where lateral diffusion of membrane domains is possible. Lipid rafts are described as plasma membrane compartments highly enriched in cholesterol, sphingolipids, and phospholipids containing saturated fatty acids (Figure 1) that support different functions of the cell, such as signal transduction [24,26,27]. By norm, the lipid rafts are defined as membrane subdomains enriched in cholesterol and sphingolipids containing saturated acyl chains as represented in Figure 1 [1,24]. The idea of rafts derives from the floating property promoted by the sphingolipids' enrichment in the outer leaflet of the membrane (Figure 1) [28].

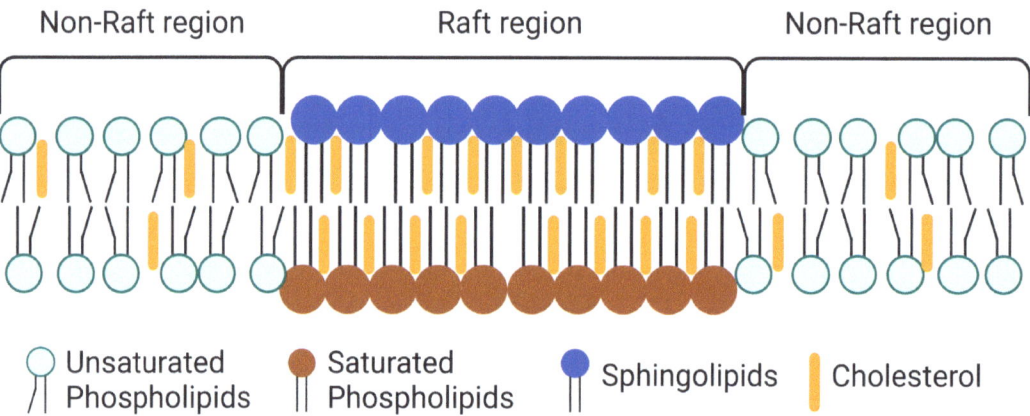

Figure 1. Representation of the lipidic distribution in the lipid raft and non-lipid raft regions of the cell membrane. Sphingolipids are enriched in the outer leaflet of the raft region, along with saturated phospholipids present in the inner leaflet. Lipid rafts present a more packed organization than non-raft regions. Figure created with BioRender.com.

The frontier between floating membrane domains and larger and more stable membrane subdomains is not clear. Lipid rafts can vary from highly transient domains to larger and more stable structures [29]. In this sense, the extent of lipid raft enlargement depends on the organism, cell type, and composition of the raft [30]. In eukaryotic cells, lateral compartmentalization of the plasma membrane into microdomains has been described, and yeast cells present very well-defined membrane compartments [30]. The membrane compartmentalization into subdomains is crucial for the physiological functions of the cell [31], in accordance, the structure of these domains is distinct depending on the cell specialization [32–34]. Nevertheless, the compartmentalization mechanisms are complex and still need to be better understood, with a variety of possibilities for membrane subdomains to co-exist, such as stable domains, transient compartments, or nanodomains [31].

In many mammalian cells, caveolae are the most abundant membrane subdomains [35]. They were first reported in 1955 [36] and are also considered a sub-type of lipid raft in the form of small flask-shaped invaginations due to the presence of caveolin [37–39]. Although lipid rafts have similar components and comparable functions, they are more diverse in terms of size and considered more dynamic than caveolae [40]. Caveolae, on the contrary, are considered stable structures in the plasma membrane [41].

The physical-chemical characteristics of caveolae facilitate their identification by electron microscopy, while the existence of lipid rafts in living cells remains to be clearly demonstrated [40]. The direct observation of lipid rafts that would clarify the existence of these structures in living organisms is challenging due to their nanoscale dimensions and limited lifetime. For this reason, some authors are critical of the concept of lipid rafts [42,43] and the methods used to study these domains are discussed [44]. Yet, scientific advances are being made in this field [45] and a collection of fluorescent lipid probes that preferentially partition into raft and non-raft domains has been suggested recently [46].

Despite the doubts of the scientific community about the appropriate nomenclature of membrane raft-like domains and methodological limitations to proof the existence of lipid rafts, from the perspective of Sevcsik and Schütz (2015), the concept of lipid rafts is defended until methodological evidence is clarified [42]. Having this discussion in mind and the common properties shared by the different membrane raft-like domains, the reader will be guided throughout this review on the use of the general term "lipid rafts" as an umbrella for the different nomenclatures that include rafts, detergent-resistant membranes (DRMs), and caveolae [1,42].

2.2. Properties of Lipid Rafts and Composition

The lipid rafts, which originate from the interactions between sterols and saturated lipids, form a liquid-ordered phase that is tightly packed, distinct from the typical disordered lipid phase regarding flexibility and permeability [24]. Regen (2020) presented lipid rafts with a central role for cholesterol in promoting favorable or repelling interactions depending on the lipid with which cholesterol interacts, i.e., high-melting lipids or low-melting lipids, respectively [47]. Moreover, the lipid composition of these rafts was described as being different between the exoplasmic and cytoplasmic leaflet faces. Cholesterol and sphingolipids are described as being present in the outer face, while cholesterol and phospholipids are in the inner leaflet of these microdomains (Figure 1) [48]. The difference in lipids' function is justified by the difference in lipids' function, with the phospholipids forming the lipid bilayer and the sphingolipids modulating fundamental cell processes such as apoptosis [49]. Furthermore, there is a correlation between the complexity of membrane composition, properties, and functions. The presence of sphingolipids and sterols in eukaryotic cell membranes makes vesicular trafficking possible, impacting the establishment and maintenance of distinct organelles [50].

In general, cholesterol is an essential player in the different types of lipid rafts. The deprivation of cholesterol reduced the number of caveolae in the cell, showing its essential role in the formation of these structures [51], but its relevance doesn't stop here. Its key role in the cell requires its synthesis, homeostasis, and efflux to be maintained through a free cholesterol concentration gradient between the endoplasmic reticulum and the plasma membrane that is preserved by a tight feedback control mechanism [52]. Moreover, intracellular cholesterol trafficking regulates membrane rafts and consequent cell signaling [52,53]. To investigate the effect of cholesterol in lipid rafts' cellular mechanisms, different chemical agents are used as methodological approaches to experimentally remove cholesterol. One example of these cholesterol-depleting agents is nystatin, as described in [54], but methyl-ß-cyclodextrin is probably one of the most commonly used to test the presence or function of a protein in the cell microdomains [55–58].

A well-described lipid specific to membrane rafts is the GM1 glycosphingolipids or ganglioside [59,60], which is highly relevant for the function of diverse signalosomes [61]. The GM1 glycosphingolipids are cellular receptors for the cholera toxin B-subunit (CTxB) [62], a protein widely investigated and associated with lipid rafts [63]. This relationship makes CTxB a lipid raft marker extensively used in studies of membrane biology and biophysics [19,64]. In the laboratory led by Professor Carlos Gutierrez-Merino, CTxB was useful to demonstrate the clustering of plasma membrane-bound cytochrome b5 reductase within "lipid raft" microdomains in neurons in vitro and the cerebellum cortex of adult rats [65,66]. In more recent works developed by other groups, the presence of GM1 gangliosides near specific neuronal proteins is starting to be revealed as an interfering factor for their function [67,68].

The lipid rafts are also composed of membrane proteins that can be recruited by different molecular mechanisms, such as post-translational modifications like palmitoylation or protein-protein/lipid interactions, among others [69]. Moreover, the cooperation between lipids and proteins is essential for membrane organization. For example, some proteins, like cytoskeletal components, can regulate lipid domains, or, on the other hand, protein oligomerization can contribute to the clustering and stabilization of raft domains, as reviewed by [43]. As described before, a specific type of raft is known as caveolae ("little caves"), containing caveolin proteins and forming the innermost layer of the caveolar coat [39,70]. Caveolae form invaginations enriched in cholesterol, sphingolipids, and lipid-modified proteins such as H-Ras, with the caveolins being suggested to act as concentration and organization agents of these domains [71]. Other proteins were also reported to be enriched on lipid rafts, and in the specific case of flotillin, it was described as stabilizing caveolin-1 [71,72]. For better comprehension, in 2003, a study identified three different types of proteins: raft proteins, raft-associated proteins, and nonspecific proteins [73]. Proteins like flotillins and caveolin-1 were identified as raft and raft-associated proteins [73]. Moreover, another work reviewed the properties and functions of permanent raft-resident proteins and temporary raft-resident proteins [69]. Again, the structural proteins caveolins and flotillins were identified as permanent raft-resident proteins, while other proteins like TNF receptor 1 and NADPH oxidase were identified as temporary raft-resident proteins [69].

At the experimental level, having proteins identified by different studies as characteristic of lipid rafts allows us to use them as lipid raft markers in DRMs. DRMs are considered representative of membrane lipid rafts [1] since their obtention takes advantage of the lipid rafts' insolubility in non-ionic detergents at 4 °C and the consequent use of sucrose-density gradients [74]. This methodological approach was used in the laboratory of Professor Carlos Gutiérrez-Merino to investigate the presence of functional proteins in the membrane microdomains of cultured cerebellar granule neurons [58,75–78]. But fluorescence methods, such as Foster resonance energy transfer (FRET) and high-resolution microscopic techniques, are useful when studying lipid rafts [45,46,52]. These tools allow for carrying out studies related to signal transduction and cellular responses associated with lipid rafts, which can be considered a technical challenge due to the nanoscale of these cellular structures, estimated to be 5–80 nm [52].

2.3. Lipid Rafts as Platforms for Signal Transduction in Cells

As described in Section 2.1, despite the immensity of works on lipid rafts, their existence, nature, and function in vivo are still an open question for some authors [43], due to their dynamic nature and small occurrence scale [52]. Although their relevance for cell function has been proposed since the first reports of lipid rafts [27], there is accumulating evidence for their existence and role in cell biology [52].

It is expected that the presence of proteins in lipid rafts in nanoscale dimensions favors the ability of lipid raft components to respond to diverse stimuli [52]. For example, proteins such as calcium channels, transporters, and redox proteins were identified in lipid raft microdomains of cerebellar granule cells [75–79]. These nanodomains were suggested to act as "calcium micro-chip-like structures," forming a focalized redox/calcium integrative structure for fast and efficient cross-talk between calcium and redox signaling in neurons [77], which can be highly relevant to avoid distortion of cytoskeleton-linked lipid raft structures more prone to oxidation such as actin [80]. Additionally, the removal of cholesterol impacted cytosolic calcium homeostasis, leading cells to a pro-apoptotic state, showing that the proximity between the investigated proteins guarantees their function in cell signaling [58]. Indeed, the consequences of removing cholesterol and having non-functional proteins because they are dissociated from lipid rafts have long been described [48]. These physiological advantages are representative of the cellular benefit of membrane compartmentalization generated by the lipid rafts, but other works widely reflect the effect of lipid rafts in cell signaling [1,81]. And, new cellular mechanisms associated with raft membranes are being continuously described, such as inflammation [53], tyrosine kinase receptor, T cell antigen receptor, and estrogenic signaling [82–84], as well as signaling associated with cancer [3,85,86]. In the next section, a detailed description is provided for the cellular mechanisms associated with lipid rafts.

3. Lipid Rafts in Cell Signaling and Disease

Cell maintenance and proper functioning rely on the different intra and extra-cellular processes, their flux, equilibrium, and control. And lipid raft-like domains are described as contributing to different cellular processes as described previously [1,53,81–84].

3.1. Calcium and Redox Signaling in Neurodegeneration

Different studies investigated the importance of lipid rafts in neurodegeneration, some pointing to neuroprotective effects while others pointed to neuropathological consequences. In this sense, different points of view are reflected in [87] and a reconfiguration of membrane rafts was proposed as a strategy to counteract mechanisms associated with Alzheimer's disease (AD), Parkinson's disease, and amyotrophic lateral sclerosis [88]. For example, effects on the aggregation of amyloid and on the processing of the amyloid precursor protein associated with lipid rafts have been reported [17,89]. Nevertheless, how chemical toxicants can affect these mechanisms is not yet known. Recently, DTT was shown to provoke loss of the postsynaptic density protein 95, a protein reported in complexes of raft and postsynaptic proteins [90] and this effect was related to altered levels of the amyloid precursor protein [91].

In terms of understanding the disrupting effects of oxidative and nitrosative stress in lipid rafts, they are well described in neuroimmune disorders [92]. In the neuronal cell line N27, the disruption of lipid rafts blocked androgen-induced oxidative stress in cells by decreasing the localization of the membrane androgen receptor in lipid rafts [54]. In this case, as in another study with brain endothelial cells [16], the production of reactive oxygen species (ROS) was ascribed to raft-localized NADPH oxidase, a superoxide-producing enzyme. On the contrary, lipid rafts in cerebellar granule neurons were described as ROS generation points since they cluster the cytochrome b5 reductase, leading to exaggerated plasma membrane-focalized superoxide anion production and oxidative stress-mediated apoptosis [66,78]. This same protein was found close to lipid raft regions in adult rat cerebellum neurons [65]. Additionally, in primary fibroblasts from familial AD patients, the amyloid beta oligomers were recruited to membrane rafts leading to lipid peroxidation and deregulation of calcium homeostasis [93]. A similar effect was observed in cerebellar granule neurons, where the cytosolic calcium homeostasis was affected by the binding of amyloid-calmodulin complexes to lipid rafts [94]. Indeed, calcium deregulation is implicated in neurodegeneration [95–97] and, in different neurons, the removal of cholesterol affected the calcium homeostasis controlled by different calcium proteins, leading, in the case of cerebellar granule neurons, to apoptosis [58,98,99]. This interplay between oxidative stress and calcium homeostasis in neurons related to lipid rafts is described by different authors [77,99]. Thus, if we consider that the amyloid precursor protein and amyloid peptides occur in the membrane rafts that are implicated in nitrosative processes and modulation of calcium signaling in different neurons [17,89,94], the relevance of these structures—allowing the interplay between both signaling actors—in neurodegeneration and other pathologies deserves further investigation.

3.2. Inflammation and Atherosclerosis

Another example of lipid rafts' relevance in cell signaling is their implication in TNFα-mediated signaling. A study showed that cholesterol sequestration from lipid rafts inhibits the activation of the nuclear factor kappa-light chain-enhancer of activated B cells (NF-κB) pathway and therefore induces the switch of TNFα-mediated responses toward apoptosis [100]. Moreover, the effects on TRL4 signaling in macrophages are also influenced by lipid rafts. There are different mechanisms by which lipid raft perturbations—including intracellular and extracellular cholesterol trafficking—regulate the innate immune response [53]. Recently, in the context of neuroinflammation and pain processing, the concept of inflammaraft was proposed to represent the lipid raft platforms that initiate an inflammatory response [101]. These membrane microdomains function as a framework for inflammatory signaling, containing receptors and signaling molecules such as TRL4, ion channels, and enzymes [101].

Exposure to ambient and diesel exhaust particulate matter (PM) and heavy metals like lead and mercury induces inflammation and endothelial/vascular dysfunction, which is associated with altered vasoconstriction/vasorelaxation and the development of atherosclerosis and cardiovascular diseases [5,12,14]. Noteworthy, proteins controlling Ca^{2+} signaling and the endothelial nitric oxide synthase (eNOS or NOS3) are localized in caveolae of endothelial cells and play central roles in regulating blood pressure and flow, angiogenesis, and vascular inflammation [14,16,102,103]. In these cells, when cytosolic or local microdomain calcium levels rise, calcium-calmodulin activates NOS3 and nitric oxide production by displacing the enzyme from caveolin-1 [14,103]. At the disease level, a review explored the relevance of the plasma membrane microdomains in the inflammation associated with atherosclerosis [104]. Moreover, in vivo evidence highlights the significance of lipid rafts [56,57] and inflammarafts were observed in nonfoamy macrophages in atherosclerotic lesions [105].

3.3. Immune Regulation

The plasma membrane microdomains play an important role in immune regulation. One example is the requirement of lipid rafts for target internalization by the platelet IgG Fc receptor (FcγRIIa). Although the receptor activities are independent of the receptor localization [106].

In T and B cell lines, the lipid rafts are also required for the recruitment of different components of the death-inducing signaling complex (DISC), allowing efficient Fas signaling and apoptosis [107]. Also in T cells, the lipid rafts were shown to be implicated in the induction of apoptosis through the clustering of DISC protein components [108]. Moreover, the disruption of lipid rafts suppressed the drug-induced DISC assembly and apoptosis [108]. Regarding the effects of disrupting lipid rafts in T cells, it was shown that it affected T cell receptor (TCR) signaling [83] and receptor nanoclusters could be involved in enhanced memory sensitivity compared with naive T cells [109]. Indeed, a study revealed that T cell responses to TCR stimulation will depend on the level of lipid ordering in the plasma membrane. The authors observed that high membrane order promoted T cell proliferation, while low membrane order derives from insensitive T cells [110].

The deregulation of T and B cell signaling can conduct to autoimmune diseases. Diverse studies point to the relevance of the lipid raft signaling platform in unbridled T cell responses in systemic lupus erythematosus (SLE). The T cells of SLE patients showed increased expression of the raft-associated GM1 [111] and different lipid raft compositions were associated with higher and frontloaded calcium responses [112]. Moreover, B lymphocytes of SLE patients showed altered expression of kinases and phosphatases and altered interaction with lipid rafts or translocation into these microdomains [113].

In the case of autoimmune rheumatic disease, a study investigated ex vivo primary human CD4$^+$ T cells, observing that the response to TCR stimulation depends on the ordering of the lipid membrane. This study identified that the patients' T cells showed a distinct membrane order when compared with the T cells of healthy volunteers [110]. And a recent study highlights the relevance of cholesterol-dependent membrane order in CD4$^+$ T cell signaling [114].

Another interesting example of the rafts' involvement in disease is the study case of raftlin, an abundant protein in the lipid rafts of B cells and long known as essential for the functioning of these lipid rafts and the associated B-cell antigen receptor signaling [115]. The fact that the development of chronic rhinosinusitis with nasal polyps is related to the deficiency of raftlin in the nasal polyp tissue [116] points to the critical role of lipid raft integrity in this tissue and disease.

3.4. Hormone Signaling

The thyrotropin receptor's (TSHR) functions are regulated by lipid rafts [117]. And these receptors are key regulators for thyroid growth and function, and interaction with G proteins results in different cellular responses such as hormone synthesis and secretion but also cell proliferation or survival. In a cell model, thyrotropin increased the TSHR localization in plasma membrane rafts, apparently necessary for the subsequent internalization of the receptor [19]. Moreover, the same mechanism of lipid raft-mediated hormone signaling is described for the luteinizing hormone receptors. In this sense, the translocation of the hormone-occupied luteinizing hormone receptors into lipid rafts was reported as an optimizing condition for signaling [118].

The receptor tyrosine kinases, which also play a relevant role as hormone receptors, are associated with different cellular processes after ligand binding. It should be recalled that several environmental toxicants behave as endocrine disruptors, and some effects may involve G protein-coupled receptors [4,119] and/or signal-transducing protein kinases associated with lipid rafts—Src, MAPKs, JAK2, and LRRK2 (as detailed in Section 4). The clustering of receptors and related kinases into the different lipid raft types along with the affected signaling pathways is widely described, and a review is recommended for further details [82]. In the same way, the nongenomic effects of estrogens were also described as being related to the presence of estrogen receptor (ER) subpopulations in lipid rafts [84]. The activation of these plasma membrane ER triggers rapid cell responses, while the classic effects mediated by intracellular ER take a few hours [84].

The interaction of estrogen with the ER located in signalosomes mainly present in lipid rafts is described as conducting preventive mechanisms counteracting AD [120]. Indeed, the malfunction of ER-signalosomes was also discussed in menopause conditions [121]. More recently, the same group showed a slight increase in six proteins associated with the ER-signalosome—including ERalpha, caveolin-1, and flotillin—in the preclinical stages of AD [122]. In addition to neurons, ERalfa or ERbeta have been found at caveola/lipid rafts or associated with raft proteins in endothelial cells, vascular smooth muscle cells, cardiomyocytes, platelets, lymphocytes, and cancer cells [84].

The ERalfa at membrane caveolae associates with G proteins, NOS3, Src kinases, phosphoinositide 3-kinase (PI3K)/Akt, JAK/STAT, and MAPKs [84]. This cluster of proteins partially coincides with the rafts-associated protein network further described in Section 4 and can underlie changes in cytosolic calcium and cAMP levels, dysregulation of nitric oxide production, and MAPK, PI3K, JAK/STAT, or Src/STAT pathway activation, processes implicated in environmental toxicants' exposure, inflammation, and carcinogenesis [4,5,11,12,123,124]. These ER signalosome complexes could allow estrogen disruptors targeting lipid rafts to modify hormone signaling without direct interference with receptor-hormone binding.

A membrane androgen receptor (AR45) has also been found in the plasma membrane rafts of neuronal, prostate, and Sertoli cells [54]. In N27 neurons, AR45 is associated with caveolin-1 and NADPH oxidase, and under oxidative conditions, testosterone amplified cell stress and activated caspase-3 in a cholesterol-dependent way. Furthermore, the disruption of lipid rafts was reported to decrease membrane androgen receptors and their internalization [54].

3.5. Cell Communication

Also in cell communication processes, the lipid rafts reveal themselves to be essential either by favoring exosome uptake or biogenesis [125,126] or by influencing the co-localization of connexin-43 with caveolin-1 [127].

Indeed, connexin-43 allows direct cell-cell communication through participation in gap junctions and is also suggested to take part in cellular fine-tuned regulation mechanisms like cell cycle regulation [128] which highlights the role of lipid rafts in these mechanisms. Moreover, the spatiotemporal dimensions are becoming increasingly relevant to understanding membrane trafficking mechanisms, and lipid rafts are one of the players in the automation of these biological processes [2].

3.6. Cell Death and Cancer

Additionally, and complementary to the role of cholesterol described earlier, the depletion of this sterol can also affect apoptosis and proliferation mechanisms since it activates a protein responsible for the maintenance of cellular pH, the Na+/H+ exchanger 1 (NHE-1). In this case, cholesterol depletion is associated with a relocation of the protein outside the microdomains, leading to its activation [129]. But from the therapeutic perspective of cell signaling, cholesterol was shown to play a critical role in the resistance of glioblastoma cells to temozolomide. The cell viability of non-resistant U251 cells increased by decreasing intracellular cholesterol, whereas the addition of cholesterol decreased cell viability [130,131]. This effect occurred via the accumulation and activation of a protein of the tumor necrosis factor receptor family—death receptor 5—in the lipid rafts that affect cell death mechanisms via caspase signaling [131].

Other apoptotic and anti-apoptotic signaling pathways were also described as being triggered by lipid rafts [132]. The apoptotic signaling dependent on lipid rafts can derive from the receptors and channels embedded in the plasma membrane, such as Fas, CD5, CD20, and Trpc-1, or via protein kinase proteins like Akt (or PKB), JNK, Src kinases, and protein kinase C (PKC) family proteins [132]. Lipid rafts are implicated in the operation of different signaling mechanisms regulating cancer cell survival, death, invasion, and metastasis [85,86]. It is especially impressive that lipid rafts were revealed to be essential to promoting or inhibiting the different cell signaling pathways associated with distinct stages of metastasis, such as angiogenesis, epithelial-to-mesenchymal transition, migration, transendothelial migration, cell death, and adhesion [3].

4. Effects of Environmental Toxicants in Lipid Rafts Organization and Signaling

Considering the high relevance of lipid rafts in cell signaling and disease, how environmental toxicants affect such cellular mechanisms deserves to be explored.

If we look at the Gene Ontology (GO) database, 109 proteins are listed in the "Plasma membrane raft" class of Cellular Component (GO:0044853). And, as expected, these proteins are associated with a great diversity of cellular and molecular functions, including responses to chemical stimuli and cellular stress.

Under the scope of this work, by refining the list of proteins to those classified in the biological process "Cellular response to chemical stress" (GO:0062197), the protein association network shown in Figure 2 could be obtained. The more enriched KEGG pathway is the vascular endothelial growth factor (VEGF) signaling pathway—proteins Src, MAPK1, and 3 (also known as ERK2 and 1, respectively), PTGS2, and NOS3—a pathway tightly connected to angiogenesis, the permeability of endothelial cells, and tumor growth. Also to be noted, the network contains several protein kinases, components of the mitogen-activated protein kinase (MAPK), and other important signal transduction pathways controlling a variety of biological processes, including cytoskeletal arrangements, regulation of cell fate, and immune response. Hence, the proteins identified in this network seem to be probable mediators of cellular responses to toxic chemicals targeting plasma membrane rafts. Indeed, as discussed in the next sections, some of these proteins were described as involved in the cellular effects of environmental toxicants. But other proteins, the lipids present in lipid raft-like domains, and the lipid rafts themselves are also described as targets of environmental toxicants. At the end of this section, Figure 3 compiles a schematic overview of the reported evidence found in the literature and distributed along the next subsections.

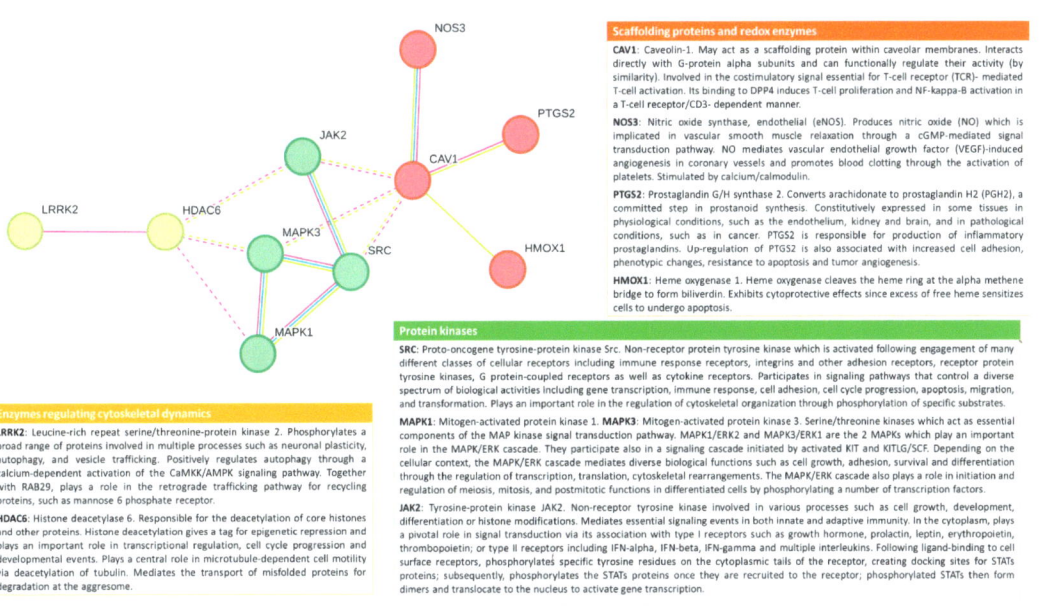

Figure 2. Interaction network of the proteins closely related to membrane lipid rafts and involved in cellular responses to chemical stress. The network was generated with STRING https://string-db.org (accessed on 15 April 2023) entering proteins classified simultaneously in Gene Ontology (GO) "Plasma membrane raft" cellular component (GO:0044853) and Biological Process "Cellular response to chemical stress" (GO:0062197). Physical subnetwork (edges indicate physical association) of proteins with a minimum Interaction score of 0.400. Different colors represent the three clusters of proteins obtained by both K-means and MCL clustering methods. The protein descriptions were adapted from UniProtKB https://www.uniprot.org (accessed on 15 April 2023).

4.1. Accumulation of Environmental Toxicants in Lipid Rafts and Associated Cellular Effects

Being the cell membrane a barrier between extracellular and intracellular space, it is expected that lipophilic organic compounds accumulate in this lipidic environment (Figure 3). A study showed that lipophilic hydrocarbons accumulate in the lipid membrane, affecting the structure and properties of the membrane [133]. In liposomes, the pesticides 1,1,1-trichloro-2,2-bis(p-chlorophenyl)-ethane (DDT) and lindane were found to intercalate between the fatty acyl chains of membrane phospholipids [134,135]. Moreover, another study investigating 240 organic compounds showed that partition coefficients for membrane lipids are higher when compared to the partition coefficient for storage lipids [136]. And specifically, in the case of PAHs, it was shown that depending on the compound investigated, it could mix or not with phospholipid monolayers. B[a]P, among others, was shown to incorporate into the membrane [137]. But other cases of toxic accumulation in the plasma membrane were described, such as the case of 2,4,6-trinitrotoluene (TNT) and its metabolites [138]. Toxicant metabolites, even if more hydrophilic than the parent molecules, can be incorporated into lipid membranes and modify lipid-lipid and lipid-protein interactions. For instance, 1-hydroxypyrene, the main metabolite of pyrene and a biomarker of PAH exposure, occupies the water-inaccessible interior of liposomes, apparently residing in a quite rigid environment [139].

Studies with clear evidence for the accumulation of environmental toxicants on the lipid raft domains of cell membranes are scarce. The enrichment of lipid rafts on toxic species can occur by binding to proteins, as proposed for copper ion complexation by amyloid in neuronal lipid rafts [89]. Another study demonstrated the accumulation of PCB77 in the caveolae-rich fraction [102] and further studies revealed that exposure to PCB77 strongly impacts vascular inflammation mechanisms [102,140]. Interestingly, in both studies, caveolin-1 silencing attenuates the effects provoked by PCB77 either in vitro or in vivo [102,140]. There was an increase in MCP-1 cytokine levels in endothelial cells exposed to PCB77 [140]. Depicting the molecular mechanism implicated in the increase of MCP-1 levels produced by PCB77, different pathways such as the aryl hydrocarbon receptor (AhR), p38, and JNK signaling were identified [140]. Moreover, PCB77 provoked an increase in caveolin-1 and CYP1A1 levels in the same cells, showing that PCB77 promoted the binding of the AhR to caveolin-1 [102].

AhR is a transcription factor activated by several major environmental toxicants, such as dioxins, some PAHs, pesticides, and PCBs, regulating the transcription of CYP450 enzymes (e.g., CYP1A1) and matrix metalloproteinases (MMP), among other genes [141]. However, the relevance of AhR non-genomic functions has been discussed, namely the modulation of cytosolic calcium and caveolin-1 distribution [4,14,142]. In line with the data above on endothelial cells, a subpopulation of AhR could be found in caveolin-1 DRMs from fibroblasts and hepatoma cells, and the two proteins could immunoprecipitate each other [142]. Moreover, AhR expression promoted the localization of caveolin-1 at fibroblasts' DRMs, playing an important role in controlling cell adhesion and migration. Mechanistically, a non-canonical AhR signaling pathway has been proposed to activate c-Src, at least in response to dioxin (Figure 3), and c-Src activity participates in the regulation of caveolin-1 expression and phosphorylation [14,141,142].

Oxidative stress was also associated with PCB77 exposure [102,140]. The aggregation of PCBs into lipid rafts and induction of oxidative stress has been previously suggested, as well as antioxidant compounds that could protect against the damaging effects of PCBs [143,144]. PCB-induced oxidative stress can be related to the inhibition of nuclear factor (erythroid-derived 2)-like 2 (Nrf2) pathways, which are important for the induction of antioxidant genes like heme oxygenase-1 (HMOX1). Caveolin-1 silencing increased Nrf2 transcriptional activity in PCB126-incubated cells, and endothelial cells from caveolin-1$^{-/-}$ mice treated with PCB126 showed higher expression of antioxidant genes [145].

The same group observed that disruption of caveolae attenuated the B[a]P-induced expression of the intercellular adhesion molecule-1 (ICAM-1), again revealing a pro-inflammatory mechanism involving AhR signaling dependent on caveolae [146]. Thus far, the accumulation of B[a]P in lipid rafts is not clearly evident. Therefore, this type of evidence regarding the accumulation of environmental toxicants in lipid rafts would amplify the perception of the relevance of these lipid structures in environmental toxicology.

4.2. Alterations in Rafts' Lipid Composition and Associated Cellular Effects

4.2.1. Disruption of Lipid Rafts

Alteration of lipid raft properties and composition by environmental toxicants has been reported in different studies [18,19,55,147].

A concrete effect on lipid rafts was described for iron associated with silica exposure in macrophages, where disruption of lipid rafts was observed together with an increase in superoxide, lipid oxidation, and cytokine production [55]. Iron chelators inhibited all the effects, and an inhibitor of phospholipase C (PLC) blocked cytokine production. The authors proposed that in the presence of a low noncytotoxic concentration of silica, iron prompted lipid oxidation, disrupting lipid rafts, and signaling to produce cytokines by way of PLC and NF-kB. The NF-kB is an essential regulator of inflammation and innate immunity, controlling the transcription of a variety of effectors including cytokines, ICAM-1, and cyclooxygenase-2 (coded by the PTGS2 gene, Figure 2).

Lipid oxidation and oxidative stress were also observed in lipid raft fractions from both the cerebral cortex of mice and neuronal cell models of AD exposed to airborne PM with pro-amyloidogenic activity [17]. Pointing to the critical role of the oxidative modifications, the PM triggered rapid increases in nitric oxide and hydroxynonenal in the cells, and the antioxidant N-acetyl-cysteine attenuated the PM-induced increase in lipid raft amyloidogenesis [17].

The effect of B[a]P in membrane remodeling was investigated by using rat liver F258 epithelial cells, revealing modification of lipid rafts [18]. Previously, the authors described that B[a]P affected membrane fluidity, inducing apoptosis [148] and a deeper research design showed that exposure to this toxicant changed the cellular distribution of the ganglioside-GM1, altered fatty acid composition, and decreased the cholesterol content of lipid rafts in different cell types [18,149]. This effect could be explained by the reduced expression of 3-hydroxy-3-methylglutaryl-CoA reductase (HMG-CoA reductase), observed with as low as 50 nM of B[a]P [18], since HMG-CoA reductase catalyzes the rate-limiting step of cholesterol synthesis [150]. Moreover, the authors went further, and the experimental results obtained suggest that AhR and CYP1 pathways are implicated in the membrane remodeling triggered by B[a]P [18]. Indeed, the toxicity of this compound is closely linked to the activation of the AhR and metabolization by CYP450 enzymes [4]. Furthermore, the membrane remodeling by B[a]P was considered an apoptosis-inducing intracellular alkalinization event [18] that was then shown to be related to the relocation of NHE-1 from lipid rafts promoted by B[a]P [151]. This alkalinization event was prevented by docosahexaenoic acid (DHA) and eicosapentaenoic acid (EPA), which showed to act as protector agents precisely by affecting B[a]P effects at the plasma membrane and NHE-1 activity [152].

B[a]P was also suggested as a destabilizing agent of lipid raft structure [147]. By using rat hepatocytes, 100 nM of B[a]P provoked diffuse staining of the ganglioside-GM1 compared to a no-treatment situation, but supplying cells with cholesterol counteracted the B[a]P effect. Moreover, the addition of cholesterol also inhibited further cellular effects of B[a]P such as decreased cell viability and ATP content. Additionally, B[a]P provoked lipid oxidation that was then reversed by a lipid raft disrupter [147]. Furthermore, the authors observed that B[a]P effects were aggravated by further exposing the cells to ethanol and that both toxicants triggered the permeabilization of lysosomes through the plasma membrane [147]. The effect of B[a]P exposure on the decrease of membrane cholesterol was also reported in human macrophages, where lipid raft stability is affected along with their activation mechanism [15]. Finally, the effect of B[a]P on membrane dynamics and lipid components was recently investigated in vivo [22]. In the lung tissue of B[a]P-exposed animals, it was observed a decrease in the levels of cholesterol, glycolipids, microviscosity, and anisotropy, together with an increase in total lipids and phospholipids [22]. Additionally, alterations in membrane fluidity, polarization, and order of membrane were also described in lung tissue [22].

4.2.2. Alterations in Membrane Lipids

Together with disruption, changes in the membrane order and levels of raft-related lipids are also reported after exposures to other organic and inorganic pollutants. By incorporating into the bilayer, DTT decreased the phase transition temperature of model membranes [134,135] and depleted rafts of their phosphoglycolipid and cholesterol contents [19]. In Wistar rats, it was observed that aluminum treatment caused disorganization of the lipid bilayer in erythrocytes [153]. PCB52 is described in two different studies for its effect on cell membrane fluidity, either by increasing it in mouse thymocytes [154], or by decreasing it in cerebellar granule cells [155]. Moreover, exposure of DU145 cells to 1 microM of the pesticide aldrin led to a decrease in phospholipids and sphingolipids, whereas aroclor 1254 (PCB 82) and chlorpyrifos caused an increase in certain phospholipids and glycosphingolipids in the chloroform and methanol extracts [156]. On a different front, exposure to the anti-cancer cardiotoxic drug doxorubicin downregulated the HMG-CoA reductase in cancer cells, as previously reported for B[a]P [18], with the consequent reduction of cholesterol and lipid rafts [157]. These actions of doxorubicin were closely connected to the inactivation of the epidermal growth factor receptor (EGFR)/Src signaling pathway and activation of caspase-3, effects that were ameliorated by cholesterol supplementation. Interestingly, other work observed doxorubicin-induced caspase-3 activation in association with lipid oxidation and NADPH oxidase activation [158], similar to the reported for B[a]P and PM organic mixtures [4,147,159]. These environmental toxicants and others are ligands of AhR that, in turn, can activate membrane NADPH oxidase [4,141].

The membrane raft-associated AhR discussed before and their possible functions as signaling mediators, in addition to being transcription factors, might play important roles in fibroblasts, hepatocytes, and endothelial cells' responses to dioxin-like pollutants, especially under conditions of membrane cholesterol deficit [14,142]. A dichloromethane extract of diesel exhaust particles, containing the PAHs phenanthrene, fluoranthene, pyrene, and chrysene, among other organic compounds, was found to disorder the plasma membrane of human microvascular endothelial cells, an effect that was prevented with cholesterol supplementation of the media [14]. The same extract and others with more lipophilic compounds triggered a rapid increase in intracellular calcium, which was substantially reduced when AhR was pharmacologically inhibited or knocked down via siRNA. However, the fast kinetics of this response are inconsistent with a mechanism of transcriptional regulation and can only be explained by a nongenomic AhR signaling pathway. Functional interaction of the rafts-associated AhR with caveolin-1 and Src signaling [14,141,142] indicates that caveolin-1, cytosolic calcium, NADPH oxidases, and Src kinases can transduce the destabilization of cholesterol-rich plasma membrane domains by organic toxicants (Figure 3). In neurons, the strongly hydrophobic pesticide rotenone also induced a fast cytosolic calcium increase, but by way of specific calcium channels expressed in these cells at membrane rafts [13,77].

4.2.3. Alterations in the Levels of Raft-Related Lipids

In humans, it is well established that cadmium, lead, and mercury exposures increase serum cholesterol levels [12]. Correlations were also detected between blood concentrations of arsenic and mercury, and especially manganese and zinc, with alterations in the levels of plasmenyl phospholipids and sphingomyelin [160]. A metabolomic study of mice exposed to PM also uncovered alterations in the blood levels of glycerol (phospho)lipids, sphingolipids, and lysophospholipids and in pathways involved in the metabolism of fatty acids and sterols, among other critical metabolites and hormones [20].

However, how these changes in lipid levels reflect in cell membrane lipid rafts has yet to be investigated. In one study, exposure to manganese induced apoptosis in PC12 cells together with an alteration of the lipidic profile of the DRMs regarding their composition on phosphatidylinositol, phosphatidylcholine, and sphingomyelin [161]. Concerning changes of lipids in membrane rafts, a recent study revealed that electronic cigarette smoke in A549 provoked alterations in the levels of phosphatidylcholines, phosphatidylserine, and sphingomyelin, among others, in lipid raft fractions [21]. Moreover, the addition of nicotine exacerbated the differences in lipid raft composition [21].

4.3. Alterations in Rafts' Proteome and Associated Cellular Effects

Following the rationale of the previous section for the effects of environmental toxicants on the lipid composition of lipid rafts, in this section, the evidence for the effect of environmental toxicants on the protein composition of lipid rafts will be presented together with associated cellular effects.

4.3.1. Alterations in Lipid Raft-Associated Proteins

A recent study using red blood cells reported that mercury exposure leads to alterations in flotillin-2 levels, detected by electrophoresis of total membrane proteins [23]. This is highly relevant because in these cells, the protein flotillin-2 is reported as one of the major protein components of lipid rafts [162]. Moreover, at the structural level, the authors propose that mercury exposure could provoke membrane fragmentation of red blood cells [23], since flotillin-2 is responsible for membrane stability and is recognized to facilitate the association of protein complexes at the interface between membrane and cytosol [163]. Interestingly, exposure to copper was also described as having an effect on the distribution of flotillin-2 in the lipid rafts of neuroblastoma cells [89].

Another example of alterations in rafts' proteomes is the displacement of proteins from these membrane regions, as occurs for occluding in human brain endothelial cells exposed to the industrial chemical 2,2',4,4',5,5'-hexachlorobiphenyl, also known as PCB153 [164]. The cellular mechanism by which this displacement occurs is related to PCB153-induced dephosphorylation of the threonine residues of occluding via activation of protein phosphatase 2A (PP2A) and MMP-2 [164]. In this cell model, MMP-2 activity was detected in lipid rafts and increased after PCB153 incubation. More importantly, MMP-2 inhibition prevented PCB153-induced loss of occluding from tight junctions and disruption of lipid raft assembly associated with endothelial barrier function (Figure 3). Other polychlorinated chemicals induce MMP-2 release by prostate cancer cells [156].

Exposure of CHO-K1 cells transfected with TSHR to the pesticide DDT abrogated the co-localization between the TSHR and lipid rafts, with consequences for receptor internalization [19]. Interestingly, the actions of DDT were not unspecific, as a lipophilic compound structurally related to DDT (diphenylethylene) did not mimic DDT's effects. Also, the exposure of macrophages to B[a]P was reported to provoke a displacement of the CD32 protein from lipid rafts to non-lipid raft fractions, affecting macrophage effector functions [15] (Figure 3). Other authors showed that secondhand smoke depleted the expression of the cystic fibrosis transmembrane conductance regulator and lipid-raft-associated activity, a potential mechanism suggested for impaired phagocytosis [165]. Similar effects were observed for the SH-SY5Y human neuroblastoma cells incubated with copper ions, where a decrease of the γ-secretase protein in lipid rafts and activity was observed [89].

4.3.2. Recruitment and Aggregation of Proteins in Lipid Rafts

Recently, exposure to vanadium (IV) compounds was revealed to promote aggregation and accumulation of the luteinizing hormone receptors in the plasma membrane of CHO cells, with the formation of clusters containing these receptors [119]. One of the compounds—bis(maltolato)oxovanadium(IV)—also provoked lipid packing. Indeed, exposure to these compounds was previously reported to produce similar effects in RBL-2H3 cells regarding lipid packing and insulin receptors [166].

The exposure to traffic-related PM revealed that it altered the processing of amyloid precursor protein in lipid raft fractions from in vivo and in vitro samples [17]. On hepatoma Hepa1c1c7 cells, the effect of B[a]P—a cigarette smoke and PM component—provoked changes in the membrane localization of flotillin-1 and the displacement of connexin-2 from lipid rafts [149]. Indeed, the recruitment of signaling proteins into lipid rafts after exposure to cigarette smoke extract or PM is not a surprise. In human lung fibroblasts, the recruitment of the death-inducing signaling complex into lipid rafts was reported after exposure to cigarette smoke extract [167]. In human alveolar epithelial cells, exposure to tire debris organic extracts—described to contain PM10 and PM2.5 [168]—resulted in an increase in lipid rafts and caveolae markers flotillin-1, caveolin-1, and CD55 in the prepared DRMs [169]. Also in these fractions, an increase in the levels of HMOX1 was observed after exposure to these extracts [169], a protein already signaled in Figure 2. Interestingly, a decade later, in the same cell line—A549—similar effects were observed for exposure to cigarette smoke extract or e-cigarette vapor condensate. This exposure provoked an increment in the expression of the lipid raft proteins caveolin-1, -2, and flotillin-1 [170]. It was observed that exposure of A549 cells to cigarette extract promoted the recruitment of inflammation-related proteins—NLRP10 and NLRP12—into the lipid rafts, as well as the interaction of NLRP12 with caveolin-1 [170]. In addition, e-cigarette smoke with or without nicotine promoted the formation of protein complexes associated with inflammation containing TRL4, NOD-1, and caveolin-1 in the lipid rafts [21]. A study investigating the effect of nicotine on macrophages highlighted the increase in nicotinic acetylcholine receptor expression and accumulation in lipid rafts and the consequent activation of the NLRP3 inflammasome [56]. Moreover, the disruption of lipid rafts by methyl-β-cyclodextrin reduced the accumulation of these receptors in lipid rafts and inflammasome activation [56]. Having in mind that inflammatory signaling is a common response to environmental pollutants, the effects of airborne PM and organic pollutants on the dynamics of inflammasome proteins in lipid rafts deserve further investigation.

4.3.3. Activation of Other Signaling Pathways

Lipid rafts were reported as a structural scenario for the PCB153-induced phosphorylation of JAK and Src kinases and upregulation of cell adhesion molecules (CAMs) that affect leukocyte infiltration in brain endothelial cells [16]. In this study, cholesterol depletion blocked the lipid raft-dependent NADPH oxidase/JAK/EGFR signaling mechanism triggered by PCB153. Nevertheless, silencing caveolin-1 didn't affect the upregulation of CAMs, indicating that caveolae are not a condition for the PCB153-induced phosphorylation mechanisms [16]. Remarkably, occludin co-immunoprecipitated with PP2A and caveolin-1, and the displacement of occludin from DRMs and increased permeability of endothelial cells were substantially reduced when PP2A activity was inhibited [164]. Therefore, the Src/PP2A described in other settings [171] might participate in the early toxic actions of PCB153 at membrane rafts (Figure 3).

Lipid rafts are also implicated in the signaling pathway associated with the TCR by favoring the co-localization of the TCR, of the linker for activation of T cells (LAT), and of the LCK [172]. This last one is a protein of the Src family that, after stimulation of TCR, is activated and favors a phosphorylation cascade involving ZAP70 and LAT, which, as a consequence, recruits PLC to rafts [173]. In this case, exposure of T lymphocytes to ethanol resulted in an inhibition of the co-localization of LCK, ZAP70, LAT, and PLC in plasma membrane lipid rafts essential for TCR signaling and consequent expression of interleukin-2 [173].

More recently, a study reinforced the role of G protein-coupled receptor (GPCR) activation by toxicants through lipid raft regions. In CHO cells, an increase in intracellular cAMP was observed after exposure to vanadium compounds, which is complementary to the aggregation of luteinizing hormone receptors in clusters, as described previously [119]. In addition to the luteinizing hormone receptor and TSHR already mentioned, there are GPCRs for a variety of peptide hormones, lipid mediators of inflammation, and biogenic amines (e.g., adrenaline), among other ligands, and GPCRs are commonly palmitoylated and located at cholesterol-rich domains of the plasma membrane [174,175]. In this regard, the β-adrenoceptor has been implicated in the PAH-induced increase of intracellular calcium concentration [176], and the beta-blocker carvedilol attenuates B[a]P toxicity [177]. GPCRs transduce the signal primarily by the cAMP/protein kinase A and the phosphatidylinositol/PLC/PKC pathways, incorporating calcium/calmodulin, ROS, and nitric oxide signaling, so their possible modulation by environmental toxicants warrants more extensive studies.

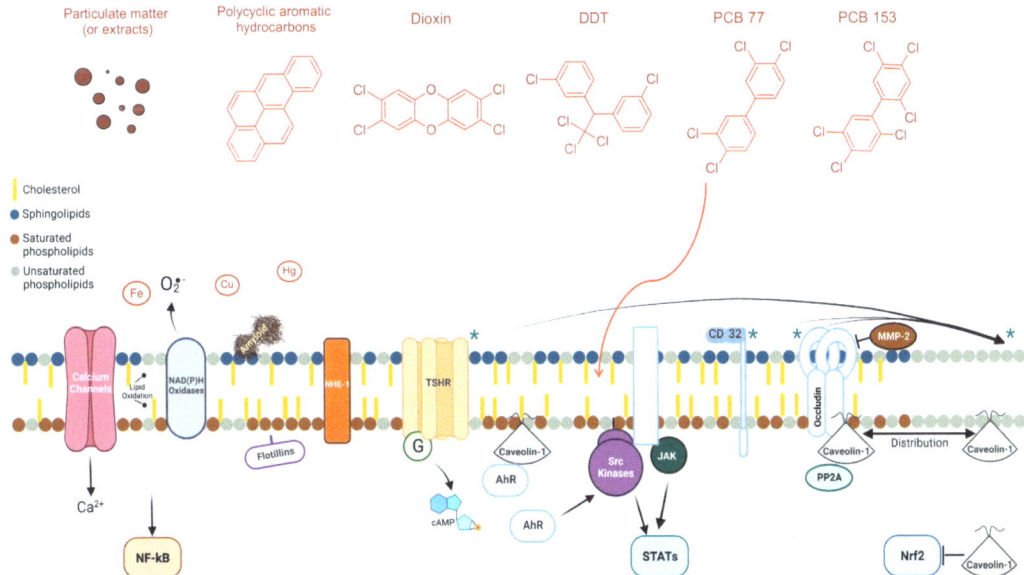

Figure 3. Membrane lipid rafts components and associated signaling pathways implicated in the cellular effects of environmental toxicants. The proteins marked with an asterisk (*) are distributed between raft and non-raft domains, and environmental toxicants were described to displace them from lipid rafts. Abbreviations: AhR, Aryl hydrocarbon receptor; cAMP, Cyclic adenosine monophosphate; DDT, 1,1,1-trichloro-2,2-bis(p-chlorophenyl)-ethane; G, G proteins; JAK, Janus kinase; MMP2, Matrix metalloproteinase-2; NF-kB, factor nuclear kappa B; NHE-1, Na+/H+ exchanger 1; Nrf2, Nuclear factor (erythroid-derived 2)-like 2; PCB, Polychlorinated biphenyl; PP2A, Protein phosphatase 2A; Src, Proto-oncogene tyrosine-protein kinase; STATs, signal transducer and activator of transcription; TSHR, thyrotropin receptor. Figure created with BioRender.com.

5. Conclusions and Future Perspectives

The evidence collected throughout this work points to the role of lipid rafts as targets of environmental toxicants—such as PM, PAHs, PCBs, pesticides, and metal ions, among others—unleashing cell signaling mechanisms consequent to toxic exposure. The identified triggering mechanisms may be toxicant-specific, while other mechanisms are common to different toxicants. Considering this, some suggestions for future research are given:

- When studying the effect of a toxicant in lipid rafts, several effects can be considered for research since they have already been reported to be common to different toxicant exposures. They include alteration of lipid raft composition (lipids and proteins), alteration of cholesterol content and membrane fluidity, recruitment or displacement of proteins from these membrane domains, and oxidative stress.
- The accumulation of toxicants in lipid rafts is not a clear point, with only PCB77 being reported to accumulate in these membrane domains [102]. Nevertheless, if similar behavior could be demonstrated for additional toxicants, it would strengthen the relevance of these lipid structures in environmental toxicology.
- The effect of environmental toxicants on inflammatory processes deserves to be further investigated, considering that inflammatory signaling is a common response to environmental pollutants [5], with some responses dependent on inflammarafts [101], and activation of inflammasomes [56].
- In the case of exposure to B[a]P, alteration of GM1 and raft protein localization is reported. With this in mind, investigating the effect of other environmental toxicants on the distribution of GM1 can be highly interesting if we consider that the location

of GM1 near membrane channels affects their activity [67,68]. Moreover, the effect of B[a]P on the relocation of NHE-1 outside lipid rafts, with consequences for its apoptotic function [151], may be translated to other toxicants.
- The activation of a specific GPCR type via membrane clustering after exposure to vanadium [119], together with the wide range of ligands binding to these receptors and the vast signaling associated, makes these receptors a potential trigger for environmental toxicants, but whether this depends on lipid raft structure is a hypothesis that deserves to be studied.
- Another research dimension to be explored is how environmental toxicants can interfere with the interplay of different signals coming from proteins associated with lipid rafts. For example, the lipid rafts are near enzymatic systems producing ROS, like NADPH oxidases and nitric oxide synthases [16,66,78]. This gains even more relevance if we consider that different environmental toxicants are ligands of AhR, leading to activation of membrane NADPH oxidases [4,141].
- AhR is a reported target of PCBs, PAHs, PM, and persistent organic pollutants [140,141,146] and the non-canonical AhR signaling pathway [14,141,142] deserves to be explored for the effects of additional environmental toxicants. More specific data is needed to understand how membrane rafts/caveola modulate the activity of transcription factors like AhR and Nrf2, which are highly implicated in the cellular effects of environmental toxicants.
- Finally, to address the role of lipid rafts in triggering a specific cellular mechanism after any toxic exposure, it is important to employ different cell models expressing different membrane receptors and signaling components at lipid rafts since signaling differences were identified in this work. For example, in endothelial cells, the toxicant effects described to be associated with lipid rafts are changes in Nrf2 signaling, an increase in MCP-1 associated with AhR, p38, and JNK signaling pathways, and the displacement of occludin from lipid rafts is also described [140,145,164]. Nevertheless, in neurons, the involvement of lipid rafts in oxidative stress and the increase of cell calcium are potential cellular mechanisms affected by exposure to harmful compounds [13,17,77].

Information on the effect of environmental toxicants in lipid rafts and associated cell signaling mechanisms is compiled in this article, and to the best of our knowledge, this is the first review approaching the effect of environmental toxicants on lipid raft signaling. The collected data endorse that membrane raft-like domains can function as hubs for the regulation of toxic cellular mechanisms triggered by these harmful chemical agents. Therefore, this concept can provide meaningful insights into the comprehension of environmental toxicants' molecular effects at the cellular level.

Author Contributions: Conceptualization, D.M.-d.-S. and R.L.; investigation, D.M.-d.-S. and R.L.; writing—original draft preparation, D.M.-d.-S.; writing—review and editing, D.M.-d.-S. and R.L.; visualization, D.M.-d.-S. and R.L. All authors have read and agreed to the published version of the manuscript.

Funding: This research was funded by Fundação para a Ciência e Tecnologia, LA/P/0045/2020 (ALiCE), UIDB/50020/2020 and UIDP/50020/2020 (LSRE-LCM), funded by national funds through FCT/MCTES (PIDDAC).

Data Availability Statement: Data is contained within the article.

Conflicts of Interest: The authors declare no conflict of interest.

References

1. Simons, K.; Toomre, D. Lipid Rafts and Signal Transduction. *Nat. Rev. Mol. Cell Biol.* **2000**, *1*, 31–39. [CrossRef] [PubMed]
2. Placidi, G.; Campa, C.C. Deliver on Time or Pay the Fine: Scheduling in Membrane Trafficking. *Int. J. Mol. Sci.* **2021**, *22*, 11773. [CrossRef] [PubMed]
3. Greenlee, J.D.; Subramanian, T.; Liu, K.; King, M.R. Rafting down the Metastatic Cascade: The Role of Lipid Rafts in Cancer Metastasis, Cell Death, and Clinical Outcomes. *Cancer Res.* **2021**, *81*, 815–817. [CrossRef] [PubMed]
4. Lagoa, R.; Marques-da-Silva, D.; Diniz, M.; Daglia, M.; Bishayee, A. Molecular Mechanisms Linking Environmental Toxicants to Cancer Development: Significance for Protective Interventions with Polyphenols. *Semin. Cancer Biol.* **2022**, *80*, 118–144. [CrossRef]

5. Marques-da-Silva, D.; Videira, P.A.; Lagoa, R. Registered Human Trials Addressing Environmental and Occupational Toxicant Exposures: Scoping Review of Immunological Markers and Protective Strategies. *Environ. Toxicol. Pharmacol.* **2022**, *93*, 103886. [CrossRef]
6. Aminov, Z.; Haase, R.F.; Pavuk, M.; Carpenter, D.O. Analysis of the Effects of Exposure to Polychlorinated Biphenyls and Chlorinated Pesticides on Serum Lipid Levels in Residents of Anniston, Alabama. *Environ. Health* **2013**, *12*, 108. [CrossRef]
7. Adetona, A.M.; Adetona, O.; Gogal, R.M.; Diaz-Sanchez, D.; Rathbun, S.L.; Naeher, L.P. Impact of Work Task-Related Acute Occupational Smoke Exposures on Select Proinflammatory Immune Parameters in Wildland Firefighters. *J. Occup. Environ. Med.* **2017**, *59*, 679–690. [CrossRef]
8. Goyal, T.; Mitra, P.; Singh, P.; Ghosh, R.; Sharma, S.; Sharma, P. Association of MicroRNA Expression with Changes in Immune Markers in Workers with Cadmium Exposure. *Chemosphere* **2021**, *274*, 129615. [CrossRef]
9. Parks, C.G.; Santos, A.d.S.E.; Lerro, C.C.; DellaValle, C.T.; Ward, M.H.; Alavanja, M.C.; Berndt, S.I.; Beane Freeman, L.E.; Sandler, D.P.; Hofmann, J.N. Lifetime Pesticide Use and Antinuclear Antibodies in Male Farmers from the Agricultural Health Study. *Front. Immunol.* **2019**, *10*, 1476. [CrossRef]
10. Rider, C.F.; Carlsten, C. Air Pollution and DNA Methylation: Effects of Exposure in Humans. *Clin. Epigenetics* **2019**, *11*, 131. [CrossRef]
11. Rubini, E.; Minacori, M.; Paglia, G.; Macone, A.; Chichiarelli, S.; Altieri, F.; Eufemi, M. Tomato and Olive Bioactive Compounds: A Natural Shield against the Cellular Effects Induced by β-Hexachlorocyclohexane-Activated Signaling Pathways. *Molecules* **2021**, *26*, 7135. [CrossRef] [PubMed]
12. Renu, K.; Mukherjee, A.G.; Wanjari, U.R.; Vinayagam, S.; Veeraraghavan, V.P.; Vellingiri, B.; George, A.; Lagoa, R.; Sattu, K.; Dey, A.; et al. Misuse of Cardiac Lipid upon Exposure to Toxic Trace Elements—A Focused Review. *Molecules* **2022**, *27*, 5657. [CrossRef] [PubMed]
13. Fortalezas, S.; Marques-da-Silva, D.; Gutierrez-Merino, C. Creatine Protects Against Cytosolic Calcium Dysregulation, Mitochondrial Depolarization and Increase of Reactive Oxygen Species Production in Rotenone-Induced Cell Death of Cerebellar Granule Neurons. *Neurotox. Res.* **2018**, *34*, 717–732. [CrossRef] [PubMed]
14. Brinchmann, B.C.; Le Ferrec, E.; Podechard, N.; Lagadic-Gossmann, D.; Shoji, K.F.; Penna, A.; Kukowski, K. Lipophilic Chemicals from Diesel Exhaust Particles Trigger Calcium Response in Human Endothelial Cells via Aryl Hydrocarbon Receptor Non-Genomic Signalling. *Int. J. Mol. Sci.* **2018**, *19*, 1429. [CrossRef]
15. Clark, R.S.; Pellom, S.T.; Booker, B.; Ramesh, A.; Zhang, T.; Shanker, A.; Maguire, M.; Juarez, P.D.; Patricia, M.J.; Langston, M.A.; et al. Validation of Research Trajectory 1 of an Exposome Framework: Exposure to Benzo(a)Pyrene Confers Enhanced Susceptibility to Bacterial Infection. *Environ. Res.* **2016**, *146*, 173–184. [CrossRef]
16. Eum, S.Y.; Andras, I.; Hennig, B.; Toborek, M. NADPH Oxidase and Lipid Raft-Associated Redox Signaling Are Required for PCB153-Induced Upregulation of Cell Adhesion Molecules in Human Brain Endothelial Cells. *Toxicol. Appl. Pharmacol.* **2009**, *240*, 299–305. [CrossRef]
17. Cacciottolo, M.; Morgan, T.E.; Saffari, A.A.; Shirmohammadi, F.; Forman, H.J.; Sioutas, C.; Finch, C.E. Traffic-Related Air Pollutants (TRAP-PM) Promote Neuronal Amyloidogenesis through Oxidative Damage to Lipid Rafts. *Free Radic. Biol. Med.* **2020**, *147*, 242–251. [CrossRef]
18. Tekpli, X.; Rissel, M.; Huc, L.; Catheline, D.; Sergent, O.; Rioux, V.; Legrand, P.; Holme, J.A.; Dimanche-Boitrel, M.T.; Lagadic-Gossmann, D. Membrane Remodeling, an Early Event in Benzo[α]Pyrene-Induced Apoptosis. *Toxicol. Appl. Pharmacol.* **2010**, *243*, 68–76. [CrossRef]
19. De Gregorio, F.; Pellegrino, M.; Picchietti, S.; Belardinelli, M.C.; Taddei, A.R.; Fausto, A.M.; Rossi, M.; Maggio, R.; Giorgi, F. The Insecticide 1,1,1-Trichloro-2,2-Bis(p-Chlorophenyl) Ethane (DDT) Alters the Membrane Raft Location of the TSH Receptor Stably Expressed in Chinese Hamster Ovary Cells. *Toxicol. Appl. Pharmacol.* **2011**, *253*, 121–129. [CrossRef]
20. Xu, Y.; Wang, W.; Zhou, J.; Chen, M.; Huang, X.; Zhu, Y.; Xie, X.; Li, W.; Zhang, Y.; Kan, H.; et al. Metabolomics Analysis of a Mouse Model for Chronic Exposure to Ambient PM2.5. *Environ. Pollut.* **2019**, *247*, 953–963. [CrossRef]
21. Singh, D.P.; Begum, R.; Kaur, G.; Bagam, P.; Kambiranda, D.; Singh, R.; Batra, S. E-Cig Vapor Condensate Alters Proteome and Lipid Profiles of Membrane Rafts: Impact on Inflammatory Responses in A549 Cells. *Cell Biol. Toxicol.* **2021**, *37*, 773–793. [CrossRef] [PubMed]
22. Bhardwaj, P.; Kumar, M.; Dhatwalia, S.K.; Garg, M.L.; Dhawan, D.K. Acetyl-11-Keto-β-Boswellic Acid Modulates Membrane Dynamics in Benzo(a)Pyrene-Induced Lung Carcinogenesis. *Mol. Cell. Biochem.* **2019**, *460*, 17–27. [CrossRef] [PubMed]
23. Notariale, R.; Längst, E.; Perrone, P.; Crettaz, D.; Prudent, M.; Manna, C. Effect of Mercury on Membrane Proteins Anionic Transport and Cell Morphology in Human Erythrocytes. *Cell. Physiol. Biochem.* **2022**, *56*, 500–513. [CrossRef]
24. Brown, D.A.; London, E. Structure and Origin of Ordered Lipid Domains in Biological Membranes. *J. Membr. Biol.* **1998**, *164*, 103–114. [CrossRef]
25. Hjort Ipsen, J.; Karlström, G.; Mourtisen, O.G.; Wennerström, H.; Zuckermann, M.J. Phase Equilibria in the Phosphatidylcholine-Cholesterol System. *BBA—Biomembr.* **1987**, *905*, 162–172. [CrossRef] [PubMed]
26. Pike, L.J. Lipid Rafts: Bringing Order to Chaos. *J. Lipid Res.* **2003**, *44*, 655–667. [CrossRef]
27. Simons, K.; Ikonen, E. Functional Rafts in Cell Membranes. *Nature* **1997**, *387*, 569–572. [CrossRef]
28. Waheed, A.A.; Freed, E.O. The Role of Lipids in Retroviral Replication. In *Retrovirus-Cell Interactions*; Parent, L.J., Ed.; Academic Press: Cambridge, MA, USA, 2018; pp. 353–399. [CrossRef]

29. Shankar, J.; Boscher, C.; Nabi, I.R. Caveolin-1, Galectin-3 and Lipid Raft Domains in Cancer Cell Signalling. *Essays Biochem.* **2015**, *57*, 189–201. [CrossRef]
30. Bartlett, K.; Kim, K. Insight into Tor2, a Budding Yeast Microdomain Protein. *Eur. J. Cell Biol.* **2014**, *93*, 87–97. [CrossRef]
31. Krapf, D. Compartmentalization of the Plasma Membrane. *Curr. Opin. Cell Biol.* **2018**, *53*, 15–21. [CrossRef]
32. Godoy, V.; Riquelme, G. Distinct Lipid Rafts in Subdomains from Human Placental Apical Syncytiotrophoblast Membranes. *J. Membr. Biol.* **2008**, *224*, 21–31. [CrossRef] [PubMed]
33. Toledo, A.; Huang, Z.; Coleman, J.L.; London, E.; Benach, J.L. Lipid Rafts Can Form in the Inner and Outer Membranes of Borrelia Burgdorferi and Have Different Properties and Associated Proteins. *Mol. Microbiol.* **2018**, *108*, 63. [CrossRef] [PubMed]
34. Blouin, C.M.; Prado, C.; Takane, K.K.; Lasnier, F.; Garcia-Ocana, A.; Ferré, P.; Dugail, I.; Hajduch, E. Plasma Membrane Subdomain Compartmentalization Contributes to Distinct Mechanisms of Ceramide Action on Insulin Signaling. *Diabetes* **2010**, *59*, 600–610. [CrossRef] [PubMed]
35. Parton, R.G. Caveolae: Structure, Function, and Relationship to Disease. *Annu. Rev. Cell Dev. Biol.* **2018**, *34*, 111–136. [CrossRef]
36. Yamada, E. The Fine Structure of the Fall Bladder Epithelium of the Mouse. *J. Biophys. Biochem. Cytol.* **1955**, *1*, 445. [CrossRef]
37. Razani, B.; Woodman, S.E.; Lisanti, M.P. Caveolae: From Cell Biology to Animal Physiology. *Pharmacol. Rev.* **2002**, *54*, 431–467. [CrossRef]
38. Martinez-Outschoorn, U.E.; Sotgia, F.; Lisanti, M.P. Caveolae and Signalling in Cancer. *Nat. Rev. Cancer* **2015**, *15*, 225–237. [CrossRef]
39. Hansen, C.G.; Nichols, B.J. Exploring the Caves: Cavins, Caveolins and Caveolae. *Trends Cell Biol.* **2010**, *20*, 177–186. [CrossRef]
40. Filippini, A.; D'alessio, A. Caveolae and Lipid Rafts in Endothelium: Valuable Organelles for Multiple Functions. *Biomolecules* **2020**, *10*, 1218. [CrossRef]
41. Parton, R.G.; Tillu, V.A.; Collins, B.M. Caveolae. *Curr. Biol.* **2018**, *28*, R402–R405. [CrossRef]
42. Sevcsik, E.; Schütz, G.J. With or without Rafts? Alternative Views on Cell Membranes. *BioEssays* **2016**, *38*, 129–139. [CrossRef] [PubMed]
43. Levental, I.; Levental, K.R.; Heberle, F.A. Lipid Rafts: Controversies Resolved, Mysteries Remain. *Trends Cell Biol.* **2020**, *30*, 341–353. [CrossRef] [PubMed]
44. Klotzsch, E.; Schütz, G.J. A Critical Survey of Methods to Detect Plasma Membrane Rafts. *Philos. Trans. R. Soc. B Biol. Sci.* **2013**, *368*, 20120033. [CrossRef] [PubMed]
45. Suzuki, K.G.N.; Kusumi, A. Refinement of Singer-Nicolson Fluid-Mosaic Model by Microscopy Imaging: Lipid Rafts and Actin-Induced Membrane Compartmentalization. *Biochim. Biophys. Acta—Biomembr.* **2023**, *1865*, 184093. [CrossRef]
46. Kusumi, A.; Fujiwara, T.K.; Tsunoyama, T.A.; Kasai, R.S.; Liu, A.A.; Hirosawa, K.M.; Kinoshita, M.; Matsumori, N.; Komura, N.; Ando, H.; et al. Defining Raft Domains in the Plasma Membrane. *Traffic* **2020**, *21*, 106–137. [CrossRef] [PubMed]
47. Regen, S.L. The Origin of Lipid Rafts. *Biochemistry* **2020**, *59*, 4617–4621. [CrossRef]
48. Simons, K.; Ehehalt, R. Cholesterol, Lipid Rafts, and Disease. *J. Clin. Investig.* **2002**, *110*, 597–603. [CrossRef]
49. Kraft, M.L. Sphingolipid Organization in the Plasma Membrane and the Mechanisms That Influence It. *Front. Cell Dev. Biol.* **2017**, *4*, 154. [CrossRef] [PubMed]
50. Simons, K.; Sampaio, J.L. Membrane Organization and Lipid Rafts. *Cold Spring Harb. Perspect. Biol.* **2011**, *3*, a004697. [CrossRef]
51. Chang, W.J.; Rothberg, K.G.; Kamen, B.A.; Anderson, R.G.W. Lowering the Cholesterol Content of MA104 Cells Inhibits Receptor-Mediated Transport of Folate. *J. Cell Biol.* **1992**, *118*, 63–69. [CrossRef]
52. Ouweneel, A.B.; Thomas, M.J.; Sorci-Thomas, M.G. The Ins and Outs of Lipid Rafts: Functions in Intracellular Cholesterol Homeostasis, Microparticles, and Cell Membranes. *J. Lipid Res.* **2020**, *61*, 676–686. [CrossRef] [PubMed]
53. Fessler, M.B.; Parks, J.S. Intracellular Lipid Flux and Membrane Microdomains as Organizing Principles in Inflammatory Cell Signaling. *J. Immunol.* **2011**, *187*, 1529–1535. [CrossRef] [PubMed]
54. Fadeyibi, O.; Rybalchenko, N.; Mabry, S.; Nguyen, D.H.; Cunningham, R.L. The Role of Lipid Rafts and Membrane Androgen Receptors in Androgen's Neurotoxic Effects. *J. Endocr. Soc.* **2022**, *6*, bvac030. [CrossRef]
55. Premasekharan, G.; Nguyen, K.; Contreras, J.; Ramon, V.; Leppert, V.J.; Forman, H.J. Iron-Mediated Lipid Peroxidation and Lipid Raft Disruption in Low-Dose Silica-Induced Macrophage Cytokine Production. *Free Radic. Biol. Med.* **2011**, *51*, 1184–1194. [CrossRef]
56. Duan, F.; Zeng, C.; Liu, S.; Gong, J.; Hu, J.; Li, H.; Tan, H. A1-NAchR-Mediated Signaling Through Lipid Raft Is Required for Nicotine-Induced NLRP3 Inflammasome Activation and Nicotine-Accelerated Atherosclerosis. *Front. Cell Dev. Biol.* **2021**, *9*, 724699. [CrossRef] [PubMed]
57. Liu, S.; Tao, J.; Duan, F.; Li, H.; Tan, H. HHcy Induces Pyroptosis and Atherosclerosis via the Lipid Raft-Mediated NOX-ROS-NLRP3 Inflammasome Pathway in ApoE$^{-/-}$ Mice. *Cells* **2022**, *11*, 2438. [CrossRef]
58. Fortalezas, S.; Marques-da-Silva, D.; Gutierrez-Merino, C. Methyl-β-Cyclodextrin Impairs the Phosphorylation of the B2 Subunit of L-Type Calcium Channels and Cytosolic Calcium Homeostasis in Mature Cerebellar Granule Neurons. *Int. J. Mol. Sci.* **2018**, *19*, 3667. [CrossRef]
59. Dietrich, C.; Bagatolli, L.A.; Volovyk, Z.N.; Thompson, N.L.; Levi, M.; Jacobson, K.; Gratton, E. Lipid Rafts Reconstituted in Model Membranes. *Biophys. J.* **2001**, *80*, 1417–1428. [CrossRef]
60. Palestini, P.; Calvi, C.; Conforti, E.; Daffara, R.; Botto, L.; Miserocchi, G. Compositional Changes in Lipid Microdomains of Air-Blood Barrier Plasma Membranes in Pulmonary Interstitial Edema. *J. Appl. Physiol.* **2003**, *95*, 1446–1452. [CrossRef]

61. Ledeen, R.W.; Wu, G. The Multi-Tasked Life of GM1 Ganglioside, a True Factotum of Nature. *Trends Biochem. Sci.* **2015**, *40*, 407–418. [CrossRef]
62. Van Heyningen, S. Cholera Toxin: Interaction of Subunits with Ganglioside GM1. *Science* **1974**, *183*, 656–657. [CrossRef] [PubMed]
63. Day, C.A.; Kenworthy, A.K. Functions of Cholera Toxin B-Subunit as a Raft Cross-Linker. *Essays Biochem.* **2015**, *57*, 135–145. [CrossRef] [PubMed]
64. Kenworthy, A.K.; Schmieder, S.S.; Raghunathan, K.; Tiwari, A.; Wang, T.; Kelly, C.V.; Lencer, W.I. Cholera Toxin as a Probe for Membrane Biology. *Toxins* **2021**, *13*, 543. [CrossRef] [PubMed]
65. Samhan-Arias, A.K.; López-Sánchez, C.; Marques-da-Silva, D.; Lagoa, R.; Garcia-Lopez, V.; García-Martínez, V.; Gutierrez-Merino, C. High Expression of Cytochrome b_5 Reductase Isoform 3/Cytochrome b_5 System in the Cerebellum and Pyramidal Neurons of Adult Rat Brain. *Brain Struct. Funct.* **2016**, *221*, 2147–2162. [CrossRef]
66. Samhan-Arias, A.K.; Garcia-Bereguiain, M.A.; Martin-Romero, F.J.; Gutierrez-Merino, C. Clustering of Plasma Membrane-Bound Cytochrome B5 Reductase within "lipid Raft" Microdomains of the Neuronal Plasma Membrane. *Mol. Cell. Neurosci.* **2009**, *40*, 14–26. [CrossRef]
67. Puljko, B.; Stojanović, M.; Ilic, K.; Kalanj-Bognar, S.; Mlinac-Jerkovic, K. Start Me Up: How Can Surrounding Gangliosides Affect Sodium-Potassium ATPase Activity and Steer towards Pathological Ion Imbalance in Neurons? *Biomedicines* **2022**, *10*, 1518. [CrossRef]
68. Ilic, K.; Lin, X.; Malci, A.; Stojanović, M.; Puljko, B.; Rožman, M.; Vukelić, Ž.; Heffer, M.; Montag, D.; Schnaar, R.L.; et al. Plasma Membrane Calcium ATPase-Neuroplastin Complexes Are Selectively Stabilized in GM1-Containing Lipid Rafts. *Int. J. Mol. Sci.* **2021**, *22*, 13590. [CrossRef]
69. Lucero, H.A.; Robbins, P.W. Lipid Rafts-Protein Association and the Regulation of Protein Activity. *Arch. Biochem. Biophys.* **2004**, *426*, 208–224. [CrossRef]
70. Kurzchalia, T.V.; Parton, R.G. Membrane Microdomains and Caveolae. *Curr. Opin. Cell Biol.* **1999**, *11*, 424–431. [CrossRef]
71. Galbiati, F.; Razani, B.; Lisanti, M.P. Emerging Themes in Lipid Rafts and Caveolae. *Cell* **2001**, *106*, 403–411. [CrossRef]
72. Vassilieva, E.V.; Ivanov, A.I.; Nusrat, A. Flotillin-1 Stabilizes Caveolin-1 in Intestinal Epithelial Cells. *Biochem. Biophys. Res. Commun.* **2009**, *379*, 460–465. [CrossRef]
73. Foster, L.J.; De Hoog, C.L.; Mann, M. Unbiased Quantitative Proteomics of Lipid Rafts Reveals High Specificity for Signaling Factors. *Proc. Natl. Acad. Sci. USA* **2003**, *100*, 5813–5818. [CrossRef]
74. Magee, A.I.; Parmryd, I. Detergent-Resistant Membranes and the Protein Composition of Lipid Rafts. *Genome Biol.* **2003**, *4*, 234. [CrossRef]
75. Marques-da-Silva, D.; Samhan-Arias, A.K.; Tiago, T.; Gutierrez-Merino, C. L-Type Calcium Channels and Cytochrome B_5 Reductase Are Components of Protein Complexes Tightly Associated with Lipid Rafts Microdomains of the Neuronal Plasma Membrane. *J. Proteom.* **2010**, *73*, 1502–1510. [CrossRef] [PubMed]
76. Marques-da-Silva, D.; Gutierrez-Merino, C. L-Type Voltage-Operated Calcium Channels, N-Methyl-d-Aspartate Receptors and Neuronal Nitric-Oxide Synthase Form a Calcium/Redox Nano-Transducer within Lipid Rafts. *Biochem. Biophys. Res. Commun.* **2012**, *420*, 257–262. [CrossRef]
77. Marques-da-Silva, D.; Gutierrez-Merino, C. Caveolin-Rich Lipid Rafts of the Plasma Membrane of Mature Cerebellar Granule Neurons Are Microcompartments for Calcium/Reactive Oxygen and Nitrogen Species Cross-Talk Signaling. *Cell Calcium* **2014**, *56*, 108–123. [CrossRef] [PubMed]
78. Samhan-Arias, A.K.; Marques-da-Silva, D.; Yanamala, N.; Gutierrez-Merino, C. Stimulation and Clustering of Cytochrome b 5 Reductase in Caveolin-Rich Lipid Microdomains Is an Early Event in Oxidative Stress-Mediated Apoptosis of Cerebellar Granule Neurons. *J. Proteom.* **2012**, *75*, 2934–2949. [CrossRef] [PubMed]
79. Fortalezas, S.; Poejo, J.; Samhan-Arias, A.K.; Gutierrez-Merino, C. Cholesterol-Rich Plasma Membrane Submicrodomains Can Be a Major Extramitochondrial Source of Reactive Oxygen Species in Partially Depolarized Mature Cerebellar Granule Neurons in Culture. *J. Neurophysiol. Neurol. Disord.* **2019**, *5*, 1–22.
80. Tiago, T.; Palma, P.S.; Gutierrez-Merino, C.; Aureliano, M. Peroxynitrite-Mediated Oxidative Modifications of Myosin and Implications on Structure and Function. *Free Radic. Res.* **2010**, *44*, 1317–1327. [CrossRef]
81. Gupta, N.; DeFranco, A.L. Lipid Rafts and B Cell Signaling. *Semin. Cell Dev. Biol.* **2007**, *18*, 616–626. [CrossRef]
82. Delos Santos, R.C.; Garay, C.; Antonescu, C.N. Charming Neighborhoods on the Cell Surface: Plasma Membrane Microdomains Regulate Receptor Tyrosine Kinase Signaling. *Cell. Signal.* **2015**, *27*, 1963–1976. [CrossRef]
83. Janes, P.W.; Ley, S.C.; Magee, A.I.; Kabouridis, P.S. The Role of Lipid Rafts in T Cell Antigen Receptor (TCR) Signalling. *Semin. Immunol.* **2000**, *12*, 23–34. [CrossRef] [PubMed]
84. Maselli, A.; Pierdominici, M.; Vitale, C.; Ortona, E. Membrane Lipid Rafts and Estrogenic Signalling: A Functional Role in the Modulation of Cell Homeostasis. *Apoptosis* **2015**, *20*, 671–678. [CrossRef]
85. Li, B.; Qin, Y.; Yu, X.; Xu, X.; Yu, W. Lipid Raft Involvement in Signal Transduction in Cancer Cell Survival, Cell Death and Metastasis. *Cell Prolif.* **2022**, *55*, e13167. [CrossRef] [PubMed]
86. Mollinedo, F.; Gajate, C. Lipid Rafts as Signaling Hubs in Cancer Cell Survival/Death and Invasion: Implications in Tumor Progression and Therapy. *J. Lipid Res.* **2020**, *61*, 611–635. [CrossRef] [PubMed]
87. Marin, R. Lipid Rafts as Molecular Platforms of Neuronal Toxicity and Survival: Two Sides of the Same Coin. In *Lipid Rafts: Properties and Role in Signaling*; Nils, T., Sten, J., Eds.; Nova Science Publishers: Hauppauge, NY, USA, 2018; ISBN 978-1-53613-624-1.

88. Moll, T.; Marshall, J.N.G.; Soni, N.; Zhang, S.; Cooper-Knock, J.; Shaw, P.J. Membrane Lipid Raft Homeostasis Is Directly Linked to Neurodegeneration. *Essays Biochem.* **2021**, *65*, 999–1011. [CrossRef] [PubMed]
89. Hung, Y.H.; Robb, E.L.; Voltakis, I.; Ho, M.; Evin, G.; Li, Q.X.; Culvenor, J.G.; Masters, C.L.; Cherny, R.A.; Bush, A.I. Paradoxical Condensation of Copper with Elevated β-Amyloid in Lipid Rafts under Cellular Copper Deficiency Conditions. Implications for Alzheimer Disease. *J. Biol. Chem.* **2009**, *284*, 21899–21907. [CrossRef] [PubMed]
90. Suzuki, T.; Zhang, J.; Miyazawa, S.; Liu, Q.; Farzan, M.R.; Yao, W.D. Association of Membrane Rafts and Postsynaptic Density: Proteomics, Biochemical, and Ultrastructural Analyses. *J. Neurochem.* **2011**, *119*, 64. [CrossRef]
91. Eid, A.; Mhatre-Winters, I.; Sammoura, F.M.; Edler, M.K.; von Stein, R.; Hossain, M.M.; Han, Y.; Lisci, M.; Carney, K.; Konsolaki, M.; et al. Effects of DDT on Amyloid Precursor Protein Levels and Amyloid Beta Pathology: Mechanistic Links to Alzheimer's Disease Risk. *Environ. Health Perspect.* **2022**, *130*, 87005. [CrossRef]
92. Morris, G.; Walder, K.; Puri, B.K.; Berk, M.; Maes, M. The Deleterious Effects of Oxidative and Nitrosative Stress on Palmitoylation, Membrane Lipid Rafts and Lipid-Based Cellular Signalling: New Drug Targets in Neuroimmune Disorders. *Mol. Neurobiol.* **2016**, *53*, 4638–4658. [CrossRef]
93. Evangelisti, E.; Wright, D.; Zampagni, M.; Cascella, R.; Fiorillo, C.; Bagnoli, S.; Relini, A.; Nichino, D.; Scartabelli, T.; Nacmias, B.; et al. Lipid Rafts Mediate Amyloid-Induced Calcium Dyshomeostasis and Oxidative Stress in Alzheimer's Disease. *Curr. Alzheimer Res.* **2013**, *10*, 143–153. [CrossRef] [PubMed]
94. Poejo, J.; Salazar, J.; Mata, A.M.; Gutierrez-merino, C. Binding of Amyloid β(1–42)-calmodulin Complexes to Plasma Membrane Lipid Rafts in Cerebellar Granule Neurons Alters Resting Cytosolic Calcium Homeostasis. *Int. J. Mol. Sci.* **2021**, *22*, 1984. [CrossRef]
95. Mattson, M.P.; Chan, S.L. Dysregulation of Cellular Calcium Homeostasis in Alzheimer's Disease: Bad Genes and Bad Habits. *J. Mol. Neurosci.* **2001**, *17*, 205–224. [CrossRef] [PubMed]
96. Sattler, R.; Tymianski, M. Molecular Mechanisms of Calcium-Dependent Excitotoxicity. *J. Mol. Med.* **2000**, *78*, 3–13. [CrossRef] [PubMed]
97. Choi, D.W. Calcium: Still Center-Stage in Hypoxic-Ischemic Neuronal Death. *Trends Neurosci.* **1995**, *18*, 58–60. [CrossRef]
98. Jiang, L.; Fernandes, D.; Mehta, N.; Bean, J.L.; Michaelis, M.L.; Zaidi, A. Partitioning of the Plasma Membrane Ca^{2+}-ATPase into Lipid Rafts in Primary Neurons: Effects of Cholesterol Depletion. *J. Neurochem.* **2007**, *102*, 378–388. [CrossRef]
99. Duan, W.; Zhou, J.; Li, W.; Zhou, T.; Chen, Q.; Yang, F.; Wei, T. Plasma Membrane Calcium ATPase 4b Inhibits Nitric Oxide Generation through Calcium-Induced Dynamic Interaction with Neuronal Nitric Oxide Synthase. *Protein Cell* **2013**, *4*, 286–298. [CrossRef]
100. Legler, D.F.; Micheau, O.; Doucey, M.A.; Tschopp, J.; Bron, C. Recruitment of TNF Receptor 1 to Lipid Rafts Is Essential for TNFα-Mediated NF-ĸB Activation. *Immunity* **2003**, *18*, 655–664. [CrossRef]
101. Miller, Y.I.; Navia-Pelaez, J.M.; Corr, M.; Yaksh, T.L. Lipid Rafts in Glial Cells: Role in Neuroinflammation and Pain Processing. *J. Lipid Res.* **2020**, *61*, 655–666. [CrossRef]
102. Lim, E.J.; Májková, Z.; Xu, S.; Bachas, L.; Arzuaga, X.; Smart, E.; Tseng, M.T.; Toborek, M.; Hennig, B. Coplanar Polychlorinated Biphenyl-Induced CYP1A1 Is Regulated through Caveolae Signaling in Vascular Endothelial Cells. *Chem. Biol. Interact.* **2008**, *176*, 71–78. [CrossRef]
103. Shihata, W.A.; Michell, D.L.; Andrews, K.L.; Chin-Dusting, J.P.F. Caveolae: A Role in Endothelial Inflammation and Mechanotransduction? *Front. Physiol.* **2016**, *7*, 628. [CrossRef]
104. Sorci-Thomas, M.G.; Thomas, M.J. Microdomains, Inflammation, and Atherosclerosis. *Circ. Res.* **2016**, *118*, 679–691. [CrossRef] [PubMed]
105. Navia-Pelaez, J.M.; Agatisa-Boyle, C.; Choi, S.-H.; Sak Kim, Y.; Li, S.; Alekseeva, E.; Weldy, K.; Miller, Y.I. Differential Expression of Inflammarafts in Macrophage Foam Cells and in Nonfoamy Macrophages in Atherosclerotic Lesions. *Arterioscler. Thromb. Vasc. Biol.* **2023**, *43*, 323–329. [CrossRef] [PubMed]
106. Vieth, J.A.; Kim, M.K.; Glaser, D.; Stiles, K.; Schreiber, A.D.; Worth, R.G. FcγRIIa Requires Lipid Rafts, but Not Co-Localization into Rafts, for Effector Function. *Inflamm. Res.* **2013**, *62*, 37–43. [CrossRef] [PubMed]
107. Scheel-Toellner, D.; Wang, K.; Singh, R.; Majeed, S.; Raza, K.; Curnow, S.J.; Salmon, M.; Lord, J.M. The Death-Inducing Signalling Complex Is Recruited to Lipid Rafts in Fas-Induced Apoptosis. *Biochem. Biophys. Res. Commun.* **2002**, *297*, 876–879. [CrossRef]
108. Gajate, C.; Gonzalez-Camacho, F.; Mollinedo, F. Involvement of Raft Aggregates Enriched in Fas/CD95 Death-Inducing Signaling Complex in the Antileukemic Action of Edelfosine in Jurkat Cells. *PLoS ONE* **2009**, *4*, e5044. [CrossRef]
109. Molnár, E.; Swamy, M.; Holzer, M.; Beck-García, K.; Worch, R.; Thiele, C.; Guigas, G.; Boye, K.; Luescher, I.F.; Schwille, P.; et al. Cholesterol and Sphingomyelin Drive Ligand-Independent T-Cell Antigen Receptor Nanoclustering. *J. Biol. Chem.* **2012**, *287*, 42664–42674. [CrossRef]
110. Miguel, L.; Owen, D.M.; Lim, C.; Liebig, C.; Evans, J.; Magee, A.I.; Jury, E.C. Primary Human CD4 + T Cells Have Diverse Levels of Membrane Lipid Order That Correlate with Their Function. *J. Immunol.* **2011**, *186*, 3505–3516. [CrossRef]
111. Jury, E.C.; Kabouridis, P.S.; Flores-Borja, F.; Mageed, R.A.; Isenberg, D.A. Altered Lipid Raft–Associated Signaling and Ganglioside Expression in T Lymphocytes from Patients with Systemic Lupus Erythematosus. *J. Clin. Investig.* **2004**, *113*, 1176–1187. [CrossRef]
112. Krishnan, S.; Nambiar, M.P.; Warke, V.G.; Fisher, C.U.; Mitchell, J.; Delaney, N.; Tsokos, G.C. Alterations in Lipid Raft Composition and Dynamics Contribute to Abnormal T Cell Responses in Systemic Lupus Erythematosus. *J. Immunol.* **2004**, *172*, 7821–7831. [CrossRef]

113. Flores-Borja, F.; Kabouridis, P.S.; Jury, E.C.; Isenberg, D.A.; Mageed, R.A. Altered Lipid Raft-Associated Proximal Signaling and Translocation of CD45 Tyrosine Phosphatase in B Lymphocytes from Patients with Systemic Lupus Erythematosus. *Arthritis Rheum.* **2007**, *56*, 291–302. [CrossRef] [PubMed]
114. Sengupta, S.; Karsalia, R.; Morrissey, A.; Bamezai, A.K. Cholesterol-Dependent Plasma Membrane Order (Lo) Is Critical for Antigen-Specific Clonal Expansion of CD4+ T Cells. *Sci. Rep.* **2021**, *11*, 13970. [CrossRef] [PubMed]
115. Saeki, K.; Miura, Y.; Aki, D.; Kurosaki, T.; Yoshimura, A. The B Cell-Specific Major Raft Protein, Raftlin, Is Necessary for the Integrity of Lipid Raft and BCR Signal Transduction. *EMBO J.* **2003**, *22*, 3015–3026. [CrossRef] [PubMed]
116. Kumbul, Y.Ç.; Yasan, H.; Okur, E.; Tüz, M.; Sivrice, M.E.; Akın, V.; Şirin, F.B.; Doğan Kıran, E. The Role of Raftlin in the Pathogenesis of Chronic Rhinosinusitis with Nasal Polyps. *Eur. Arch. Oto-Rhino-Laryngol.* **2022**, *279*, 3519–3523. [CrossRef]
117. Latif, R.; Ando, T.; Davies, T.F. Lipid Rafts Are Triage Centers for Multimeric and Monomeric Thyrotropin Receptor Regulation. *Endocrinology* **2007**, *148*, 3164–3175. [CrossRef]
118. Smith, S.M.L.; Lei, Y.; Liu, J.; Cahill, M.E.; Hagen, G.M.; Barisas, B.G.; Roess, D.A. Luteinizing Hormone Receptors Translocate to Plasma Membrane Microdomains after Binding of Human Chorionic Gonadotropin. *Endocrinology* **2006**, *147*, 1789–1795. [CrossRef]
119. Althumairy, D.; Murakami, H.A.; Zhang, D.; Barisas, B.G.; Roess, D.A.; Crans, D.C. Effects of Vanadium(IV) Compounds on Plasma Membrane Lipids Lead to G Protein-Coupled Receptor Signal Transduction. *J. Inorg. Biochem.* **2020**, *203*, 110873. [CrossRef]
120. Marin, R.; Diaz, M. Estrogen Interactions with Lipid Rafts Related to Neuroprotection. Impact of Brain Ageing and Menopause. *Front. Neurosci.* **2018**, *12*, 128. [CrossRef]
121. Canerina-Amaro, A.; Hernandez-Abad, L.G.; Ferrer, I.; Quinto-Alemany, D.; Mesa-Herrera, F.; Ferri, C.; Puertas-Avendaño, R.A.; Diaz, M.; Marin, R. Lipid Raft ER Signalosome Malfunctions in Menopause and Alzheimer's Disease. *Front. Biosci.—Sch.* **2017**, *9*, 111–126. [CrossRef]
122. Mesa-Herrera, F.; Marín, R.; Torrealba, E.; Santos, G.; Díaz, M. Neuronal ER-Signalosome Proteins as Early Biomarkers in Prodromal Alzheimer's Disease Independent of Amyloid-β Production and Tau Phosphorylation. *Front. Mol. Neurosci.* **2022**, *15*, 879146. [CrossRef]
123. Marques-Da-Silva, D.; Rodrigues, J.R.; Lagoa, R. Anthocyanins, Effects in Mitochondria and Metabolism. In *Mitochondrial Physiology and Vegetal Molecules Therapeutic Potential of Natural Compounds on Mitochondrial Health*; de Oliveira, M.R., Ed.; Academic Press: Cambridge, MA, USA, 2021; pp. 267–300. [CrossRef]
124. Ghanbari-Movahed, M.; Shafiee, S.; Burcher, J.T.; Lagoa, R.; Farzaei, M.H.; Bishayee, A. Anticancer Potential of Apigenin and Isovitexin with Focus on Oncogenic Metabolism in Cancer Stem Cells. *Metabolites* **2023**, *13*, 404. [CrossRef] [PubMed]
125. Svensson, K.J.; Christianson, H.C.; Wittrup, A.; Bourseau-Guilmain, E.; Lindqvist, E.; Svensson, L.M.; Mörgelin, M.; Belting, M. Exosome Uptake Depends on ERK1/2-Heat Shock Protein 27 Signaling and Lipid Raft-Mediated Endocytosis Negatively Regulated by Caveolin-1. *J. Biol. Chem.* **2013**, *288*, 17713–17724. [CrossRef]
126. Skryabin, G.O.; Komelkov, A.V.; Savelyeva, E.E.; Tchevkina, E.M. Lipid Rafts in Exosome Biogenesis. *Biochemistry* **2020**, *85*, 177–191. [CrossRef] [PubMed]
127. Schubert, A.L.; Schubert, W.; Spray, D.C.; Lisanti, M.P. Connexin Family Members Target to Lipid Raft Domains and Interact with Caveolin-1. *Biochemistry* **2002**, *41*, 5754–5764. [CrossRef] [PubMed]
128. Martins-Marques, T.; Ribeiro-Rodrigues, T.; Batista-Almeida, D.; Aasen, T.; Kwak, B.R.; Girao, H. Biological Functions of Connexin43 Beyond Intercellular Communication. *Trends Cell Biol.* **2019**, *29*, 835–847. [CrossRef]
129. Tekpli, X.; Huc, L.; Lacroix, J.; Rissel, M.; Poët, M.; Noël, J.; Dimanche-Boitrel, M.T.; Counillon, L.; Lagadic-Gossmann, D. Regulation of Na+/H+ Exchanger 1 Allosteric Balance by Its Localization in Cholesterol- and Caveolin-Rich Membrane Microdomains. *J. Cell. Physiol.* **2008**, *216*, 207–220. [CrossRef]
130. Casaburi, I.; Chimento, A.; De Luca, A.; Nocito, M.; Sculco, S.; Avena, P.; Trotta, F.; Rago, V.; Sirianni, R.; Pezzi, V. Cholesterol as an Endogenous ERRα Agonist: A New Perspective to Cancer Treatment. *Front. Endocrinol.* **2018**, *9*, 525. [CrossRef]
131. Yamamoto, Y.; Tomiyama, A.; Sasaki, N.; Yamaguchi, H.; Shirakihara, T.; Nakashima, K.; Kumagai, K.; Takeuchi, S.; Toyooka, T.; Otani, N.; et al. Intracellular Cholesterol Level Regulates Sensitivity of Glioblastoma Cells against Temozolomide-Induced Cell Death by Modulation of Caspase-8 Activation via Death Receptor 5-Accumulation and Activation in the Plasma Membrane Lipid Raft. *Biochem. Biophys. Res. Commun.* **2018**, *495*, 1292–1299. [CrossRef]
132. George, K.S.; Wu, S. Lipid Raft: A Floating Island of Death or Survival. *Toxicol. Appl. Pharmacol.* **2012**, *259*, 311–319. [CrossRef]
133. Sikkema, J.; de Bont, J.A.; Poolman, B. Mechanisms of Membrane Toxicity of Hydrocarbons. *Microbiol. Rev.* **1995**, *59*, 201–222. [CrossRef]
134. Buff, K.; Berndt, J. Interaction of DDT (1,1,1-Trichloro-2,2-BIS(p-Chlorophenyl)-Ethane with Liposomal Phospholipids. *BBA—Biomembr.* **1981**, *643*, 205–212. [CrossRef] [PubMed]
135. Antunes-Madeira, M.C.; Madeira, V.M.C. Membrane Fluidity as Affected by the Organochlorine Insecticide DDT. *BBA—Biomembr.* **1990**, *1023*, 469–474. [CrossRef] [PubMed]
136. Endo, S.; Escher, B.I.; Goss, K.U. Capacities of Membrane Lipids to Accumulate Neutral Organic Chemicals. *Environ. Sci. Technol.* **2011**, *45*, 5912–5921. [CrossRef] [PubMed]
137. Broniatowski, M.; Binczycka, M.; Wójcik, A.; Flasiński, M.; Wydro, P. Polycyclic Aromatic Hydrocarbons in Model Bacterial Membranes—Langmuir Monolayer Studies. *Biochim. Biophys. Acta—Biomembr.* **2017**, *1859*, 2402–2412. [CrossRef]

138. Yang, H.; Li, H.; Liu, L.; Zhou, Y.; Long, X. Molecular Simulation Studies on the Interactions of 2,4,6-Trinitrotoluene and Its Metabolites with Lipid Membranes. *J. Phys. Chem. B* **2019**, *123*, 6481–6491. [CrossRef]
139. Subuddhi, U.; Mishra, A.K. Prototropism of 1-Hydroxypyrene in Liposome Suspensions: Implications towards Fluorescence Probing of Lipid Bilayers in Alkaline Medium. *Photochem. Photobiol. Sci.* **2006**, *5*, 283–290. [CrossRef]
140. Majkova, Z.; Smart, E.; Toborek, M.; Hennig, B. Up-Regulation of Endothelial Monocyte Chemoattractant Protein-1 by Coplanar PCB77 Is Caveolin-1-Dependent. *Toxicol. Appl. Pharmacol.* **2009**, *237*, 1–7. [CrossRef]
141. Vogel, C.F.A.; Van Winkle, L.S.; Esser, C.; Haarmann-Stemmann, T. The Aryl Hydrocarbon Receptor as a Target of Environmental Stressors—Implications for Pollution Mediated Stress and Inflammatory Responses. *Redox Biol.* **2020**, *34*, 101530. [CrossRef]
142. Rey-Barroso, J.; Alvarez-Barrientos, A.; Rico-Leo, E.; Contador-Troca, M.; Carvajal-Gonzalez, J.M.; Echarri, A.; Del Pozo, M.A.; Fernandez-Salguero, P.M. The Dioxin Receptor Modulates Caveolin-1 Mobilization during Directional Migration: Role of Cholesterol. *Cell Commun. Signal.* **2014**, *12*, 57. [CrossRef]
143. Hennig, B.; Reiterer, G.; Majkova, Z.; Oesterling, E.; Meerarani, P.; Toborek, M. Modification of Environmental Toxicity by Nutrients. Implications in Atherosclerosis. *Cardiovasc. Toxicol.* **2005**, *5*, 153–160. [CrossRef]
144. Ramadass, P.; Meerarani, P.; Toborek, M.; Robertson, L.W.; Hennig, B. Dietary Flavonoids Modulate PCB-Induced Oxidative Stress, CYP1A1 Induction, and AhR-DNA Binding Activity in Vascular Endothelial Cells. *Toxicol. Sci.* **2003**, *76*, 212–219. [CrossRef] [PubMed]
145. Petriello, M.C.; Han, S.G.; Newsome, B.J.; Hennig, B. PCB 126 Toxicity Is Modulated by Cross-Talk between Caveolae and Nrf2 Signaling. *Toxicol. Appl. Pharmacol.* **2014**, *277*, 192–199. [CrossRef] [PubMed]
146. Oesterling, E.; Toborek, M.; Hennig, B. Benzo[a]Pyrene Induces Intercellular Adhesion Molecule-1 through a Caveolae and Aryl Hydrocarbon Receptor Mediated Pathway. *Toxicol. Appl. Pharmacol.* **2008**, *232*, 309–316. [CrossRef] [PubMed]
147. Collin, A.; Hardonnière, K.; Chevanne, M.; Vuillemin, J.; Podechard, N.; Burel, A.; Dimanche-Boitrel, M.T.; Lagadic-Gossmann, D.; Sergent, O. Cooperative Interaction of Benzo[a]Pyrene and Ethanol on Plasma Membrane Remodeling Is Responsible for Enhanced Oxidative Stress and Cell Death in Primary Rat Hepatocytes. *Free Radic. Biol. Med.* **2014**, *72*, 11–22. [CrossRef]
148. Gorria, M.; Tekpli, X.; Sergent, O.; Huc, L.; Gaboriau, F.; Rissel, M.; Chevanne, M.; Dimanche-Boitrel, M.-T.; Lagadic-Gossmann, D. Membrane Fluidity Changes Are Associated with Benzo[a]Pyrene-Induced Apoptosis in F258 Cells: Protection by Exogenous Cholesterol. *Ann. N. Y. Acad. Sci.* **2006**, *1090*, 108–112. [CrossRef]
149. Tekpli, X.; Rivedal, E.; Gorria, M.; Landvik, N.E.; Rissel, M.; Dimanche-Boitrel, M.T.; Baffet, G.; Holme, J.A.; Lagadic-Gossmann, D. The B[a]P-Increased Intercellular Communication via Translocation of Connexin-43 into Gap Junctions Reduces Apoptosis. *Toxicol. Appl. Pharmacol.* **2010**, *242*, 231–240. [CrossRef]
150. Goldstein, J.L.; Brown, M.S. Regulation of the Mevalonate Pathway. *Nature* **1990**, *343*, 425–430. [CrossRef]
151. Tekpli, X.; Huc, L.; Sergent, O.; Dendelé, B.; Dimanche-Boitrel, M.T.; Holme, J.A.; Lagadic-Gossmann, D. NHE-1 Relocation Outside Cholesterol-Rich Membrane Microdomains Is Associated with Its Benzo[a]Pyrene-Related Apoptotic Function. *Cell. Physiol. Biochem.* **2012**, *29*, 657–666. [CrossRef]
152. Dendelé, B.; Tekpli, X.; Hardonnière, K.; Holme, J.A.; Debure, L.; Catheline, D.; Arlt, V.M.; Nagy, E.; Phillips, D.H.; Øvrebø, S.; et al. Protective Action of N-3 Fatty Acids on Benzo[a]Pyrene-Induced Apoptosis through the Plasma Membrane Remodeling-Dependent NHE1 Pathway. *Chem. Biol. Interact.* **2014**, *207*, 41–51. [CrossRef]
153. Bazzoni, G.B.; Bollini, A.N.; Hernández, G.N.; Contini, M.D.C.; Chiarotto, M.M.; Rasia, M.L. In Vivo Effect of Aluminium upon the Physical Properties of the Erythrocyte Membrane. *J. Inorg. Biochem.* **2005**, *99*, 822–827. [CrossRef]
154. Yilmaz, B.; Sandal, S.; Chen, C.H.; Carpenter, D.O. Effects of PCB 52 and PCB 77 on Cell Viability, $[Ca^{2+}]$ i Levels and Membrane Fluidity in Mouse Thymocytes. *Toxicology* **2006**, *217*, 184–193. [CrossRef] [PubMed]
155. Tan, Y. Ortho-Substituted but Not Coplanar PCBs Rapidly Kill Cerebellar Granule Cells. *Toxicol. Sci.* **2004**, *79*, 147–156. [CrossRef]
156. Bedia, C.; Dalmau, N.; Jaumot, J.; Tauler, R. Phenotypic Malignant Changes and Untargeted Lipidomic Analysis of Long-Term Exposed Prostate Cancer Cells to Endocrine Disruptors. *Environ. Res.* **2015**, *140*, 18–31. [CrossRef] [PubMed]
157. Yun, U.J.; Lee, J.H.; Shim, J.; Yoon, K.; Goh, S.H.; Yi, E.H.; Ye, S.K.; Lee, J.S.; Lee, H.; Park, J.; et al. Anti-Cancer Effect of Doxorubicin Is Mediated by Downregulation of HMG-Co A Reductase via Inhibition of EGFR/Src Pathway. *Lab. Investig.* **2019**, *99*, 1157–1172. [CrossRef]
158. Lagoa, R.; Gañán, C.; López-Sánchez, C.; García-Martínez, V.; Gutierrez-Merino, C. The Decrease of NAD(P)H:Quinone Oxidoreductase 1 Activity and Increase of ROS Production by NADPH Oxidases Are Early Biomarkers in Doxorubicin Cardiotoxicity. *Biomarkers* **2014**, *19*, 142–153. [CrossRef]
159. Busso, I.T.; Silva, G.B.; Carreras, H.A. Organic Compounds Present in Airborne Particles Stimulate Superoxide Production and DNA Fragmentation: Role of NOX and Xanthine Oxidase in Animal Tissues. *Environ. Sci. Pollut. Res.* **2016**, *23*, 16653–16660. [CrossRef]
160. Kim, C.; Ashrap, P.; Watkins, D.J.; Mukherjee, B.; Rosario-Pabón, Z.Y.; Vélez-Vega, C.M.; Alshawabkeh, A.N.; Cordero, J.F.; Meeker, J.D. Maternal Metals/Metalloid Blood Levels Are Associated with Lipidomic Profiles Among Pregnant Women in Puerto Rico. *Front. Public Health* **2022**, *9*, 2248. [CrossRef] [PubMed]
161. Corsetto, P.A.; Ferrara, G.; Buratta, S.; Urbanelli, L.; Montorfano, G.; Gambelunghe, A.; Chiaradia, E.; Magini, A.; Roderi, P.; Colombo, I.; et al. Changes in Lipid Composition during Manganese-Induced Apoptosis in PC12 Cells. *Neurochem. Res.* **2016**, *41*, 258–269. [CrossRef]

162. Salzer, U.; Prohaska, R. Stomatin, Flotillin-1, and Flotillin-2 Are Major Integral Proteins of Erythrocyte Lipid Rafts. *Blood* **2001**, *97*, 1141–1143. [CrossRef]
163. Kwiatkowska, K.; Matveichuk, O.V.; Fronk, J.; Ciesielska, A. Flotillins: At the Intersection of Protein S-Palmitoylation and Lipid-Mediated Signaling. *Int. J. Mol. Sci.* **2020**, *21*, 2283. [CrossRef]
164. Eum, S.Y.; Jaraki, D.; András, I.E.; Toborek, M. Lipid Rafts Regulate PCB153-Induced Disruption of Occludin and Brain Endothelial Barrier Function through Protein Phosphatase 2A and Matrix Metalloproteinase-2. *Toxicol. Appl. Pharmacol.* **2015**, *287*, 258–266. [CrossRef] [PubMed]
165. Ni, I.; Ji, C.; Vij, N. Second-Hand Cigarette Smoke Impairs Bacterial Phagocytosis in Macrophages by Modulating CFTR Dependent Lipid-Rafts. *PLoS ONE* **2015**, *10*, e0121200. [CrossRef] [PubMed]
166. Winter, P.W.; Al-Qatati, A.; Wolf-Ringwall, A.L.; Schoeberl, S.; Chatterjee, P.B.; Barisas, B.G.; Roess, D.A.; Crans, D.C. The Anti-Diabetic Bis(Maltolato)Oxovanadium(Iv) Decreases Lipid Order While Increasing Insulin Receptor Localization in Membrane Microdomains. *Dalt. Trans.* **2012**, *41*, 6419–6430. [CrossRef] [PubMed]
167. Park, J.-W.; Kim, H.P.; Lee, S.-J.; Wang, X.; Wang, Y.; Ifedigbo, E.; Watkins, S.C.; Ohba, M.; Ryter, S.W.; Vyas, Y.M.; et al. Protein Kinase Cα and ζ Differentially Regulate Death-Inducing Signaling Complex Formation in Cigarette Smoke Extract-Induced Apoptosis. *J. Immunol.* **2008**, *180*, 4668–4678. [CrossRef]
168. Tappe, M.; Null, V. Requirements for Tires from the Environmental View Point. In Proceedings of the Tire Technology Expo Conference, Hamburg, Germany, 18–20 May 2002.
169. Beretta, E.; Gualtieri, M.; Botto, L.; Palestini, P.; Miserocchi, G.; Camatini, M. Organic Extract of Tire Debris Causes Localized Damage in the Plasma Membrane of Human Lung Epithelial Cells. *Toxicol. Lett.* **2007**, *173*, 191–200. [CrossRef]
170. Singh, D.P.; Kaur, G.; Bagam, P.; Pinkston, R.; Batra, S. Membrane Microdomains Regulate NLRP10- and NLRP12-Dependent Signalling in A549 Cells Challenged with Cigarette Smoke Extract. *Arch. Toxicol.* **2018**, *92*, 1767–1783. [CrossRef]
171. Fedida-Metula, S.; Feldman, B.; Koshelev, V.; Levin-Gromiko, U.; Voronov, E.; Fishman, D. Lipid Rafts Couple Store-Operated Ca^{2+} Entry to Constitutive Activation of PKB/Akt in a Ca^{2+}/Calmodulin-, Src- and PP2A-Mediated Pathway and Promote Melanoma Tumor Growth. *Carcinogenesis* **2012**, *33*, 740–750. [CrossRef]
172. Janes, P.W.; Ley, S.C.; Magee, A.I. Aggregation of Lipid Rafts Accompanies Signaling via the T Cell Antigen Receptor. *J. Cell Biol.* **1999**, *147*, 447–461. [CrossRef]
173. Ghare, S.; Patil, M.; Hote, P.; Suttles, J.; McClain, C.; Barve, S.; Joshi-Barve, S. Ethanol Inhibits Lipid Raft-Mediated TCR Signaling and IL-2 Expression: Potential Mechanism of Alcohol-Induced Immune Suppression. *Alcohol. Clin. Exp. Res.* **2011**, *35*, 1435–1444. [CrossRef]
174. Goddard, A.D.; Watts, A. Regulation of G Protein-Coupled Receptors by Palmitoylation and Cholesterol. *BMC Biol.* **2012**, *10*, 27. [CrossRef]
175. Zheng, H.; Pearsall, E.A.; Hurst, D.P.; Zhang, Y.; Chu, J.; Zhou, Y.; Reggio, P.H.; Loh, H.H.; Law, P.Y. Palmitoylation and Membrane Cholesterol Stabilize μ-Opioid Receptor Homodimerization and G Protein Coupling. *BMC Cell Biol.* **2012**, *13*, 6. [CrossRef] [PubMed]
176. Le Ferrec, E.; Øvrevik, J. G-Protein Coupled Receptors (GPCR) and Environmental Exposure. Consequences for Cell Metabolism Using the β-Adrenoceptors as Example. *Curr. Opin. Toxicol.* **2018**, *8*, 14–19. [CrossRef]
177. Shahid, A.; Chen, M.; Lin, C.; Andresen, B.T.; Parsa, C.; Orlando, R.; Huang, Y. The β-Blocker Carvedilol Prevents Benzo(a)Pyrene-Induced Lung Toxicity, Inflammation and Carcinogenesis. *Cancers* **2023**, *15*, 583. [CrossRef] [PubMed]

Disclaimer/Publisher's Note: The statements, opinions and data contained in all publications are solely those of the individual author(s) and contributor(s) and not of MDPI and/or the editor(s). MDPI and/or the editor(s) disclaim responsibility for any injury to people or property resulting from any ideas, methods, instructions or products referred to in the content.

Membrane Lipid Derivatives: Roles of Arachidonic Acid and Its Metabolites in Pancreatic Physiology and Pathophysiology

Cándido Ortiz-Placín [†], Alba Castillejo-Rufo [†], Matías Estarás and Antonio González *

Instituto de Biomarcadores de Patologías Moleculares, Departamento de Fisiología, Universidad de Extremadura, 10003 Cáceres, Spain; coplacin@unex.es (C.O.-P.); alcasru@unex.es (A.C.-R.); meh@unex.es (M.E.)

* Correspondence: agmateos@unex.es; Tel.: +34-927-251377; Fax: + 34-927-257110
† These authors contributed equally to this work.

Abstract: One of the most important constituents of the cell membrane is arachidonic acid. Lipids forming part of the cellular membrane can be metabolized in a variety of cellular types of the body by a family of enzymes termed phospholipases: phospholipase A2, phospholipase C and phospholipase D. Phospholipase A2 is considered the most important enzyme type for the release of arachidonic acid. The latter is subsequently subjected to metabolization via different enzymes. Three enzymatic pathways, involving the enzymes cyclooxygenase, lipoxygenase and cytochrome P450, transform the lipid derivative into several bioactive compounds. Arachidonic acid itself plays a role as an intracellular signaling molecule. Additionally, its derivatives play critical roles in cell physiology and, moreover, are involved in the development of disease. Its metabolites comprise, predominantly, prostaglandins, thromboxanes, leukotrienes and hydroxyeicosatetraenoic acids. Their involvement in cellular responses leading to inflammation and/or cancer development is subject to intense study. This manuscript reviews the findings on the involvement of the membrane lipid derivative arachidonic acid and its metabolites in the development of pancreatitis, diabetes and/or pancreatic cancer.

Keywords: arachidonic acid; cancer; inflammation; fibrosis; pancreas; stroma

1. Introduction

This work is an invited review that covers interesting findings on the involvement of the membrane lipid derivative arachidonic acid and its metabolites in the development of pancreatic diseases such as pancreatitis, diabetes and/or pancreatic cancer. Released from the constituent lipids of the cellular membrane, arachidonic acid is metabolized by major enzymes, which yields a subfamily of derivatives with important functions in cell physiology and pathophysiology, either in an autocrine, paracrine or endocrine manner. In this regard, the so-called tumor microenvironment (TME) has been signaled as an important cause of pancreatic disease. Specifically, the TME plays a critical role in cancer proliferation, invasion, metastasis and resistance to radiotherapy and chemotherapy. Because the relationship between inflammation and cancer is close, the role of the stroma and the putative cell-to-cell intercommunication in the pathophysiology of the pancreatic gland has been extensively analyzed. This research tries to summarize the advances made in the involvement of membrane lipid derivatives in pancreatic physiology and focuses its attention on the usefulness of arachidonic acid (AA) metabolism for the diagnosis, prevention and/or treatment of pancreatic disorders.

2. Arachidonic Acid Metabolism in the Pancreas

Lipid-derived messengers are well-known mediators of intracellular signaling. One of the most important constituents of biological membranes is AA, a polyunsaturated 20 carbon fatty acid (PUFA). Due to the presence of four double bonds in its molecule,

AA can interact with oxygen molecules in order to generate several bioactive compounds such as eicosanoids and isoprostanes [1]. Normally, membrane-embedded lipids can be metabolized in a variety of cellular types of the body by a family of enzymes termed phospholipases. These enzymes are mostly responsible for the release of AA from glycerophospholipids located within the cellular membrane. Three types of phospholipases have been described: phospholipase A2 (PLA$_2$), phospholipase C (PLC) and phospholipase D (PLD). PLA$_2$ is considered the most important enzyme type for the metabolization of AA. It recognizes the sn-2 acyl bond within the membrane phospholipids and releases AA and lysophospholipids in a single step [2–4]. The mentioned enzyme comprises six subtypes, which are known as cytosolic PLA$_2$, calcium-independent PLA$_2$, secreted PLA$_2$, lysosomal PLA$_2$, platelet-activating factor acetyl-hydrolases and adipose-specific PLA$_2$ [5,6]. AA exerts a pivotal role as a messenger in the cell physiology [7]. In addition to its role as an intracellular signal, AA also acts as a precursor for eicosanoid synthesis. The latter, in turn, also plays biological roles in the body, including the pancreas [8,9]. In this context, AA can be metabolized via three possible enzymatic pathways, through the enzymes cyclooxygenase (COX), lipoxygenase (LOX) and cytochrome P450 (CYP450) [10].

COX is also known as a prostaglandin endoperoxide synthase and is a type of oxidoreductase enzyme. Two isoforms of COX exist, termed COX-1 and COX-2. COX-1 is constitutively expressed in nearly all tissue and carries out normal (physiological) functions. COX-2 is inducible. The inducing stimuli include pro-inflammatory cytokines and growth factors. Consequently, COX-2 has been signaled to play a key role in inflammation and the control of cell growth [11]. COX-2 is highly expressed in a variety of cancers, where it exerts pleiotropic and multifaceted functions, which are considered responsible for, or critical contributors to, the genesis and/or promotion of carcinogenesis and cancer cell resistance [12]. COX generate prostanoids (20-carbon fatty acids), including prostaglandins (PGs) and thromboxanes (TXs). AA is firstly cyclized and oxygenated by COX. This step forms a cyclic endoperoxide derivative, prostaglandin G2 (PGG2). The hydroperoxyl group of PGG2 is also rapidly reduced by COX to produce hydroxyl-prostaglandin H2 (PGH2) [13]. PGH2 is later metabolized by various downstream enzymes, such as prostaglandin synthases and isomerases, leading to the generation of other specific PGs in the pancreas, such as prostaglandin E2 (PGE2—the most abundant PG in humans), prostaglandin D2 (PGD2), prostaglandin F1 alpha (PGF1α) and prostacyclin or PGI2. COX isoform derivatives have a preference for downstream PG synthases/isomerases. However, this coupling is not exclusive. For example, COX-1-derived PGH2 pairs mainly with PGF synthase, thromboxane synthase and cytosolic PGE synthase. Meanwhile, COX-2-derived PGH2 feeds mostly with PGI synthase and microsomal PGE synthase [14–16]. PGs exert their effects by activating membrane-linked G-protein receptors and have several different effects, depending on the specific PG and the cell type [17]. Another COX isoform has been found, COX-3, which is produced by the splicing of COX-1. However, its expression in the pancreas has not been properly studied yet. The only information that we could find refers to the study by Persaud et al. [18], who signal that this form of COX is not expressed in pancreatic β cells. Likewise, PGH2 can be metabolized to TXA2 by the TXA2 synthase. The latter is a highly unstable compound; its half-life is approximately 30 s. Thus, it is spontaneously hydrolyzed to thromboxane B2 (TXB2) [15,19]. TXB2 or its derivates, 2,3-dinor-TXB2 and 11-dehydro-TXB2, can be used as parameters for TXA2 production, whose increase is associated with pancreatic diseases [20–22].

LOX comprises a group of dioxygenases that catalyze the peroxidation of PUFAs, mainly linoleic acid (LA) or AA, in the presence of molecular oxygen [23]. The LOX family is classified according to the carbon atom that is oxygenated. Four types of LOX have described: 5-lipoxygenase (5-LOX), 8-lipoxygenase (8-LOX), 12-lipoxygenase (12-LOX) and 15-lipoxygenase type 1 and 2 (15-LOX-1 and 15-LOX-2). However, the main enzymes expressed in humans are 5-LOX (called leukocyte 5-LOX), 12-LOX (also known as platelet 12-LOX and leukocyte 12-LOX, respectively) and 15-LOX [3,24]. Generally, these enzymes synthesize active metabolites such as leukotrienes (LTs), lipoxins (LXs), hepoxillins (HOs) and hydroxy-eicosatetraenoic acids (HETEs) [25], which could act in an autocrine, paracrine and/or endocrine manner [26]. LOX enzymes generate the forms 5-, 8-, 12- or 15- hydroperoxyl-eicosatetraenoic acids (HpETEs), which are reduced by glutathione peroxidase (GPx) to the hydroxy forms (5-, 8-, 12-, 15-HETE), respectively [3,25]. However, the major sites on which AA is oxygenated are represented by the 5-, 12- and 15-positions. Therefore, in this review, we will focus on 5-LOX, 12-LOX and 15-LOX, which have been indicated to play important roles in the development and progression of human cancers, including pancreatic cancer, while 8-LOX has not been properly studied in the pancreas yet [10,24,27].

Firstly, 5-LOX generates 5-HpEPES from AA, which is a precursor for the synthesis of leukotrienes A4 (LTA4), 5-HEPEs and lipoxins (LXA4 and LXB4) [14]. LTA4 is an unstable metabolite that might be converted into LTB4 by LTA4 hydrolase. Then, LTB4 is conjugated with glutathione by glutathione S-transferase (GST) in order to produce LTC4, LTD4 and LTE4 [24]. With regard to the 12-LOX pathway, the metabolite generated from AA is termed 12-HpETES, which is further reduced to the more stable form 12-HETE. In addition, 12-HETE could lead to the generation of HO forms, such as 8-hydroxy-11,12-epoxy-eicosatetraenoic acid (HxA3) and 10-hydroxy-11,12-epoxy-eicosatrienoic acid (HxB3). Finally, the 15-LOX enzyme is subdivided into two subtypes, 15-LOX-1 and 15-LOX-2, which may have pro- or antitumorigenic activity depending on the isoforms. Moreover, 15-LOX-1 metabolizes AA to 3-hydroxy-octadecadienoic acid (13-HODE) and 15-HETE, while 15-LOX-2 mainly produces 15-HETE. Then, 15-HETE, which is a substrate for 5-LOX, is rapidly converted to LXA4 and LXB4 [28].

CYP450 consists of a group of membrane-bound hemoproteins with enzymatic activity that detoxify xenobiotics and exert key roles in cellular metabolism and homeostasis. CYP450 can be transcriptionally activated by different xenobiotics and endogenous substrates and its expression can be modulated by hormones and growth factors [29]. The CYP family is composed of numerous subclasses, giving rise to more than 6000 different enzymes. However, the CYP enzymes that catalyze AA are those with omega-hydroxylases and epoxidase activity. The former enzymes provide HETEs from AA and the latter produce epoxides and epoxyeicosatrienoic acids (EETs). The best known HETEs are 6-, 12-, 17-, 18-, 19- and 20-HETE. Some HETEs synthesized by CYP450 can be transformed subsequently by LOX [30]. CYP450 epoxygenases generate four EETs: 5,6-EET; 8,9-EET; 11,12-EET; and 14,15-EET. Stereoisomers exist for each of the four EET regioisomers, each of which may exert different effects [31]. CYP450 2J2 (CYP2J2) is the primary extrahepatic enzyme that processes AA to produce EETs in human [32]. These EETs have functions of their own, such as promoting angiogenesis and cell migration and cancer. In addition, EETs are rapidly metabolized by epoxide hydrolases to form dihydroxyeicosatrienoic acids (DHETs), which also exhibit diverse cellular functions [33–35]. The rapid transformation of EETs into DHETs has made it necessary to inhibit or delete epoxide hydroxylase to analyze the effects of EETs [36].

In summary, all these enzymes convert AA into different metabolites that will be involved in cellular fates. Among them, PGs, TXs, LTs and HETEs are the major metabolites generated from AA that are responsible for cellular responses [3]. Figure 1 provides a schematic representation of the bioactive eicosanoids derived from the AA pathway.

Finally, the activation of cell membrane receptors for pancreatic secretagogues, such as cholecystokinin, is linked to PLA_2 and to AA metabolism and, hence, modulates pancreatic function [18,37]. Furthermore, the overstimulation of pancreatic cells with secretagogues has been related to pancreatic disease [38,39]. Thus, either unbalanced secretagogue stimulation or the arrival of noxious agents may alter signaling in pancreatic cells, which has been related to the onset of pancreatic diseases such as inflammation and cancer [40–45].

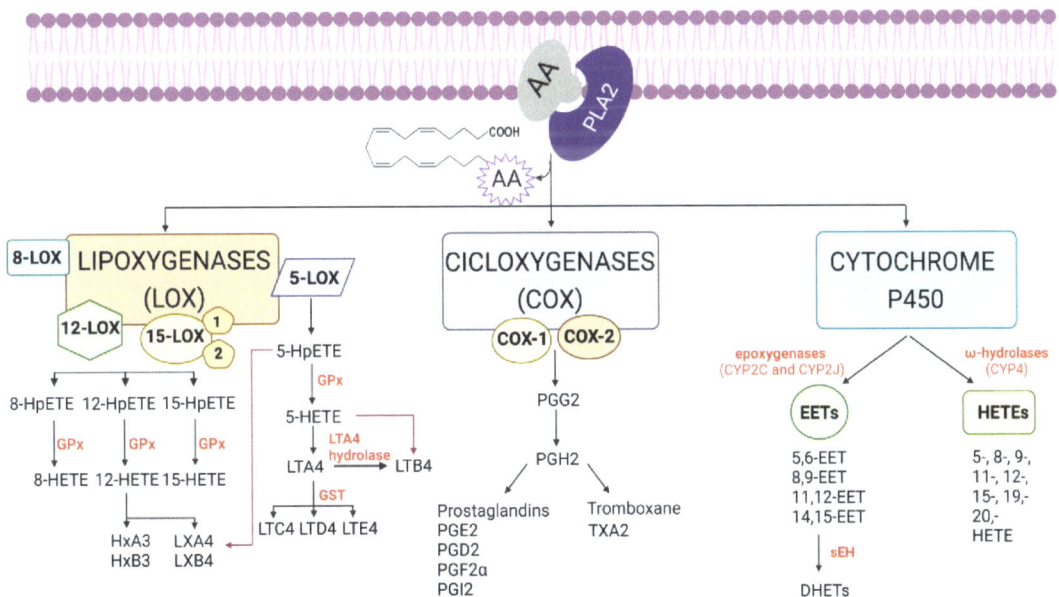

Figure 1. Schematic representation of the bioactive eicosanoids derived from arachidonic acid (AA) pathway. AA is mainly metabolized by three types of enzymes: cyclooxygenases (COX), lipoxygenases (LOX) and cytochrome P450 (CYP450). First, AA, which forms part of the phospholipids of the biological membrane, is released by phospholipase A2 (PLA$_2$). Then, COX, LOX and/or CYP450 enzymes act on the free AA to generate a cascade of prostaglandins (PGs), thromboxanes (TXs), a series of hydroxyeicosatetraenoic acids (HETEs), leukotrienes (LTs), lipoxins (LXs) hepoxilins (HOs) and epoxyeicosatrienoics acids (EETs). Finally, the effect of each bioactive eicosanoid will depend on the specific receptor that it binds to (HpETE: hydroperoxy-eicosatetraenoic acid; GPx: glutathione peroxidase; GST: glutathione S-transferase; HxA3: 8-hydroxy-11,12-epoxy-eicosatetraenoic acid; HxB3: 10-hydroxy-11,12-epoxy-eicosatrienoic acid; sEH: soluble epoxidehydrolase; DHETs: dihydroxyepoxyeicosatrienoic acid). Created with BioRender.com (accessed on 17 May 2023).

In line with the above-reported information, AA and its metabolites, as well as associated genes, could be used for prognostication and therapeutic aspects of pancreatic diseases. For example, an impaired serum fatty acid composition has been associated with primary insulin autoimmunity, on the basis that higher palmitoleic acid, cis-vaccenic, arachidonic, docosapentaenoic and docosahexaenoic acids decrease the risk, whereas higher α-linoleic acid and arachidonic:docosahexaenoic and n-6:n-3 acid ratios increase the risk [46]. Similarly, the lipidomic profiling of serum and pancreatic fluid can be used for the detection of chronic pancreatitis, a disease in which the serum and/or pancreatic fluid levels of oxidized fatty acids are elevated [47]. With regard to prognosis and therapy, signaling via 12-lipoxygenase-Gpr31 has been proposed to be required for pancreatic organogenesis in the zebrafish. This was based on the observation that 12-LOX-generated metabolites of AA increased sharply during organogenesis stages and that either the depletion or inhibition of 12-LOX impaired exocrine pancreas growth and the generation of insulin-producing β cells [48]. Additionally, the feedback modulation of glucose-induced insulin secretion by AA metabolites has been reported. In this context, the stimulation of insulin release by glucose may trigger a negative feedback loop via the local release of an inhibitor of β cell function. One or more metabolites of AA could be involved. Hence, the development of selective inhibitors of AA metabolism might be used in the therapy of impaired β cell function [49]. Moreover, the endocannabinoid system, which is reported as a lipid signaling system, comprises endogenous cannabis-like ligands that are derived from AA—for example, 2-arachidonoylglycerol. These signaling molecules bind to G-protein-coupled receptors, termed CB1 and CB2. The receptor for CB1 is widely distributed in the body, including the pancreas, where it could be coupled to the functional regulation of the gland and could represent a therapeutical approach [50]. Last but not least, suppression of the 5-LOX gene could be involved in the activation of apoptosis in pancreatic tumor cell lines in response to triptolide. These results suggest that the inhibition of AA metabolism by the 5-LOX pathway is associated with the antiproliferation activity of the mentioned drug, exhibiting clinical therapeutic value for patients with pancreatic cancer [51].

3. Arachidonic Acid and Calcium Signaling in the Pancreas

Calcium (Ca^{2+}) is a universal intracellular messenger that, in addition, exhibits enormous versatility. As such, Ca^{2+} serves as a powerful tool to control a wide array of processes—for example, proliferation, growth and development, learning and memory, muscle contraction, fertilization and/or secretion (enzymes and hormones). Nevertheless, impairment of its control may lead to undesirable effects, which might result in cell transformation and/or cell death [52].

As in other tissues and organs, Ca^{2+} is a critical intracellular messenger in pancreatic cell physiology [53]. Moreover, impairment of Ca^{2+} homeostasis is of critical relevance for pancreatic diseases, such as inflammation and cancer [54,55]. Attention has been paid to how genetic alterations can conduct Ca^{2+} signaling pathways, in the sense that mutations or the impaired expression of critical proteins that are involved in the control of the intracellular Ca^{2+} concentration could lead to the deregulation of Ca^{2+}-dependent effectors and, as a consequence, to the impairment of the mechanisms that control the cell's fate. Of major relevance is the way in which the impairment of Ca^{2+} homeostasis might influence a cell´s behavior to promote enhanced proliferation, survival and invasion, which are all pathophysiological hallmarks of cancer [56,57].

Interestingly, the involvement of AA metabolism and Ca^{2+} signaling in the pancreas has been reported. The release of Ca^{2+} from its intracellular stores depends on the activation of different intracellular pathways by the gut hormone cholecystokinin, which may bind to low- and/or high-affinity receptors. The latter would be linked to the activation of PLA_2 cascades. The products of the mentioned enzyme, AA and/or its metabolites, might modulate Ca^{2+} signals and, hence, the pancreatic physiology. Specifically, AA modulated the propagation of Ca^{2+} waves in pancreatic acinar cells, reducing the speed of propagation of Ca^{2+} signals [37,58,59]. Moreover, endogenously generated AA inhibited polyphosphoinositide synthesis and blocked agonist-induced inositol trisphosphate synthesis and Ca^{2+} mobilization in healthy cells [8].

On the contrary, AA might behave differentially in tumoral/transformed cells. In the study by Wu et al., the authors signaled that the AA pathway was involved in the increase in the intracellular Ca^{2+} concentration in pancreatic cancer cells. In the research, it was suggested that the metabolites of arachidonic acid were not involved in AA-mediated Ca^{2+} release. Rather, AA itself was responsible for their observation [60]. In rat pancreatic β cells, AA released Ca^{2+} from intracellular stores, an effect that was not observed in response to the analogue eicosatetraynoic acid. This further confirmed that AA metabolism was not required for Ca^{2+} mobilization [9]. Similarly, the analogue of AA arachidonyltrifluoromethyl ketone increased cytosolic Ca^{2+} in HIT insulinoma cells, which contributed to insulin secretion [61]. Thus, the effects of AA on cell physiology and its consequences might depend on the cellular type and on its status.

4. Role of Arachidonic Acid in Pancreatitis and Diabetes

As mentioned above, not only AA itself but its metabolization into different derivatives might be involved in major inflammatory responses in different tissues and organs, including the pancreas. Pancreatitis is a multifactorial disease that may be caused by the activation of different inflammatory mediators. Gallstones, smoking and alcohol consumption are well-established risk factors that may induce pancreatitis [62,63], but there are other factors contributing to the development of inflammation within the gland, including certain drugs such as mesalazine, azathioprine and simvastatine [64]. Additionally, post-endoscopic retrograde cholangiopancreatography has also been considered a potential risk factor that might induce pancreatitis as a common complication [65], in a similar way to pancreaticoduodenectomy [66]. Alteration of the immune response induced by gene mutations and/or environmental factors has also been considered a determinant of pancreatic damage [67]. All these factors might be related to the inappropriate intrapancreatic activation and release of pancreatic hydrolases. This could represent a pathogenetic mechanism of autodigestion of the gland that might lead to the onset of pancreatic inflammation [68]. The underlying cause responsible for the impairment of enzyme secretion could involve intracellular Ca^{2+} accumulation and concomitant oxidative stress [69–71]. The relationship between AA and Ca^{2+} signaling has been studied (see above).

In general, a major consensus points towards AA derivatives as being responsible for inflammation. COX, LOX and/or CYP450 produce metabolites that, to a variable extent, are involved in cell damage [72,73]. In fact, the levels of leukotriene B4 (LTB4), 15 hydroxyeicosatetraenoic acid (15-HETE), 6-keto prostaglandin F1 alpha (6-keto PGF1α), thromboxane B2 (TXB2) and prostaglandin E2 (PGE2) were increased in pancreatic tissue upon the induction of acute pancreatitis [20].

As previously reported, there are two genes encoding two COX isoenzymes. COX-1 is expressed constitutively in the cell and appears to regulate many normal physiologic functions. Conversely, COX-2 is inducible. Various growth factors, endotoxins, mitogens and tumor agents lead to an increase in its expression [74]. Activation of COX-2 has been signaled to mediate the inflammatory response. As such, COX-2 might be involved in the progression of inflammatory disease and in the development of chronic pancreatitis and/or diabetes [75]. COX-1 and COX-2 catalyze the formation of prostaglandins (PGs), thromboxanes (TXs) and levuloglandins [12]. The work carried out by Huang et al. showed that the expression of COX-2 in transgenic mice induced progressive changes in the pancreas, which included pancreas enlargement, inflammation, collagen deposition and acinar-to-ductal metaplasia [76]. Indeed, the success of anti-inflammatory drugs has been linked to their ability to inhibit COX-2 at the sites of damage and to a decrease in inflammation [77,78].

The generation of PGE2 through the COX pathway was considered a significant factor involved in β cell dysfunction and destruction and contributed to the pathogenesis of diabetes [3]. PGE2 is upregulated in diabetes and induces cell damage. Blockade of its receptor EP3 promoted β cell proliferation and survival via activation of the transcription factor nuclear factor E2-related factor 2 (Nrf2) [24]. AA metabolization led to the generation of PGE2 and TXB2, which activated the pro-inflammatory pathways nuclear factor kappa-light-chain-enhancer of activated B cells (NFκB) and Janus kinase (JAK)/signal transducer and activator of transcription 3 (STAT3) [79].

The induction of pancreatitis was related to increases in the levels of PGE2, PGD2 and TBX2, among others, in the gland [80]. High levels of PGE2 were detected in Sprague-Dawley rats upon the induction of acute necrotizing pancreatitis. Lipid peroxidation, together with edema, inflammation, bleeding and necrosis, was observed. The histopathologic severity was decreased by n-3 fatty acids, which was explained by the inhibition of PGE2 [81]. PGE2 modulated the activation of tumor necrosis factor alpha (TNF-α) in rat pancreatic lobules, an effect probably mediated by the activation of protein kinase A. This was interpreted as a putative mechanism that might explain the COX-2-dependent propagation of pancreatic inflammation [82]. Similarly, increased levels of PGE2 and TNF-α were detected in a cell line and animal models of severe acute pancreatitis. Meanwhile, 2-acetoxy-5-(2-4-(trifluoromethyl)-phenethylamino)-benzoic acid exhibited antioxidative and anti-inflammatory activity and diminished serum amylase and lipase levels and pancreatic wet weights, thereby inducing significant tissue-protective effects [83]. Rofecoxib, a selective COX-2 inhibitor, diminished PGE2 levels and collagen and transforming growth factor β (TGFβ) synthesis in an animal model of chronic pancreatitis. All the effects reported were related to the diminished infiltration of macrophages [84].

Apart from prostaglandins, leukotrienes also may be involved in the onset of pancreatic damage. LOX is a family of iron-containing dioxygenases that catalyze the formation of bioactive HETE metabolites from polyunsaturated fatty acids such as linoleic acid and AA [85]. These enzymes comprise six isoforms, which are expressed in different types of cells and tissues, such as immune, epithelial and tumor cells. LOX displays a wide range of functions, which include inflammation and tumorigenesis. The major end products of their activity are termed leukotrienes [86]. It should be pointed out that lipoxins have an important role in cancer cells. Lipoxins have anti-inflammatory effects, which decrease the chronic inflammation in the damaged tissue. This action takes place when these molecules bind to G-protein-coupled lipoxin A4 receptor (ALX)/formyl peptide receptor (FPR2). On the one hand, lipoxins may interact with many cells of the immune system, such as neutrophils, macrophages and T and B cells. On the other hand, these molecules also might regulate the levels of several transcription factors, such as NFκB factor [87]. Specifically, it has been shown that LXA4 is able to reduce cell proliferation, to inhibit cell invasion and to suppress tumor growth, therefore exhibiting anti-inflammatory properties in cancer. For this reason, it is important to evaluate its putative use in the treatment of cancer [25].

Caerulein, a pancreatic secretagogue, or intraductal bile acids, are common tools used to induce pancreatitis. Both of them increased the production of LTB4 in mice pancreatic acinar cells. In the study, a marked increase in the level of 5-LOX was observed [88]. The administration of LTB4 induced pancreatic damage, evidenced by pancreatic edema, neutrophil infiltration and necrosis [89]. LTB4 induced polymorphonuclear leucocyte accumulation in response to the generation of oxygen free radicals in an experimental rat model of pancreatic inflammation. The LTB4 inhibitor MK-886 exhibited protective effects [90]. The 5-LOX inhibitor zileuton repressed blood biomarkers of neutrophil activation and attenuated pancreatic tissue damage in a rat model [91]. Zafirlukast, a leukotriene receptor antagonist, improved histopathological parameters in the pancreas of rats subjected to acute pancreatitis [92].

Moreover, 12-lipoxygenase (12-LOX) has also been involved in the development of diabetes [26]. Increases in the levels of 12- and 15-HETE followed increases in the expression of 12/15-LOX and were accompanied by islet dysfunction and insulin resistance [93]. Leukotrienes inhibited glucose-induced insulin release, thereby altering endocrine pancreas functioning [94]. Zafirlukast also proved to be a potential candidate for a therapeutic intervention in diabetes, since it enhanced insulin secretion and prompted the activation of Ca^{2+}/calmodulin-dependent protein kinase II and extracellular signal-regulated kinase signaling. Zafirlukast treatment further resulted in a significant drop in glucose levels [95].

CYP450 is a group of enzymes that are differentiated by a number for the isoform or individual enzyme (e.g., CYP1A1, CYP2D6) [96]. The major site of CYP expression is the liver [97]. These enzymes convert AA to four EETs that exhibit various biological effects, especially in the cardiovascular system [32]. There is some evidence for the involvement of CYP in pancreatic β cell dysfunction. CYP1A1 and CYP1B1 have been signaled to be involved in glucose homeostasis, insulin resistance and diabetes development [98]. EETs play an important role in insulin and glucagon secretion. Moreover, 5,6-EET was found to increase insulin release, while 8,9-, 11,12- or 14,15-EET stimulated glucagon production [99]. Loss of epoxide hydroxylase, an enzyme that degrades EETs, significantly reduced hyperglycemia in streptozotocin-treated mice and increased glucose-dependent insulin secretion and reduced apoptosis in pancreatic β cells [36]. An association between the CYP27B1 and CYP24A1 gene polymorphisms and type 1 diabetes has been reported [100]. However, to our knowledge, studies on the involvement of CYP in pancreatitis are currently lacking.

In general, it is accepted that the inhibition of the AA pathway and/or blockade of its metabolites will undoubtedly protect the pancreas against inflammation. In this context, knockout of the co-chaperone protein St13 exacerbated fatty replacement and fibrosis in a model of chronic pancreatitis. Therefore, it was suggested that St13 was functionally activated in acinar cells and exerted protection against inflammation, via regulation of the AA pathway [101].

Although the majority of the studies reviewed point toward the deleterious actions of AA metabolism, protective actions of AA have been reported in the pancreas. AA restored the antioxidant status to a normal range in an experimental animal model of diabetes mellitus. The study suggested that AA exerted protective actions in pancreatic β cells against alloxan-induced diabetes by attenuating oxidative stress [102]. The AA present in ARASCO oil was related to protective actions in the pancreas. Indeed, ARASCO oil, which was identified as a source of AA, diminished hyperglycemia, restored insulin sensitivity, suppressed inflammation and reversed the altered antioxidant status in streptozotocin-induced diabetes mellitus [103]. In a similar way, a decrease in PGE2 was correlated with an increase in tissue damage in alcohol-fed rats. Conversely, there was an inverse correlation between PGE2 levels and fibrogenesis. Because of these observations, the authors of this research suggested that endogenous PGE2 plays a protective role in alcohol-induced injury in the pancreas [104]. All this suggests the possibility, mentioned earlier in this manuscript, that the effects of AA on cell physiology and its consequences may vary from cell to cell and also may depend on the cellular state.

5. Arachidonic Acid's Involvement in Pancreatic Cancer Development

The relationship between inflammation and cancer is widely accepted [105], including in pancreatic cancer [106]. In fact, both COX-2 and 5-lipoxygenase (5-LOX) are upregulated in different types of cancer, including pancreatic cancer. It is generally accepted that the metabolization of AA by these two enzymes leads to the formation of eicosanoids that directly contribute to pancreatic cancer cell proliferation, whereas the inhibition of the mentioned enzymes abrogates cancer cell proliferation [107].

The COX-2 enzyme appears to be overexpressed in a number of cancers and, as such, its products might play critical roles in carcinogenesis [108]. In fact, COX-2 activation has been related to an increase in cell proliferation and survival and the inhibition of the pro-apoptotic pathway, thereby resulting in tumor angiogenesis, invasion and metastasis [109]. Thus, the inhibition of COX-2 has received increasing attention as a useful tool for the prevention and treatment of cancer [110–112]. Drugs that blocked COX enzymes inhibited pancreatic cancer growth both in vitro and in vivo and induced cell death through the activation of apoptosis [113]. Omura et al. [114] suggested that COX-2-derived PG are used by cancer cells to proliferate and that the inhibition of its import from the extracellular medium via the blockade of multidrug-resistance-associated proteins abrogated pancreatic cancer growth. Likewise, the expression of PG biosynthetic pathway enzymes in mucinous pancreatic cysts has been detected. Additionally, the levels of COX-2 and cPLA$_2$ were increased in the epithelia of mucinous pancreatic cysts [115]. Concomitant activation of COX-2 and K-Ras(G12D) accelerated the progression of pancreatic intraepithelial lesions, which involved components of the neurogenic locus notch homolog protein 1 (Notch1) [116]. The expression of COX-2 was increased in a number of resection specimens of pancreatic ductal adenocarcinoma (PDCA). Synergistic increases were also detected in the expression of the tumor protein p53 [117]. The latter consists of a gene that codes a protein (p53) that plays a key role in controlling cell division and cell death and, hence, is pivotal to cancer cell growth and the development of the disease [118]. Therefore, the inhibition of COX-2 and/or PLA$_2$ might help to prevent the progression of tumor cell growth and cancer development [115]. A decrease in both cell proliferation and PG levels was related to the improved turnover of preneoplastic lesions in the pancreas [119]. The COX inhibitor ibuprofen exerted modulating effects in pancreatic cancers experimentally induced in hamsters [4].

With respect to LOX enzymes, evidence also exists that signals their involvement in pancreatic cancer development. Expression of both 5-LOX and 12-LOX has been detected in pancreatic cancer tissue [113] and cell lines, including PANC-1, AsPC-1 and MiaPaCa2 cells. The expression of the receptor of the downstream 5-LOX metabolite, leukotriene

B4, was also increased [120]. LOX metabolites stimulated the growth of the tumor cells, whereas their inhibition markedly inhibited pancreatic cancer cell proliferation [113]. Similarly, growth inhibition and apoptosis in human pancreatic cell lines were noticed upon the downregulation of 5-LOX expression, as well as in the production of its downstream product LTB4 [51]. Meanwhile, 15-LOX-1 expression and activity were suggested to exert antitumorigenic effects in pancreatic cancer. Interestingly, 15-LOX-1 was found to be strongly present in normal ductal cells, tubular complexes and centro-acinar cells, whereas no staining was noted in tumor cells. These observations suggested that 15-LOX-1 expression might be lost during pancreatic cancer development [121]. The lichen (symbiotic partnership of a fungus and an alga) metabolites protolichesterinic acid, lobaric acid and baeomycesic acid exhibited antiproliferative effects against twelve different human cancer cell lines, including the pancreatic cancer cell lines Capan-1, Capan-2 and PANC-1. All three compounds had in vitro 5-LOX inhibitory activity, whereas protolichesterinic and lobaric acid inhibited 12-LOX [122]. Zyflo, a selective inhibitor of 5-LOX, diminished the incidence and the sizes of carcinomas in a model of pancreatic cancer induced in Syrian hamsters. Additionally, the activity of several antioxidant enzymes was increased and the concentration of products of lipid peroxidation was decreased. Thus, it was suggested that the inhibition of 5-LOX might be useful to decrease tumor growth in advanced pancreatic cancer [123]. Moreover, Zyflo also diminished liver metastasis in pancreatic cancer [124]. Another compound, termed triptolide, induced apoptosis that was related to the inhibition of the 5-LOX pathway in SW1990 pancreatic cancer cells in vitro. Conversely, overexpression of 5-LOX or the exogenous administration of LTB4 made cells more resistant [51]. The work carried out by Tersey et al. showed that 12-LOX promoted inflammation and increased the production of reactive oxygen species, through the p38 mitogen-activated protein kinase (p38 MAPK) and NFκB pathway [125]. Therefore, 5-HETE and 12-HETE metabolites might promote cancer growth via activation of the p44/42 and PI3/Akt mitogen-activated protein kinase pathways [27].

CYP450s are considered another group of enzymes related to AA metabolism that play a key role in carcinogenesis. They represent a superfamily of enzymes that catalyze the oxidation of lipids, steroids and drugs [126]. Several CYP enzymes metabolically activate procarcinogens [127]. The expression of the form CYP2J2 is increased in various human tumor cells and its metabolites are suggested to be involved in the development of human cancers [32]. CYP2J2 is overexpressed in PDAC, and its metabolites downstream of AA, specifically 8,9-EET, could inhibit ferroptosis in the pancreatic tumor line PANC-1 [34]. CYP450-2E1 (CYP2E1) was induced by ethanol consumption and was related to consequent toxicity, including carcinogenesis in the gastrointestinal tract [128]. The expression of certain CYP4 isoforms has been detected at significantly high levels in PDAC tissue, suggesting a role in the development of the disease [126]. The role of this enzyme system in the pathogenesis of chronic inflammatory and malignant pancreatic diseases has been confirmed by other studies. Compared to the normal pancreas, the expression of CYPs was increased in a number of pancreatic cancer samples [129]. CYP2A6, a metabolic enzyme that activates several procarcinogens, which include dietary and tobacco-specific nitrosamines, has been linked to pancreatic cancer. Consistent with this, high levels of CYP2A6 activity were detected in patients suffering from pancreatic cancer [130].

6. Arachidonic Acid and Stroma: Interplay in the Tissue Microenvironment

The stroma comprises the cells, components and structures that support and give form to organs, glands and/or tissues in the body. The stroma is mainly composed of connective tissue, blood vessels, lymphatic vessels and nerves. It provides the conditions for the normal functioning of the cells present in a certain tissue or organ [131]. Replacement of the exocrine parenchyma (i.e., the tissue formed by the cells that carry out an essential function) by fibrous tissue is a major characteristic of chronic pancreatitis and pancreatic cancer [76].

The tumor microenvironment (TME) is defined as the environment and/or conditions that surround a population of cells that form a tumor [132]. This environment includes blood vessels, immune cells, fibroblasts, stellate cells, signaling molecules, respiratory gases and the extracellular matrix, all of which participate as constituents of the stroma [133]. In cancer, the stroma plays an important role in contributing to the development of malignant cells [131]. The cells and their surroundings establish a close relationship, i.e., a bidirectional interaction is constantly ongoing "indoors". This creates favorable conditions that will confer upon tumor cells the capability for active proliferation and growth, invasion and metastasis, which are all hallmarks of malignancy [134].

As previously reported, inflammation within the tumor microenvironment is a hallmark of cancer and is accepted as a major characteristic of carcinogens. The participation of AA´s metabolites has been investigated. Its products, and the metabolism of related fatty acids, which include prostaglandins, leukotrienes, lipoxins and epoxyeicosanoids, exhibit a critical ability to regulate inflammation. It is therefore expected that the resolution of inflammation might be a valuable tool to prevent malignant transformation [135]. Moreover, it has been suggested that targeting the enzymes, such as PLA_2, COX and LOX, would lead to the achievement of beneficial outcomes in cancer therapy [136].

The role of stromal sources of PG for pancreatic cancers has been demonstrated. Overexpression of COX-2 is a factor that links chronic inflammation with metaplastic and neoplastic changes in various tissues, including the exocrine pancreas. Indeed, elevated expression is associated with worse outcomes. The COX-2 product PGE2 acts through a receptor termed EP4, which has been found to be upregulated in cancer. Activation of this receptor supports cell proliferation, migration, invasion and metastasis through the activation of multiple signaling pathways, including extracellular signal-regulated kinase (ERK), cyclic adenosine monophosphate/protein kinase A (cAMP/PKA), phosphoinositide 3-kinase/protein kinase B (PI3K/AKT) and NFκB [137]. Stimulation of pancreatic cancer cells with PGE2 led to the secretion of fibroblast growth factor 1 (FGF1). This was related to the enhanced proliferation of cancer-associated fibroblasts and increased expression of vascular endothelial growth factor A (VEGF-A) [138]. In a transgenic murine model, cellular atypia and a loss of normal cell/tissue organization were observed. A diet containing celecoxib, a COX-2 inhibitor, prevented the development of an abnormal pancreatic phenotype [139]. Profibrogenic factors were upregulated in transgenic mice expressing COX-2 [76]. Another study reported that COX-1 expression was not detected in various pancreatic cancer cells and some of them also lacked COX-2 expression. This led the researchers to suspect that such cancers rely on exogenous sources of PG. Interestingly, fibroblasts expressing COX-1 and COX-2 might be a source of PG, which would be used by pancreatic cancer cells, allowing them to grow and to proliferate [114]. Pancreatic stellate cells (PSC) contribute, in addition to fibroblasts, as a source of fibrotic stroma [140]. Moreover, other components of the TME, such as the peripherical blood mononuclear cells, are able to produce PG [141]. A correlation between the levels of COX-2 and its product PGE2 and the extent of pancreatic fibrosis has been suggested. PGE2 stimulated the proliferation, migration and invasion of PSC. Furthermore, PGE2 increased the expression of extracellular matrix genes [142]. The peroxisome proliferator-activated receptor gamma (PPAR-γ) is a ligand-activated transcription factor that controls inflammation, in addition to growth and differentiation. In PSC, activation of this transcription factor inhibited cell proliferation and the synthesis of collagen [143]. Melatonin, the main product of the pineal gland, exhibits several pharmacological properties, including anti-inflammatory effects. In this context, this indolamine reduced the expression of COX-2 though the inhibition of NFκB signaling in pancreatic stellate cells subjected to hypoxia [144]. Melatonin has shown a significant antifibrotic role in the pancreas and some of its effects may be mediated by its anti-inflammatory actions exerted by modulating COX-2 expression. One of the characteristics of the pancreatic tumor microenvironment is the exclusion or poor infiltration of T cells [145]. This is one of the main reasons that pancreatic tumors are often refractory to immunotherapy. The production of PGE2 by the metabolization of AA via

COX-2 appears to have an immunosuppressive effect, by which T cells are excluded from the tumor focus [146]. A similar observation was made by Zhang et al., who observed that the inhibition of COX-2 by apricoxib alone or in combination with anti-VEGF therapy increased the infiltration of CD8+ T cells in PDAC in vivo models [147].

Among the six different isoforms of LOX that have been described, 5-LOX is the most vital enzyme for the synthesis of leukotrienes. Evidence exists that relates 5-LOX to tumors [23]. Leukotriene signaling contributes to the active tumor microenvironment, promoting tumor growth and resistance to therapy [148]. Metabolites generated by 5-LOX from AA, such as 5-hydroxyeicosatetraenoic acid (5-HETE) and a variety of leukotrienes, have been suggested to act as mediators of inflammation in pathological states, leading to cancer. Furthermore, upregulation of the expression of 5-LOX has been associated with increased tumorigenesis. Pathways activated by 5-LOX may interact with the tumor microenvironment and can participate actively during the development and progression of a tumor [149]. Moreover, 5-LOX and the prostaglandin E synthase-1 (PGES-1) play an important role in the immune evasion evoked by tumor associated macrophages, which constrains the action of the antitumoral natural killer T cells [150].

Increased expression of 12-LOX and elevated levels of its metabolite 12-(S)-HETE were found in fibroblasts, one of the major nonmalignant cell types present in the stroma of pancreatic ductal adenocarcinoma (PDAC). This fact conferred upon fibroblasts the capability to transfer AA derivatives to tumor cells, which would be used for their proliferative needs [151]. However, not all metabolites of LOX exhibit fibrogenic effects. LXA4, a derivative metabolite of AA generated via LOX, inhibited the differentiation of PSC into a myofibroblast phenotype and reduced the proliferation and migration of pancreatic cancer cells evoked by PSC [152].

In addition to AA metabolism, CYP450 enzymes also are involved in the metabolism of drugs, foreign chemicals, cholesterol, steroids and other major lipids. This primarily takes place in the liver and in the gastrointestinal tract. However, evidence also exists that suggests that this occurs within the tumor microenvironment [153]. CYP450-derived AA epoxides, termed epoxyeicosatrienoic acids (EETs), also play a certain role in the promotion of the growth of certain tumors [154].

7. Discussion and Conclusions

As stated above, the relationship between inflammation and cancer is close. The existing literature covers a wide range of studies that show that isoenzymes of both COX and LOX are upregulated in different types of cancer, including pancreatic cancer. Less is known about the role of CYP450. Table 1 contains information about the functions of different metabolites of AA in pancreatitis, diabetes and pancreatic cancer The mentioned enzymes mainly convert AA into PGs, TXs, LTs and HETEs. These lipid-derived messengers are well-known mediators of intra- and intercellular signaling and are involved in cellular responses and fates. In this context, the role of the stroma and the putative cell-to-cell intercommunication in the pathophysiology of pancreatic diseases exhibits major relevance. The effect of certain inhibitors of the enzymes involved in AA metabolism is summarized in Table 2.

The stroma provides the conditions for the normal functioning of the cells present in a certain tissue or organ. Inflammation within the TME is a hallmark of cancer and is accepted as a major characteristic of carcinogens. Consequently, the stroma plays an important role in terms of a contribution to the development of malignant cells. In this context, the modulation of AA and the pathways regulated by its metabolites might be a valuable tool to prevent malignant transformation.

Table 1. AA metabolites and its effects related to pancreatic diseases.

Diseases	AA Metabolism Pathway	Metabolite	Effect	Reference
DIABETES	COX pathway	PGE2	- β cell damage, dysfunction and final cell destruction in a murine model - Activates ERK, NFκB and JNK/STAT3 proinflammatory pathways in isolated rat pancreatic acini - Endogenous PGE2 acts as a protector against alcohol-induced injury in alcohol-fed rats	[3,79,104]
		TXB2	- Activates NFκB and JNK/STAT3 proinflammatory pathway in isolated rat pancreatic acini	[79]
	LOX pathway	12, 15-HETE	- Generates islet dysfunction and insulin resistance in prediabetic mice	[93]
	CYP-450 pathway	5,6-EET	- Increases insulin secretion from isolated rat pancreatic islets	[99]
		8,9-, 11,12- or 14,15-EET	- Increases glucagon secretion from isolated rat pancreatic islets	[99]
	COX pathway	TXB2, PGE2, 6-ketoPGF1α and PGD2	- High levels observed in chronic pancreatitis induced in rats, responsible for inflammation	[20,80]
		PGE2	- High levels observed in induced-acute pancreatitis, which produced edema, lipid peroxidation, inflammation, bleeding and pancreatic necrosis in animal models	[79,81,83]
		PGE2	- Promotes the activation of TNF-α in rat pancreatic acinar cells	[82]

Table 1. *Cont.*

Diseases	AA Metabolism Pathway	Metabolite	Effect	Reference
PANCREATITIS	LOX pathway	LTB4 and 15-HETE	- Elevated levels have been observed in chronic pancreatitis in rats	[20]
		Lipoxins (LXs)	- Acts as anti-inflammatory mediator in the damage of tissue - Regulation of the expression of several transcription factors such as NFκB, EGR1, PPARγ, AP-1 in animal models - Interacts with many cells in both the innate and adaptive immune systems	[87]
		LTB4	- Generation of pancreatic edema, neutrophil infiltration and necrosis in rat pancreas - Produces polymorphonuclear leucocyte accumulation induced by oxygen free radicals in rats	[89,90]
PANCREATIC CANCER	COX pathway	PGE2	- Increases the cell proliferation of pancreatic tumor cells (MiaPaCa2) - Leads to FGF1 secretion by PANC-2 and this factor enhances proliferation of cancer-associated fibroblasts (CAFs) - Stimulates proliferation and migration of human PSC; also boosts the expression of extracellular matrix genes - Regulates the profibrotic activity of human PSC via EP4 receptor - Immunosuppressive effect that excludes T cells from pancreatic tumoral mass in human PDA	[114,138,142, 146]
	LOX pathway	LXA4	- Inhibits the differentiation of human PSC into a CAF-like myofibroblast phenotype - Reduces the migration and growth of human pancreatic cell line - Decreases the growth of 3D heterospheroids of human PSC and PANC-1	[152]
		5,12-HETE	- Activation of the p44/42 and PI3/Akt pathway in cancer cells	[27]

Table 1. Cont.

Diseases	AA Metabolism Pathway	Metabolite	Effect	Reference
	CYP-450 pathway	8,9-ETE	- Inhibit ferroptosis in the tumor line PANC-1	[34]
		20-HETE	- Overexpression in cancer promotes angiogenesis and metastasis via MMP activation in human pancreatic specimens	[126]

The table contains information about the functions of different metabolites of AA in pancreatitis, diabetes and pancreatic cancer. The metabolite is mentioned, in addition to the effects reported by researchers (reference include).

Table 2. Inhibitors of AA pathway and their effects on cell physiology.

Inhibitor	AA Metabolism Pathway	Therapeutic Target	Effector Function	Reference
Rofecoxib		COX-2	- Decreases PGE2 levels, collagen and TGFβ synthesis in a rat model	[84]
Apricoxib		COX-2	- Alone or combined with anti-VEGF, reduced the infiltration of CD8+ T cells in PDAC in vivo models	[147]
Melatonin		COX-2	- Decreases the expression of COX-2 via inhibition of NFκB pathway in rat PSC treated under hypoxia - Anti-inflammatory and antifibrotic actions in rat PSC	[144,145]
5-aminosalicylic acid (compound of mesalazine)	COX pathway	COX-2	- Inhibits PGE2 expression and NF-α- and IL-1β-induced COX-2 expression - Increases pancreatic duct permeability - Increases the risk of pancreatitis	[64]
Nimesulide		COX-2	- Reduced level of PGE2 and tumor angiogenesis in nude mice model (in vivo study)	[107]
Ibuprofen		COX	- Inhibits the development of pancreatic carcinogenesis induced in hamsters	[4]
Celecoxib		COX-2	- Prevents the development of abnormal pancreatic phenotype in mice	[139]

Table 2. Cont.

Inhibitor	AA Metabolism Pathway	Therapeutic Target	Effector Function	Reference
MK-886	LOX pathway	5-LOX activating protein (FLAP)	- Inhibitor of LT synthesis because it prevents the translocation of 5-LOX to the cell membrane in rats - Protective effects against pancreatic inflammation in cancer in animal models	[4,90,107]
Zileuton		5-LOX	- Reduces pancreatic damage and neutrophil activation in rat tissue	[91]
Zafirlukast		Leukotriene receptor antagonist	- Increases the pancreatitis histopathological parameters and necrosis in rats - Enhances insulin secretion in mice	[92,95]
Zyflo		5-LOX	- Increases the activity of antioxidant enzymes and reduces the concentration of lipid peroxidation in hamsters	[123,124]
Triptolide		5-LOX	- Cytotoxic effect on human pancreatic cell lines; induces apoptosis and reduces LTB4 production	[51]
Protolichesterinic acid and lobaric acid		5, 12-LOX	- Antiproliferative effects on pancreatic tumor cell lines Capan-1, Capan-2 and PANC-1	[122]

The table summarizes the effects of certain inhibitors of the enzymes involved in AA metabolism. The enzyme involved is mentioned, in addition to the effect induced on the cell type, as reported by scientists in their research (reference is cited).

In conclusion, AA exhibits a role as an intracellular signal. Moreover, AA also acts as a precursor for eicosanoid synthesis, which further amplifies the actions of AA in terms of extending its actions to the surrounding cells. Cell communication within the TME depicts major relevance for cancer development and growth, and AA's derivatives exhibit potential roles in the development of the disease. A summary of the main findings on the involvement of AA metabolization in the pancreatic tumor microenvironment is given in Figure 2.

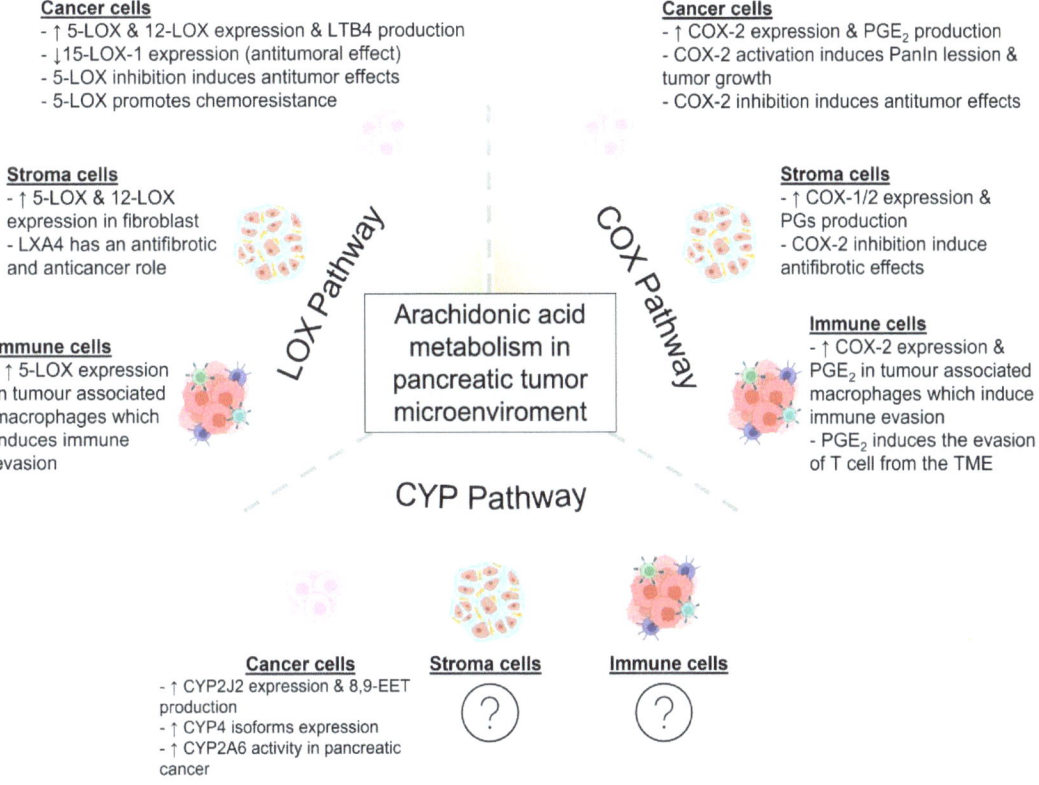

Figure 2. Metabolism of arachidonic acid in the pancreatic tumor microenvironment. The cells that form the pancreatic tumor microenvironment can metabolize arachidonic acid (AA) by the action of cyclooxygenases (COX), lipoxygenases (LOX) or cytochrome P450 (CYP450). These pathways give rise to different metabolites that can promote or diminish tumor development and growth. In this figure, the main findings on AA metabolization within the pancreatic tumor microenvironment are summarized (8,9-EET: 8,9-epoxyeicosatrienoic acid; COX: cyclooxygenase; LOX: lipoxygenase; CYP: cytochrome, LTB4: leukotriene B4; LXA4: lipoxin A4; PanIN: pancreatic intraepithelial neoplasia; PGE2: prostaglandin E2; PGs: prostaglandins; TME: tumor microenvironment). Created with BioRender.com (accessed on 17 May 2023).

8. Future Directions

In contrast to the wide variety of research focused on the involvement of COX and LOX in cancer development, fewer studies exist regarding the functions in carcinogenesis of CYP450. Therefore, further studies will be needed to shed more light on the role of CYP450 in pancreatic cancer development and/or progression. Additionally, although the majority of the studies reviewed point toward the deleterious actions of AA metabolism, protective actions of AA in the pancreas have been suggested, which need to be explored.

Author Contributions: C.O.-P. wrote parts of the manuscript; designed the figures; and revised, corrected and approved the submitted version of the manuscript. A.C.-R. wrote parts of the manuscript; designed the figures; and revised, corrected and approved the submitted version of the manuscript. M.E. wrote parts of the manuscript; designed the figures; and revised, corrected and approved the submitted version of the manuscript. A.G. designed the first draft; wrote parts of the manuscript; and revised, corrected and approved the submitted version of the manuscript. All authors have read and agreed to the published version of the manuscript.

Funding: Funding for the studies was provided by Junta de Extremadura—FEDER (GR21037). Matias Estaras was awarded a grant from the Valhondo Calaff Foundation. Candido Ortiz was awarded a grant from the Spanish Association Against Cancer (AECC). The contract for Alba Castillejo-Rufo was funded by Servicio Extremeño de Empleo (SEXPE, TE-0028-21). The funding sources had no role in the study design; in the collection, analysis and interpretation of data; in the writing of the report; or in the decision to submit the paper for publication.

Conflicts of Interest: The authors declare that there is no conflict of interest. All authors contributed to the preparation of this work and revised and approved the published version of the manuscript.

References

1. Hanna, V.S.; Hafez, E.A.A. Synopsis of arachidonic acid metabolism: A review. *J. Adv. Res.* **2018**, *11*, 23–32. [CrossRef] [PubMed]
2. Zhang, M.; Xiang, R.; Glorieux, C.; Huang, P. PLA2G2A Phospholipase Promotes Fatty Acid Synthesis and Energy Metabolism in Pancreatic Cancer Cells with K-ras Mutation. *Int. J. Mol. Sci.* **2022**, *23*, 11721. [CrossRef] [PubMed]
3. Luo, P.; Wang, M.-H. Eicosanoids, β-cell function, and diabetes. *Prostaglandins Other Lipid Mediat.* **2011**, *95*, 1–10. [CrossRef] [PubMed]
4. Schuller, H.M.; Zhang, L.; Weddle, D.L.; Castonguay, A.; Walker, K.; Miller, M.S. The cyclooxygenase inhibitor ibuprofen and the FLAP inhibitor MK886 inhibit pancreatic carcinogenesis induced in hamsters by transplacental exposure to ethanol and the tobacco carcinogen NNK. *J. Cancer Res. Clin. Oncol.* **2002**, *128*, 525–532. [CrossRef]
5. Murakami, M.; Nakatani, Y.; Atsumi, G.-I.; Inoue, K.; Kudo, I. Regulatory Functions of Phospholipase A2. *Crit. Rev. Immunol.* **2017**, *37*, 127–195. [CrossRef] [PubMed]
6. Peng, Z.; Chang, Y.; Fan, J.; Ji, W.; Su, C. Phospholipase A2 superfamily in cancer. *Cancer Lett.* **2021**, *497*, 165–177. [CrossRef]
7. Turunen, P.M.; Putula, J.; Kukkonen, J.P. Filtration assay for arachidonic acid release. *Anal. Biochem.* **2010**, *407*, 233–236. [CrossRef]
8. Chaudhry, A.; Rubin, R.P. Mediators of Ca2(+)-dependent secretion. *Environ. Health Perspect.* **1990**, *84*, 35–39. [CrossRef]
9. Yeung-Yam-Wah, V.; Lee, A.K.; Tse, A. Arachidonic acid mobilizes Ca^{2+} from the endoplasmic reticulum and an acidic store in rat pancreatic β cells. *Cell Calcium* **2012**, *51*, 140–148. [CrossRef]
10. Ding, X.-Z.; Hennig, R.; Adrian, T.E. Lipoxygenase and cyclooxygenase metabolism: New insights in treatment and chemoprevention of pancreatic cancer. *Mol. Cancer* **2003**, *2*, 10. [CrossRef]
11. Vane, J.R.; Bakhle, Y.S.; Botting, R.M. Cyclooxygenases 1 and 2. *Annu. Rev. Pharmacol. Toxicol.* **1998**, *38*, 97–120. [CrossRef] [PubMed]
12. Fitzpatrick, F.A. Cyclooxygenase enzymes: Regulation and function. *Curr. Pharm. Des.* **2004**, *10*, 577–588. [CrossRef] [PubMed]
13. Simmons, D.L.; Botting, R.M.; Hla, T. Cyclooxygenase isozymes: The biology of prostaglandin synthesis and inhibition. *Pharmacol. Rev.* **2004**, *56*, 387–437. [CrossRef] [PubMed]
14. Wang, B.; Wu, L.; Chen, J.; Dong, L.; Chen, C.; Wen, Z.; Hu, J.; Fleming, I.; Wang, D.W. Metabolism pathways of arachidonic acids: Mechanisms and potential therapeutic targets. *Signal Transduct. Target. Ther.* **2021**, *6*, 94. [CrossRef] [PubMed]
15. Rong, Y.; Ren, J.; Song, W.; Xiang, R.; Ge, Y.; Lu, W.; Fu, T. Resveratrol Suppresses Severe Acute Pancreatitis-Induced Microcirculation Disturbance through Targeting SIRT1-FOXO1 Axis. *Oxid. Med. Cell. Longev.* **2021**, *2021*, 8891544. [CrossRef] [PubMed]
16. Park, J.Y.; Pillinger, M.H.; Abramson, S.B. Prostaglandin E2 synthesis and secretion: The role of PGE2 synthases. *Clin. Immunol.* **2006**, *119*, 229–240. [CrossRef] [PubMed]
17. Narumiya, S.; Fitzgerald, G.A. Genetic and pharmacological analysis of prostanoid receptor function. *J. Clin. Investig.* **2001**, *108*, 25–30. [CrossRef]
18. Persaud, S.J.; Muller, D.; Belin, V.D.; Kitsou-Mylona, I.; Asare-Anane, H.; Papadimitriou, A.; Burns, C.J.; Huang, G.C.; Amiel, S.A.; Jones, P.M. The role of arachidonic acid and its metabolites in insulin secretion from human islets of langerhans. *Diabetes* **2007**, *56*, 197–203. [CrossRef]
19. Ashton, A.W.; Zhang, Y.; Cazzolli, R.; Honn, K.V. The Role and Regulation of Thromboxane A2 Signaling in Cancer-Trojan Horses and Misdirection. *Molecules* **2022**, *27*, 6234. [CrossRef]
20. Closa, D.; Rosello-Catafau, J.; Hotter, G.; Bulbena, O.; Fernandez-Cruz, L.; Gelpi, E. Cyclooxygenase and lipoxygenase metabolism in sodium taurocholate induced acute hemorrhagic pancreatitis in rats. *Prostaglandins* **1993**, *45*, 315–322. [CrossRef]
21. Katori, M.; Kawamura, M.; Sawada, M. 11-Dehydro-TXB2 and 2,3-dinor-TXB2 as new parameters of TXA2 generation. *Nihon Rinsho* **1992**, *50*, 349–354. [PubMed]
22. Lasserre, B.; Navarro-Delmasure, C.; Chanh, A.P.H.; Catala, J.; Hollande, E. Modifications in the TXA2and PGI2plasma levels and some other biochemical parameters during the initiation and development of non-insulin-dependent diabetes mellitus (NIDDM) syndrome in the rabbit. *Prostaglandins Leukot. Essent. Fat. Acids* **2000**, *62*, 285–291. [CrossRef] [PubMed]
23. Merchant, N.; Bhaskar, L.V.K.S.; Momin, S.; Sujatha, P.; Reddy, A.B.M.; Nagaraju, G.P. 5-Lipoxygenase: Its involvement in gastrointestinal malignancies. *Crit. Rev. Oncol. Hematol.* **2018**, *127*, 50–55. [CrossRef] [PubMed]
24. Bosma, K.J.; Andrei, S.R.; Katz, L.S.; Smith, A.A.; Dunn, J.C.; Ricciardi, V.F.; Ramirez, M.A.; Baumel-Alterzon, S.; Pace, W.A.; Carroll, D.T.; et al. Pharmacological blockade of the EP3 prostaglandin E2 receptor in the setting of type 2 diabetes enhances β-cell proliferation and identity and relieves oxidative damage. *Mol. Metab.* **2021**, *54*, 101347. [CrossRef]

25. Borin, T.F.; Angara, K.; Rashid, M.H.; Achyut, B.R.; Arbab, A.S. Arachidonic Acid Metabolite as a Novel Therapeutic Target in Breast Cancer Metastasis. *Int. J. Mol. Sci.* **2017**, *18*, 2661. [CrossRef]
26. Dobrian, A.D.; Morris, M.A.; Taylor-Fishwick, D.A.; Holman, T.R.; Imai, Y.; Mirmira, R.G.; Nadler, J.L. Role of the 12-lipoxygenase pathway in diabetes pathogenesis and complications. *Pharmacol. Ther.* **2019**, *195*, 100–110. [CrossRef] [PubMed]
27. Zhou, G.-X.; Ding, X.-L.; Wu, S.-B.; Zhang, H.-F.; Cao, W.; Qu, L.-S.; Zhang, H. Inhibition of 5-lipoxygenase triggers apoptosis in pancreatic cancer cells. *Oncol. Rep.* **2015**, *33*, 661–668. [CrossRef]
28. Wang, T.; Fu, X.; Chen, Q.; Patra, J.K.; Wang, D.; Wang, Z.; Gai, Z. Arachidonic Acid Metabolism and Kidney Inflammation. *Int. J. Mol. Sci.* **2019**, *20*, 3683. [CrossRef]
29. Manikandan, P.; Nagini, S. Cytochrome P450 Structure, Function and Clinical Significance: A Review. *Curr. Drug Targets* **2018**, *19*, 38–54. [CrossRef]
30. Gubbala, V.B.; Jytosana, N.; Trinh, V.Q.; Maurer, H.C.; Naeem, R.F.; Lytle, N.K.; Ma, Z.; Zhao, S.; Lin, W.; Han, H.; et al. Eicosanoids in the pancreatic tumor microenvironment—A multicellular, multifaceted progression. *Gastro Hep Adv.* **2022**, *1*, 682–697. [CrossRef]
31. Kiss, L.; Bier, J.; Röder, Y.; Weissmann, N.; Grimminger, F.; Seeger, W. Direct and simultaneous profiling of epoxyeicosatrienoic acid enantiomers by capillary tandem column chiral-phase liquid chromatography with dual online photodiode array and tandem mass spectrometric detection. *Anal. Bioanal. Chem.* **2008**, *392*, 717–726. [CrossRef] [PubMed]
32. Xu, M.; Ju, W.; Hao, H.; Wang, G.; Li, P. Cytochrome P450 2J2: Distribution, function, regulation, genetic polymorphisms and clinical significance. *Drug Metab. Rev.* **2013**, *45*, 311–352. [CrossRef] [PubMed]
33. Panigrahy, D.; Greene, E.R.; Pozzi, A.; Wang, D.W.; Zeldin, D.C. EET signaling in cancer. *Cancer Metastasis Rev.* **2011**, *30*, 525–540. [CrossRef] [PubMed]
34. Tao, P.; Jiang, Y.; Wang, H.; Gao, G. CYP2J2-produced epoxyeicosatrienoic acids contribute to the ferroptosis resistance of pancreatic ductal adenocarcinoma in a PPARγ-dependent manner. *Zhong Nan Da Xue Xue Bao Yi Xue Ban J. Cent. South Univ. Med. Sci.* **2021**, *46*, 932–941. [CrossRef]
35. Frömel, T.; Naeem, Z.; Pirzeh, L.; Fleming, I. Cytochrome P450-derived fatty acid epoxides and diols in angiogenesis and stem cell biology. *Pharmacol. Ther.* **2022**, *234*, 108049. [CrossRef]
36. Luo, P.; Chang, H.-H.; Zhou, Y.; Zhang, S.; Hwang, S.H.; Morisseau, C.; Wang, C.-Y.; Inscho, E.W.; Hammock, B.D.; Wang, M.-H. Inhibition or deletion of soluble epoxide hydrolase prevents hyperglycemia, promotes insulin secretion, and reduces islet apoptosis. *J. Pharmacol. Exp. Ther.* **2010**, *334*, 430–438. [CrossRef]
37. Schulz, I.; Krause, E.; González, A.; Göbel, A.; Sternfeld, L.; Schmid, A. Agonist-stimulated pathways of calcium signaling in pancreatic acinar cells. *Biol. Chem.* **1999**, *380*, 903–908. [CrossRef]
38. Nadella, S.; Ciofoaia, V.; Cao, H.; Kallakury, B.; Tucker, R.D.; Smith, J.P. Cholecystokinin Receptor Antagonist Therapy Decreases Inflammation and Fibrosis in Chronic Pancreatitis. *Dig. Dis. Sci.* **2020**, *65*, 1376–1384. [CrossRef]
39. Smith, J.P.; Solomon, T.E. Cholecystokinin and pancreatic cancer: The chicken or the egg? *Am. J. Physiol. Gastrointest. Liver Physiol.* **2014**, *306*, G91–G101. [CrossRef]
40. Del Castillo-Vaquero, A.; Salido, G.M.; González, A. Increased calcium influx in the presence of ethanol in mouse pancreatic acinar cells. *Int. J. Exp. Pathol.* **2010**, *91*, 114–124. [CrossRef]
41. Tapia, J.A.; Salido, G.M.; González, A. Ethanol consumption as inductor of pancreatitis. *World J. Gastrointest. Pharmacol. Ther.* **2010**, *1*, 3–8. [CrossRef] [PubMed]
42. Gitto, S.B.; Nakkina, S.P.; Beardsley, J.M.; Parikh, J.G.; Altomare, D.A. Induction of pancreatitis in mice with susceptibility to pancreatic cancer. *Methods Cell Biol.* **2022**, *168*, 139–159. [CrossRef] [PubMed]
43. Minaga, K.; Watanabe, T.; Kamata, K.; Kudo, M.; Strober, W. A Mouse Model of Acute and Chronic Pancreatitis. *Curr. Protoc.* **2022**, *2*, e422. [CrossRef] [PubMed]
44. Trulsson, L.M.; Gasslander, T.; Svanvik, J. Cholecystokinin-8-induced hypoplasia of the rat pancreas: Influence of nitric oxide on cell proliferation and programmed cell death. *Basic Clin. Pharmacol. Toxicol.* **2004**, *95*, 183–190. [CrossRef] [PubMed]
45. Wang, H.H.; Portincasa, P.; Wang, D.Q.-H. Update on the Molecular Mechanisms Underlying the Effect of Cholecystokinin and Cholecystokinin-1 Receptor on the Formation of Cholesterol Gallstones. *Curr. Med. Chem.* **2019**, *26*, 3407–3423. [CrossRef]
46. Niinistö, S.; Takkinen, H.-M.; Erlund, I.; Ahonen, S.; Toppari, J.; Ilonen, J.; Veijola, R.; Knip, M.; Vaarala, O.; Virtanen, S.M. Fatty acid status in infancy is associated with the risk of type 1 diabetes-associated autoimmunity. *Diabetologia* **2017**, *60*, 1223–1233. [CrossRef]
47. Stevens, T.; Berk, M.P.; Lopez, R.; Chung, Y.-M.; Zhang, R.; Parsi, M.A.; Bronner, M.P.; Feldstein, A.E. Lipidomic profiling of serum and pancreatic fluid in chronic pancreatitis. *Pancreas* **2012**, *41*, 518–522. [CrossRef]
48. Hernandez-Perez, M.; Kulkarni, A.; Samala, N.; Sorrell, C.; El, K.; Haider, I.; Aleem, A.M.; Holman, T.R.; Rai, G.; Tersey, S.A.; et al. A 12-lipoxygenase-Gpr31 signaling axis is required for pancreatic organogenesis in the zebrafish. *FASEB J. Off. Publ. Fed. Am. Soc. Exp. Biol.* **2020**, *34*, 14850–14862. [CrossRef]
49. Metz, S.A. Feedback modulation of glucose-induced insulin secretion by arachidonic acid metabolites: Possible molecular mechanisms and relevance to diabetes mellitus. *Prostaglandins Med.* **1981**, *7*, 581–589. [CrossRef]
50. Mouslech, Z.; Valla, V. Endocannabinoid system: An overview of its potential in current medical practice. *Neuro Endocrinol. Lett.* **2009**, *30*, 153–179.
51. Zhou, G.X.; Ding, X.L.; Huang, J.F.; Zhang, H.; Wu, S.B. Suppression of 5-lipoxygenase gene is involved in triptolide-induced apoptosis in pancreatic tumor cell lines. *Biochim. Biophys. Acta* **2007**, *1770*, 1021–1027. [CrossRef] [PubMed]

52. Berridge, M.J.; Lipp, P.; Bootman, M.D. The versatility and universality of calcium signalling. *Nat. Rev. Mol. Cell Biol.* **2000**, *1*, 11–21. [CrossRef] [PubMed]
53. Schulz, I.; Stolze, H.H. The exocrine pancreas: The role of secretagogues, cyclic nucleotides, and calcium in enzyme secretion. *Annu. Rev. Physiol.* **1980**, *42*, 127–156. [CrossRef] [PubMed]
54. Crottès, D.; Lin, Y.-H.T.; Peters, C.J.; Gilchrist, J.M.; Wiita, A.P.; Jan, Y.N.; Jan, L.Y. TMEM16A controls EGF-induced calcium signaling implicated in pancreatic cancer prognosis. *Proc. Natl. Acad. Sci. USA* **2019**, *116*, 13026–13035. [CrossRef]
55. Yang, F.; Wang, Y.; Sternfeld, L.; Rodriguez, J.A.; Ross, C.; Hayden, M.R.; Carriere, F.; Liu, G.; Schulz, I. The role of free fatty acids, pancreatic lipase and Ca^{2+} signalling in injury of isolated acinar cells and pancreatitis model in lipoprotein lipase-deficient mice. *Acta Physiol.* **2009**, *195*, 13–28. [CrossRef]
56. Bettaieb, L.; Brulé, M.; Chomy, A.; Diedro, M.; Fruit, M.; Happernegg, E.; Heni, L.; Horochowska, A.; Housseini, M.; Klouyovo, K.; et al. Ca^{2+} Signaling and Its Potential Targeting in Pancreatic Ductal Carcinoma. *Cancers* **2021**, *13*, 3085. [CrossRef]
57. Kutschat, A.P.; Johnsen, S.A.; Hamdan, F.H. Store-Operated Calcium Entry: Shaping the Transcriptional and Epigenetic Landscape in Pancreatic Cancer. *Cells* **2021**, *10*, 966. [CrossRef]
58. Siegel, G.; Sternfeld, L.; Gonzalez, A.; Schulz, I.; Schmid, A. Arachidonic acid modulates the spatiotemporal characteristics of agonist-evoked Ca^{2+} waves in mouse pancreatic acinar cells. *J. Biol. Chem.* **2001**, *276*, 16986–16991. [CrossRef]
59. González, A.; Schmid, A.; Sternfeld, L.; Krause, E.; Salido, G.M.; Schulz, I. Cholecystokinin-evoked Ca^{2+} waves in isolated mouse pancreatic acinar cells are modulated by activation of cytosolic phospholipase A_2, phospholipase D, and protein kinase C. *Biochem. Biophys. Res. Commun.* **1999**, *261*, 726–733. [CrossRef]
60. Wu, L.; Katz, S.; Brown, G.R. Inositol 1,4,5-trisphosphate-, GTP-, arachidonic acid- and thapsigargin-mediated intracellular calcium movement in PANC-1 microsomes. *Cell Calcium* **1994**, *15*, 228–240. [CrossRef]
61. Stickle, D.; Ramanadham, S.; Turk, J. Effects of arachidonyltrifluoromethyl ketone on cytosolic [Ca^{2+}] in HIT insulinoma cells. *J. Lipid Mediat. Cell Signal.* **1997**, *17*, 65–70. [CrossRef] [PubMed]
62. Lankisch, P.G.; Apte, M.; Banks, P.A. Acute pancreatitis. *Lancet* **2015**, *386*, 85–96. [CrossRef] [PubMed]
63. Ye, X.; Lu, G.; Huai, J.; Ding, J. Impact of smoking on the risk of pancreatitis: A systematic review and meta-analysis. *PLoS ONE* **2015**, *10*, e0124075. [CrossRef] [PubMed]
64. Nitsche, C.J.; Jamieson, N.; Lerch, M.M.; Mayerle, J.V. Drug induced pancreatitis. *Best Pract. Res. Clin. Gastroenterol.* **2010**, *24*, 143–155. [CrossRef]
65. Pekgöz, M. Post-endoscopic retrograde cholangiopancreatography pancreatitis: A systematic review for prevention and treatment. *World J. Gastroenterol.* **2019**, *25*, 4019–4042. [CrossRef]
66. Yen, H.-H.; Ho, T.-W.; Wu, C.-H.; Kuo, T.-C.; Wu, J.-M.; Yang, C.-Y.; Tien, Y.-W. Late acute pancreatitis after pancreaticoduodenectomy: Incidence, outcome, and risk factors. *J. Hepatobiliary Pancreat. Sci.* **2019**, *26*, 109–116. [CrossRef]
67. Uomo, G.; Manes, G. Risk factors of chronic pancreatitis. *Dig. Dis.* **2007**, *25*, 282–284. [CrossRef]
68. Geokas, M.C.; Baltaxe, H.A.; Banks, P.A.; Silva, J.J.; Frey, C.F. Acute pancreatitis. *Ann. Intern. Med.* **1985**, *103*, 86–100. [CrossRef]
69. González, A.; Schmid, A.; Salido, G.M.; Camello, P.J.; Pariente, J.A. XOD-catalyzed ROS generation mobilizes calcium from intracellular stores in mouse pancreatic acinar cells. *Cell. Signal.* **2002**, *14*, 153–159. [CrossRef]
70. González, A.; Granados, M.P.; Salido, G.M.; Pariente, J.A. H_2O_2-induced changes in mitochondrial activity in isolated mouse pancreatic acinar cells. *Mol. Cell. Biochem.* **2005**, *269*, 165–173. [CrossRef]
71. Rivera-Barreno, R.; del Castillo-Vaquero, A.; Salido, G.M.; Gonzalez, A. Effect of cinnamtannin B-1 on cholecystokinin-8-evoked responses in mouse pancreatic acinar cells. *Clin. Exp. Pharmacol. Physiol.* **2010**, *37*, 980–988. [CrossRef] [PubMed]
72. Nevalainen, T.J.; Hietaranta, A.J.; Gronroos, J.M. Phospholipase A2 in acute pancreatitis: New biochemical and pathological aspects. *Hepato-Gastroenterology* **1999**, *46*, 2731–2735. [PubMed]
73. Lei, X.; Barbour, S.E.; Ramanadham, S. Group VIA Ca^{2+}-independent phospholipase A_2 (iPLA2beta) and its role in beta-cell programmed cell death. *Biochimie* **2010**, *92*, 627–637. [CrossRef] [PubMed]
74. Süleyman, H.; Demircan, B.; Karagöz, Y. Anti-inflammatory and side effects of cyclooxygenase inhibitors. *Pharmacol. Rep.* **2007**, *59*, 247–258.
75. Schlosser, W.; Schlosser, S.; Ramadani, M.; Gansauge, F.; Gansauge, S.; Beger, H.-G. Cyclooxygenase-2 is overexpressed in chronic pancreatitis. *Pancreas* **2002**, *25*, 26–30. [CrossRef]
76. Huang, H.; Chen, J.; Peng, L.; Yao, Y.; Deng, D.; Zhang, Y.; Liu, Y.; Wang, H.; Li, Z.; Bi, Y.; et al. Transgenic expression of cyclooxygenase-2 in pancreatic acinar cells induces chronic pancreatitis. *Am. J. Physiol. Gastrointest. Liver Physiol.* **2019**, *316*, G179–G186. [CrossRef]
77. Polito, F.; Bitto, A.; Irrera, N.; Squadrito, F.; Fazzari, C.; Minutoli, L.; Altavilla, D. Flavocoxid, a dual inhibitor of cyclooxygenase-2 and 5-lipoxygenase, reduces pancreatic damage in an experimental model of acute pancreatitis. *Br. J. Pharmacol.* **2010**, *161*, 1002–1011. [CrossRef]
78. Warner, T.D.; Mitchell, J.A. Cyclooxygenases: New forms, new inhibitors, and lessons from the clinic. *FASEB J. Off. Publ. Fed. Am. Soc. Exp. Biol.* **2004**, *18*, 790–804. [CrossRef]
79. Mateu, A.; Ramudo, L.; Manso, M.A.; De Dios, I. Cross-talk between TLR4 and PPARγ pathways in the arachidonic acid-induced inflammatory response in pancreatic acini. *Int. J. Biochem. Cell Biol.* **2015**, *69*, 132–141. [CrossRef]
80. Zhou, W.; Levine, B.A.; Olson, M.S. Lipid mediator production in acute and chronic pancreatitis in the rat. *J. Surg. Res.* **1994**, *56*, 37–44. [CrossRef]

81. Kilian, M.; Gregor, J.I.; Heukamp, I.; Wagner, C.; Walz, M.K.; Schimke, I.; Kristiansen, G.; Wenger, F.A. Early inhibition of prostaglandin synthesis by n-3 fatty acids determinates histologic severity of necrotizing pancreatitis. *Pancreas* **2009**, *38*, 436–441. [CrossRef] [PubMed]
82. Sun, L.-K.; Reding, T.; Bain, M.; Heikenwalder, M.; Bimmler, D.; Graf, R. Prostaglandin E$_2$ modulates TNF-alpha-induced MCP-1 synthesis in pancreatic acinar cells in a PKA-dependent manner. *Am. J. Physiol. Gastrointest. Liver Physiol.* **2007**, *293*, G1196–G1204. [CrossRef] [PubMed]
83. Lee, J.H.; An, C.S.; Yun, B.S.; Kang, K.S.; Lee, Y.A.; Won, S.M.; Gwag, B.J.; Cho, S.I.; Hahm, K.-B. Prevention effects of ND-07, a novel drug candidate with a potent antioxidative action and anti-inflammatory action, in animal models of severe acute pancreatitis. *Eur. J. Pharmacol.* **2012**, *687*, 28–38. [CrossRef] [PubMed]
84. Reding, T.; Bimmler, D.; Perren, A.; Sun, L.-K.; Fortunato, F.; Storni, F.; Graf, R. A selective COX-2 inhibitor suppresses chronic pancreatitis in an animal model (WBN/Kob rats): Significant reduction of macrophage infiltration and fibrosis. *Gut* **2006**, *55*, 1165–1173. [CrossRef]
85. Luci, D.K.; Jameson, J.B., 2nd; Yasgar, A.; Diaz, G.; Joshi, N.; Kantz, A.; Markham, K.; Perry, S.; Kuhn, N.; Yeung, J.; et al. Synthesis and structure-activity relationship studies of 4-((2-hydroxy-3-methoxybenzyl)amino)benzenesulfonamide derivatives as potent and selective inhibitors of 12-lipoxygenase. *J. Med. Chem.* **2014**, *57*, 495–506. [CrossRef] [PubMed]
86. Mashima, R.; Okuyama, T. The role of lipoxygenases in pathophysiology; new insights and future perspectives. *Redox Biol.* **2015**, *6*, 297–310. [CrossRef]
87. Chandrasekharan, J.A.; Sharma-Walia, N. Lipoxins: Nature's way to resolve inflammation. *J. Inflamm. Res.* **2015**, *8*, 181–192. [CrossRef]
88. Shahid, R.A.; Vigna, S.R.; Layne, A.C.; Romac, J.M.-J.; Liddle, R.A. Acinar Cell Production of Leukotriene B$_4$ Contributes to Development of Neurogenic Pancreatitis in Mice. *Cell. Mol. Gastroenterol. Hepatol.* **2015**, *1*, 75–86. [CrossRef]
89. Vigna, S.R.; Shahid, R.A.; Nathan, J.D.; McVey, D.C.; Liddle, R.A. Leukotriene B4 mediates inflammation via TRPV1 in duct obstruction-induced pancreatitis in rats. *Pancreas* **2011**, *40*, 708–714. [CrossRef]
90. Hotter, G.; Closa, D.; Prats, N.; Pi, F.; Gelpí, E.; Roselló-Catafau, J. Free radical enhancement promotes leucocyte recruitment through a PAF and LTB4 dependent mechanism. *Free Radic. Biol. Med.* **1997**, *22*, 947–954. [CrossRef]
91. Liao, D.; Qian, B.; Zhang, Y.; Wu, K.; Xu, M. Inhibition of 5-lipoxygenase represses neutrophils activation and activates apoptosis in pancreatic tissues during acute necrotizing pancreatitis. *Biochem. Biophys. Res. Commun.* **2018**, *498*, 79–85. [CrossRef] [PubMed]
92. Oruc, N.; Yukselen, V.; Ozutemiz, A.O.; Yuce, G.; Celik, H.A.; Musoglu, A.; Batur, Y. Leukotriene receptor antagonism in experimental acute pancreatitis in rats. *Eur. J. Gastroenterol. Hepatol.* **2004**, *16*, 383–388. [CrossRef] [PubMed]
93. Dobrian, A.D.; Huyck, R.W.; Glenn, L.; Gottipati, V.; Haynes, B.A.; Hansson, G.I.; Marley, A.; McPheat, W.L.; Nadler, J.L. Activation of the 12/15 lipoxygenase pathway accompanies metabolic decline in db/db pre-diabetic mice. *Prostaglandins Other Lipid Mediat.* **2018**, *136*, 23–32. [CrossRef] [PubMed]
94. Pek, S.B.; Nathan, M.H. Role of eicosanoids in biosynthesis and secretion of insulin. *Diabete Metab.* **1994**, *20*, 146–149.
95. Hwang, H.-J.; Park, K.-S.; Choi, J.H.; Cocco, L.; Jang, H.-J.; Suh, P.-G. Zafirlukast promotes insulin secretion by increasing calcium influx through L-type calcium channels. *J. Cell. Physiol.* **2018**, *233*, 8701–8710. [CrossRef]
96. McDonnell, A.M.; Dang, C.H. Basic review of the cytochrome p450 system. *J. Adv. Pract. Oncol.* **2013**, *4*, 263–268. [CrossRef]
97. Sarlis, N.J.; Gourgiotis, L. Hormonal effects on drug metabolism through the CYP system: Perspectives on their potential significance in the era of pharmacogenomics. *Curr. Drug Targets Immune Endocr. Metab. Disord.* **2005**, *5*, 439–448. [CrossRef]
98. Sayed, T.S.; Maayah, Z.H.; Zeidan, H.A.; Agouni, A.; Korashy, H.M. Insight into the physiological and pathological roles of the aryl hydrocarbon receptor pathway in glucose homeostasis, insulin resistance, and diabetes development. *Cell. Mol. Biol. Lett.* **2022**, *27*, 103. [CrossRef]
99. Falck, J.R.; Manna, S.; Moltz, J.; Chacos, N.; Capdevila, J. Epoxyeicosatrienoic acids stimulate glucagon and insulin release from isolated rat pancreatic islets. *Biochem. Biophys. Res. Commun.* **1983**, *114*, 743–749. [CrossRef]
100. Bailey, R.; Cooper, J.D.; Zeitels, L.; Smyth, D.J.; Yang, J.H.M.; Walker, N.M.; Hyppönen, E.; Dunger, D.B.; Ramos-Lopez, E.; Badenhoop, K.; et al. Association of the vitamin D metabolism gene *CYP27B1* with type 1 diabetes. *Diabetes* **2007**, *56*, 2616–2621. [CrossRef]
101. Cao, R.-C.; Yang, W.-J.; Xiao, W.; Zhou, L.; Tan, J.-H.; Wang, M.; Zhou, Z.-T.; Chen, H.-J.; Xu, J.; Chen, X.-M.; et al. St13 protects against disordered acinar cell arachidonic acid pathway in chronic pancreatitis. *J. Transl. Med.* **2022**, *20*, 218. [CrossRef] [PubMed]
102. Suresh, Y.; Das, U.N. Differential effect of saturated, monounsaturated, and polyunsaturated fatty acids on alloxan-induced diabetes mellitus. *Prostaglandins, Leukot. Essent. Fat. Acids* **2006**, *74*, 199–213. [CrossRef] [PubMed]
103. Gundala, N.K.V.; Das, U.N. Arachidonic acid–rich ARASCO oil has anti-inflammatory and antidiabetic actions against streptozotocin + high fat diet induced diabetes mellitus in Wistar rats. *Nutrition* **2019**, *66*, 203–218. [CrossRef] [PubMed]
104. Siegmund, E.; Weber, H.; Kasper, M.; Jonas, L. Role of PGE2 in the development of pancreatic injury induced by chronic alcohol feeding in rats. *Pancreatol. Off. J. Int. Assoc. Pancreatol.* **2003**, *3*, 26–35. [CrossRef] [PubMed]
105. Shadhu, K.; Xi, C. Inflammation and pancreatic cancer: An updated review. *Saudi J. Gastroenterol. Off. J. Saudi Gastroenterol. Assoc.* **2019**, *25*, 3–13. [CrossRef]
106. Ling, S.; Feng, T.; Jia, K.; Tian, Y.; Li, Y. Inflammation to cancer: The molecular biology in the pancreas (Review). *Oncol. Lett.* **2014**, *7*, 1747–1754. [CrossRef]

107. Knab, L.M.; Grippo, P.J.; Bentrem, D.J. Involvement of eicosanoids in the pathogenesis of pancreatic cancer: The roles of cyclooxygenase-2 and 5-lipoxygenase. *World J. Gastroenterol.* **2014**, *20*, 10729–10739. [CrossRef]
108. Subongkot, S.; Frame, D.; Leslie, W.; Drajer, D. Selective cyclooxygenase-2 inhibition: A target in cancer prevention and treatment. *Pharmacotherapy* **2003**, *23*, 9–28. [CrossRef]
109. Sarkar, F.H.; Adsule, S.; Li, Y.; Padhye, S. Back to the future: COX-2 inhibitors for chemoprevention and cancer therapy. *Mini Rev. Med. Chem.* **2007**, *7*, 599–608. [CrossRef]
110. Grossman, H.B. Selective COX-2 inhibitors as chemopreventive and therapeutic agents. *Drugs Today* **2003**, *39*, 203–212. [CrossRef]
111. Anderson, W.F.; Umar, A.; Hawk, E.T. Cyclooxygenase inhibition in cancer prevention and treatment. *Expert Opin. Pharmacother.* **2003**, *4*, 2193–2204. [CrossRef] [PubMed]
112. Stratton, M.S.; Alberts, D.S. Current application of selective COX-2 inhibitors in cancer prevention and treatment. *Oncology* **2002**, *16*, 37–51. [PubMed]
113. Ding, X.-Z.; Tong, W.-G.; Adrian, T.E. Cyclooxygenases and lipoxygenases as potential targets for treatment of pancreatic cancer. *Pancreatol. Off. J. Int. Assoc. Pancreatol.* **2001**, *1*, 291–299. [CrossRef] [PubMed]
114. Omura, N.; Griffith, M.; Vincent, A.; Li, A.; Hong, S.-M.; Walter, K.; Borges, M.; Goggins, M. Cyclooxygenase-deficient pancreatic cancer cells use exogenous sources of prostaglandins. *Mol. Cancer Res.* **2010**, *8*, 821–832. [CrossRef]
115. Mensah, E.T.; Smyrk, T.; Zhang, L.; Bick, B.; Wood-Wentz, C.M.; Buttar, N.; Chari, S.T.; Gleeson, F.C.; Kendrick, M.; Levy, M.; et al. Cyclooxygenase-2 and Cytosolic Phospholipase A2 Are Overexpressed in Mucinous Pancreatic Cysts. *Clin. Transl. Gastroenterol.* **2019**, *10*, e00028. [CrossRef]
116. Chiblak, S.; Steinbauer, B.; Pohl-Arnold, A.; Kucher, D.; Abdollahi, A.; Schwager, C.; Höft, B.; Esposito, I.; Müller-Decker, K. K-Ras and cyclooxygenase-2 coactivation augments intraductal papillary mucinous neoplasm and Notch1 mimicking human pancreas lesions. *Sci. Rep.* **2016**, *6*, 29455. [CrossRef]
117. Hermanova, M.; Trna, J.; Nenutil, R.; Dite, P.; Kala, Z. Expression of COX-2 is associated with accumulation of p53 in pancreatic cancer: Analysis of COX-2 and p53 expression in premalignant and malignant ductal pancreatic lesions. *Eur. J. Gastroenterol. Hepatol.* **2008**, *20*, 732–739. [CrossRef]
118. Kim, M.P.; Li, X.; Deng, J.; Zhang, Y.; Dai, B.; Allton, K.L.; Hughes, T.G.; Siangco, C.; Augustine, J.J.; Kang, Y.; et al. Oncogenic KRAS Recruits an Expansive Transcriptional Network through Mutant p53 to Drive Pancreatic Cancer Metastasis. *Cancer Discov.* **2021**, *11*, 2094–2111. [CrossRef]
119. Appel, M.J.; Woutersen, R.A. Modulation of growth and cell turnover of preoplastic lesions and of prostaglandin levels in rat pancreas by dietary fish oil. *Carcinogenesis* **1994**, *15*, 2107–2112. [CrossRef]
120. Hennig, R.; Ding, X.-Z.; Tong, W.-G.; Schneider, M.B.; Standop, J.; Friess, H.; Büchler, M.W.; Pour, P.M.; Adrian, T.E. 5-Lipoxygenase and leukotriene B_4 receptor are expressed in human pancreatic cancers but not in pancreatic ducts in normal tissue. *Am. J. Pathol.* **2002**, *161*, 421–428. [CrossRef]
121. Hennig, R.; Kehl, T.; Noor, S.; Ding, X.-Z.; Rao, S.M.; Bergmann, F.; Fürstenberger, G.; Büchler, M.W.; Friess, H.; Krieg, P.; et al. 15-lipoxygenase-1 production is lost in pancreatic cancer and overexpression of the gene inhibits tumor cell growth. *Neoplasia* **2007**, *9*, 917–926. [CrossRef] [PubMed]
122. Haraldsdóttir, S.; Guolaugsdóttir, E.; Ingólfsdóttir, K.; Ogmundsdóttir, H.M. Anti-proliferative effects of lichen-derived lipoxygenase inhibitors on twelve human cancer cell lines of different tissue origin in vitro. *Planta Med.* **2004**, *70*, 1098–1100. [CrossRef] [PubMed]
123. Wenger, F.A.; Kilian, M.; Achucarro, P.; Heinicken, D.; Schimke, I.; Guski, H.; Jacobi, C.A.; Müller, J.M. Effects of Celebrex and Zyflo on BOP-induced pancreatic cancer in Syrian hamsters. *Pancreatol. Off. J. Int. Assoc. Pancreatol.* **2002**, *2*, 54–60. [CrossRef] [PubMed]
124. Gregor, J.I.; Kilian, M.; Heukamp, I.; Kiewert, C.; Kristiansen, G.; Schimke, I.; Walz, M.K.; Jacobi, C.A.; Wenger, F.A. Effects of selective COX-2 and 5-LOX inhibition on prostaglandin and leukotriene synthesis in ductal pancreatic cancer in Syrian hamster. *Prostaglandins Leukot. Essent. Fat. Acids* **2005**, *73*, 89–97. [CrossRef] [PubMed]
125. Tersey, S.A.; Bolanis, E.; Holman, T.R.; Maloney, D.J.; Nadler, J.L.; Mirmira, R.G. Minireview: 12-Lipoxygenase and Islet β-Cell Dysfunction in Diabetes. *Mol. Endocrinol.* **2015**, *29*, 791–800. [CrossRef] [PubMed]
126. Gandhi, A.V.; Saxena, S.; Relles, D.; Sarosiek, K.; Kang, C.Y.; Chipitsyna, G.; Sendecki, J.A.; Yeo, C.J.; Arafat, H.A. Differential expression of cytochrome P450 omega-hydroxylase isoforms and their association with clinicopathological features in pancreatic ductal adenocarcinoma. *Ann. Surg. Oncol.* **2013**, *20*, S636–S643. [CrossRef]
127. Agundez, J.A.G. Cytochrome P450 gene polymorphism and cancer. *Curr. Drug Metab.* **2004**, *5*, 211–224. [CrossRef]
128. Song, B.-J.; Abdelmegeed, M.A.; Cho, Y.-E.; Akbar, M.; Rhim, J.S.; Song, M.-K.; Hardwick, J.P. Contributing Roles of CYP2E1 and Other Cytochrome P450 Isoforms in Alcohol-Related Tissue Injury and Carcinogenesis. *Adv. Exp. Med. Biol.* **2019**, *1164*, 73–87. [CrossRef]
129. Standop, J.; Schneider, M.; Ulrich, A.; Büchler, M.W.; Pour, P.M. Differences in immunohistochemical expression of xenobiotic-metabolizing enzymes between normal pancreas, chronic pancreatitis and pancreatic cancer. *Toxicol. Pathol.* **2003**, *31*, 506–513. [CrossRef]
130. Kadlubar, S.; Anderson, J.P.; Sweeney, C.; Gross, M.D.; Lang, N.P.; Kadlubar, F.F.; Anderson, K.E. Phenotypic CYP2A6 variation and the risk of pancreatic cancer. *JOP* **2009**, *10*, 263–270.
131. De Wever, O.; Mareel, M. Role of tissue stroma in cancer cell invasion. *J. Pathol.* **2003**, *200*, 429–447. [CrossRef] [PubMed]

132. Gola, M.; Sejda, A.; Godlewski, J.; Cieślak, M.; Starzyńska, A. Neural Component of the Tumor Microenvironment in Pancreatic Ductal Adenocarcinoma. *Cancers* **2022**, *14*, 5246. [CrossRef] [PubMed]
133. Hughes, R.; Snook, A.E.; Mueller, A.C. The poorly immunogenic tumor microenvironment of pancreatic cancer: The impact of radiation therapy, and strategies targeting resistance. *Immunotherapy* **2022**, *14*, 1393–1405. [CrossRef] [PubMed]
134. Liu, X.; Iovanna, J.; Santofimia-Castaño, P. Stroma-targeting strategies in pancreatic cancer: A double-edged sword. *J. Physiol. Biochem.* **2023**, *79*, 213–222. [CrossRef]
135. Fishbein, A.; Hammock, B.D.; Serhan, C.N.; Panigrahy, D. Carcinogenesis: Failure of resolution of inflammation? *Pharmacol. Ther.* **2021**, *218*, 107670. [CrossRef]
136. Kim, W.; Son, B.; Lee, S.; Do, H.; Youn, B. Targeting the enzymes involved in arachidonic acid metabolism to improve radiotherapy. *Cancer Metastasis Rev.* **2018**, *37*, 213–225. [CrossRef]
137. Ching, M.M.; Reader, J.; Fulton, A.M. Eicosanoids in Cancer: Prostaglandin E_2 Receptor 4 in Cancer Therapeutics and Immunotherapy. *Front. Pharmacol.* **2020**, *11*, 819. [CrossRef]
138. Bu, L.; Yonemura, A.; Yasuda-Yoshihara, N.; Uchihara, T.; Ismagulov, G.; Takasugi, S.; Yasuda, T.; Okamoto, Y.; Kitamura, F.; Akiyama, T.; et al. Tumor microenvironmental 15-PGDH depletion promotes fibrotic tumor formation and angiogenesis in pancreatic cancer. *Cancer Sci.* **2022**, *113*, 3579–3592. [CrossRef]
139. Colby, J.K.; Klein, R.D.; McArthur, M.J.; Conti, C.J.; Kiguchi, K.; Kawamoto, T.; Riggs, P.K.; Pavone, A.I.; Sawicki, J.; Fischer, S.M. Progressive metaplastic and dysplastic changes in mouse pancreas induced by cyclooxygenase-2 overexpression. *Neoplasia* **2008**, *10*, 782–796. [CrossRef]
140. Estaras, M.; Ortiz-Placin, C.; Castillejo-Rufo, A.; Fernandez-Bermejo, M.; Blanco, G.; Mateos, J.M.; Vara, D.; Gonzalez-Cordero, P.L.; Chamizo, S.; Lopez, D.; et al. Melatonin controls cell proliferation and modulates mitochondrial physiology in pancreatic stellate cells. *J. Physiol. Biochem.* **2023**, *79*, 235–249. [CrossRef]
141. Grekova, S.P.; Angelova, A.; Daeffler, L.; Raykov, Z. Pancreatic Cancer Cell Lines Can Induce Prostaglandin E2 Production from Human Blood Mononuclear Cells. *J. Oncol.* **2011**, *2011*, 741868. [CrossRef] [PubMed]
142. Charo, C.; Holla, V.; Arumugam, T.; Hwang, R.; Yang, P.; Dubois, R.N.; Menter, D.G.; Logsdon, C.D.; Ramachandran, V. Prostaglandin E2 Regulates Pancreatic Stellate Cell Activity via the EP4 Receptor. *Pancreas* **2013**, *42*, 467–474. [CrossRef] [PubMed]
143. Masamune, A.; Kikuta, K.; Satoh, M.; Sakai, Y.; Satoh, A.; Shimosegawa, T. Ligands of peroxisome proliferator-activated receptor-gamma block activation of pancreatic stellate cells. *J. Biol. Chem.* **2002**, *277*, 141–147. [CrossRef] [PubMed]
144. Estaras, M.; Gonzalez-Portillo, M.R.; Martinez, R.; Garcia, A.; Estevez, M.; Fernandez-Bermejo, M.; Mateos, J.M.; Vara, D.; Blanco-Fernández, G.; Lopez-Guerra, D.; et al. Melatonin Modulates the Antioxidant Defenses and the Expression of Proinflammatory Mediators in Pancreatic Stellate Cells Subjected to Hypoxia. *Antioxidants* **2021**, *10*, 577. [CrossRef]
145. Morrison, A.H.; Byrne, K.T.; Vonderheide, R.H. Immunotherapy and Prevention of Pancreatic Cancer. *Trends Cancer* **2018**, *4*, 418–428. [CrossRef]
146. Markosyan, N.; Li, J.; Sun, Y.H.; Richman, L.P.; Lin, J.H.; Yan, F.; Quinones, L.; Sela, Y.; Yamazoe, T.; Gordon, N.; et al. Tumor cell–intrinsic EPHA2 suppresses antitumor immunity by regulating PTGS2 (COX-2). *J. Clin. Investig.* **2019**, *129*, 3594–3609. [CrossRef]
147. Zhang, Y.; Kirane, A.; Huang, H.; Sorrelle, N.B.; Burrows, F.J.; Dellinger, M.T.; Brekken, R.A. Cyclooxygenase-2 Inhibition Potentiates the Efficacy of Vascular Endothelial Growth Factor Blockade and Promotes an Immune Stimulatory Microenvironment in Preclinical Models of Pancreatic Cancer. *Mol. Cancer Res.* **2019**, *17*, 348–355. [CrossRef]
148. Tian, W.; Jiang, X.; Kim, D.; Guan, T.; Nicolls, M.R.; Rockson, S.G. Leukotrienes in Tumor-Associated Inflammation. *Front. Pharmacol.* **2020**, *11*, 1289. [CrossRef]
149. Moore, G.Y.; Pidgeon, G.P. Cross-Talk between Cancer Cells and the Tumour Microenvironment: The Role of the 5-Lipoxygenase Pathway. *Int. J. Mol. Sci.* **2017**, *18*, 236. [CrossRef]
150. Janakiram, N.B.; Mohammed, A.; Bryant, T.; Ritchie, R.; Stratton, N.; Jackson, L.; Lightfoot, S.; Benbrook, D.M.; Asch, A.S.; Lang, M.L.; et al. Loss of natural killer T cells promotes pancreatic cancer in LSL-Kras$^{G12D/+}$ mice. *Immunology* **2017**, *152*, 36–51. [CrossRef]
151. Sarsour, E.H.; Son, J.M.; Kalen, A.L.; Xiao, W.; Du, J.; Alexander, M.S.; O'Leary, B.R.; Cullen, J.J.; Goswami, P.C. Arachidonate 12-lipoxygenase and 12-hydroxyeicosatetraenoic acid contribute to stromal aging-induced progression of pancreatic cancer. *J. Biol. Chem.* **2020**, *295*, 6946–6957. [CrossRef] [PubMed]
152. Schnittert, J.; Heinrich, M.A.; Kuninty, P.R.; Storm, G.; Prakash, J. Reprogramming tumor stroma using an endogenous lipid lipoxin A4 to treat pancreatic cancer. *Cancer Lett.* **2018**, *420*, 247–258. [CrossRef] [PubMed]
153. Rooney, P.H.; Telfer, C.; McFadyen, M.C.E.; Melvin, W.T.; Murray, G.I. The role of cytochrome P450 in cytotoxic bioactivation: Future therapeutic directions. *Curr. Cancer Drug Targets* **2004**, *4*, 257–265. [CrossRef] [PubMed]
154. Guo, Z.; Johnson, V.; Barrera, J.; Porras, M.; Hinojosa, D.; Hernández, I.; McGarrah, P.; Potter, D.A. Targeting cytochrome P450-dependent cancer cell mitochondria: Cancer associated CYPs and where to find them. *Cancer Metastasis Rev.* **2018**, *37*, 409–423. [CrossRef] [PubMed]

Disclaimer/Publisher's Note: The statements, opinions and data contained in all publications are solely those of the individual author(s) and contributor(s) and not of MDPI and/or the editor(s). MDPI and/or the editor(s) disclaim responsibility for any injury to people or property resulting from any ideas, methods, instructions or products referred to in the content.

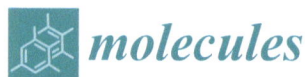 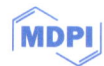

Article

Cardiolipin Membranes Promote Cytochrome *c* Transformation of Polycyclic Aromatic Hydrocarbons and Their In Vivo Metabolites

João Lopes [1,2,3], Dorinda Marques-da-Silva [1,2,3], Paula A. Videira [4,5], Alejandro K. Samhan-Arias [6,7] and Ricardo Lagoa [1,2,3,4,5,*]

[1] School of Technology and Management, Polytechnic Institute of Leiria, Morro do Lena-Alto do Vieiro, 2411-901 Leiria, Portugal; joao.m.lopes@ipleiria.pt (J.L.); dorinda.silva@ipleiria.pt (D.M.-d.-S.)
[2] Laboratory of Separation and Reaction Engineering-Laboratory of Catalysis and Materials (LSRE-LCM), School of Management and Technology, Polytechnic Institute of Leiria, 2411-901 Leiria, Portugal
[3] Associate Laboratory in Chemical Engineering (ALiCE), Faculty of Engineering, University of Porto, Rua Dr. Roberto Frias, 4200-465 Porto, Portugal
[4] Applied Molecular Biosciences Unit (UCIBIO), NOVA School of Science and Technology, NOVA University of Lisbon, 2829-516 Caparica, Portugal; p.videira@fct.unl.pt
[5] Institute for Health and Bioeconomy (i4HB), NOVA School of Science and Technology, NOVA University of Lisbon, 2829-516 Caparica, Portugal
[6] Department of Biochemistry, Autonoma University of Madrid (UAM), C/Arturo Duperier 4, 28029 Madrid, Spain; alejandro.samhan@uam.es
[7] Institute for Biomedical Research 'Sols-Morreale' (CSIC-UAM), C/Arturo Duperier 4, 28029 Madrid, Spain
* Correspondence: ricardo.lagoa@ipleiria.pt

Abstract: The catalytic properties of cytochrome *c* (C*c*) have captured great interest in respect to mitochondrial physiology and apoptosis, and hold potential for novel enzymatic bioremediation systems. Nevertheless, its contribution to the metabolism of environmental toxicants remains unstudied. Human exposure to polycyclic aromatic hydrocarbons (PAHs) has been associated with impactful diseases, and animal models have unveiled concerning signs of PAHs' toxicity to mitochondria. In this work, a series of eight PAHs with ionization potentials between 7.2 and 8.1 eV were used to challenge the catalytic ability of C*c* and to evaluate the effect of vesicles containing cardiolipin mimicking mitochondrial membranes activating the peroxidase activity of C*c*. With moderate levels of H_2O_2 and at pH 7.0, C*c* catalyzed the oxidation of toxic PAHs, such as benzo[a]pyrene, anthracene, and benzo[a]anthracene, and the cardiolipin-containing membranes clearly increased the PAH conversions. Our results also demonstrate for the first time that C*c* and C*c*–cardiolipin complexes efficiently transformed the PAH metabolites 2-hydroxynaphthalene and 1-hydroxypyrene. In comparison to horseradish peroxidase, C*c* was shown to reach more potent oxidizing states and react with PAHs with ionization potentials up to 7.70 eV, including pyrene and acenaphthene. Spectral assays indicated that anthracene binds to C*c*, and docking simulations proposed possible binding sites positioning anthracene for oxidation. The results give support to the participation of C*c* in the metabolism of PAHs, especially in mitochondria, and encourage further investigation of the molecular interaction between PAHs and C*c*.

Keywords: environmental toxicology; hemeproteins; ionization potential threshold; lipid membrane; mutagenesis; oxidative damage; peroxidases; pollutants; pseudo-peroxidases; radical cations

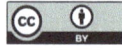

1. Introduction

Polycyclic aromatic hydrocarbons (PAHs) constitute a large group of hazardous organic compounds containing two or more fused benzene rings. These compounds emerge in the environment through the release of petroleum products and the incomplete combustion of coal, biomass, and other sources of organic carbon [1,2].

Humans are exposed to PAHs through inhalation, ingestion, and skin contact by way of air particulate matter, vehicle exhaust, cigarette smoke, and foods, among other specific exposures [2–5]. Certain professional groups, such as firefighters and coke oven workers, face elevated PAH exposure [5–7].

Epidemiological and experimental studies underscore the association between PAH exposure and pathologies, particularly cancers and cardiovascular diseases [3,8–11]. Benzo[a]pyrene (BaP) is a recognized carcinogen, whereas other PAHs like naphthalene, anthracene, benzo[a]anthracene (BaA), and benzo[b]fluoranthene (BbF) are classified as potentially carcinogenic to humans [12]. In a recent cohort study, a positive association between dietary PAH intake (BaP, chrysene, BaA, and BbF) and lung/tracheal cancer mortality risk was reported [3]. There are also increasing concerns regarding the neurotoxicity of PAHs, especially in children and occupationally exposed professionals [6,7].

While BaP carcinogenicity is closely related to DNA adduct formation, the overall of toxicity PAHs is associated with oxidative stress, inflammation, mitochondrial damage, and apoptosis [9,13–15]. There is growing attention to the involvement of mitochondria in the toxicity of environmental contaminants [8], with studies revealing mtDNA damage, stimulation of mitochondrial apoptosis, and reduced ATP production in animals exposed to BaP and acenaphthene [14–16]. Also, mice exposed to BaP showed decreased antioxidants in mitochondria, as well as reduced Krebs cycle enzymes activities, in an organ-independent manner [17]. In cells, low levels of BaP were enough to affect the mitochondrial membrane potential and ATP levels [18]. In other studies, air particulate matter was detected inside cells associated with membrane structures like mitochondria [19], and lipophilic PAHs effectively incorporated into phospholipid membranes [20,21], including those containing cardiolipin (CL), a phospholipid characteristic of bacterial and mitochondrial membranes [22]. Hence, PAHs and their metabolites in cells are probably available to interact with mitochondrial components, especially with membrane-associated lipids and proteins.

The current understanding of the human metabolism of PAHs underlines the contribution of cytochrome P450 (CYP450) monooxygenase or peroxidase activities, combined with epoxide hydrolase and aldo–keto reductase enzymes, in the generation of diverse hydroxylated, epoxide, and quinone PAH derivatives [8,9,21]. Although the precise role of each enzyme in the biotransformation of the different PAHs remains elusive, the toxicological relevance of the in vivo generation of PAH metabolites is well established. Actually, hydroxylated PAHs (HO-PAHs) in urine are commonly used as biomarkers of human PAH exposure [2,5,6,10,11]. The low-molecular-weight metabolites (HO-naphthalene forms) are found at the highest concentrations, and the most abundant is 2-hydroxynaphthalene [2,5,10]. However, the urinary levels of 1-hydroxypyrene among other HO-PAHs were found to be augmented significantly in firefighters after training exercises [5]. Furthermore, hydroxynaphthalenes, hydroxyfluorenes, and 1-hydroxypyrene are the PAH metabolites presenting a closer association to cardiovascular disorders [10,11]. In occupationally exposed individuals, neurological alterations were correlated to the levels of 2-hydroxynaphthalene [6] and 1-hydroxypyrene [7].

In addition to CYP450, several microbial and plant peroxidases were demonstrated to catalyze oxidative modifications of PAHs, attracting interest for their potential ecological and biotechnological relevance [23,24]. However, other hemeproteins like cytochrome *c* (C*c*), more recognized for other biological roles, can also display peroxidase activity, at least under certain activating conditions [24,25]. The pseudo-peroxidase or peroxidase-like activity of C*c* towards organic compounds has been reported [26], including the oxidation of sulfur heterocyclic compounds [27] and PAHs [28]. More specifically, horse C*c* was described to oxidize anthracene, pyrene, and BaP in the presence of 1 mM H_2O_2 at pH 6.1 [28]. However, the catalytic abilities of C*c* towards PAHs seem inferior to other peroxidases and CYP450 [29], and do not enable an attack of oxidant-resistant compounds (with very high ionization potential) like phenanthrene and naphthalene [28]. Nevertheless, the catalytic activities measured with anthracene and pyrene suggest that C*c* could oxidize other intermediate resistant PAHs, namely, acenaphthene, contrary to that reported [28]. Moreover, from a toxicological perspective, it is unclear if Cc can have a significant role in the transformation of PAHs or their metabolites under moderate H_2O_2 levels and pHs more representative of biological conditions.

In cells, Cc is present in the mitochondrial intermembrane space and anchors to the mitochondrial inner membrane, being an essential component of the electron transport chain. In addition, extensive binding to CL in mitochondrial membranes under apoptotic conditions enables the massive release of Cc into the cytosol, where it can interact with a variety of other targets [30,31]. The CLs (1,3-bis(sn-3'-phosphatidyl)-sn-glycerol) are a group of anionic phospholipids found in the plasma membrane of bacteria and in the inner mitochondrial membranes of eukaryotic cells [30]. Interestingly, exposure to different organic pollutants has caused a huge increase in some CL species in cells [32].

The interaction of Cc with CL, and the subsequent formation of Cc-CL complexes, induces structural changes that affect the heme Fe coordination and increase the peroxidase activity of Cc [30,33–35]. Previous work has shown that in the presence of CL-containing phospholipid membranes and sub-millimolar concentrations of H_2O_2, the peroxidase activity of Cc can increase by more than one order of magnitude when measured with standard peroxidase substrates [34–36]. Yet, the potential relevance of free or CL-complexed Cc in the metabolism of environmental toxicants has not been given attention.

Cc binding to vesicles containing CL, as a model of mitochondrial membranes, was described to decrease the Cc reduction potential [E^0 of Fe(III)/Fe(II) redox couple] by about 350–400 mV, to approximately −170 mV [33], which is well within the range of typical peroxidases [23]. For example, horseradish peroxidase (HRP) can oxidize several PAHs to DNA-binding radical cations [37]. Thus, we hypothesized that CL-containing membranes could promote the Cc-catalyzed transformation of PAHs, and Cc might participate in the metabolism of these compounds. Preliminary studies with BbF and an azo dye pointed out that CL vesicles indeed accelerated their Cc-mediated oxidation by H_2O_2, as published by our group in a conference abstract [38].

The aims of the present work were to investigate the catalytic ability of Cc to transform PAHs and metabolites, and to evaluate the effect of CL membranes in that process. For this study, eight PAHs with two to five rings, including compounds of top toxicological relevance, were selected along with two common HO-PAH metabolites. Table S1 of the Supplementary Materials comprises a list of the CAS number, molecular weight, log $K_{o/w}$, water solubility, and ionization potential of the 10 studied compounds.

2. Results and Discussion

To investigate the ability of Cc to transform toxicologically relevant PAHs, we conducted assays at pH 7.0 with a protein concentration of 1 µM, except in the study of comparison to HRP, and always in the presence of H_2O_2 at 100 µM, as specified in the Methods Section 3.4. The impact of CL-containing membranes on the activity was tested with small unilamellar vesicles (SUVs), formed from a mixture of phosphatidylcholine (PC) and CL, which mimic mitochondrial membranes, activating the peroxidase activity of Cc [33–36].

The assay mixtures were incubated for 24 h and at the end the reaction media was extracted with hexane for HPLC analysis. Two extraction procedures were employed, essentially differing in the number of extraction runs, as described in Section 3.5. The procedure with two extraction runs was optimized in our laboratory for the complete recovery of different PAHs with three to five benzene rings. In the present work, the efficiency of this procedure was assessed with the smaller and less hydrophobic (log $K_{o/w}$ < 5) compounds studied, naphthalene, acenaphthene, anthracene, and pyrene; and the two HO-PAH metabolites. The results showed that the recovery was superior to 94% for all those compounds, except for 2-hydroxynaphthalene. For this metabolite (log $K_{o/w}$ = 2.7), it was necessary to extend the extraction procedure to four runs, achieving a higher efficiency of 80 ± 8%. For the more hydrophobic and less water-soluble PAHs (log $K_{o/w}$ > 5, see

Table S1), an efficiency of extraction close to 100% was expected and the shorter two-runs procedure was followed.

2.1. Transformation of Polycyclic Aromatic Hydrocarbons by Cytochrome c

The initial set of assays focused on three PAHs—naphthalene (2 rings), pyrene (4 rings), and BaP (5 rings)—encompassing wide differences in the molecular weight and ionization potential (Table S1). In addition to reaction mixtures with Cc alone (in the absence of phospholipids), parallel assays were carried out with Cc in the presence of phospholipid SUVs: vesicles composed only of PC, and others of PC and CL in a 4:1 ratio (Section 3.2).

The results in Figure 1 and Table 1 show that Cc was unable to catalyze any significant transformation of naphthalene in the conditions of the assays, but it catalyzed the conversion of pyrene and BaP into two or more products each. In the case of naphthalene, small decreases in the chromatographic peak of the PAH were measured from the assays containing Cc relative to the controls without protein, as presented in Figure 1A, but the differences were not significant (Table 1). Furthermore, the chromatograms from these assays did not reveal a consistent generation of any product of the reaction. Yet, as observed in the chromatograms (see at tR approx. 2 and 5 min, Figure 1A), small peaks were occasionally present in the analysis of assay media containing Cc and naphthalene, but they were not constant throughout the study.

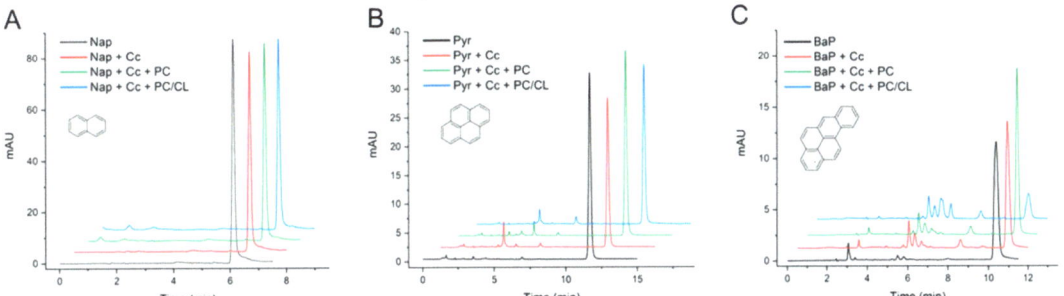

Figure 1. HPLC chromatograms of naphthalene (**A**), pyrene (**B**), and benzo[a]pyrene (**C**) transformation assays by cytochrome c (Cc) in the absence and in the presence of PC and PC/CL small unilamellar vesicles. Chromatograms are shown for controls of each compound (1 mg/L) incubated in the absence of Cc, of the compound with Cc 0.01 mg/mL, and with and without PC and PC/CL vesicles (200 µM). All assay media included 100 µM H_2O_2 in 20 mM phosphate buffer pH 7.0 and were incubated for 24 h at 37 °C. The chromatograms are displaced in the vertical and horizontal axes for better observation. The chromatograms shown are representative results of triplicate assays for each reaction condition. The molecular structures of the compounds are depicted.

On the contrary, Cc catalyzed the transformation of pyrene and BaP with the generation of reaction products clearly distinguishable in the chromatograms (Figure 1B,C). When PC vesicles were present in the reaction media, the conversion of these PAHs was not substantially affected, but the SUVs containing CL greatly increased the Cc-catalyzed transformation of BaP (Figure 1C and Table 1). In the presence of the PC/CL vesicles, the conversion of BaP reached almost 70% and gave rise to six detectable reaction products (see tR from 5 to 8 min in Figure 1C).

The quantification of the degree of transformation, as presented in Table 1, revealed the efficiency of Cc in the conversion of BaP in the presence of CL membranes. Several additional control assays were carried out with BaP to rule out PAH transformation by some non-catalyzed reaction with H_2O_2 and/or the lipids. As presented in Table S2, the BaP measured in the samples after incubations showed no significant alterations, and the chromatograms did not reveal the formation of any reaction products. These results clarify that the enzyme-independent oxidation of BaP by H_2O_2 is negligible, even in the presence of the PC/CL vesicles. In addition, the hypothesis that PC/CL lipids could react with BaP in the presence of Cc by some mechanism cumulative to H_2O_2 oxidation was discarded.

Table 1. Summary of the transformation of polycyclic aromatic hydrocarbons and metabolites catalyzed by cytochrome c (Cc) in the absence and presence of phospholipid membranes (PC-phosphatidylcholine; PC/CL- phosphatidylcholine and cardiolipin 4:1 mixture). The reaction media contained the PAHs at an initial concentration of 1 mg/L in 20 mM phosphate buffer (pH 7.0), Cc at 0.01 mg/mL, and H_2O_2 at 100 µM. When lipid membranes (small unilamellar vesicles) were present, the total phospholipid concentration was 200 µM. After 24 h incubations (or 4 h when indicated) at 37 °C, reaction media was analyzed by using HPLC. The area of the chromatographic peak corresponding to the remaining parent compound was compared to the results from parallel control assays (no Cc), which were taken as 100%. The data presented are the mean ± SE from triplicate assays.

Compound	Lipid Membranes	Area Relative to Control (%)
Naphthalene	Absent	90 ± 9
	PC	82 ± 10
	PC/CL	91 ± 10
Pyrene	Absent	79 ± 4 [1]
	PC	105 ± 5 [1]
	PC/CL	89 ± 3 [1]
Benzo[a]pyrene	Absent	105 ± 13 [1]
	PC	99 ± 16 [1]
	PC/CL	29 ± 13
Acenaphthene	Absent	93 ± 12 [1]
	PC/CL	155 ± 22 [1]
Anthracene	Absent	79 ± 21 [1]
	PC/CL	39 ± 14
Benzo[a]anthracene	Absent	65 ± 7
	PC/CL	48 ± 4
Chrysene	Absent	91 ± 12
	PC/CL	109 ± 9
Benzo[b]fluoranthene	Absent	91 ± 4
	PC/CL	79 ± 6 [1]
2-Hydroxynaphthalene (t = 4 h)	Absent	87 ± 9 [1]
	PC/CL	76 ± 12
1-Hydroxypyrene (t = 4 h)	Absent	41 ± 4
	PC/CL	20 ± 4

[1] In spite of the small decreases in the peak area of the parent compound (variation < 20%), reaction products were constantly detected in the chromatograms, and/or larger conversions were evident with longer incubation times.

The differential effect of the PC and PC/CL membranes on the peroxidase activity of Cc is in line with previous data on the Cc-catalyzed transformation of methyl orange [38] and prototypical peroxidase substrates [34–36]. While Cc does not interact specifically with PC, and the peroxidase activity is thus not altered, the binding to CL triggers alterations in the conformation of the polypeptide chain that reflect in the redox reactivity of the heme group and favor the peroxidase activity of Cc [25,33,34,36].

It should be noted that CL-induced activation of the peroxidase activity of Cc has been shown with relatively polar substrates, namely 2,2′-azino-bis-(3-ethylbenzothiazoline-6-sulphonate (ABTS), Amplex Red, guaiacol, and etoposide [25,34–36], which are all chemical species considerably different from the highly hydrophobic PAHs now studied.

Back to the PC membranes, a plausible effect of their presence in the reaction media is to sequester the lipophilic PAHs and limit their availability to reaction with Cc in solution. Although this effect is out of the interest of the present work, it explains why the conversion of pyrene eventually seems to decrease in the presence of these lipid membranes (Table 1). In any case, there was no relevant reason to continue experiments with the PC vesicles.

At this point, it was important to extend the study and evaluate the effect of the CL-containing membranes with a larger series of PAHs. Table 1 summarizes the quantification of the changes observed in the assays with five more PAHs: acenaphthene, anthracene, BaA, chrysene, and BbF. Representative chromatograms from the assays are presented in Figure 2, and for BbF in the abstract published before [38]. The results clearly indicate that Cc was unable to transform chrysene, whereas it catalyzed the conversion of the other PAHs into two or more products each. Moreover, the vesicles made of a mixture of PC and CL enhanced the Cc-mediated transformations, as evidenced by the decrease in the chromatographic peaks of the original PAH and/or by the notable emergence of reaction product peaks repeatedly observed in the chromatograms.

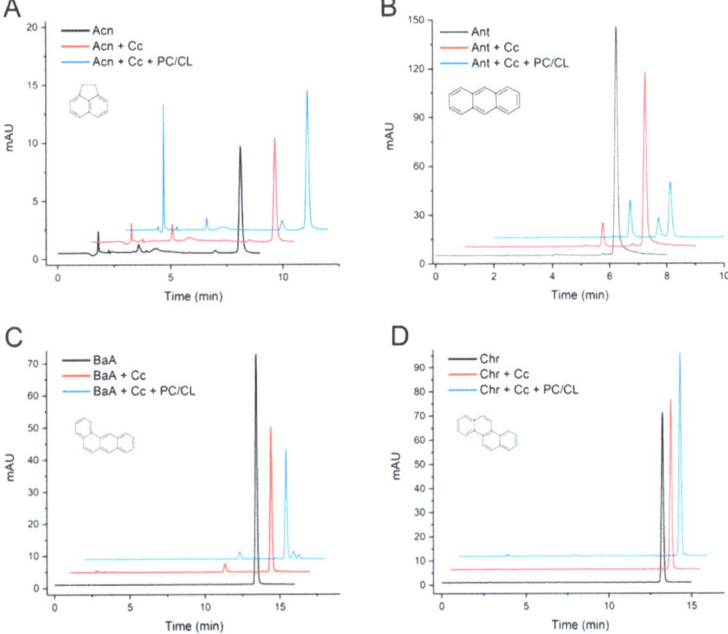

Figure 2. HPLC chromatograms of acenaphthene (**A**), anthracene (**B**), benzo[a]anthracene (**C**), and chrysene (**D**) transformation assays by cytochrome c (Cc) in the absence and in the presence of PC/CL small unilamellar vesicles. Chromatograms are shown for controls of each compound (1 mg/L) incubated in the absence of Cc, the compound with Cc 0.01 mg/mL, and with and without PC/CL vesicles (200 µM). All assay media included 100 µM H$_2$O$_2$ in 20 mM phosphate buffer pH 7.0 and were incubated for 24h at 37 °C. The chromatograms are displaced in the vertical and horizontal axes for better observation. The chromatograms shown are representative results of triplicate assays for each reaction condition. The molecular structures of the compounds are depicted.

Regarding the products, it is worth commenting that low-molecular-weight acenaphthene gave rise to a prominent peak with very low tR, indicative of a highly hydrophilic product nearly not retained by the C18 column, in addition to two other peaks with longer tRs (Figure 2A). Except in the case of BaA (Figure 2C), all the detected reaction products of the PAHs had a shorter tR than the parent compounds, following the probable hypothesis that they are quinone and hydroxylated forms of the PAHs.

It is reasonable to assume that Cc reacts with the PAHs as described for other heme peroxidases like CYP450, HRP, and prostaglandin H synthase (PGHS, or cyclooxygenase). In these enzymes, the PAHs transfer one electron to the peroxide-activated enzyme with

Fe in a highly oxidized form [24,25,29,37,39]. The produced PAH radical cations are reactive electrophilic species that can rapidly undergo further oxidations by oxygen to form quinones and hydroxylated PAHs, but in biological systems they can also bind to DNA and form DNA adducts [37,39].

In the case of pyrene, the product detected with a tR of 5 min (Figure 1B) is probably a mono-hydroxylated form of pyrene, since 1-hydroxypyrene was observed in our analyses with the same tR as that presented in Section 2.3. However, the dynamics and identification of the products and intermediates generated in the reaction systems are out of the scope of the present work and require further analytical studies.

Overall, the assays presented in this section add novel and significant data about the ability of Cc to catalyze the transformation of PAHs and how it is amplified in the presence of CL membranes. A previous study reported that Cc catalyzed the H_2O_2-triggered oxidation of anthracene, pyrene, and BaP, but not of acenaphthene, chrysene, naphthalene, or other PAHs with very high ionization potentials, indicating their strong resistance to oxidation [28]. Our results generally confirm the previous report, except for concerning acenaphthene. It is worth noting that our assays at pH 7.0 also indicate the low activity of Cc towards acenaphthene, and the demonstration of the actual reaction is supported by the appearance of reaction products (and the results at pH 5.0 presented in the next section) so it could easily go unnoticed without a full examination of the chromatographic results. More significantly, the present work demonstrates that Cc can catalyze the transformation of several important PAHs, including those not previously studied, BaA and BbF, under less-favorable yet closer-to-physiological conditions, namely with H_2O_2 at sub-millimolar levels and at pH 7.0.

Moreover, the degree of Cc-mediated conversions of PAHs of major toxicological relevance, such as BaP, anthracene, BaA, and BbF, are even more extended in the presence of phospholipid vesicles analogous to cell mitochondrial membranes. When compared to other peroxidases and CYP450, Cc was illustrated to have a low catalytic activity for PAH oxidation [29]. However, the present data at neutral pH and in the presence of CL-containing membranes indicate that Cc and Cc-CL complexes might reach oxidizing potencies towards critical PAHs similar to or higher than common peroxidases.

2.2. Comparison of Cytochrome c with Horseradish Peroxidase and Determination of the Ionization Potential Threshold of Cytochrome c

The ability of peroxidases to oxidize PAHs has been correlated with the ionization potentials of the compounds, i.e., the energy necessary to remove an electron from the neutral PAH molecule to generate a cation radical [23,24,37,39]. The prototypical plant peroxidase HRP is accepted as able to oxidize PAHs with an ionization potential of up to 7.2 eV (BaP), but it is not effective towards anthracene (7.4 eV), nor pyrene ($\geq$7.5 eV) or sturdier compounds [37]. An ionization potential threshold of 7.35 eV was assumed for HRP, as well as for PGHS [39], which are inferior to some other peroxidases [23], but there is no such estimation for the peroxidase forms of Cc.

Table S1 lists the ionization potentials of the PAHs studied herein [40]. Naphthalene and phenanthrene are common PAHs with very high ionization potentials ($\geq$8.0 eV), making these compounds very resistant to biodegradation [24]. So, it is not surprising that neither HRP [37] nor the peroxidase activity of Cc are sufficiently potent to oxidize naphthalene, even in the presence of CL membranes (Figure 1A). On the same basis, the ability of both HRP [37] and Cc to transform BaP (Figure 1C) can be justified by the relatively low ionization potential of this PAH (Table S1). However, Cc in the free form and, especially, when complexed to CL transformed anthracene and BaA in sizable extensions (Figure 2B,C). These results suggest that Cc has an ionization potential threshold superior to HRP, which did not oxidize anthracene, pyrene, or BaA [37]. Reinforcing that hypothesis, the $E^0[Fe(III)/Fe(II)]$ of approximately -0.17 V reported for Cc-CL complexes [33] is superior to the values close to -0.3 V attributed to HRP [24]. Still, some doubts could be raised since our results with acenaphthene at pH 7.0 are contradictory to those previously reported for C*c* [28]; furthermore, acenaphthene and chrysene have not been tested before with HRP [37].

Therefore, a set of transformation assays were performed to further assess the ability of HRP and C*c* to oxidize PAHs with intermediate-to-high ionization potentials: BaP, anthracene, pyrene, acenaphthene, and chrysene (values from 7.17 to 7.74 eV in Table S1). These assays were carried out at pH 5.0, a condition known to promote peroxidase activity [25,26], and with a higher concentration of catalyst to favor extended and clearly recognizable transformations.

The results confirmed the ability of both HRP and C*c* to catalyze the reaction of BaP with H_2O_2, and also that only C*c* can transform anthracene and pyrene. As shown in Figure 3A,B, acenaphthene and pyrene were substantially transformed by C*c* in the conditions of these assays. However, none of the catalysts showed enough oxidizing potency to attack chrysene (Figure 3C), despite the favorable pH and concentrations used. The conversion degrees quantified for each catalyst are represented in Figure 3D, showing the compounds ordered by increasing ionization potential. In addition to the confirmation of the cut-off of HRP between BaP and anthracene, the results of C*c* exhibit quite a good correlation with the ionization potentials, and a sharp threshold can be determined. Since C*c* was able to oxidize PAHs with ionization potentials up to 7.70 eV (acenaphthene), but not with 7.74 eV (chrysene), an ionization potential threshold of 7.70 eV can be concluded for the peroxidase activity of C*c*. This oxidizing potency is more characteristic of fungal ligninolytic peroxidases and less of plant peroxidases like HRP [23,24,29], implying the possibility of using C*c* for novel industrial and bioremediation applications.

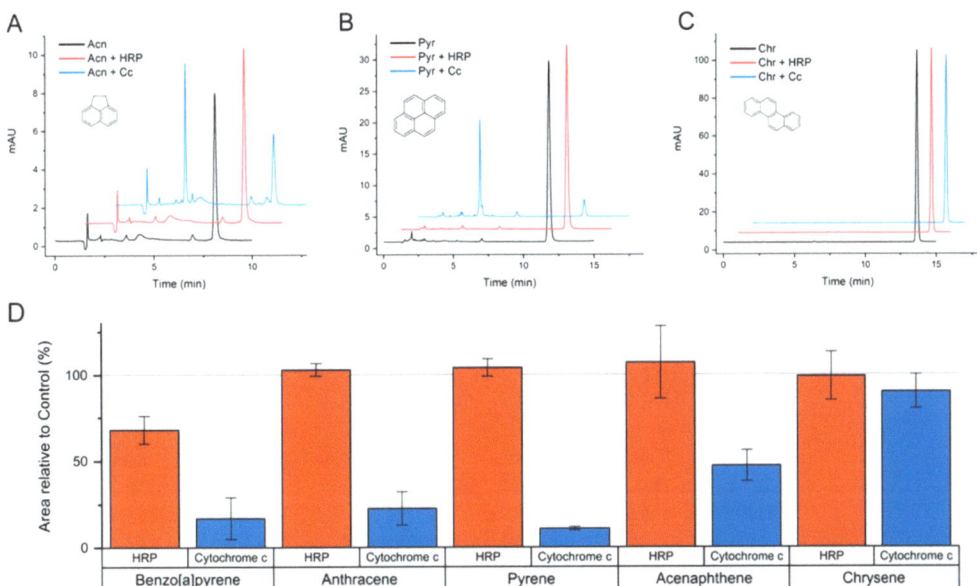

Figure 3. Transformation of acenaphthene (**A**), pyrene (**B**), chrysene (**C**), and other PAHs (**D**) catalyzed by horseradish peroxidase (HRP) and cytochrome *c* (C*c*) at pH 5.0. The reaction media contained the PAHs at an initial concentration of 1 mg/L in 100 mM acetate buffer, HRP at 0.2 µg/mL or C*c* at 0.1 mg/mL, and H_2O_2 at 100 µM. After 24 h incubations at 37 °C, the reaction media was analyzed by HPLC. The area of the chromatographic peak corresponding to the remaining parent compound was compared to the results from parallel control assays (no protein), which were taken as 100%. The mean ± SE of the data from triplicate assays are represented in panel D for the PAHs tested and ordered by increasing ionization potential. The chromatograms shown in (**A**–**C**) are representative results of triplicate assays for each compound (molecular structures depicted) and each catalyst.

2.3. Transformation of Polycyclic Aromatic Hydrocarbons Metabolites by Cytochrome c

Facing the capacity of Cc to modify PAHs, we decided to investigate if it could also transform their hydroxylated forms, which are well known in vivo metabolites and biomarkers of PAH exposure. Two HO-PAHs were selected for study, 2-hydroxynaphthalene and 1-hydroxypyrene, one low- and one high-molecular-weight metabolite that are frequently measured in greater levels in exposed individuals [2,5,10] and associated with pathological alterations [6,7,10,11].

The initial assays carried out with 24 h incubations proved that Cc catalyzed the transformation of both HO-PAHs. However, as shown in Figure S1 of the Supplementary Material, extensive conversions occurred, even in the absence of SUVs, so the effect of CL could not be clearly determined. A different group of assays was then carried out by incubations of 4 h (Figure 4). With this shorter time, the conversion of 2-hydroxynaphthalene was small, approximately 10%, but in the presence of the CL-containing vesicles it reached 24% (Table 1). The results at 4 and 24 h show that 1-hydroxypyrene is more efficiently converted than 2-hydroxynaphthalene (Figures 4B and S1B). Also, with 1-hydroxypyrene, the CL membranes increased the conversion degree from 59% to 80% (Table 1).

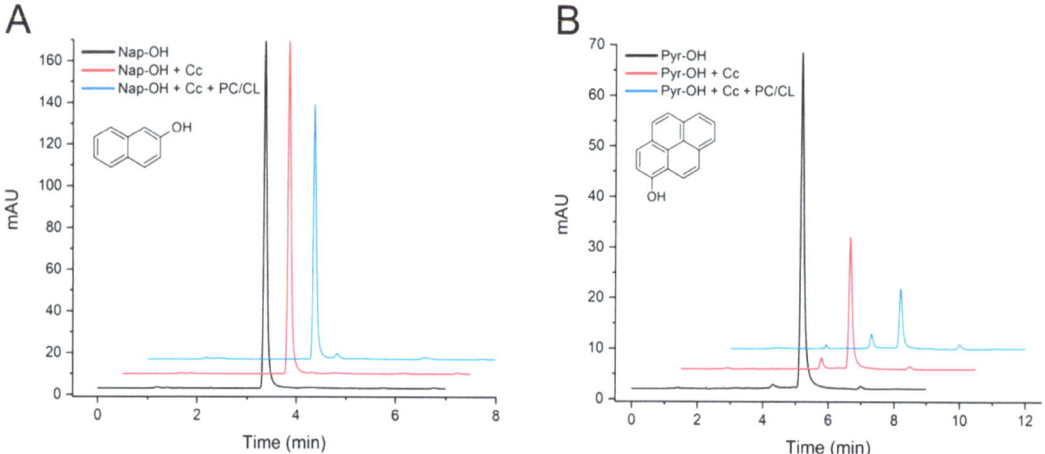

Figure 4. HPLC chromatograms of 2-hydroxynaphthalene (**A**) and 1-hydroxypyrene (**B**) transformation assays by cytochrome c (Cc) in the absence and in the presence of PC/CL small unilamellar vesicles. Chromatograms are shown for controls of each compound (1 mg/L) incubated in the absence of Cc, the compound with Cc 0.01 mg/mL, and with and without PC/CL vesicles (200 µM). All assay media included 100 µM H_2O_2 in 20 mM phosphate buffer pH 7.0 and were incubated for 4 h at 37 °C. The chromatograms are displaced in the vertical and horizontal axes for better observation. The chromatograms shown are representative results of triplicate assays for each reaction condition. The molecular structures of the compounds are depicted.

As mentioned before, 1-hydroxypyrene was observed in the analyses with a tR of 5 min, and a reaction product was detected approximately 1 min before (Figure 4B). These tRs coincide with two of the products generated in the assays with pyrene (Figure 1B), suggesting that some initial products of PAH oxidation can be further transformed by Cc.

In the mitochondria of healthy cells, it is assumed that most Cc is free and only a minor fraction is tightly bound to the inner mitochondrial membrane [41]. However, events that alter the distribution of CL in the mitochondrial membranes can vary the proportion of free to membrane-bound Cc, and during apoptosis quantities of Cc are released to the cytosol. It should be noted that small pools of Cc also appear in the cytosol of non-apoptotic cells [31]. Moreover, Cc can be present in the extracellular milieu, and elevated levels of circulating Cc were detected in conditions associated with mitochondrial damage like heart and liver disease [41]. Therefore, considering the novel data presented in this work, free and lipid-associated Cc can play an important role in the metabolism of PAHs and HO-PAHs, especially in the mitochondria, but also in the cytosol and outside the cells in specific conditions. The relatively high ionization potential cut-off and efficiency towards dangerous PAHs like BaP, anthracene, and BaA indicate that Cc can contribute to the generation of reactive metabolites and to the toxicity of PAHs in mitochondria [14–17].

2.4. Spectral Studies of Cytochrome c in the Presence of Polycyclic Aromatic Hydrocarbons

It is well accepted that Cc reacts with small molecules in solution by outer-sphere electron-transfer processes via the exposed heme edge, although alternative mechanisms of redox reaction involving binding to the protein and/or different electron migration pathways have been discussed [31]. It is also recognized that Cc has binding sites with significant affinity for lipids and amphiphilic molecules [34–36], so it is questionable as to whether the PAHs directly interact with Cc.

This hypothesis was tested by examining the effect of the PAHs in the absorption spectra of Cc in solution in the same buffered media at pH 7.0 of the transformation assays presented in Sections 2.1 and 2.3. The spectra of Cc (ferriCc) exhibited the characteristic heme absorption bands, namely the Soret band with a peak at 409 (or 410) nm in the UV-Vis region (Figure 5A) and the charge-transfer (CT) band in the near-infrared at 695 nm (Figure 5B). All the PAHs and HO-PAHs were tested, but anthracene was the only one that consistently induced a greater change in the Cc spectra. Representative UV-Vis spectra of Cc with and without anthracene are given in Figure 5A. Spectra from the studies with the remaining nine compounds are presented in Figure S2. Additional assays of prolonged incubations of Cc with anthracene discarded the hypothesis that the decrease in the Soret band augmented with time.

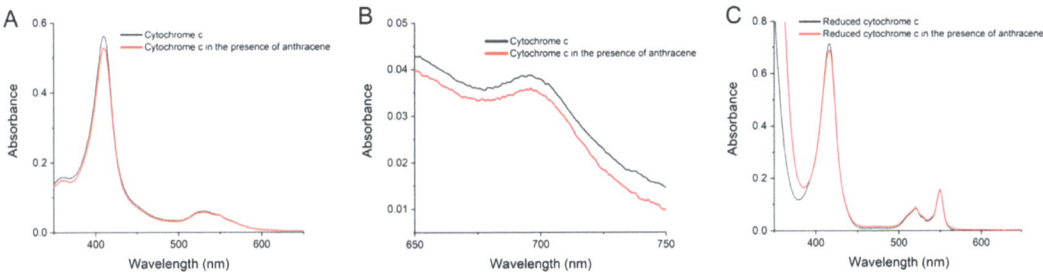

Figure 5. Spectra of cytochrome c (Cc) in the UV-visible region (**A,C**) and in the near-infrared region (**B**) in the absence and in the presence of anthracene. The concentration of Cc was 5 µM in panels (**A,C**), and 50 µM in (**B**) in 20 mM phosphate buffer pH 7.0. Anthracene was added to the Cc solutions reaching equimolar concentrations, and spectra were collected after 2 min of incubation. In panel (**C**), Cc in the absence and in the presence of anthracene was reduced with dithionite, as indicated in the Methods.

The CT band is lost when Cc is reduced to ferroCc or when ligands disturb the coordination of the heme Fe to the methionine-80 residue in the polypeptide chain [34,36]. As shown in Figure 5B, anthracene caused no significant changes in the shape or intensity of this band. The reduction in Cc also provokes a red shift of the Soret band and the appearance of 520 and 550 nm bands [33,36], as observed in Figure 5C for Cc reduced with dithionite (ferroCc). However, the spectra of ferriCc incubated with anthracene (Figure 5A) or with the other compounds (Figure S2) did not give any sign of such alterations, not even with the HO-PAHs. Instead, the Soret band of ferroCc showed a slight decay after incubation with anthracene (Figure 5C), like the one observed with ferriCc (Figure 5A).

In this context, it is relevant to notice that, in a previous study, dibenzothiophene interaction with Cc also caused a small decrease in the Soret band of the protein, which was registered in the absence of H_2O_2 to avoid any possible redox reaction [27]. In this work with several organosulfur compounds, H_2O_2 oxidation of dibenzothiophene was efficiently catalyzed by C*c*. Remarkably, our transformation assays and a previous work [28] point out that C*c* has a relatively high catalytic activity with anthracene.

The present results from the spectral studies indicate that the PAHs do not cause large alterations in the structure of C*c*. However, at least anthracene binds to C*c* in a way that slightly affects the heme environment and, thus, might contribute to the catalytic mechanism.

2.5. Prediction of Anthracene Docking to Cytochrome c

Taking into account the results from the spectral studies with anthracene and that this important prototypical PAH was efficiently transformed by C*c* (Figure 2B), the binding of anthracene was investigated by docking simulations.

The molecular docking to horse heart C*c* was computed with AutodockVina to predict models for the interaction of anthracene (Table 2 and Figure 6). The results pointed out that anthracene can interact with C*c* in different locations (Table 2). Our docking analysis suggests three possible binding sites with very similar probabilities based on the binding energy (Table 2). Anthracene was able to bind to site 1, defined by amino acid residues Lys5, Lys8, Ile9, and Glu90, with a binding energy of −5.2 kcal/mol. We also found that it was able to bind to site 2, defined by amino acid residues Lys27, Thr28, Phe46, Thr47, and Lys79, with a binding energy of −5.0 kcal/mol, and site 3, defined by amino acid residues Glu92 and Ile95, with a binding energy of −5.4 kcal/mol.

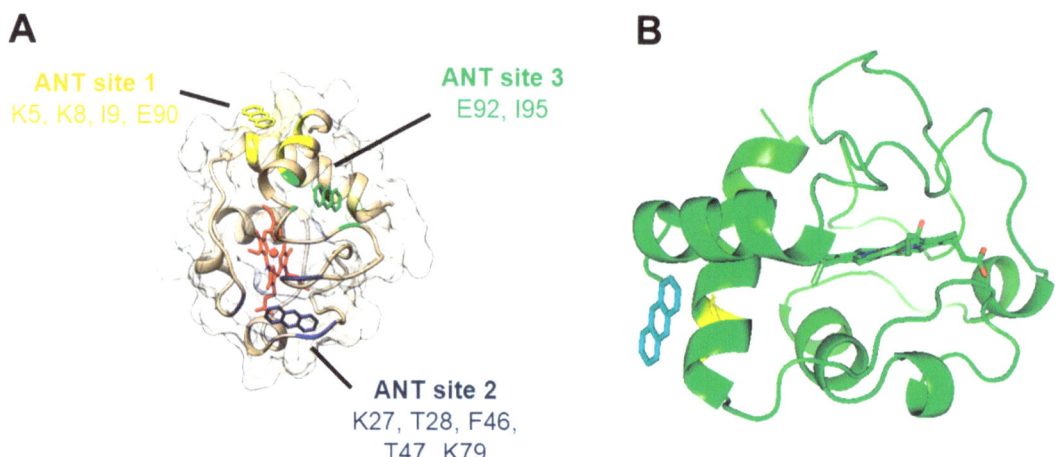

Figure 6. Docking of anthracene to cytochrome *c* (PDB 1HRC) as predicted by molecular simulations: (**A**) General view of the three predicted binding sites of anthracene to cytochrome *c*. Cytochrome *c* backbone and surface are shown in light brown, and the heme group in red. Anthracene molecules interacting with its modeled binding sites 1, 2, and 3 are shown in yellow, dark blue, and green, respectively. (**B**) Detail of the first pose of the top-ranked models of anthracene docked at cytochrome *c* (site 1). The location of an anthracene molecule (labeled in blue) interacting with cytochrome *c* (backbone and heme in green) is depicted in relation to the location of cytochrome *c*'s Glu90 residue (labeled in yellow).

Table 2. Binding sites of anthracene to cytochrome *c* (PDB 1HRC) predicted by docking simulations.

Cluster	Binding Energy (kcal/mol)	Interacting Residues
Site 1 named as ANT 1	−5.2	Lys5, Lys8, Ile9, Glu90
Site 2 named as ANT 2	−5.0	Lys27, Thr28, Phe46, Thr47, Lys79
Site 3 named as ANT3	−5.4	Glu92, Ile95

As depicted in Figure 6A, anthracene does not interact directly with the heme group, but the three predicted binding sites are close to or in regions connected to the heme. Therefore, the binding of anthracene might eventually induce a small alteration in the conformation of Cc sufficient to affect the heme environment, as suggested by the spectral studies (Figure 5A).

It should be noted that some of the residues pointed to interact with anthracene (Table 2) have been implicated in important biological functions of Cc. Lys27 is part of the so-called L-binding site of CL, and the residues 5, 8, and 9 are in very close proximity to this CL binding site [42]. Similarly, Lys27 is one of the several lysine residues involved in Cc interaction with apoptotic protease-activating factor-1 (Apaf-1) in the formation of the apoptosome [43]. However, there are other binding sites for CL under debate, and the L site includes more than 15 residues [42], while Apaf-1 binding also involves other residues like Lys72, which is more accepted as critical [43]. Therefore, a significant interference of anthracene with these Cc functions seems unlikely.

Site 1 for anthracene captured our attention since several high-ranked poses at this site were returned from the (triplicate) docking experiments and, in another study, Glu90 was directly involved in the binding of imidazole-substituted fatty acids that inhibit the peroxidase activity of Cc complexes [35]. The molecular docking of these inhibitors proposed their binding to the Glu90 region at the entrance of a hydrophobic channel, directing the molecules to the proximity of the heme group. The top-ranked pose of anthracene at site 1 is shown in Figure 6B.

However, Lys79 (site 2) has also been implicated in the binding of Cc redox partners, both proteins and small molecules, for the efficient electron transfer from or to Cc [31,44], which eventually occurs through the Tyr48 located very close to the heme group [45]. It is tempting to speculate that PAH binding to site 1 or 2 disposes the molecules for electron subtraction by Cc, but more molecular details are needed in the future to fully understand the redox reactions of PAHs and Cc.

3. Materials and Methods

3.1. Chemicals

The commercial suppliers of the PAH reagents used, along with the respective catalog number and purity, are listed in Table S1 of the Supplementary Material. The stock solutions of the PAHs were prepared at concentrations of 100 or 200 mg/L in acetonitrile.

The Cc (from equine heart, cat. no. C2506) was obtained from Sigma-Aldrich, Algés, Portugal, as well as HRP (cat. no. P6782). Diethylenetriaminepentaacetic acid (DTPA) was from Merck, Darmstadt, Germany (cat. no. D6518, purity $\geq$ 99%) and hexane from Fisher Chemical, Geel, Belgium (H/0355/17, $\geq$99%); PC was from Tokyo Chemical Industry, Tokyo, Japan (D4250) and tetraoleoyl CL from Avanti, Alabaster, AL, USA (710335P). All other chemicals used were HPLC or analytical-grade reagents.

3.2. Phospolipid Membranes

SUVs composed of PC or mixtures of PC with CL at a 4:1 molar ratio were obtained as described in [36]. Briefly, chloroform solutions of the phospholipids were dried and resuspended in 20 mM sodium phosphate buffer (pH 7.0, supplemented with 100 µM DTPA) to a final concentration of 10 mM. Just before the catalysis assays, SUVs were prepared by sonication of 200 µL aliquots (in ice) of the phospholipid suspension, employing a titanium-microtip-equipped Hielscher UP100H sonicator until clarity of the suspension was achieved.

3.3. Cytochrome c Solutions and Spectral Studies

Stock solutions of Cc were routinely prepared in distilled water and, just before the assays, diluted in the corresponding buffer. The concentration in the stock solutions was quantified after reduction with sodium dithionite and by using the extinction coefficient $\varepsilon(550 \text{ nm}) = 27.6 \text{ mM}^{-1} \text{ cm}^{-1}$.

The absorption spectra of Cc in 20 mM sodium phosphate buffer (pH 7.0) were collected using a Varian Cary 50 UV-Vis spectrophotometer. The protein concentration was 5 or 50 µM, as indicated in the figure captions. The effect of the equimolar concentration of each PAH was assessed by the direct addition of small volumes to the Cc solution and collection of the spectra approximately 2 min after gentle homogenization of the mixtures. The absorbance of the compounds registered in the same wavelength range was subtracted from the spectra of the mixtures. For the spectra of reduced Cc, the addition of a small amount of sodium dithionite was enough to reduce the protein heme in a few seconds, as is performed in a common procedure [33,36].

3.4. Peroxidase-Catalyzed Reaction Assays

For the catalytic assays of Cc at pH 7.0, the PAHs and metabolites were diluted in 20 mM sodium phosphate buffer (pH 7.0, supplemented with 100 µM DTPA) to a concentration of 1 mg/L. Depending on the compound, this mass concentration corresponds to between 4 and 8 µM. Since the stock solutions of the compounds were in acetonitrile, the reaction media contained up to 1% (v/v) of this solvent. Cc was added at a concentration of 0.0125 mg/mL (1 µM), and H_2O_2 at 100 µM. Immediately after, the reaction tubes were tightly sealed and incubated in the absence of light at 37 °C for 24 h. Incubations of 4 h with the HO-PAHs were also carried out. In the assays with lipid membranes, the SUVs were added in a concentration of 200 µM for the total volume of the reaction media, before the addition of Cc and H_2O_2.

The studies with Cc and HRP at pH 5.0 followed the same procedure as above, except for that the reaction media was 100 mM sodium acetate buffer, and the protein concentrations were Cc 0.1 mg/mL and HRP 0.2 µg/mL. These concentrations corresponded to 0.9 and 93 mU of peroxidase activity/mL (ABTS substrate), respectively.

In all sets of the assays, control tubes without the addition of any of the proteins were run in parallel to account for the actual PAH concentration in the reaction media.

3.5. HPLC Analysis

At the end of the incubations, hexane extracts of the reaction media were prepared for analysis by reverse-phase HPLC. Two extraction procedures were employed, differing in the number of hexane extraction runs. For the shorter method, a total of 1 mL of hexane was added in two 500 µL runs to 1 mL of reaction media, with 30 s of vigorous stirring in each run (protected from light). The two organic phases were collected after each run and combined for posterior HPLC analysis. This procedure was followed in the assays of all the compounds, except for 2-hydroxynaphthalene. For this less hydrophobic HO-PAH, an extended procedure with 4 extraction runs was employed. Starting with the 1 mL of reaction media, a first volume of 400 µL of hexane was added, followed by 1 min vigorous stirring and 1 min resting before the organic phase was collected. Two more 400 µL runs and one 300 µL run were carried out, and the combined 1.5 mL hexane extract was subsequently analyzed. The extraction efficiency of these procedures was assessed by measuring the recovery of the compounds from standards in phosphate buffer extracted and analyzed by HPLC as applied to the assay samples.

The HPLC analysis of the extracts was carried out in an Agilent 1100 system equipped with a C18 column by using a mobile phase of acetonitrile and water (85:15) at a 1 mL/min flux [46]. Two C18 columns were used in different periods of the work, a Zorbax Eclipse Plus (Santa Clara, CA, USA) and a Knauer Eurospher II (Berlin, Germany). The UV detection wavelengths were 220 nm for naphthalene; 251 nm for anthracene; 240 nm for pyrene; 266 nm for BaP and chrysene; 288 nm for BaA; 256 nm for BbF; 224 nm for acenaphthene and 2-hydroxynaphthalene; and 242 nm for 1-hydroxypyrene. The linearity of the response signal in the range of PAH concentrations measured in the assays was assessed based on the calibration curves obtained with standards of each of the compounds in hexane.

3.6. Molecular Docking of Anthracene to Cytochrome c

For the simulations, the file with an sdf extension containing the molecular structure of anthracene was downloaded from Zinc12 (ZINC01586329) [47] and transformed into files with extension mol2 using Openbabel 2.3.1 [48]. This tool was also used to minimize the structure of the ligand by applying the steepest descent algorithm, MMFF94 force field, and 50,000 steps for fitting after adding hydrogens to the molecule. We used Autodock Tools 4 (ver. 1.5.6) [49] to prepare the molecule as ligands for docking analysis. We visualized and set the torsion parameters, and then saved the file with the extension pdbqt for its submission for docking analysis. The molecular structure of Cc was downloaded from the Protein Data bank (PDB file: 1HRC), which corresponds to the high-resolution three-dimensional structure of horse heart Cc. For docking preparation, water molecules were removed from the structure, hydrogens were added (polar only), and Kollmand charges were added using Autodock Tools 4. The prepared file for docking was saved as a pdbqt file. The grid for the docking analysis was structured as follows: center x = 46.839, center y = 23.029, center z = 5.505 with a box size of: 52 for x, 52 for y and 52 for z.

The docking analysis was performed with AutodockVina 1.1.2 and the previously indicated files for the receptor (PDB:1HRC.pdbqt) and the ligand (anthracene.pdbqt) [50] by using the previously indicated grid for Cc and an exhaustiveness value of 9. The top 10 ranked poses associated with models of the ligand–Cc complex were visually analyzed using UCSF Chimera 1.15 [51] and clustered by homology. The binding site for anthracene was defined and selected based on the residues making contact and clashing with the ligand within a distance of 0.1 Å. We gathered similar poses together in subclusters for each experiment. Each experiment was performed in triplicate. A cluster was defined as the set of residues present in subclusters in all the performed individual experiments. The lowest energy value of the top-ranked pose present in a subcluster forming a cluster was selected as the energy value for the selected cluster.

4. Conclusions

PAHs are metabolized by three major pathways that generate reactive intermediates able to cause DNA mutations and oxidative damage to other biomolecules: (1) the CYP450/epoxide hydrolase pathway that produces epoxides; (2) aldo–keto reductases that lead to the formation of redox cycling PAH o-quinones; and (3) peroxidases that produce PAH radical cations which, in spite of being short-lived, can react with DNA, RNA, proteins, and lipids [8,9,21]. In addition to CYP450 peroxidase activity, other peroxidases like PGHS were implicated in the one-electron oxidation of PAHs to produce radical cations that react with DNA and cause mutations [21,37,39].

The results in this work indicate that Cc is another possible source of PAH radical cations, which has special implications for the mitochondrial toxicity of PAHs. With moderate levels of H_2O_2 and at pH 7.0, Cc catalyzes the oxidation of toxic PAHs, such as BaP, anthracene, BaA, and BbF, and does so more efficiently in the presence of CL-containing membranes. Future research should evaluate the genotoxic potential of the oxidized PAHs produced by Cc. Also demonstrated for the first time, Cc and Cc-CL complexes were able to transform important HO-PAHs metabolites, suggesting that Cc might participate in different steps of the metabolism of PAHs.

In a direct comparison with the canonical peroxidase HRP, Cc was shown to reach more potent oxidizing states and react with PAHs with intermediate ionization potential, namely pyrene and acenaphthene, which are not attacked by HRP. The PAHs with an ionization potential of up to 7.70 eV were transformed by Cc, and more extensively in the presence of CL membranes or at pH 5.0. However, chrysene (7.74 eV) was not oxidized, even in the presence of CL; therefore, the ionization potential threshold of the peroxidase activity of Cc is 7.70 eV.

Spectral studies indicate that, at least, anthracene binds to Cc, but none of the 10 PAHs/HO-PAHs studied were found to cause substantial alterations in the protein structure. The docking simulations proposed three possible binding sites of anthracene to C*c*, requiring further investigation to provide a full comprehension of the molecular interactions between PAHs and C*c*.

Supplementary Materials: The following supporting information can be downloaded at: https://www.mdpi.com/article/10.3390/molecules29051129/s1, Table S1: Polycyclic aromatic hydrocarbons studied in this work; Table S2: Control assays of benzo[a]pyrene transformation in the absence of cytochrome *c* or in the absence of H_2O_2; Figure S1: HPLC chromatograms of 2-hydroxynaphthalene and 1-hydroxypyrene transformation assays (24 h); Figure S2: UV-Vis absorption spectrum of cytochrome *c* in the presence of naphthalene, acenaphthene, pyrene, benzo[a]anthracene, chrysene, benzo[a]pyrene, benzo[b]fluoranthene, 2-hydroxynaphthalene and 1-hydroxypyrene.

Author Contributions: Investigation, J.L., D.M.-d.-S., A.K.S.-A. and R.L.; writing—original draft preparation, D.M.-d.-S., A.K.S.-A. and R.L.; writing—review and editing, P.A.V. and R.L. All authors have read and agreed to the published version of the manuscript.

Funding: This research was funded by Fundação para a Ciência e Tecnologia (FCT—Portugal) through the project PTDC/BIA-MIB/31864/2017. It was also supported by national funds through FCT/MCTES (PIDDAC) to research units: UCIBIO, UIDB/04378/2020 (DOI: 10.54499/UIDB/04378/2020) and UIDP/04378/2020 (DOI: 10.54499/UIDP/04378/2020); i4HB, LA/P/0140/2020 (DOI: 10.54499/LA/P/0140/2020); LSRE-LCM, UIDB/50020/2020 (DOI: 10.54499/UIDB/50020/2020) and UIDP/50020/2020 (DOI: 10.54499/UIDP/50020/2020); and ALiCE, LA/P/0045/2020 (DOI: 10.54499/LA/P/0045/2020). J.L. is presently supported by a PhD scholarship from FCT-Portugal, reference 2023.04204.BD.

Institutional Review Board Statement: Not applicable.

Informed Consent Statement: Not applicable.

Data Availability Statement: The data are presented within the article and available from the authors (R.L.) on request.

Acknowledgments: J.L. is grateful to LSRE-LCM-Polytechnic Institute of Leiria for the fellowship that enabled the conclusion of this work and to FCT-Portugal for the recently awarded PhD fellowship.

Conflicts of Interest: The authors declare no conflict of interest.

References

1. Zhang, Y.; Cheng, D.; Lei, Y.; Song, J.; Xia, J. Spatiotemporal Distribution of Polycyclic Aromatic Hydrocarbons in Sediments of a Typical River Located in the Loess Plateau, China: Influence of Human Activities and Land-Use Changes. *J. Hazard. Mater.* **2022**, *424*, 127744. [CrossRef]
2. Iamiceli, A.L.; Abate, V.; Bena, A.; De Filippis, S.P.; De Luca, S.; Iacovella, N.; Farina, E.; Gandini, M.; Orengia, M.; De Felip, E.; et al. The Longitudinal Biomonitoring of Residents Living near the Waste Incinerator of Turin: Polycyclic Aromatic Hydrocarbon Metabolites after Three Years from the Plant Start-Up. *Environ. Pollut.* **2022**, *314*, 120199. [CrossRef]
3. Marques, C.; Fiolet, T.; Frenoy, P.; Severi, G.; Mancini, F.R. Association between Polycyclic Aromatic Hydrocarbons (PAH) Dietary Exposure and Mortality Risk in the E3N Cohort. *Sci. Total Environ.* **2022**, *840*, 156626. [CrossRef] [PubMed]
4. Silva, J.; Marques-da-Silva, D.; Lagoa, R. Reassessment of the Experimental Skin Permeability Coefficients of Polycyclic Aromatic Hydrocarbons and Organophosphorus Pesticides. *Environ. Toxicol. Pharmacol.* **2021**, *86*, 103671. [CrossRef] [PubMed]
5. Fent, K.W.; Toennis, C.; Sammons, D.; Robertson, S.; Bertke, S.; Calafat, A.M.; Pleil, J.D.; Geer Wallace, M.A.; Kerber, S.; Smith, D.L.; et al. Firefighters' and Instructors' Absorption of PAHs and Benzene during Training Exercises. *Int. J. Hyg. Environ. Health* **2019**, *222*, 991–1000. [CrossRef] [PubMed]
6. Kim, Y.T.; Kim, W.; Bae, M.; Choi, J.E.; Kim, M.J.; Oh, S.S.; Park, K.S.; Park, S.; Lee, S.K.; Koh, S.B.; et al. The Effect of Polycyclic Aromatic Hydrocarbons on Changes in the Brain Structure of Firefighters: An Analysis Using Data from the Firefighters Research on Enhancement of Safety & Health Study. *Sci. Total Environ.* **2022**, *816*, 151655. [CrossRef] [PubMed]
7. Qiu, C.; Peng, B.; Cheng, S.; Xia, Y.; Tu, B. The Effect of Occupational Exposure to Benzo[a]Pyrene on Neurobehavioral Function in Coke Oven Workers. *Am. J. Ind. Med.* **2013**, *56*, 347–355. [CrossRef] [PubMed]
8. Lagoa, R.; Marques-da-Silva, D.; Diniz, M.; Daglia, M.; Bishayee, A. Molecular Mechanisms Linking Environmental Toxicants to Cancer Development: Significance for Protective Interventions with Polyphenols. *Semin. Cancer Biol.* **2022**, *80*, 118–144. [CrossRef] [PubMed]
9. Bukowska, B.; Duchnowicz, P. Molecular Mechanisms of Action of Selected Substances Involved in the Reduction of Benzo[a]Pyrene-Induced Oxidative Stress. *Molecules* **2022**, *27*, 1379. [CrossRef]
10. Alshaarawy, O.; Elbaz, H.A.; Andrew, M.E. The Association of Urinary Polycyclic Aromatic Hydrocarbon Biomarkers and Cardiovascular Disease in the US Population. *Environ. Int.* **2016**, *89–90*, 174–178. [CrossRef]

11. Lu, L.; Ni, R. Association between Polycyclic Aromatic Hydrocarbon Exposure and Hypertension among the U.S. Adults in the NHANES 2003–2016: A Cross-Sectional Study. *Environ. Res.* **2023**, *217*, 114907. [CrossRef]
12. IARC Website. Available online: https://monographs.iarc.who.int/ (accessed on 3 December 2023).
13. Marques-da-Silva, D.; Videira, P.A.; Lagoa, R. Registered Human Trials Addressing Environmental and Occupational Toxicant Exposures: Scoping Review of Immunological Markers and Protective Strategies. *Environ. Toxicol. Pharmacol.* **2022**, *93*, 103886. [CrossRef]
14. Ge, J.; Hao, R.; Rong, X.; Dou, Q.P.; Tan, X.; Li, G.; Li, F.; Li, D. Secoisolariciresinol Diglucoside Mitigates Benzo[a]Pyrene-Induced Liver and Kidney Toxicity in Mice via MiR-101a/MKP-1-Mediated P38 and ERK Pathway. *Food Chem. Toxicol.* **2022**, *159*, 112733. [CrossRef]
15. Zhang, J.; Wang, K.; Guo, J.; Huang, Y.; Wei, Y.; Jia, K.; Peng, Y.; Lu, H. Study on the Mechanism of Liver Toxicity Induced by Acenaphthene in Zebrafish. *Ecotoxicol. Environ. Saf.* **2023**, *249*, 114441. [CrossRef]
16. Kozal, J.S.; Jayasundara, N.; Massarsky, A.; Lindberg, C.D.; Oliveri, A.N.; Cooper, E.M.; Levin, E.D.; Meyer, J.N.; Giulio, R.T.D. Mitochondrial Dysfunction and Oxidative Stress Contribute to Cross-Generational Toxicity of Benzo(a)Pyrene in Danio Rerio. *Aquat. Toxicol.* **2023**, *263*, 106658. [CrossRef]
17. Ji, X.; Li, Y.; He, J.; Shah, W.; Xue, X.; Feng, G.; Zhang, H.; Gao, M. Depletion of Mitochondrial Enzyme System in Liver, Lung, Brain, Stomach and Kidney Induced by Benzo(a)Pyrene. *Environ. Toxicol. Pharmacol.* **2016**, *43*, 83–93. [CrossRef]
18. Omidian, K.; Rafiei, H.; Bandy, B. Increased Mitochondrial Content and Function by Resveratrol and Select Flavonoids Protects against Benzo[a]Pyrene-Induced Bioenergetic Dysfunction and ROS Generation in a Cell Model of Neoplastic Transformation. *Free Radic. Biol. Med.* **2020**, *152*, 767–775. [CrossRef] [PubMed]
19. Loxham, M.; Morgan-Walsh, R.J.; Cooper, M.J.; Blume, C.; Swindle, E.J.; Dennison, P.; Howarth, P. The Effects on Bronchial Epithelial Mucociliary Cultures of Coarse, Fine, and Ultrafine Particulate Matter from an Underground Railway Station. *Toxicol. Sci.* **2015**, *145*, 98–107. [CrossRef] [PubMed]
20. Marques-da-Silva, D.; Lagoa, R. Rafting on the Evidence for Lipid Raft-like Domains as Hubs Triggering Environmental Toxicants' Cellular Effects. *Molecules* **2023**, *28*, 6598. [CrossRef]
21. Stading, R.; Gastelum, G.; Chu, C.; Jiang, W.; Moorthy, B. Molecular Mechanisms of Pulmonary Carcinogenesis by Polycyclic Aromatic Hydrocarbons (PAHs): Implications for Human Lung Cancer. *Semin. Cancer Biol.* **2021**, *76*, 3–16. [CrossRef] [PubMed]
22. Broniatowski, M.; Binczycka, M.; Wójcik, A.; Flasiński, M.; Wydro, P. Polycyclic Aromatic Hydrocarbons in Model Bacterial Membranes—Langmuir Monolayer Studies. *Biochim. Biophys. Acta Biomembr.* **2017**, *1859*, 2402–2412. [CrossRef] [PubMed]
23. Ayala, M. Redox Potential of Peroxidases. In *Biocatalysis Based on Heme Peroxidases*; Torres, E., Ayala, M., Eds.; Springer: Berlin/Heidelberg, Germany, 2010; pp. 61–77, ISBN 9783642126260.
24. Lopes, J.M.; Marques-da-Silva, D.; Videira, P.; Lagoa, R. Comparison of Laccases and Hemeproteins Systems in Bioremediation of Organic Pollutants. *Curr. Protein Pept. Sci.* **2022**, *23*, 402–423. [CrossRef] [PubMed]
25. Vlasova, I.I. Peroxidase Activity of Human Hemoproteins: Keeping the Fire under Control. *Molecules* **2018**, *23*, 2561. [CrossRef] [PubMed]
26. Radi, R.; Thomson, L.; Rubbo, H.; Prodanov, E. Cytochrome C-Catalyzed Oxidation of Organic Molecules by Hydrogen Peroxide. *Arch. Biochem. Biophys.* **1991**, *288*, 112–117. [CrossRef] [PubMed]
27. Vazquez-Duhalt, R.; Westlake, D.W.S.; Fedorak, P.M. Cytochrome c as a Biocatalyst for the Oxidation of Thiophenes and Organosulfides. *Enzyme Microb. Technol.* **1993**, *15*, 494–499. [CrossRef]
28. Tinoco, R.; Vazquez-Duhalt, R. Chemical Modification of Cytochrome C Improves Their Catalytic Properties in Oxidation of Polycyclic Aromatic Hydrocarbons. *Enzyme Microb. Technol.* **1998**, *22*, 8–12. [CrossRef]
29. Torres, E.; Bustos-Jaimes, I.; Le Borgne, S. Potential Use of Oxidative Enzymes for the Detoxification of Organic Pollutants. *Appl. Catal. B Environ.* **2003**, *46*, 1–15. [CrossRef]
30. Díaz-Quintana, A.; Pérez-Mejías, G.; Guerra-Castellano, A.; De la Rosa, M.; Díaz-Moreno, I. Wheel and Deal in the Mitochondrial Inner Membranes: The Tale of Cytochrome c and Cardiolipin. *Oxid. Med. Cell. Longev.* **2020**, *2020*, 813405. [CrossRef]
31. Lagoa, R.; Gutierrez-Merino, C. Cytochrome c Reducing Agents and Antiapoptotic Action of Antioxidants. In *Cytochrome c: Roles and Therapeutic Implications*; Arias, N., Ed.; Nova Science Publishers: New York, NY, USA, 2019; pp. 1–49, ISBN 978-1-53614-907-4.
32. Bedia, C.; Dalmau, N.; Jaumot, J.; Tauler, R. Phenotypic Malignant Changes and Untargeted Lipidomic Analysis of Long-Term Exposed Prostate Cancer Cells to Endocrine Disruptors. *Environ. Res.* **2015**, *140*, 18–31. [CrossRef]
33. Basova, L.V.; Kurnikov, I.V.; Wang, L.; Ritov, V.B.; Belikova, N.A.; Vlasova, I.I.; Pacheco, A.A.; Winnica, D.E.; Peterson, J.; Bayir, H.; et al. Cardiolipin Switch in Mitochondria: Shutting off the Reduction of Cytochrome c and Turning on the Peroxidase Activity. *Biochemistry* **2007**, *46*, 3423–3434. [CrossRef]
34. Hanske, J.; Toffey, J.R.; Morenz, A.M.; Bonilla, A.J.; Schiavoni, K.H.; Pletneva, E.V. Conformational Properties of Cardiolipin-Bound Cytochrome C. *Proc. Natl. Acad. Sci. USA* **2012**, *109*, 125–130. [CrossRef]
35. Atkinson, J.; Kapralov, A.A.; Yanamala, N.; Tyurina, Y.Y.; Amoscato, A.A.; Pearce, L.; Peterson, J.; Huang, Z.; Jiang, J.; Samhan-Arias, A.K.; et al. A Mitochondria-Targeted Inhibitor of Cytochrome c Peroxidase Mitigates Radiation-Induced Death. *Nat. Commun.* **2011**, *2*, 497. [CrossRef] [PubMed]
36. Lagoa, R.; Samhan-Arias, A.; Gutierrez-Merino, C. Correlation between the Potency of Flavonoids for Cytochrome c Reduction and Inhibition of Cardiolipin-Induced Peroxidase Activity. *BioFactors* **2017**, *43*, 451–468. [CrossRef] [PubMed]

37. Cavalieri, E.; Rogan, E. Role of Radical Cations in Aromatic Hydrocarbon Carcinogenesis. *Environ. Health Perspect.* **1985**, *64*, 69–84. [CrossRef] [PubMed]
38. Lopes, J.M.; Marques-da-Silva, D.; Videira, P.A.; Lagoa, R. Use of Lipid Vesicles for Revealing the Potential Contribution of Cytochrome C in the Metabolism of Environmental Toxicants. *Med. Sci. Forum* **2022**, *11*, 6. [CrossRef]
39. Devanesan, P.; Rogan, E.; Cavalieri, E. The Relationship between Ionization Potential and Prostaglandin H Synthase-Catalyzed Binding of Aromatic Hydrocarbons to DNA. *Chem. Biol. Interact.* **1987**, *61*, 89–95. [CrossRef] [PubMed]
40. Lee, M.L.; Hites, R.A. Mixed Charge Exchange-Chemical Ionization Mass Spectrometry of Polycyclic Aromatic Hydrocarbons. *J. Am. Chem. Soc.* **1977**, *99*, 2008–2009. [CrossRef]
41. Fiorucci, L.; Sinibaldi, F.; Chimenti, M.; Perricone, R.; Santucci, R. Cytochrome c as a Clinical Biomarker in Diseases Characterized by Cell Apoptosis. In *Cytochrome c: Roles and Therapeutic Implications*; Arias, N., Ed.; Nova Science Publishers: New York, NY, USA, 2019; pp. 119–147, ISBN 978-1-53614-907-4.
42. Mohammadyani, D.; Yanamala, N.; Samhan-Arias, A.K.; Kapralov, A.A.; Stepanov, G.; Nuar, N.; Planas-Iglesias, J.; Sanghera, N.; Kagan, V.E.; Klein-Seetharaman, J. Structural Characterization of Cardiolipin-Driven Activation of Cytochrome c into a Peroxidase and Membrane Perturbation. *Biochim. Biophys. Acta. Biomembr.* **2018**, *1860*, 1057–1068. [CrossRef]
43. Yadav, N.; Gogada, R.; O'Malley, J.; Gundampati, R.K.; Jayanthi, S.; Hashmi, S.; Lella, R.; Zhang, D.; Wang, J.; Kumar, R.; et al. Molecular Insights on Cytochrome c and Nucleotide Regulation of Apoptosome Function and Its Implication in Cancer. *Biochim. Biophys. Acta Mol. Cell Res.* **2020**, *1867*, 118573. [CrossRef]
44. Volkov, A.N.; van Nuland, N.A.J. Electron Transfer Interactome of Cytochrome C. *PLoS Comput. Biol.* **2012**, *8*, e1002807. [CrossRef]
45. Kapralov, A.A.; Yanamala, N.; Tyurina, Y.Y.; Castro, L.; Samhan-Arias, A.; Vladimirov, Y.A.; Maeda, A.; Weitz, A.A.; Peterson, J.; Mylnikov, D.; et al. Topography of Tyrosine Residues and Their Involvement in Peroxidation of Polyunsaturated Cardiolipin in Cytochrome c/Cardiolipin Peroxidase Complexes. *Biochim. Biophys. Acta Biomembr.* **2011**, *1808*, 2147–2155. [CrossRef] [PubMed]
46. Marques-da-Silva, D.; Lopes, J.M.; Correia, I.; Silva, J.S.; Lagoa, R. Removal of Hydrophobic Organic Pollutants and Copper by Alginate-Based and Polycaprolactone Materials. *Processes* **2022**, *10*, 2300. [CrossRef]
47. Irwin, J.J.; Shoichet, B.K. ZINC—A Free Database of Commercially Available Compounds for Virtual Screening. *J. Chem. Inf. Model.* **2005**, *45*, 177. [CrossRef] [PubMed]
48. O'Boyle, N.M.; Banck, M.; James, C.A.; Morley, C.; Vandermeersch, T.; Hutchison, G.R. Open Babel: An Open Chemical Toolbox. *J. Cheminform.* **2011**, *3*, 33. [CrossRef] [PubMed]
49. Morris, G.M.; Ruth, H.; Lindstrom, W.; Sanner, M.F.; Belew, R.K.; Goodsell, D.S.; Olson, A.J. AutoDock4 and AutoDockTools4: Automated Docking with Selective Receptor Flexibility. *J. Comput. Chem.* **2009**, *30*, 2785–2791. [CrossRef]
50. Trott, O.; Olson, A.J. AutoDock Vina: Improving the Speed and Accuracy of Docking with a New Scoring Function, Efficient Optimization, and Multithreading. *J. Comput. Chem.* **2010**, *31*, 455–461. [CrossRef]
51. Pettersen, E.F.; Goddard, T.D.; Huang, C.C.; Couch, G.S.; Greenblatt, D.M.; Meng, E.C.; Ferrin, T.E. UCSF Chimera—A Visualization System for Exploratory Research and Analysis. *J. Comput. Chem.* **2004**, *25*, 1605–1612. [CrossRef]

Disclaimer/Publisher's Note: The statements, opinions and data contained in all publications are solely those of the individual author(s) and contributor(s) and not of MDPI and/or the editor(s). MDPI and/or the editor(s) disclaim responsibility for any injury to people or property resulting from any ideas, methods, instructions or products referred to in the content.

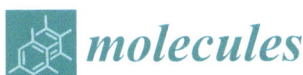

Article

Hexa-Histidine, a Peptide with Versatile Applications in the Study of Amyloid-β(1–42) Molecular Mechanisms of Action

Jairo Salazar [1,*], Alejandro K. Samhan-Arias [2,3] and Carlos Gutierrez-Merino [4,*]

1. Departamento de Química, Universidad Nacional Autónoma de Nicaragua-León, León 21000, Nicaragua
2. Departamento de Bioquímica, Universidad Autónoma de Madrid (UAM), C\Arzobispo Morcillo 4, 28029 Madrid, Spain; alejandro.samhan@uam.es
3. Instituto de Investigaciones Biomédicas 'Alberto Sols' (CSIC-UAM), C\Arturo Duperier 4, 28029 Madrid, Spain
4. Instituto de Biomarcadores de Patologías Moleculares, Universidad de Extremadura, 06006 Badajoz, Spain
* Correspondence: jairochemsalazar@gmail.com (J.S.); biocgm@gmail.com (C.G.-M.)

Abstract: Amyloid β (Aβ) oligomers are the most neurotoxic forms of Aβ, and Aβ(1–42) is the prevalent Aβ peptide found in the amyloid plaques of Alzheimer's disease patients. Aβ(25–35) is the shortest peptide that retains the toxicity of Aβ(1–42). Aβ oligomers bind to calmodulin (CaM) and calbindin-D28k with dissociation constants in the nanomolar Aβ(1–42) concentration range. Aβ and histidine-rich proteins have a high affinity for transition metal ions Cu^{2+}, Fe^{3+} and Zn^{2+}. In this work, we show that the fluorescence of Aβ(1–42) HiLyte™-Fluor555 can be used to monitor hexa-histidine peptide (His_6) interaction with Aβ(1–42). The formation of His_6/Aβ(1–42) complexes is also supported by docking results yielded by the MDockPeP Server. Also, we found that micromolar concentrations of His_6 block the increase in the fluorescence of Aβ(1–42) HiLyte™-Fluor555 produced by its interaction with the proteins CaM and calbindin-D28k. In addition, we found that the His_6-tag provides a high-affinity site for the binding of Aβ(1–42) and Aβ(25–35) peptides to the human recombinant cytochrome b_5 reductase, and sensitizes this enzyme to inhibition by these peptides. In conclusion, our results suggest that a His_6-tag could provide a valuable new tool to experimentally direct the action of neurotoxic Aβ peptides toward selected cellular targets.

Keywords: amyloid β(1–42); amyloid β(25–35); hexa-histidine; calmodulin; calbindin-D28k; hexa-histidine-tag; recombinant cytochrome b_5 reductase; fluorescence; fluorescence resonance energy transfer

Citation: Salazar, J.; Samhan-Arias, A.K.; Gutierrez-Merino, C. Hexa-Histidine, a Peptide with Versatile Applications in the Study of Amyloid-β(1–42) Molecular Mechanisms of Action. *Molecules* **2023**, *28*, 7138. https://doi.org/10.3390/molecules28207138

Academic Editor: Tibor Páli

Received: 19 September 2023
Revised: 10 October 2023
Accepted: 13 October 2023
Published: 17 October 2023

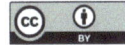

Copyright: © 2023 by the authors. Licensee MDPI, Basel, Switzerland. This article is an open access article distributed under the terms and conditions of the Creative Commons Attribution (CC BY) license (https://creativecommons.org/licenses/by/4.0/).

1. Introduction

Amyloid β (Aβ) peptides are a hallmark of Alzheimer's disease (AD). Aβ(1–42) is the prevalent Aβ peptide found in the amyloid plaques of AD patients [1]. Owing to the high affinity of Aβ(1–42) for Cu^{2+}, Fe^{3+} and Zn^{2+}, these metal ions are accumulated in Aβ plaques [2]. Despite the fact that Aβ plaques are cytotoxic, it has been proposed that Aβ plaques could serve as reservoirs to assemble small Aβ oligomers [3]. Aβ oligomers are the main neurotoxic forms of Aβ and have been linked to AD pathogenesis [4–11]. Furthermore, it has been shown that intraneuronal Aβ accumulation precedes the appearance of amyloid plaques or tangles in transgenic mice models of AD [6,12–14]. Aβ(25–35) is the shortest peptide that retains the toxicity of the full-length Aβ(1–42) peptide [15], and it has been suggested to be the biologically active region of Aβ(1–42) [16,17].

Aβ peptides bind to ganglioside-clustered raft-like membrane microdomains, which foster the formation of Aβ oligomers and fibrils in a cholesterol-dependent manner [18–22]. Indeed, dimeric nonfibrillar Aβ has been shown to accumulate in lipid rafts in the Tg2576 mouse model of AD [23], and exogenous oligomeric Aβ applied to neurons in culture concentrates in lipid rafts [24]. Moreover, plasma membrane lipid rafts play an active role in extracellular Aβ uptake and internalization in neurons [25]. After the uptake of extracellular Aβ(1–42) into neurons, the intracellular aggregates elicit neuronal damage and neurotoxicity [8,9,26,27]. Intracellular targets of Aβ(1–42) oligomers have been identified in the cytosol and subcellular organelles like the endoplasmic reticulum (ER) and mitochondria [28–30]. Of particular relevance are the intracellular targets of Aβ(1–42) oligomers that bind nanomolar concentrations of Aβ peptides, because concentrations of non-fibrillar Aβ peptides within the nanomolar range have been reported in the brain [31–33], and the critical concentration that induces Aβ(1–42) fibrillization lies in the submicromolar range [34,35]. Until now, dissociation constants lower than 10 nM have been reported for the complexes between Aβ peptides and a few intracellular proteins expressed in brain neurons, namely calmodulin (CaM) [36], cellular prion protein [37], glycogen synthase kinase 3α [38], tau [39], calbindin-D28k [40] and STIM1 [30]. However, in neurons, the concentration of CaM is in the micromolar range, which is orders of magnitude higher than the concentration of the other competing proteins in neurons listed above, with the exception of calbindin-D28k. Nevertheless, it is to be noted that, although calbindin-D28k is abundant throughout the central nervous system, including pyramidal hippocampal neurons and cortical neurons [41], the dissociation constant of the Aβ(1–42)/calbindin-D28k complex is around 10-fold higher than that of the Aβ(1–42)/CaM complex [40]. Due to this, CaM binds a large fraction of intracellular Aβ(1–42) in the nanomolar concentration range [27].

As CaM binds Aβ(1–42) and Aβ(25–35) peptides with very high affinity, i.e., with a dissociation constant $\approx$1 nM [36]. In a previous work, we used CaM as a template protein for the design of an antagonist peptide of Aβ(1–42) using docking approaches [40]. Fluorescence assays with Aβ(1–42) HiLyte^{TM}-Fluor555 confirmed that this peptide efficiently inhibits the interaction between Aβ(1–42) and CaM [40]. Interestingly, the peptide designed to bind the 25–35 amino acid residues of Aβ(1–42) was experimentally found to also be a potent inhibitor of the interaction between Aβ(1–42) and calbindin-D28k [40], pointing out that the same amino acid domain of Aβ(1–42) is involved in its complexation with both CaM and calbindin-D28k. This bears a special relevance in AD, since these proteins play important roles in neuronal calcium signaling and the dysregulation of intracellular calcium homeostasis, and alterations of neuronal excitability have been shown to mediate Aβ neurotoxicity [42–45]. On the other hand, it is known that several endogenous neuropeptides can antagonize the actions of Aβ, both in animal models [46–48] and in cell cultures [49,50]. Therefore, the search for novel peptides that binds Aβ with high affinity can shed light on the research of endogenous neuropeptides with neuroprotection actions against Aβ. Histidine-rich proteins have a high affinity for Cu^{2+}, Fe^{3+} and Zn^{2+} [51–53], like Aβ(1–42) [2,54]. Thus, polyhistidine motifs or peptides are good candidates as Aβ(1–42) antagonists and putative novel therapeutic agents in AD. Moreover, it has been noted that the hexa-histidine binding by monoclonal antibody C706, which recognizes the human Aβ peptide, mimics Aβ recognition [55].

In this work, we report that the fluorescence of Aβ(1–42) HiLyte^{TM}-Fluor555 (dye covalently bound to ASP1 of Aβ) monitors hexa-histidine peptide (His_6) interaction with Aβ(1–42) and the inhibition of the interaction between Aβ(1–42) and the proteins CaM and calbindin-D28k. Also, we found that the presence of a C-terminal His_6-tag in human recombinant cytochrome b_5 reductase (Cb5R) sensitizes its enzymatic activity to modulation by submicromolar Aβ(1–42) concentrations. In this work, we have used human recombinant Cb5R because the cytochrome b_5 (Cb_5)/Cb5R system has a relevant role in lipid metabolism, which is significantly altered in AD [56,57].

2. Results

2.1. Hexa-Histidine (His_6) Interacts with Aβ(1–42) HiLyte^{TM}-Fluor555

The addition of submicromolar concentrations of His_6 to a solution of 10 nM Aβ(1–42) HiLyte^{TM}-Fluor555 increases the fluorescence intensity of the labelled peptide (Figure 1A). The kinetics of the increase in fluorescence, which monitors the interaction between His_6 and Aβ(1–42) HiLyte^{TM}-Fluor555, has an initial slower phase of 1–2 min and reaches a maximum of 8 ± 2% with a half-time of approximately 10 min. Although the kinetics are slightly faster with 0.25 μM of His$_6$, the large overlap between the kinetic traces obtained with 0.1 and 0.25 μM of His$_6$ points out that at the latter concentration, no new complexes are being formed. The results of titration with His$_6$ shown in Figure 1B confirm the saturation of the maximum fluorescence change at a concentration of 0.1 μM of His$_6$. The small value of the maximum fluorescence change indicates that His$_6$ interaction with Aβ(1–42) elicits only a small change in the microenvironment of the HiLyte^{TM}-Fluor555 dye, which is bound to ASP1 of Aβ(1–42). The short initial lag phase suggests that conformational changes in His$_6$ and/or Aβ(1–42) HiLyte^{TM}-Fluor555 are needed for a better coupling between both molecules. The dependence upon the His$_6$ concentration of the increase in fluorescence intensity at 2000 s of the kinetic of the increase in fluorescence is shown in Figure 1B. Taking into account that the noise of the fluorescence signal introduces an error close to ±2% in the differences between fluorescence intensity readings, the 50% of the maximum fluorescence change is reached with a concentration of ≈50–60 nM of His$_6$, i.e., the saturation of the fluorescence change is observed at ratios ≥10 molecules of His$_6$ per Aβ(1–42) HiLyte^{TM}-Fluor555 monomer.

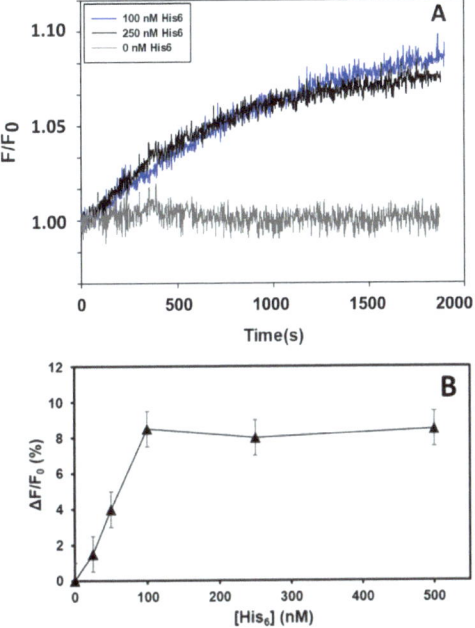

Figure 1. The fluorescence of Aβ(1–42) HiLyte^{TM}-Fluor555 monitors its interaction with His$_6$. (**A**) Kinetics of the increase in Aβ(1–42) HiLyte^{TM}-Fluor555 fluorescence induced by the addition of His$_6$. For a more direct evaluation of the magnitude of the increase in the fluorescence, the results are presented as the ratio between the fluorescence intensity at different times (F) and the fluorescence intensity at time 0 (F_0). The kinetic traces shown are the means of triplicate experiments performed with 10 nM Aβ(1–42) HiLyte^{TM}-Fluor555 and the concentrations of His$_6$ indicated in the figure, which was added at time 0. The kinetic trace in gray color is the control with the addition of only the buffer in which His$_6$ is prepared (0 His$_6$). (**B**) Dependence upon the His$_6$ concentration of the increase in the fluorescence intensity of Aβ(1–42) HiLyte^{TM}-Fluor555 at the end of the kinetic of increase in fluorescence. Other experimental conditions used for these fluorescence measurements are given in Section 4.

The experimental results shown above prompted us to perform docking between His$_6$ and/or Aβ(1–42). The analysis of docking has been performed using the MDockPeP Server, as indicated in Section 4. The structure of Aβ(1–42) registered with PDB ID: 1IYT in UniPro

Databank has been selected for this docking work due to the following reasons: (1) at the concentration of 10 nM used in these experiments, the Aβ(1–42) peptide must be largely in the monomeric state because the dissociation constant for Aβ(1–42) dimers is similar to that reported for Aβ(1–40) dimers, i.e., around 198 ± 43 nM [58], and (2) we found in a previous work that this structure of the Aβ(1–42) monomer is a good template structure for the design of an efficient peptide antagonist for the interaction between Aβ(1–42) and CaM [40]. The results generated 10 possible structural models for the complex formation, which can be grouped into three clusters, as shown in Table 1 and Supplementary Tables.

Table 1. Interacting interfaces for the complex formation between His$_6$ and Aβ peptides obtained via molecular docking simulation.

Cluster	Involved Receptor Residues on the Interaction (Aβ Peptide)	Involved Ligand Residues on the Interaction (His$_6$ Peptide)	Binding Energy $\Delta^i G$ (kcal/mol)
Cluster 1	LYS16, LEU1, PHE20, LA21, VAL24, GLY25, LYS2, ILE31, LEU34, MET35,	HIS1, HIS3, HIS4, HIS5, HIS6	−6.8
Cluster 2	GLU3, HIS6, ASP7, TYR10, HIS14	HIS1, HIS2, HIS6	−4.8
Cluster 3	GLY9, VAL18	HIS1, HIS2, HIS6	−2.6

In cluster 1, His$_6$ interacts with the Aβ(1–42) domain close to the NH$_2$-terminus and involves the short α-helix and the part of the long α-helix near the structural tilt of this peptide. Cluster 1 gathers models 1, 4, 7 and 8 and presents an estimated free energy for the complex formation of −6.8 kcal/mol, which is that found for the lowest energy model of the cluster (model 7) (Figure 2, cluster 1). The interacting interface in cluster 1 comprises the following amino acid residues of the Aβ peptide: LYS16, LEU1, PHE20, ALA21, VAL24, GLY25, LYS2, ILE31, LEU34 and MET35 and HIS1, HIS3, HIS4, HIS5 and HIS6 residues of the His$_6$ peptide. Buried surface area/accessible solvent area ratio allowed us to rank those amino acid residues with higher participation in the interaction with Aβ peptide: VAL24 > ALA21 > GLY25 > LEU34 > PHE20 > MET35 > LEU17 > ILE31 > LYS28 > LYS16 and a similar participation for the HIS1, HIS3, HIS4, HIS5 and HIS6 of the His$_6$ peptide. Several H-bonds and salt bridges were found in models from cluster 1 but without sharing the same amino acid residues among themselves (Supplementary Table S1).

Cluster 2 is the second most probable cluster and is representative of another four of the ten most probable outcomes generated using the MDockPeP Server. In cluster 2, His$_6$ interacts with the Aβ(1–42) domain close to the COOH-terminus. Cluster 2 gathers models 2, 5, 9 and 10. Analysis with PDBePisa estimated free energy for the complex formation of −4.8 kcal/mol, which is that found for the lowest energy model of the cluster (model 9) (Figure 2, cluster 2). The interacting interface in cluster 2 comprises the following amino acid residues of the Aβ peptide: GLU3, HIS6, ASP7, TYR10, HIS14 and HIS1, HIS2, HIS6 residues of the His$_6$ peptide. Buried surface area/accessible solvent area ratio allowed us to rank those amino acid residues with higher participation in the interaction with Aβ peptide: TYR10 > HIS6 > GLU3 > HIS14 > ASP7 and similar participation for the HIS1, HIS2 and HIS6 of the His$_6$ peptide. Several H-bonds and salt bridges were also found in models from cluster 2, but as also accounting for cluster 1, they did not share similarities among themselves (Supplementary Table S2). A third cluster was found based on models sharing similarities in their interaction. Cluster 3 is representative of two of the ten most probable structures generated using the MDockPeP Server and predicts that His$_6$ may also interact with the long α-helix part closer to the COOH-terminus of Aβ(1–42). Cluster 3 gathers models 3 and 6. Analysis with PDBePisa estimated free energy for the complex formation of −2.6 kcal/mol, which is that found for the lowest energy model of the cluster (model 3) (Figure 2, cluster 3). The interacting interface in cluster 3 comprises the GLY9 and VAL184 amino acid residues of Aβ peptide and HIS1, HIS2, HIS6 residues of the His$_6$ peptide. Buried surface area/ accessible solvent area ratio indicates that both amino acid residues of Aβ peptide (GLY9 and VAL184) participate similarly in the interaction with the His$_6$ peptide and Aβ peptide. Several H-bonds and salt bridges were also found in models from cluster 3 without sharing similarities among themselves (Supplementary Table S3).

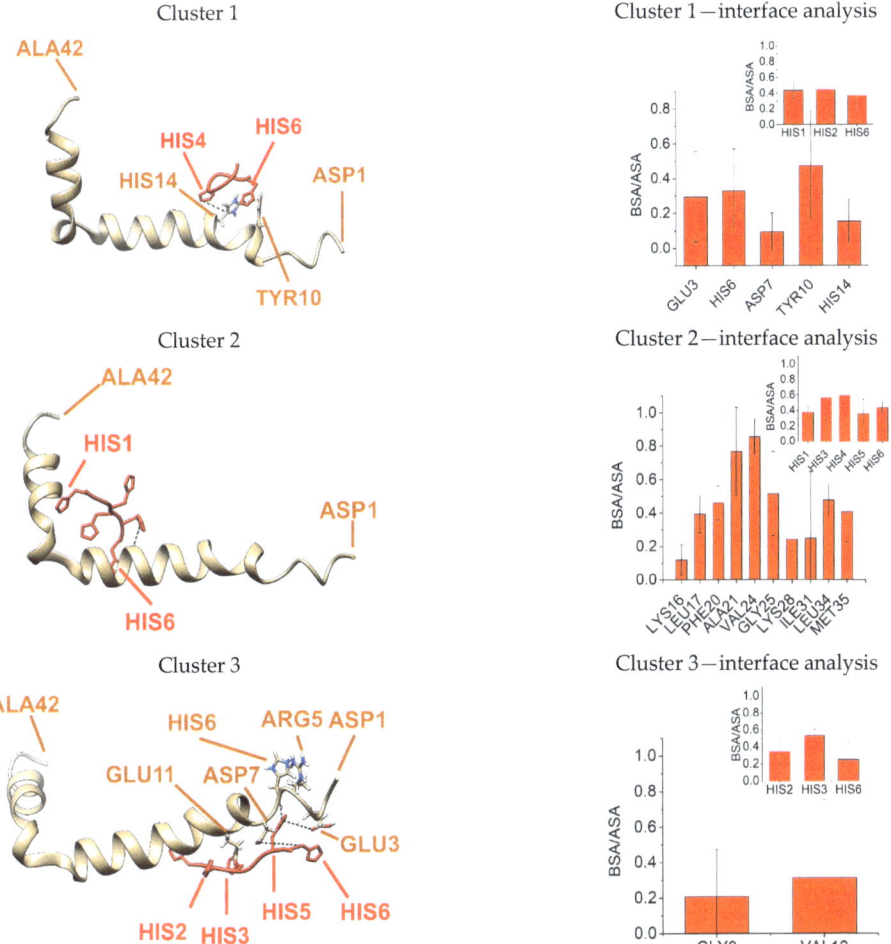

Figure 2. Clusters of the structures generated using the MDockPeP Server for the complex between 1His$_6$ and the structure of Aβ(1–42) registered with PDB ID: 1IYT in UniPro Databank analyzed with PDBePISA. Aβ(1–42) backbone is shown in brown and 1His$_6$ peptide is shown in red for the representative models with the lowest estimated binding energy of cluster1, cluster 2 and cluster 3, model 7, model 9 and model 3, respectively. H-bonds between amino acids of both structures are shown as a dotted black line.

We can summarize that the analysis in silico allows us to predict large conformational plasticity in the His$_6$/Aβ(1–42) complex, suggesting that the predominant conformation of this complex could be strongly affected by its microenvironment. In addition, docking results raise the possibility that the Aβ(1–42) monomer can bind up to 2–3 molecules of His$_6$.

2.2. His_6 Antagonizes the Interaction of Aβ(1–42) HiLyte^{TM}-Fluor555 with CaM and Calbindin D28k

In previous works, we have shown that Aβ(1–42) binds with high affinity to CaM and calbindin-D28k [36,40]. Since model 1 predicts a strong interaction of His_6 with the domain of Aβ(1–42) more directly involved in its interaction with CaM and calbindin-D28k, in this work, we have experimentally assessed the possibility that His_6 could antagonize the interaction of Aβ(1–42) with these proteins.

The kinetics of the interaction of the fluorescence derivative of Aβ(1–42), Aβ(1–42) HiLyte^{TM}-Fluor555, with CaM and calbindin-D28k can be monitored by the fluorescence intensity changes of the dye HiLyte^{TM}-Fluor555 [40]. A preincubation of 15 min with His_6 was included in the experimental design to prevent a distortion of the kinetics of fluorescence increase produced by CaM or calbindin-D28k by the change of fluorescence elicited by His_6. Figure 3 shows that His_6 attenuates the increase in fluorescence intensity Aβ(1–42) HiLyte^{TM}-Fluor555 after adding either calbindin-D28k or CaM. This is an effect dependent upon the concentration of His_6. As shown in Figure 3, the maximum change of the fluorescence intensity and the rate of the kinetic process are decreased by His_6, albeit with different efficacy. These results yield His_6 concentrations for a 50% attenuation of the maximum change of fluorescence intensity of ≈0.1 and 1 μM for the interaction of Aβ(1–42) with calbindin-D28k and CaM, respectively. Therefore, His_6 behaves as an antagonist of the interaction of Aβ(1–42) with these proteins, although with different potency in the submicromolar-to-micromolar concentration range.

2.3. Submicromolar Concentrations of Aβ Peptides Inhibit the Reduction in Cb_5 Catalyzed by Purified Recombinant His_6-Tagged Cb5R, and No Inhibition Is Observed after Deletion of the His_6-Tag

In order to evaluate the ability of His_6 to sensitize proteins to Aβ peptides, we have used human recombinant Cb5R with a His_6-tag covalently linked to the NH_2-terminus amino acid, expressed and purified as described in Section 4. The NADH-dependent reduction in Cb_5 has been measured, following protocols used in previous works, as indicated in Section 4.

Representative kinetic traces of the rate of NADH-dependent reduction in Cb_5 are presented in Figure 4A. A specific activity of 7.9 ± 0.7 μmoles of the reduced Cb_5/min/mg of Cb5R at 25 °C has been calculated from initial rate measurements for the samples of human recombinant C-terminal His_6-tagged Cb5R. Also, the kinetic traces shown in Figure 4A highlight the potent inhibition of this activity by nanomolar Aβ(1–42) concentrations. As up to 2 μM of Aβ(1–42), the highest concentration tested in this work, we have not detected any alteration of the absorbance spectrum of Cb_5, the possibility that this inhibition could be due to an Aβ(1–42)-induced conformational change in the microenvironment of the heme group of Cb_5 can be discarded. Moreover, the inhibition is seen from the first absorbance measurements after the addition of Aβ(1–42), implying its rapid binding to the inhibitory site in the Cb5R. Indeed, the observed inhibition was the same without or with up to 30 min preincubation of the Cb5R with 50 and 100 nM of Aβ(1–42). Next, we removed the His_6-tag from human recombinant Cb5R as described in detail in Section 4. We found that the addition of up to 2 μM of Aβ(1–42) and of Aβ(25–35) does not produce a statistically significant inhibition of the rate of NADH-dependent reduction in Cb_5 by human recombinant Cb5R minus a His_6-tag, i.e., less than 10% inhibition. Of note, a 2 micromolar concentration of Aβ(1–42) oligomers is higher than those that can be expected intracellularly in AD, since the induction of fibrillization only requires submicromolar concentrations of Aβ(1–42) [34,35].

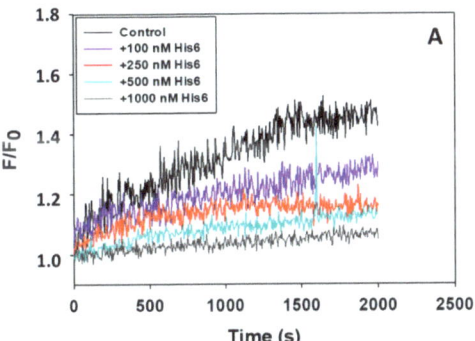

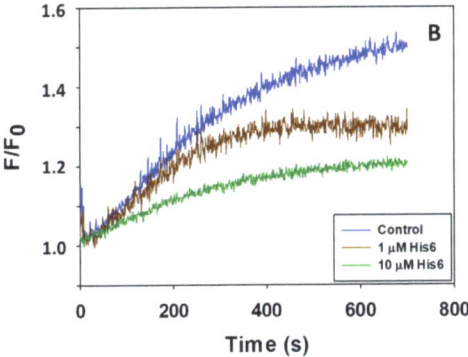

Figure 3. The peptide His$_6$ antagonizes the interaction of Aβ(1–42) with calbindin-D28k and CaM. (**A**) Effect of increasing concentrations of His$_6$ on the kinetics at an increase of 10 nM Aβ(1–42) HiLyte^{TM}-Fluor555 fluorescence after adding 5 nM calbindin-D28k at time 0. (**B**) Effect of increasing concentrations of His$_6$ on the kinetics at an increase of 10 nM Aβ(1–42) HiLyte^{TM}-Fluor555 fluorescence after adding 5 nM CaM at time 0. The results are presented as the ratio between the fluorescence intensity at different times (F) and the fluorescence intensity at time 0 (F$_0$), and the kinetic traces shown in this figure are the means of experiments performed in triplicate. The color code used for the assayed concentrations of His$_6$ is given in the inset of the figures. Other experimental conditions used for these fluorescence measurements are given in Section 4.

The results of the dependence upon the concentration of Aβ(1–42) and Aβ(25–35) of the inhibition of the NADH-dependent reduction in Cb$_5$ by human recombinant Cb5R with a His$_6$-tag are shown in Figure 4B. These results showed that Aβ(1–42) and Aβ(25–35) are equally potent as inhibitors of this activity, without statistically significant differences between both datasets. The inhibitory effect is specific of neurotoxic Aβ peptides, because a peptide with a random sequence of the 42 amino acids of Aβ (scrambled Aβ), which has been found non-toxic in previous works [27,30], does not inhibit this activity (Figure 4B). The results of inhibition by Aβ(1–42) and Aβ(25–35) fit well to the equation for one inhibitor binding site, with an inhibition constant (Ki) between 50 and 60 nM of Aβ monomers, and maximum inhibition (Imax) between 75 and 80%. Of note, this Ki value is nearly 10-fold higher than the Cb5R concentration used in these assays, and, therefore, the contribution of the peptide bound to Cb5R to the total Aβ concentration is lower than 10% at half of the saturation of the inhibition curve.

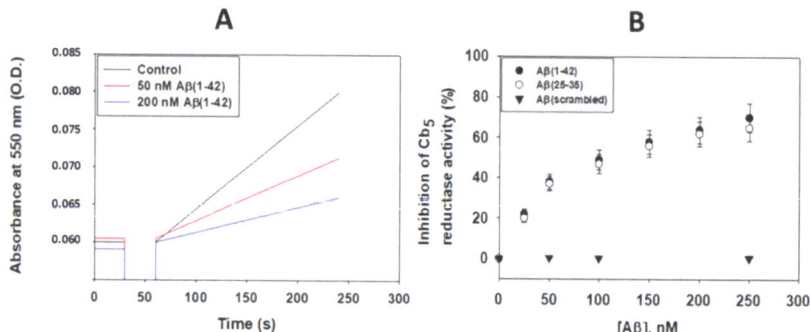

Figure 4. Aβ(1–42) and Aβ(25–35) inhibit the NADH-dependent Cb$_5$ reductase activity of the human recombinant Cb5R with a His$_6$-tag. (**A**) Kinetics of Cb$_5$ reduction by the human recombinant Cb5R with a His$_6$-tag in the absence and presence of 50 and 100 nM Aβ(1–42). (**B**) Dependence upon the concentration of Aβ(1–42), Aβ(25–35) and scrambled Aβ(1–42) of the inhibition of the Cb$_5$ reductase activity of the human recombinant Cb5R with a His$_6$-tag. The results shown are the means ± standard error of the mean (S.E.M.) of experiments performed in triplicate. Other experimental conditions used for these assays are given in the Section 4.7.

Combining these kinetic results, it merges the conclusion that the Cb$_5$ reductase activity of the His$_6$-tagged Cb5R is strongly sensitized to neurotoxic Aβ peptides.

2.4. The Binding of Aβ(1–42) and of Aβ(25–35) to the Human Recombinant Cb5R with a His$_6$-tag Increases the Fluorescence of Its Prosthetic Group FAD

In previous works [59,60], we have shown that the fluorescence of the prosthetic group FAD can be used to monitor conformational changes of Cb5R, which impair its catalytic activity.

In this work, we found that the addition of Aβ(1–42) and of Aβ(25–35) produces an increase in the FAD fluorescence of human recombinant Cb5R with a His$_6$-tag without a significant shift of the emission peak wavelength due to a conformational change that leads to an increase in the quantum yield of FAD bound to the Cb5R. Figure 5 shows that the FAD fluorescence increase depends on the concentration of the Aβ(1–42) and of Aβ(25–35) peptides. Moreover, both the magnitude and the dependence upon the Aβ peptide concentration of the change of FAD fluorescence are not significantly different between Aβ(1–42) and Aβ(25–35). Of note, this is an effect produced by the assayed neurotoxic peptides because up to 1 μM of "scrambled" Aβ(1–42) peptide does not elicit a statistically significant change in FAD fluorescence. The results obtained for the dependence of the increase in FAD fluorescence upon the concentration of Aβ(1–42) and of Aβ(25–35) fit well into the equation for one-site ligand–protein interaction (Figure 5). The non-linear fit of the results to this equation yields an increase of 41 ± 4% of the FAD fluorescence at saturation with these peptides, and an Aβ concentration for 50% of the effect of 75 ± 5 nM of peptide monomer. Since the concentration of Cb5R in the fluorescence assays is 32 ± 3 nM, the real free-peptide concentration at 50% saturation allows us to calculate an apparent dissociation constant ($K_{d,app}$) of 59 ± 5 nM for the complex between the Cb5R and the Aβ peptide. This $K_{d,app}$ value is within the range of values obtained for the Ki, pointing out that the binding of the Aβ peptide to this site causes the inhibition of the NADH-dependent Cb$_5$ reductase activity of the human recombinant Cb5R with a His$_6$-tag. Since the dependence of the FAD fluorescence upon the concentration of Aβ(1–42) was the same in the absence and presence of 5 μM of Cb$_5$, the possibility that Aβ could interact with the Cb$_5$ binding domain in the Cb5R can be excluded. Also, this result indicates that Aβ(1–42) does not bind to Cb$_5$, resulting in further experimental support to our conclusion derived from the lack of effect of Aβ(1–42) on the absorbance spectrum of Cb$_5$ (see above).

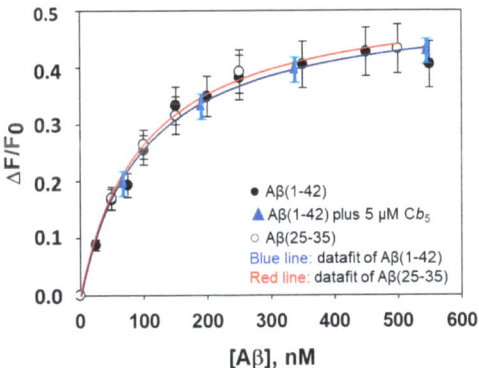

Figure 5. Dependence upon the concentration of Aβ(1–42) and Aβ(25–35) of the increase in FAD fluorescence (ΔF/F0) bound to the human recombinant Cb5R with a His$_6$-tag. There was not a significant difference between the titration of FAD fluorescence with Aβ(1–42) in the absence (filled black circles) and the presence of 5 μM Cb$_5$ (blue triangles). The lines are the results obtained via non-linear regression fit to the equation for 1:1 ligand binding site per protein molecule. The fit of the data yielded the following results: Y = −0.0095 + [0.5227 × x/(96.92 + x)] (R^2 = 0.9870) for Aβ(1–42), and Y = −0.0019 + [0.5311 × x/(99.253 + x)] (R^2 = 0.9974) for Aβ(25–35). The results shown are the means ± S.E.M. of experiments performed in triplicate. Other experimental conditions used for these fluorescence measurements are given in Section 4.

In order to further assess the interaction between Aβ(1–42) and human recombinant Cb5R with a His$_6$-tag, we have used the fluorescent derivative Aβ(1–42) HiLyte^{TM}-Fluor555. This compound can act as a fluorescence resonance energy transfer (FRET) acceptor of FAD fluorescence as illustrated by the overlap between the emission fluorescence spectrum of FAD and the absorbance spectrum (Figure 6A). Next, we calculated the distance for 50% FRET efficiency (R_0) between FAD and Aβ(1–42) HiLyte^{TM}-Fluor555 as described in Section 4, following a protocol used in previous works [61–63]. A value of 3.96×10^{-3} has been calculated for the quantum yield of FAD bound to the Cb5R (Φ_D), using as reference the quantum yield of FMN given in standard fluorescence data tables. A value of the overlap integral J(λ) of 6.0254174×10^{15} cm$^3 \cdot$M^{-1} has been calculated from the recorded emission spectrum of FAD bound to the Cb5R and the absorbance spectrum of Aβ(1–42) HiLyte^{TM}-Fluor555. An R_0 value of 2.77 nm has been obtained by applying the equation given in Section 4, assuming a random orientation between donor and acceptor.

Then, we recorded the emission spectrum of human recombinant Cb5R with a His$_6$-tag in the absence and presence of 100 nM of Aβ(1–42) HiLyte^{TM}-Fluor555 and the emission spectrum of 100 nM Aβ(1–42) HiLyte^{TM}-Fluor555 in the absence of Cb5R (Figure 6B). Next, the latter spectrum, which is due to the direct excitation of the acceptor HiLyte-Fluor555, has been subtracted to the emission spectrum of Cb5R plus 100 nM of Aβ(1–42) HiLyte^{TM}-Fluor555, and the result is shown in Figure 6C. We avoided the use of a saturating concentration of the Aβ(1–42)-induced increase in the FAD fluorescence in Cb5R shown in Figure 5 to prevent the complications of analysis coming from an excessively large peak of the HiLyte^{TM}-Fluor555 fluorescence on the overall emission spectrum. The results shown in Figure 6C indicate that 100 nM of Aβ(1–42) HiLyte^{TM}-Fluor555 produces a 45 ± 5% quenching of the peak donor FAD fluorescence at 525 nm, and a similar increase in the peak of the acceptor HiLyte^{TM}-Fluor555 fluorescence at 555 nm. Thus, FRET measurements provide an additional proof of interaction between Cb5R with a His$_6$-tag and Aβ(1–42) HiLyte^{TM}-Fluor555.

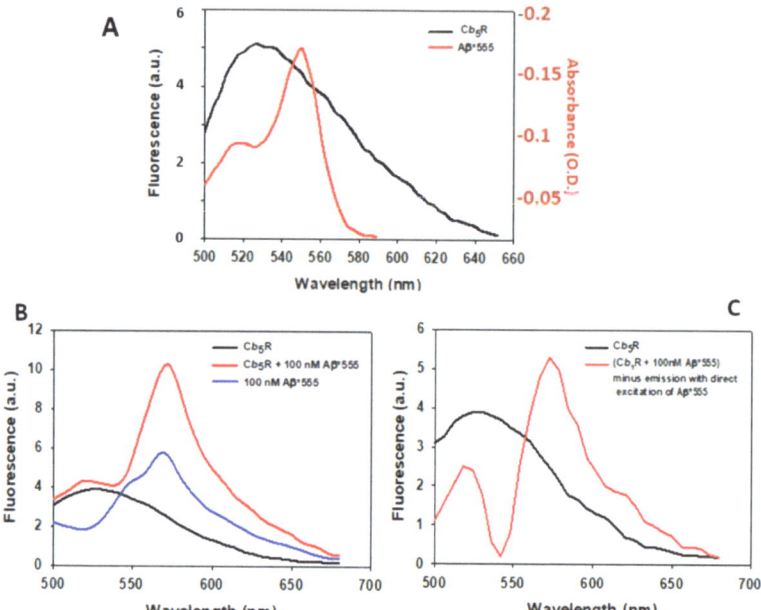

Figure 6. FRET between FAD bound to the human recombinant Cb5R with a His$_6$-tag and Aβ(1–42) HiLyte^{TM}-Fluor555. (**A**) Emission spectrum of the human recombinant Cb5R with a His$_6$-tag with an excitation wavelength of 460 nm (black line) and absorption spectrum of Aβ(1–42) HiLyte^{TM}-Fluor555 (Aβ*555, red line). (**B**) Emission spectra of the human recombinant Cb5R with a His$_6$-tag in the absence (black line) and presence of 100 nM of Aβ(1–42) HiLyte^{TM}-Fluor555 (Aβ*555) (red line), and of 100 nM Aβ(1–42) HiLyte^{TM}-Fluor555 (Aβ*555) in the absence of Cb5R (direct excitation spectrum, blue line). Excitation wavelength = 460 nm, excitation and emission slits =10 nm. (**C**) Emission spectrum of the human recombinant Cb5R with a His$_6$-tag (black line) and the result of the emission spectrum of (Cb5R plus 100 nM of Aβ(1–42) HiLyte^{TM}-Fluor555) after the subtraction of the emission spectrum of 100 nM Aβ(1–42) HiLyte^{TM}- Fluor555 in the absence of Cb5R (red line). Other experimental conditions used for these fluorescence measurements are given in Section 4.

3. Discussion

The results show the interaction between Aβ(1–42) HiLyte^{TM}-Fluor555 and submicromolar concentrations of His$_6$. Likely, this interaction will be further potentiated by transition metal ions, which bind with very high affinity to Aβ(1–42) [2,54], and, also, to His$_6$ [64]. Indeed, we cannot completely exclude that trace amounts of transition metal ions, which are present in the preparations of commercial samples of Aβ peptides and in buffers, are playing a role in the Aβ(1–42) HiLyte^{TM}-Fluor555/His6 complexes formed under our experimental conditions. The kinetics of the increase in Aβ(1–42) HiLyte^{TM}-Fluor555 fluorescence intensity after the addition of His$_6$ is a relatively slow process for this type of molecules, with a half-time of around 10 min, and an initial short lag phase within the first minute. Therefore, the kinetic results suggest the occurrence of conformational changes in the formation of a complex between Aβ(1–42) HiLyte^{TM}-Fluor555 and His$_6$. Also, it is to be noted that a concentration of 100 nM His$_6$ is almost saturating for its complexation with 10 nM Aβ(1–42) HiLyte^{TM}-Fluor555, indicating that the dissociation constant (Kd) of this complex is in the submicromolar concentration range. However, the maximum increase in the Aβ(1–42) HiLyte^{TM}-Fluor555 fluorescence intensity (<10%) is not large enough over the noise of the data to obtain a reliable Kd value for this complex from the dependence upon the His$_6$ concentration using this experimental approach.

Docking simulations provide a rational support for the formation of a complex between His_6 and $A\beta(1-42)$. The simulations performed using the CABS-dock Web Server, which do not require the input of an initial conformation of His_6, yield three-dimensional structures for this complex that can be grouped in three-classes taking into account the $A\beta(1-42)$ peptide domain directly interacting with His_6. Thus, changes in the structure of His_6 are one likely cause of the short initial lag phase of the kinetics of complex formation. On the other hand, the cluster of poses represented by cluster 1 of Figure 2, generated using docking simulations for the $His_6/A\beta(1-42)$ complex, predicts that His_6 interacts with amino acid residues 24–42 of $A\beta(1-42)$. In a previous work [40], we have shown that this domain of $A\beta(1-42)$ is the most directly involved in the formation of $A\beta(1-42)/CaM$ and $A\beta(1-42)/calbindin-D28k$ complexes. However, docking analysis predicts a relevant contribution of LYS28 and LYS16 in the case of the cluster 1 of the $His_6/A\beta(1-42)$ complex, the first cluster ranked by energy calculations, while only highly hydrophobic amino acids of $A\beta(1-42)$ are involved in the interaction interface with CaM and calbindin-D28k [40]. The contribution of electrostatic interactions and H-bonds in the interface of interaction between His_6 and $A\beta(1-42)$ is even stronger in the structures of the cluster 2 of $His_6/A\beta(1-42)$ complex, the second ranked by free energy calculations, as the buried surface area/ accessible solvent area ratio results in the following amino acid residues with higher participation in the interaction with the $A\beta$ peptide: TYR10 > HIS6 > GLU3 > HIS14 > ASP7. Also, the presence of charged amino acids ASP1, GLU3, ARG5, ASP7 and GLU11 in the $A\beta(1-42)$ domain of the interacting interface of cluster 3 of $His_6/A\beta(1-42)$ complex lends further support to the higher relevance of electrostatic interactions in the formation of this complex. Thus, docking analysis points out a higher contribution of electrostatic interactions and H-bonds in the $His_6/A\beta(1-42)$ complex than in $A\beta(1-42)/CaM$ and $A\beta(1-42)/calbindin-D28k$ complexes. Consistent with this analysis, in this work, we show that His_6 efficiently antagonizes the interaction between $A\beta(1-42)$ HiLyte^{TM}-Fluor555 and these two proteins, with concentrations for 50% effect ≤ 1 µM of His_6, values that are more than 10-fold higher than those obtained for the hydrophobic peptide VFAFAMAFML(amidated-C-terminus amino acid) in our previous work [40]. However, it is to be noted that the dye HiLyte^{TM}-Fluor555 is covalently bound to the NH_2-terminus amino acid of $A\beta(1-42)$, which is distant from the amino acid residues 24–42 of $A\beta(1-42)$. Since fluorescence measurements point out that the interaction of His_6 with $A\beta(1-42)$ HiLyte^{TM}-Fluor555 alters the microenvironment of HiLyte^{TM}-Fluor555, it is likely that the structure of the $His_6/A\beta(1-42)$ complex can be better described by a weighted combination of the three different clusters of $His_6/A\beta(1-42)$ complex shown in Figure 2 or that the molecular stoichiometry of this complex is higher than 1:1. Indeed, the cluster 2 in Figure 2, the second most probable model yielded by docking simulations, predicts the binding of His_6 to the NH_2-terminus domain of $A\beta(1-42)$. Nevertheless, the possibility of a significant generation of $3His_6/A\beta(1-42)$ complex is unlikely because of the large difference in free energies between clusters 1 and 3, and, also, because of steric hindrance between the His_6 position in clusters 2 and 3. In addition, a shift between cluster structures during the formation of the $His_6/A\beta(1-42)$ complex could provide a simple explanation for the slow kinetics of interaction between His_6 and $A\beta(1-42)$ HiLyte^{TM}-Fluor555. This is a plausible possibility because docking simulations do not yield large differences of the free energy changes predicted for the clusters 1 and 2 of the $His_6/A\beta(1-42)$ complex. Further extensive experimental studies will be required to obtain the molecular stoichiometry and structure of the $His_6/A\beta(1-42)$ complex with atomic resolution.

The high affinity of His_6 for neurotoxic $A\beta$ peptides, like $A\beta(1-42)$ and $A\beta(25-35)$, is further demonstrated by the results obtained in this work with human recombinant Cb5R with a His_6-tag. First, the inhibition of the Cb_5 reductase activity of human recombinant Cb5R with a His_6-tag by $A\beta(1-42)$ or $A\beta(25-35)$ has a Ki of 50–60 nM of $A\beta$ peptide monomers, while up to 2 µM of $A\beta(1-42)$ monomers produce less than 10% inhibition of this activity of Cb5R after removal of the His_6-tag. Second, this Ki value is not significantly different from the value of the apparent dissociation constant of the complex between

Aβ(1–42) or Aβ(25–35) and human recombinant Cb5R with a His$_6$-tag calculated from titrations with these Aβ peptides of the fluorescence of FAD, the prosthetic group of this enzyme. Since the predominant aggregation state of the Aβ(1–42) solutions used in our experimental conditions is the dimer, see Section 4, our results yield values ≤30 nM of Aβ(1–42) dimers for both Ki and $K_{d,app}$. Thus, we conclude in this work that the His$_6$-tag strongly potentiates the binding of the neurotoxic peptides Aβ(1–42) and Aβ(25–35) to the human recombinant Cb5R. In addition, our results point out that the Cb$_5$ reductase activity of the human recombinant Cb5R minus the His$_6$-tag is not significantly inhibited by up to 2 µM of Aβ(1–42) oligomers, an intracellular concentration that is unlikely to be reached within the cells because the critical concentration for the induction of Aβ(1–42) fibrillization is in the submicromolar range [34,35]. Of note, a 'scrambled' non-toxic Aβ(1–42) peptide used in previous works [27,30] does not bind to the His$_6$-tag of the human recombinant Cb5R, nor produces a significant inhibition of its activity. As the insertion of a His$_6$-tag is widely used to help with the purification of recombinant proteins, this conclusion strongly suggests removing it prior to using these recombinant proteins in studies dealing with the biochemical and biological effects of Aβ(1–42).

The large increase in the intensity of the fluorescence of its prosthetic group FAD monitors the binding of Aβ(1–42) and Aβ(25–35) to human recombinant Cb5R with a His$_6$-tag. Since the catalytic site does not overlap with the position of the His$_6$-tag bound to the NH$_2$-terminus amino acid of Cb5R, the inhibition by Aβ(1–42) or Aβ(25–35) of its Cb$_5$ reductase activity is due to a long-distance induced conformational change. Taking into account that 100 nM of Aβ(1–42) HiLyte^{TM}-Fluor555 lies between 60 and 65% of the saturating concentration of Cb5R (Figure 5), we can calculate that at a saturation by Aβ(1–42) HiLyte^{TM}-Fluor555, the quenching of the donor FAD fluorescence will rise up to 70 ± 7%. As at this concentration of Aβ(1–42), the peptide will be in equilibrium between monomers and dimers [58], we have calculated the most probable distance range between FAD and the dye HiLyte^{TM}-Fluor555 using the equation for FRET for 1 and 2 acceptors per donor with the assumption of random orientation given in Section 4. The upper distance limit of this range will be set by the case of the two acceptors HiLyte^{TM}-Fluor555 dyes, one bound to each monomer, located equidistant from the donor FAD. The calculated distances between the donor FAD group of Cb5R and the acceptor HiLyte^{TM}-Fluor555 dye covalently linked to Aβ(1–42) have been 2.35 nm and 3.1 nm for 1 or 2 equidistant acceptors, respectively. Of note, the measurements of the anisotropy of the FAD fluorescence, performed as indicated in Section 4, presented anisotropy values lower than 0.005. As noted in [65], with this low value of donor anisotropy, there is >90% probability that the above-calculated distance range is correct. In order to evaluate whether the structural coupling between the known structures of the Cb5R and Aβ(1–42) allows for the satisfaction of this requirement, we have performed docking between the soluble human erythrocytes isoform of Cb5R (PDB ID: 1UMK) and Aβ(1–42) (PDB ID: 1IYT) using the ClusPro Web Server as described in Section 4. Among the 10 model structures generated in silico, we selected the model structure of the complex between Cb5R and Aβ(1–42) shown in Figure 7, in which the Aβ(1–42) lies close to the His$_6$-tag bound to the NH$_2$-terminus amino acid of the human recombinant Cb5R. This model structure satisfies the above distance requirement between the NH$_2$-terminus amino acid of the Aβ(1–42) and FAD derived from FRET measurements, which can be estimated between 2 and 3 nm by taking into account the uncertainty of the orientation and size of the HiLyte^{TM}-Fluor555 dye in the complex. In addition, this model structure shows that the amino acids 25–35 of the Aβ(1–42) lies near the catalytic center, where the isoalloxazine ring of the FAD prosthetic group of the Cb5R is located. Also, the Cb$_5$ binding site in the Cb5R, identified in previous works [66,67], lies close to the FAD group in the protein domain located as shown below in Figure 7. The extensive overlap of the 25–35 amino acid residues of the Aβ(1–42) with the Cb$_5$ domain suggests that steric hindrance and/or an incorrect orientation of bound Cb$_5$ could account for the inhibition of the Cb$_5$ reductase activity measured in this work.

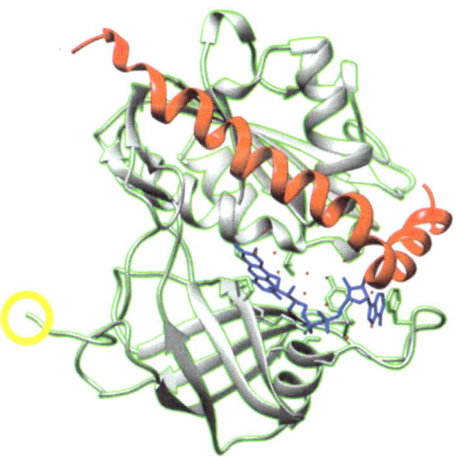

Figure 7. Simulation generated using docking between the soluble human erythrocytes isoform of Cb5R (PDB ID: 1UMK) and Aβ(1–42) (PDB ID: 1IYT) using the ClusPro Web Server. The polypeptide backbone of Cb5R is shown in gray/green, with the position of the prosthetic group FAD in blue, and the Aβ(1–42) is shown in red. The NH_2-terminus amino acid of the Cb5R is labeled with a yellow circle.

In summary, His_6 binds with high affinity to Aβ(1–42), and at micromolar concentrations antagonizes the formation of Aβ(1–42)/CaM and Aβ(1–42)/calbindin-D28k complexes. In addition, a His_6-tag provides a high-affinity site for the binding of neurotoxic Aβ(1–42) and Aβ(25–35) peptides to the human recombinant Cb5R, and sensitizes this enzyme to inhibition by these peptides. Therefore, our results suggest that a His_6-tag could be used to experimentally direct the action of neurotoxic Aβ peptides toward selected cellular targets.

4. Materials and Methods

4.1. Chemicals

Human Aβ(1–42)-HiLyte™-Fluor555 was purchased from AnaSpec (Freemont, CA, USA). Aβ(1–42), Aβ(25–35) and Aβ 'scrambled' were supplied by StabVida (Caparica, Portugal) and GenicBio Limited (Shanghai, China). His_6 was purchased from Quimigen (Madrid, Spain). Bovine brain CaM and Thrombin Clean Cleavage™ kit were purchased from Merck-Sigma-Aldrich (Madrid, Spain).

All the other chemicals used in this work were of analytical grade and supplied by Merck-Sigma-Aldrich (Madrid, Spain) and ThermoFisher Scientific (Madrid, Spain).

4.2. Preparation of Aβ(1–42) Solutions

Stock Aβ(1–42) solutions were prepared by dissolving the lyophilized peptide at 4 mg/mL in 1% NH_4OH. Later, the stock Aβ(1–42) solution was diluted in phosphate-buffered saline to a concentration of 177 μM. The aggregation state of Aβ(1–42) in the 177 μM solution has been assessed in Tricine–sodium dodecyl sulfate–polyacrylamide gel electrophoresis (SDS-PAGE) as described in our previous works [27,40]. As shown in [27,40], in this solution, dimers account for approximately 90% of Aβ(1–42) and trimers for ≤10%, while monomers and higher molecular species are almost undetectable.

4.3. Preparation of the Human Recombinant Cb5R Soluble Isoform

Clones of the soluble isoform of human Cb5R prepared in a previous work were used to express and purify the recombinant protein purified as indicated in [67]. The purified protein was aliquoted and conserved in 30% glycerol at −80 °C until use.

The C-terminal His$_6$-tag recombinant Cb5R has a thrombin-cutting site between the His$_6$-tag and the enzyme, as previously shown [67]. The His$_6$-tag was cut by overnight incubation at 4 °C with the Thrombin Clean Cleavage^{TM} kit. The recombinant Cb5R minus the His$_6$-tag was separated from the cleaved peptide via column chromatography through Sephadex G75 (1 × 25 cm), and the efficient removal of the His$_6$-tag was confirmed using SDS-PAGE (Figure 8).

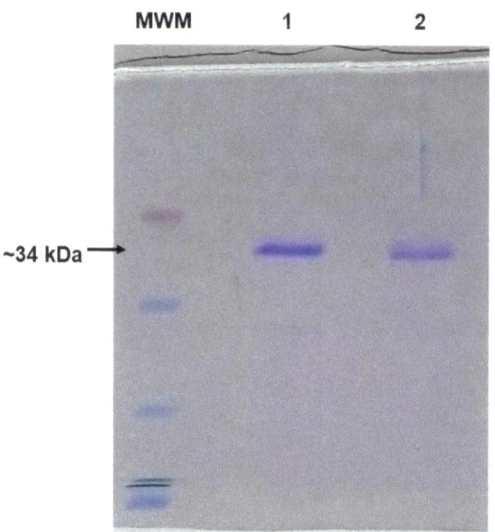

Figure 8. SDS-PAGE of human recombinant Cb5R. Lane 1: His$_6$-tagged Cb5R. Lane 2: Cb5R after the removal of His$_6$ by treatment with the Thrombin Clean Cleavage^{TM} kit and passage through a Sephadex G75 column. MWM, lane of molecular weight markers. The gel showed that the treatment with the Thrombin Clean Cleavage^{TM} kit produced the expected decrease of ~1 kDa in the molecular weight and no further proteolytic degradation of Cb5R.

The concentration of recombinant Cb5R was determined using the method of Bradford, with bovine serum albumin as standard or from absorbance measurements at 450 nm, using an extinction coefficient of 11.3 mM$^{-1}\cdot$cm^{-1} for the FAD prosthetic group [67,68].

4.4. Preparation of the Human Recombinant Calbindin-D28k and Cb$_5$

The human recombinant calbindin-D28k and soluble isoform of Cb$_5$ have been expressed and purified as described in detail in previous works [40,67,69]. The purified protein were aliquoted and conserved in 30% glycerol at −80 °C until use.

The concentration of recombinant Cb5R was determined using the method of Bradford with bovine serum albumin as standard or from absorbance measurements at 550 nm using a differential extinction coefficient between reduced and oxidized Cb$_5$ of 16.5 mM$^{-1}\cdot$cm^{-1}, as in previous works [67,69].

4.5. Measurements of His$_6$, CaM and Calbindin-D28k Interaction with Aβ(1–42) HiLyte^{TM}-Fluor555

The change of the fluorescence intensity of Aβ(1–42) HiLyte^{TM}-Fluor555 has been used to monitor its complexation with His$_6$, CaM and calbindin-D28k. Fluorescence measurements were performed using a Fluoromax+ fluorescence Spectrophotometer (Horiba Jobin Yvon IBH Ltd., Glasgow, UK) in quartz cuvettes of 1cm light pathlength with a total volume of 2.5 mL at room temperature (24–25 °C), with excitation and emission slits of 5 nm.

The measurements of the kinetics of fluorescence have been performed in buffer 50 mM N-[2-hydroxyethyl] piperazine-N'-[2-ethanesulfonic acid], 100 mM KCl and 50 µM $CaCl_2$ (pH 7.05). The cuvette was kept with magnetic stirring in the dark within the cuvette holder of the fluorimeter until stabilization of the fluorescence intensity after the addition of 10 nM Aβ(1–42) HiLyte™-Fluor555, routinely between 20 and 40 min. Then, His_6 was added to the cuvette at the concentrations indicated in the figures, and the fluorescence intensity was recorded as a function of time with excitation and emission wavelengths of 520 nm and 567 nm, respectively. His_6 was added from stock concentrated solutions prepared in the assay buffer, such that the total added volume was always lower than 10 µL. Control experiments were run by adding the same volume of the assay buffer, and showed no significant changes in the fluorescence intensity of Aβ(1–42) HiLyte™-Fluor555.

In the experiments dealing with the effect of His_6 on the kinetics of fluorescence intensity increase after the addition of 5 nM CaM or calbindin-D28k, these proteins were added after 15 min preincubation with the indicated concentration of His_6. CaM and calbindin-D28k were added from concentrated stock solutions freshly prepared in the assay buffer used in the fluorescence measurements, such that the total added volume was always lower than 10 µL.

4.6. In Silico Docking between Aβ(1–42) and His_6

These docking studies have been performed using the MDockPeP Server (https://zougrouptoolkit.missouri.edu/mdockpep/index.html), accessed on 26 November 2022. This server generates structural simulations of complexes between proteins and peptides, requiring only the input of the PDB file of the protein and the amino acids sequence of the peptide. In this work, we have used the Aβ(1–42) (PDB: 1IYT) as the protein partner. The server generates the 10 more probable poses for the complex formation, on the basis of the results after three major steps: (1) calculation of peptide conformers, in our case, of His_6; (2) global flexible sampling of the binding modes protein–peptide; and (3) score and classification of the evaluated types of bonds involved in the formation of the complex [70]. Interacting interfaces were analyzed using PDBePISA [71], access date 4–5 October 2023, and they were visualized using UCSF Chimera [72].

4.7. Titration with Aβ(1–42) and Aβ(25–35) of the NADH-Dependent Cb_5 Reductase Activity of the Cb5R

The measurements were performed with a Shimadzu UV1800 spectrophotometer at a wavelength of 550 nm in 1 mL cuvettes containing the assay buffer 20 mM phosphate/0.1 mM diethylenetriaminepentaacetic acid (pH 7), with 0.11 µg of Cb5R/mL and 5 µM of Cb_5 in the absence and presence of the concentrations of Aβ(1–42), Aβ(25–35) and 'scrambled' Aβ(1–42), indicated in the figures. The reaction was started by the addition of 0.25 mM NADH after 10 min preincubation of the Cb5R in the assay medium, and initial rates were measured during periods of time ranging between 5 and 10 min, with a less than 10% drop in the Cb_5 concentration in the assay cuvette. The Cb_5 reductase activity was calculated from the change of absorbance at 550 nm using a differential extinction coefficient between reduced and oxidized Cb_5 of 16.5 $mM^{-1} \cdot cm^{-1}$, as in previous works [67,69]. The titration of the NADH-dependent Cb_5 reductase activity of the Cb5R with the Aβ peptide was carried out by measuring in each assay cuvette the activity before and after the addition of each concentration of the Aβ peptide, in order to have an internal control of the activity in the absence of the Aβ peptide to cancel putative minor differences in Cb5R pipetting. The volume of Aβ peptide solution added ranged between 1 and 2.5 µL, pipetted from a freshly prepared solution of a prefixed concentration by dilution of aliquots of the stock solution in the assay buffer.

4.8. Titration with Aβ(1–42) and Aβ(25–35) of the FAD Fluorescence of Human Recombinant Cb5R with a His_6-Tag and FRET Analysis

The FAD fluorescence of human recombinant Cb5R with a His_6-tag (32 nM) has been measured at 25 °C with a Perkin Elmer 650-40 spectrofluorometer in quartz cuvettes of 1 cm pathlength with excitation and emission wavelengths of 460 nm and 520 nm, respectively, and excitation and emission slits of 10 nm. The assay buffer was 20 mM phosphate/0.1 mM diethylenetriaminepentaacetic acid (pH 7). We noticed that the FAD fluorescence of the recombinant enzyme displays a small but steady increase as a function of time. This indicates a weak instability of the recombinant Cb5R in these experimental conditions because its denaturation produces around a 1000-fold increase in the FAD fluorescence [67]. Due to this, the operational protocol for data acquisition was as follows: after recording the drift of the fluorescence intensity of the Cb5R in the assay buffer for 5 min, Aβ peptides were added at the concentrations indicated in the figures and the fluorescence intensity was recorded for another 5 min. The increase in fluorescence produced by each Aβ peptide concentration shown in the figures was corrected by the drift of fluorescence intensity drift recorded before the addition of the Aβ peptide.

The steady-state anisotropy of fluorescence, r_s, has been calculated from the polarization of fluorescence (P) using the equation [73]:

$$r_s = 2 \times P/(3 - P). \tag{1}$$

Polarization of fluorescence, P, was calculated using the equation:

$$P = [I_\| - G \times I_\perp]/[I_\| + G \times I_\perp], \tag{2}$$

where $I_\|$ and $I_\perp$ are the fluorescence intensities measured with parallel (0°/0°) and perpendicularly (0°/90°) oriented polarizers, respectively, and G is the correction factor for polarization characteristics of the emission monochromator [62,63,73]. A value of G of 1.04 ± 0.02 has been obtained for our fluorimeter and used in our calculations.

The distance (d) between the Cb5R prosthetic group FAD and the dye HiLyte^{TM}-Fluor555 covalently bound to Aβ(1–42), which form a donor–acceptor FRET pair, has been calculated for the cases of 1 and 2 acceptors per donor. In the case of multiple acceptors per donor, the rate constant of total FRET (k_T) is the sum of the rate constant of FRET between each donor–acceptor pair (k_i) that can be formed in the assembly [74–77]. The total FRET efficiency (E) is the sum of the FRET efficiency for each donor–acceptor pair that is possible with the geometrical constraints of the system [74–76]. For each donor–acceptor pair, we have used the equation for FRET: $E = d^{-6}/(R_0^{-6} + d^{-6})$ [62]. In this equation, E is the FRET efficiency and R_0 is the distance for 50% FRET efficiency between FAD and HiLyte^{TM}-Fluor555. The value of R_0 has been calculated in this work using the operational protocol followed from previous works for other FRET donor–acceptor pairs [61–63]. Briefly, we have applied the equation [62]:

$$R_0 = 9.7 \times 10^3 \times [K^2 \times \Phi D \times J(\lambda) \times n^{-4}]^{1/6} \times Å \tag{3}$$

with the assumption of random orientation between donor and acceptor ($K^2 = 2/3$) and the relative refraction index of an aqueous medium (n = 1.33). The quantum yield of the donor (Φ_D) and the overlap integral, $J(\lambda)$, have been calculated as indicated in Section 2 of this article.

4.9. In Silico Docking Simulation between Aβ(1–42) and Cb5R

Docking between Aβ(1–42) and Cb5R has been performed using the ClusPro server with the following PDB files: Aβ(1–42) (PDB ID: 1IYT) and Cb5R (PDB ID: 1UMK), access date 29 January 2019. The images and analysis of the model structures were built up with the UCSF Chimera software.

4.10. Statistical Analysis

All the results are means ± standard error of the mean (S.E.M.) of experiments performed, at least, in triplicate.

Supplementary Materials: The following supporting information can be downloaded at: https://www.mdpi.com/article/10.3390/molecules28207138/s1, Figure S1: PDB files of the ten most probable model structures generated using the MDockPeP Server for the His$_6$/Aβ(1–42) complex; Table S1: Supplementary Table S1; Table S2: Supplementary Table S2; Table S3: Supplementary Table S3.

Author Contributions: Conceptualization, C.G.-M. and A.K.S.-A.; methodology, J.S., A.K.S.-A. and C.G.-M.; software, J.S., A.K.S.-A. and C.G.-M.; validation, J.S., A.K.S.-A. and C.G.-M.; formal analysis, J.S. and C.G.-M.; investigation, J.S., A.K.S.-A. and C.G.-M.; resources, C.G.-M.; data curation, J.S. and C.G.-M.; writing—original draft preparation, J.S. and C.G.-M.; writing—review and editing, J.S., A.K.S.-A. and C.G.-M.; supervision, C.G.-M.; project administration, C.G.-M.; funding acquisition, C.G.-M. All authors have read and agreed to the published version of the manuscript.

Funding: This work has been supported by Grant BFU2017-85723-P of the Spanish Ministerio de Ciencia, Innovación y Universidades (Spanish National R&D program), which received co-financiation by the European Funds for Structural Development (FEDER). Jairo Salazar was supported with a Fellowship of the Spanish Fundación Carolina (Madrid, Spain).

Institutional Review Board Statement: Not applicable.

Informed Consent Statement: Not applicable.

Data Availability Statement: Data supporting the reported results can be found in the laboratory archives of the authors.

Acknowledgments: We would like to thank for the support and organization of the Special Issue dedicated to Carlos Gutiérrez-Merino: "Themed Issue in Honor of Carlos Gutiérrez Merino: Forty Years of Research Excellence in the Field of Membrane Proteins and Bioenergetics".

Conflicts of Interest: The authors declare no conflict of interest. The funders had no role in the design of the study; in the collection, analyses, or interpretation of data; in the writing of the manuscript; or in the decision to publish the results.

Abbreviations

Aβ	amyloid β peptides
AD	Alzheimer's disease
CaM	calmodulin
Cb$_5$	cytochrome b_5
Cb5R	cytochrome b_5 reductase
ER	endoplasmic reticulum
FAD	flavine adenine dinucleotide
FMN	flavine mononucleotide
FRET	fluorescence resonance energy transfer
His$_6$	hexa-histidine
$K_{d,app}$	apparent dissociation constant
K_i	inhibition constant
SDS-PAGE	sodium dodecyl sulfate polyacrylamide gel electrophoresis
S.E.M.	standard error of the mean

References

1. Younkin, S.G. The role of Aβ 42 in Alzheimer's disease. *J. Physiol. Paris* **1998**, *92*, 289–292. [CrossRef] [PubMed]
2. Lovell, M.A.; Robertson, J.D.; Teesdale, W.J.; Campbell, J.L.; Markesbery, W.R. Copper, iron and zinc in Alzheimer's disease senile plaques. *J. Neurol. Sci.* **1998**, *158*, 47–52. [CrossRef] [PubMed]
3. Mucke, L.; Selkoe, D.J. Neurotoxicity of Amyloid β-Protein: Synaptic and Network Dysfunction. *Cold Spring Harb. Perspect. Med.* **2012**, *2*, 1–18. [CrossRef] [PubMed]
4. Walsh, D.M.; Klyubin, I.; Fadeeva, J.V.; Cullen, W.K.; Anwyl, R.; Wolfe, M.S.; Rowan, M.J.; Selkoe, D.J. Naturally Secreted Oligomers of Amyloid β Protein Potently Inhibit Hippocampal Long-Term Potentiation in Vivo. *Nature* **2002**, *416*, 535–539. [CrossRef]
5. Gong, Y.; Chang, L.; Viola, K.L.; Lacor, P.N.; Lambert, M.P.; Finch, C.E.; Krafft, G.A.; Klein, W.L. Alzheimer's Disease-Affected Brain: Presence of Oligomeric Aβ Ligands (ADDLs) Suggests a Molecular Basis for Reversible Memory Loss. *Proc. Natl. Acad. Sci. USA* **2003**, *100*, 10417–10422. [CrossRef]

6. Knobloch, M.; Konietzko, U.; Krebs, D.C.; Nitsch, R.M. Intracellular Aβ and cognitive deficits precede β-amyloid deposition in transgenic arcAβ mice. *Neurobiol. Aging* **2007**, *28*, 1297–1306. [CrossRef]
7. Shankar, G.M.; Li, S.; Mehta, T.H.; Garcia-Munoz, A.; Shepardson, N.E.; Smith, I.; Brett, F.M.; Farrell, M.A.; Rowan, M.J.; Lemere, C.A.; et al. Amyloid β-Protein Dimers Isolated Directly from Alzheimer Brains Impair Synaptic Plasticity and Memory. *Nat. Med.* **2008**, *14*, 837–842. [CrossRef]
8. Hu, X.; Crick, S.L.; Bu, G.; Frieden, C.; Pappu, R.V.; Lee, J.-M. Amyloid seeds formed by cellular uptake, concentration, and aggregation of the amyloid-β peptide. *Proc. Natl. Acad. Sci. USA* **2009**, *106*, 20324–20329. [CrossRef] [PubMed]
9. Friedrich, R.P.; Tepper, K.; Rönicke, R.; Soom, M.; Westermann, M.; Reymann, K.; Kaether, C.; Fändrich, M. Mechanism of amyloid plaque formation suggests an intracellular basis of Aβ pathogenicity. *Proc. Natl. Acad. Sci. USA* **2010**, *107*, 1942–1947. [CrossRef]
10. He, Y.; Zheng, M.M.; Ma, Y.; Han, X.J.; Ma, X.Q.; Qu, C.Q.; Du, Y.F. Soluble Oligomers and Fibrillar Species of Amyloid β-Peptide Differentially Affect Cognitive Functions and Hippocampal Inflammatory Response. *Biochem. Biophys. Res. Commun.* **2012**, *429*, 125–130. [CrossRef]
11. Forny-Germano, L.; Lyra e Silva, N.M.; Batista, A.F.; Brito-Moreira, J.; Gralle, M.; Boehnke, S.E.; Coe, B.C.; Lablans, A.; Marques, S.A.; Martinez, A.M.; et al. Alzheimer's Disease-like Pathology Induced by Amyloid-β Oligomers in Nonhuman Primates. *J. Neurosci.* **2014**, *34*, 13629–13643. [CrossRef] [PubMed]
12. Wirths, O.; Multhaup, G.; Czech, C.; Blanchard, V.; Moussaoui, S.; Tremp, G.; Pradier, L.; Beyreuther, K.; Bayer, T.A. Intraneuronal Aβ accumulation precedes plaque formation in β-amyloid precursor protein and presenilin-1 double-transgenic mice. *Neurosci. Lett.* **2001**, *306*, 116–120. [CrossRef] [PubMed]
13. Oddo, S.; Caccamo, A.; Shepherd, J.D.; Murphy, M.P.; Golde, T.E.; Kayed, R.; Metherate, R.; Mattson, M.P.; Akbari, Y.; LaFerla, F.M. Triple-transgenic model of Alzheimer's disease with plaques and tangles: Intracellular Aβ and synaptic dysfunction. *Neuron* **2003**, *39*, 409–421. [CrossRef] [PubMed]
14. Oakley, H.; Cole, S.L.; Logan, S.; Maus, E.; Shao, P.; Craft, J.; Guillozet-Bongaarts, A.; Ohno, M.; Disterhoft, J.; Van Eldik, L.; et al. Intraneuronal β-amyloid aggregates, neurodegeneration, and neuron loss in transgenic mice with five familial Alzheimer's disease mutations: Potential factors in amyloid plaque formation. *J. Neurosci.* **2006**, *26*, 10129–10140. [CrossRef]
15. Millucci, L.; Ghezzi, L.; Bernardini, G.; Santucci, A. Conformations and biological activities of amyloid beta peptide 25–35. *Curr. Protein Pept. Sci.* **2010**, *11*, 54–67. [CrossRef] [PubMed]
16. Pike, C.J.; Walencewicz-Wasserman, A.J.; Kosmoski, J.; Cribbs, D.H.; Glabe, C.G.; Cotman, C.W. Structure-activity analyses of beta-amyloid peptides: Contributions of the beta 25–35 region to aggregation and neurotoxicity. *J. Neurochem.* **1995**, *64*, 253–265. [CrossRef] [PubMed]
17. Frozza, R.L.; Horn, A.P.; Hoppe, J.B.; Simão, F.; Gerhardt, D.; Comiran, R.A.; Salbego, C.G. A comparative study of beta-amyloid peptides Abeta1–42 and Abeta25–35 toxicity in organotypic hippocampal slice cultures. *Neurochem. Res.* **2009**, *34*, 295–303. [CrossRef] [PubMed]
18. Choo-Smith, L.P.; Garzon-Rodriguez, W.; Glabe, C.G.; Surewicz, W.K. Acceleration of amyloid fibril formation by specific binding of Aβ-(1–40) peptide to ganglioside containing membrane vesicles. *J. Biol. Chem.* **1997**, *272*, 22987–22990. [CrossRef]
19. Kakio, A.; Nishimoto, S.I.; Yanagisawa, K.; Kozutsumi, Y.; Matsuzaki, K. Cholesterol dependent formation of GM1 ganglioside-bound amyloid β-protein, an endogenous seed for Alzheimer amyloid. *J. Biol. Chem.* **2001**, *276*, 24985–24990. [CrossRef] [PubMed]
20. Kakio, A.; Nishimoto, S.; Yanagisawa, K.; Kozutsumi, Y.; Matsuzaki, K. Interactions of amyloid β-protein with various gangliosides in raft-like membranes: Importance of GM1 ganglioside-bound form as an endogenous seed for Alzheimer amyloid. *Biochemistry* **2002**, *41*, 7385–7390. [CrossRef]
21. Wood, W.G.; Schroeder, F.; Igbavboa, U.; Avdulov, N.A.; Chochina, S.V. Brain membrane cholesterol domains, aging and amyloid beta-peptides. *Neurobiol. Aging* **2002**, *23*, 685–694. [CrossRef] [PubMed]
22. Matsuzaki, K.; Kato, K.; Yanagisawa, K. Aβ polymerization through interaction with membrane gangliosides. *Biochim. Biophys. Acta* **2010**, *1801*, 868–877. [CrossRef] [PubMed]
23. Kawarabayashi, T.; Shoji, M.; Younkin, L.H.; Wen-Lang, L.; Dickson, D.W.; Murakami, T.; Matsubara, E.; Abe, K.; Ashe, K.H.; Younkin, S.G. Dimeric amyloid beta protein rapidly accumulates in lipid rafts followed by apolipoprotein E and phosphorylated tau accumulation in the Tg2576 mouse model of Alzheimer's disease. *J. Neurosci.* **2004**, *24*, 3801–3809. [CrossRef] [PubMed]
24. Williamson, R.; Usardi, A.; Hanger, D.P.; Anderton, B.H. Membrane-bound beta-amyloid oligomers are recruited into lipid rafts by a fyn-dependent mechanism. *FASEB J.* **2008**, *22*, 1552–1559. [CrossRef] [PubMed]
25. Lai, A.Y.; McLaurin, J.A. Mechanisms of Amyloid-Beta Peptide Uptake by Neurons: The Role of Lipid Rafts and Lipid Raft-Associated Proteins. *Int. J. Alzheimer's Dis.* **2011**, *2011*, 548380. [CrossRef]
26. Jin, S.; Kedia, N.; Illes-Toth, E.; Haralampiev, I.; Prisner, S.; Herrmann, A.; Wanker, E.E.; Bieschke, J. Amyloid-β(1–42) Aggregation Initiates Its Cellular Uptake and Cytotoxicity. *J. Biol. Chem.* **2016**, *291*, 19590–19606. [CrossRef]
27. Poejo, J.; Salazar, J.; Mata, A.M.; Gutierrez-Merino, C. Binding of Amyloid β(1–42)-Calmodulin Complexes to Plasma Membrane Lipid Rafts in Cerebellar Granule Neurons Alters Resting Cytosolic Calcium Homeostasis. *Int. J. Mol. Sci.* **2021**, *22*, 1984. [CrossRef]
28. Umeda, T.; Tomiyama, T.; Sakama, N.; Tanaka, S.; Lambert, M.P.; Klein, W.L.; Mori, H. Intraneuronal Amyloid β Oligomers Cause Cell Death Via Endoplasmic Reticulum Stress, Endosomal/Lysosomal Leakage, and Mitochondrial Dysfunction In Vivo. *J. Neurosci. Res.* **2011**, *89*, 1031–1042. [CrossRef]

29. Cha, M.Y.; Han, S.H.; Son, S.M.; Hong, H.-S.; Choi, Y.-J.; Byun, J.; Mook-Jung, I. Mitochondria-Specific Accumulation of Amyloid β Induces Mitochondrial Dysfunction Leading to Apoptotic Cell Death. *PLoS ONE* **2012**, *7*, e34929. [CrossRef]
30. Poejo, J.; Orantos-Aguilera, Y.; Martin-Romero, F.J.; Mata, A.M.; Gutierrez-Merino, C. Internalized Amyloid-β (1-42) Peptide Inhibits the Store-Operated Calcium Entry in HT-22 Cells. *Int. J. Mol. Sci.* **2022**, *23*, 12678. [CrossRef]
31. Podlisny, M.B.; Walsh, D.M.; Amarante, P.; Ostaszewski, B.L.; Stimson, E.R.; Maggio, J.E.; Teplow, D.B.; Selkoe, D.J. Oligomerization of endogenous and synthetic amyloid β-protein at nanomolar levels in cell culture and stabilization of monomer by Congo red. *Biochemistry* **1998**, *37*, 3602–3611. [CrossRef]
32. Selkoe, D.J. Alzheimer's disease: Genes, proteins, and therapy. *Physiol. Rev.* **2001**, *81*, 741–766. [CrossRef]
33. Cleary, J.P.; Walsh, D.M.; Hofmeister, J.J.; Shankar, G.M.; Kuskowski, M.A.; Selkoe, D.J.; Ashe, K.H. Natural oligomers of the amyloid-β protein specifically disrupt cognitive function. *Nat. Neurosci.* **2005**, *8*, 79–84. [CrossRef] [PubMed]
34. Hellstrand, E.; Boland, B.; Walsh, D.M.; Linse, S. Amyloid β-protein aggregation produces highly reproducible kinetic data and occurs by a two-phase process. *ACS Chem. Neurosci.* **2009**, *1*, 13–18. [CrossRef] [PubMed]
35. Hamley, I.W. The amyloid beta peptide: A chemist's perspective. Role in Alzheimer's and fibrillization. *Chem. Rev.* **2012**, *112*, 5147–5192. [CrossRef] [PubMed]
36. Corbacho, I.; Berrocal, M.; Török, K.; Mata, A.M.; Gutierrez-Merino, C. High affinity binding of amyloid β-peptide to calmodulin: Structural and functional implications. *Biochem. Biophys. Res. Commun.* **2017**, *486*, 992–997. [CrossRef]
37. Laurén, J.; Gimbel, D.A.; Nygaard, H.B.; Gilbert, J.W.; Strittmatter, S.M. Cellular prion protein mediates impairment of synaptic plasticity by amyloid-β oligomers. *Nat. Cell Biol.* **2009**, *457*, 1128–1132. [CrossRef]
38. Dunning, C.J.; McGauran, G.; Willén, K.; Gouras, G.K.; O'Connell, D.J.; Linse, S. Direct High Affinity Interaction between Aβ42 and GSK3α Stimulates Hyperphosphorylation of Tau. A New Molecular Link in Alzheimer's Disease? *ACS Chem. Neurosci.* **2015**, *7*, 161–170. [CrossRef]
39. Guo, J.-P.; Arai, T.; Miklossy, J.; McGeer, P.L. Aβ and tau form soluble complexes that may promote self-aggregation of both into the insoluble forms observed in Alzheimer's disease. *Proc. Natl. Acad. Sci. USA* **2006**, *103*, 1953–1958. [CrossRef]
40. Salazar, J.; Poejo, J.; Mata, A.M.; Samhan-Arias, A.K.; Gutierrez-Merino, C. Design and Experimental Evaluation of a Peptide Antagonist against Amyloid β(1–42) Interactions with Calmodulin and Calbindin-D28k. *Int. J. Mol. Sci.* **2022**, *23*, 2289. [CrossRef]
41. Baimbridge, K.G.; Celio, M.R.; Rogers, J.H. Calcium-binding proteins in the nervous system. *Trends Neurosci.* **1992**, *15*, 303–308. [CrossRef]
42. Kuchibhotla, K.V.; Goldman, S.T.; Lattarulo, C.R.; Wu, H.Y.; Hyman, B.T.; Bacskai, B.J. Aβ Plaques Lead to Aberrant Regulation of Calcium Homeostasis in Vivo Resulting in Structural and Functional Disruption of Neuronal Networks. *Neuron* **2008**, *59*, 214–225. [CrossRef] [PubMed]
43. Lopez, R.; Lyckman, A.; Oddo, S.; Laferla, F.M.; Querfurth, H.W.; Shtifman, A. Increased Intraneuronal Resting [Ca^{2+}] in Adult Alzheimer's Disease Mice. *J. Neurochem.* **2008**, *105*, 262–271. [CrossRef] [PubMed]
44. Berridge, M.J. Calcium Signalling and Alzheimer's Disease. *Neurochem. Res.* **2011**, *36*, 1149–1156. [CrossRef] [PubMed]
45. Poejo, J.; Salazar, J.; Mata, A.M.; Gutierrez-Merino, C. The Relevance of Amyloid β-Calmodulin Complexation in Neurons and Brain Degeneration in Alzheimer's Disease. *Int. J. Mol. Sci.* **2021**, *22*, 4976. [CrossRef]
46. dos Santos, V.V.; Santos, D.B.; Lach, G.; Rodrigues, A.L.; Farina, M.; De Lima, T.C.; Prediger, R.D. Neuropeptide Y (NPY) prevents depressive-like behavior, spatial memory deficits and oxidative stress following amyloid-β [Aβ(1–40)] administration in mice. *Behav. Brain Res.* **2013**, *244*, 107–115. [CrossRef]
47. Kang, S.; Moon, N.R.; Kim, D.S.; Kim, S.H.; Park, S. Central acylated ghrelin improves memory function and hippocampal AMPK activation and partly reverses the impairment of energy and glucose metabolism in rats infused with β-amyloid. *Peptides* **2015**, *71*, 84–93. [CrossRef]
48. Santos, V.V.; Stark, R.; Rial, D.; Silva, H.B.; Bayliss, J.A.; Lemus, M.B.; J S Davies, J.S.; Cunha, R.A.; Prediger, R.D.; Andrews, Z.B. Acyl ghrelin improves cognition, synaptic plasticity deficits and neuroinflammation following amyloid β (Aβ1-40) administration in mice. *J. Neuroendocrinol.* **2017**, *29*, 1–11. [CrossRef] [PubMed]
49. Martins, I.; Gomes, S.; Costa, R.O.; Otvos, L.; Oliveira, C.R.; Resende, R.; Pereira, C.M.F. Leptin and ghrelin prevent hippocampal dysfunction induced by Aβ oligomers. *Neuroscience* **2013**, *241*, 41–51. [CrossRef]
50. Gomes, S.; Martins, I.; Fonseca, A.C.; Oliveira, C.R.; Resende, R.; Pereira, C.M. Protective effect of leptin and ghrelin against toxicity induced by amyloid-β oligomers in a hypothalamic cell line. *J. Neuroendocrinol.* **2014**, *26*, 176–185. [CrossRef]
51. Poon, I.K.; Patel, K.K.; Davis, D.S.; Parish, C.R.; Hulett, M.D. Histidine-rich glycoprotein: The Swiss Army knife of mammalian plasma. *Blood* **2011**, *117*, 2093–2101. [CrossRef]
52. Potocki, S.; Valensinb, D.; Kozlowski, H. The specificity of interaction of Zn^{2+}, Ni^{2+} and Cu^{2+} ions with the histidine-rich domain of the TjZNT1 ZIP family transporter. *Dalton Trans.* **2014**, *43*, 10215–10223. [CrossRef] [PubMed]
53. Priebatsch, K.M.; Kvansakul, M.; Poon, I.K.; Hulett, M.D. Functional Regulation of the Plasma Protein Histidine-Rich Glycoprotein by Zn^{2+} in Settings of Tissue Injury. *Biomolecules* **2017**, *7*, 22. [CrossRef] [PubMed]
54. Atwood, C.S.; Scarpa, R.C.; Huang, X.; Moir, R.D.; Jones, W.D.; Fairlie, D.P.; Tanzi, R.E.; Bush, A.I. Characterization of copper interactions with alzheimer amyloid beta peptides: Identification of an attomolar-affinity copper binding site on amyloid beta1-42. *J. Neurochem.* **2000**, *75*, 1219–1233. [CrossRef] [PubMed]
55. Teplyakov, A.; Obmolova, G.; Canziani, G.; Zhao, Y.; Gutshall, L.; Jung, S.S.; Gilliland, G.L. His-tag binding by antibody C706 mimics β-amyloid recognition. *J. Mol. Recognit.* **2011**, *24*, 570–575. [CrossRef] [PubMed]

56. Rojo, L.; Sjöberg, M.K.; Hernández, P.; Zambrano, C.; Maccioni, R.B. Roles of cholesterol and lipids in the etiopathogenesis of Alzheimer's disease. *BioMed Res. Int.* **2006**, *2006*, 073976. [CrossRef]
57. Lee, H.J.; Korshavn, K.J.; Kochi, A.; Derrick, J.S.; Lim, M.H. Cholesterol and metal ions in Alzheimer's disease. *Chem. Soc. Rev.* **2014**, *43*, 6672–6682. [CrossRef]
58. Andreetto, E.; Yan, L.M.; Tatarek-Nossol, M.; Velkova, A.; Frank, R.; Kapurniotu, A. Identification of Hot Regions of the Aβ–IAPP Interaction Interface as High-Affinity Binding Sites in both Cross- and Self-Association. *Angew. Chem. Int. Ed.* **2010**, *49*, 3081–3085. [CrossRef]
59. Samhan-Arias, A.K.; Maia, L.B.; Cordas, C.M.; Moura, I.; Gutierrez-Merino, C.; Moura, J. Peroxidase-like activity of cytochrome b_5 is triggered upon hemichrome formation in alkaline pH. *Biochim. Biophys. Acta BBA-Proteins Proteom.* **2018**, *1866*, 373–378. [CrossRef]
60. Samhan-Arias, A.K.; Cordas, C.M.; Carepo, M.S.; Maia, L.B.; Gutierrez-Merino, C.; Moura, I.; Moura, J. Ligand accessibility to heme cytochrome b_5 coordinating sphere and enzymatic activity enhancement upon tyrosine ionization. *J. Biol. Inorg. Chem.* **2019**, *24*, 317–330. [CrossRef] [PubMed]
61. Gutierrez-Merino, C.; Molina, A.; Escudero, B.; Diez, A.; Laynez, J. Interaction of the Local Anesthetics Dibucaine and Tetracaine with Sarcoplasmic Reticulum Membranes. Differential Scanning Calorimetry and Fluorescence Studies. *Biochemistry* **1989**, *28*, 3398–3406. [CrossRef]
62. Centeno, F.; Gutierrez-Merino, C. Location of Functional Centers in the Microsomal Cytochrome P450 System. *Biochemistry* **1992**, *31*, 8473–8481. [CrossRef] [PubMed]
63. Tiago, T.; Aureliano, M.; Gutiérrez-Merino, C. Decavanadate binding to a high affinity site near the myosin catalytic centre inhibits F-actin-stimulated myosin ATPase activity. *Biochemistry* **2004**, *43*, 5551–5561. [CrossRef] [PubMed]
64. Riguero, V.; Clifford, R.; Dawley, M.; Dickson, M.; Gastfriend, B.; Thompson, C.; Wang, S.C.; O'Connor, E. Immobilized metal affinity chromatography optimization for poly-histidine tagged proteins. *J. Chromatogr. A* **2020**, *1629*, 461505. [CrossRef] [PubMed]
65. Stryer, L. Fluorescence Energy Transfer as a Spectroscopic Ruler. *Annu. Rev. Biochem.* **1978**, *47*, 819–846. [CrossRef] [PubMed]
66. Gutiérrez-Merino, C.; Martínez-Costa, O.H.; Monsalve, M.; Samhan-Arias, A.K. Structural Features of Cytochrome b_5–Cytochrome b_5 Reductase Complex Formation and Implications for the Intramolecular Dynamics of Cytochrome b_5 Reductase. *Int. J. Mol. Sci.* **2022**, *23*, 118. [CrossRef] [PubMed]
67. Samhan-Arias, A.K.; Almeida, R.M.; Ramos, S.; Cordas, C.M.; Moura, I.; Gutierrez-Merino, C.; Moura, J. Topography of human cytochrome b_5/cytochrome b_5 reductase interacting domain and redox alterations upon complex formation. *Biochim. Biophys. Acta BBA-Proteins Proteom.* **2018**, *1859*, 78–87. [CrossRef]
68. van den Berg, P.A.; Widengren, J.; Hink, M.A.; Rigler, R.; Visser, A.J. Fluorescence correlation spectroscopy of flavins and flavoenzymes: Photochemical and photophysical aspects. *Spectrochim. Acta. Part A Mol. Biomol. Spectrosc.* **2001**, *57*, 2135–2144. [CrossRef]
69. Gómez-Tabales, J.; García-Martín, E.; Agúndez, J.; Gutierrez-Merino, C. Modulation of CYP2C9 activity and hydrogen peroxide production by cytochrome b_5. *Sci. Rep.* **2020**, *10*, 15571. [CrossRef]
70. Xu, X.; Yan, C.; Zou, X. MDockPeP: An ab-initio protein-peptide docking server. *J. Comput. Chem.* **2018**, *39*, 2409–2413. [CrossRef]
71. Krissinel, E., Henrick, K. Inference of macromolecular assemblies from crystalline state. *J. Mol. Biol.* **2007**, *372*, 774–797. [CrossRef] [PubMed]
72. Pettersen, E.F.; Goddard, T.D.; Huang, C.C.; Couch, G.S.; Greenblatt, D.M.; Meng, E.C.; Ferrin, T.E. UCSF Chimera--a visualization system for exploratory research and analysis. *J. Comput. Chem.* **2004**, *25*, 1605–1612. [CrossRef] [PubMed]
73. Lakowicz, J.R. *Principles of Fluorescence Spectroscopy*, 3rd ed.; Springer: New York, NY, USA, 2010; ISBN 978-0-387-31278-1.
74. Gutiérrez-Merino, C. Quantitation of the Forster Energy Transfer for Bidimensional Systems: I) Lateral Phase Separation in Unilamellar Vesicles Formed by Binary Phospholipid Mixtures. *Biophys. Chem.* **1981**, *14*, 247–257. [CrossRef]
75. Gutiérrez-Merino, C. Quantitation of the Forster Energy Transfer for Bidimensional Systems: II) Protein Distribution and Aggregation State in Biological Membranes. *Biophys. Chem.* **1981**, *14*, 259–266. [CrossRef] [PubMed]
76. Gutiérrez-Merino, C.; Centeno, F.; García Martín, E.; Merino, J.M. Fluorescence energy transfer as a tool to locate functional sites in membrane proteins. *Biochem. Soc. Trans.* **1994**, *22*, 784–788. [CrossRef] [PubMed]
77. Gutiérrez-Merino, C.; Bonini de Romanelli, I.C.; Pietrasanta, L.I.; Barrantes, F.J. Preferential distribution of the fluorescent phospholipid probes NBD phosphatidylcholine and rhodamine phosphatidylethanolamine in the exofacial leaflet of acetylcholine receptor rich membranes from *Torpedo marmorata*. *Biochemistry* **1995**, *34*, 4846–4855. [CrossRef] [PubMed]

Disclaimer/Publisher's Note: The statements, opinions and data contained in all publications are solely those of the individual author(s) and contributor(s) and not of MDPI and/or the editor(s). MDPI and/or the editor(s) disclaim responsibility for any injury to people or property resulting from any ideas, methods, instructions or products referred to in the content.

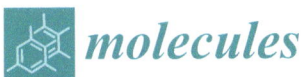

Article

Store-Operated Calcium Entry Inhibition and Plasma Membrane Calcium Pump Upregulation Contribute to the Maintenance of Resting Cytosolic Calcium Concentration in A1-like Astrocytes

Joana Poejo [1,†], María Berrocal [1,2,†], Lucía Saez [2], Carlos Gutierrez-Merino [1,*] and Ana M. Mata [1,2,*]

1. Instituto de Biomarcadores de Patologías Moleculares (IBPM), Universidad de Extremadura, 06006 Badajoz, Spain; joanapoejo86@gmail.com (J.P.); mabeca@unex.es (M.B.)
2. Departamento de Bioquímica y Biología Molecular y Genética, Facultad de Ciencias, Universidad de Extremadura, 06006 Badajoz, Spain; lucia.sm.9682@gmail.com
* Correspondence: biocgm@gmail.com (C.G.-M.); anam@unex.es (A.M.M.)
† These authors contributed equally to this work.

Abstract: Highly neurotoxic A1-reactive astrocytes have been associated with several human neurodegenerative diseases. Complement protein C3 expression is strongly upregulated in A1 astrocytes, and this protein has been shown to be a specific biomarker of these astrocytes. Several cytokines released in neurodegenerative diseases have been shown to upregulate the production of amyloid β protein precursor (APP) and neurotoxic amyloid β (Aβ) peptides in reactive astrocytes. Also, aberrant Ca^{2+} signals have been proposed as a hallmark of astrocyte functional remodeling in Alzheimer's disease mouse models. In this work, we induced the generation of A1-like reactive astrocytes after the co-treatment of U251 human astroglioma cells with a cocktail of the cytokines TNF-α, IL1-α and C1q. These A1-like astrocytes show increased production of APP and Aβ peptides compared to untreated U251 cells. Additionally, A1-like astrocytes show a $(75 \pm 10)\%$ decrease in the Ca^{2+} stored in the endoplasmic reticulum (ER), $(85 \pm 10)\%$ attenuation of Ca^{2+} entry after complete Ca^{2+} depletion of the ER, and three-fold upregulation of plasma membrane calcium pump expression, with respect to non-treated Control astrocytes. These altered intracellular Ca^{2+} dynamics allow A1-like astrocytes to efficiently counterbalance the enhanced release of Ca^{2+} from the ER, preventing a rise in the resting cytosolic Ca^{2+} concentration.

Keywords: A1 astrocytes; complement component C3; amyloid β; cytosolic calcium; intracellular calcium homeostasis; store-operated calcium entry; plasma membrane calcium pump

Citation: Poejo, J.; Berrocal, M.; Saez, L.; Gutierrez-Merino, C.; Mata, A.M. Store-Operated Calcium Entry Inhibition and Plasma Membrane Calcium Pump Upregulation Contribute to the Maintenance of Resting Cytosolic Calcium Concentration in A1-like Astrocytes. *Molecules* **2023**, *28*, 5363. https://doi.org/10.3390/molecules28145363

Academic Editor: Pietro Campiglia

Received: 6 June 2023
Revised: 30 June 2023
Accepted: 11 July 2023
Published: 12 July 2023

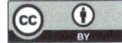

Copyright: © 2023 by the authors. Licensee MDPI, Basel, Switzerland. This article is an open access article distributed under the terms and conditions of the Creative Commons Attribution (CC BY) license (https://creativecommons.org/licenses/by/4.0/).

1. Introduction

Neuroinflammatory cytokines secreted by activated microglia in the brain can induce the generation of A1-reactive astrocytes that are highly neurotoxic [1–3]. Also, it has been reported that neurotoxic A1 astrocytes are abundant in post-mortem brain samples of the neurodegenerative diseases most prevalent in humans, like Alzheimer's and Parkinson's diseases, as well as in Huntington's disease, amyotrophic lateral sclerosis and multiple sclerosis [3]. Three cytokines secreted by activated microglia, interleukin-1α (IL-1α), tumor necrosis factor-α (TNF-α) and complement component 1q (C1q), acting together, are necessary and sufficient to induce the generation of highly neurotoxic A1 astrocytes [3]. Since astrocytes are the most abundant brain cells and are required for neuronal survival and for the maintenance of blood–brain barrier integrity [4], the production of A1 astrocytes is a harmful threat in brain degeneration. Indeed, astrocytes are increasingly viewed as critical contributors to neurological disorders [5]. A1 astrocytes can secrete pro-inflammatory mediators that induce neuroinflammation [3,5–7], which eventually lead to blood–brain barrier integrity breakdown and brain edema formation. Also, it has been proposed that A1 astrocytes secrete a yet-unknown neurotoxin that potentiates neuronal death [6]. Moreover, in a previous work, we showed that the induction of A1 astrocytes in rat brains through the intraperitoneal administration of 3-nitropropionic acid (NPA), an animal model of Huntington's disease, precedes the brain damage leading to motor neurological dysfunction in NPA-induced neurodegeneration [8]. The complement component C3 has been widely used as a specific marker of A1 astrocyte generation [3,8,9], because C3 expression is strongly upregulated in A1-reactive astrocytes.

In addition, it has been shown that reactive astrocytes induced via 2-chloroethanol poisoning can stimulate microglia polarization and microglia activation [10], leading to a feed-forward cycle that is harmful to specific brain structures. Furthermore, reactive astrocytes induced by cytokines such as interleukin-1β, TNF-α and interferon-γ have been shown to upregulate the production of amyloid β protein precursor (APP) and β-site APP-cleaving enzyme 1 (BACE1), and secrete neurotoxic amyloid β (Aβ) peptides [11–14]. In our recent work with rats treated through the intraperitoneal administration of NPA, we noticed an enhanced production of neurotoxic Aβ peptides in the brain areas displaying the generation of A1 astrocytes, namely, the striatum and hippocampus, which are also the brain regions most prone to NPA-induced degeneration [9]. The challenging possibility of an enhanced production of neurotoxic Aβ peptides in A1 astrocytes cannot be reliably concluded from our results from the animal model, and deserves to be experimentally assessed in a cell culture model.

Although astrocytes are electrically non-excitable cells, intracellular calcium signaling plays a major role in the modulation of their activities [15,16], which is critical for the activity and normal functioning of proximal neurons in the brain. As noted by [16], spontaneous astrocyte calcium transients of similar magnitude and frequency have been shown in vitro, in situ and in vivo, and these events have been suggested to facilitate the synchronization of nearby neuronal activity [17,18]. In older mice with amyloid plaques, the proportion of astrocytes with calcium oscillations has been reported to be increased, along with the amplitudes of those oscillations [19]. Indeed, aberrant Ca^{2+} signals have been proposed as a hallmark of astrocyte functional remodeling in Alzheimer's disease (AD) mouse models [19,20]. However, to the best of our knowledge, the putative changes in intracellular calcium homeostasis associated with the transformation of normal astrocytes into neurotoxic A1 astrocytes have not been reported elsewhere.

On the other hand, experimental evidence of intracellular calcium dysregulation by Aβ is now overwhelming (see [21] for a recent review). Aβ is a recognized hallmark of AD, and intraneuronal Aβ accumulation has been suggested to be an early pathological biomarker for the onset of AD [22]. Mutations in presenilins (PSENs), which contribute to over 90% of familial AD cases, can also modulate capacitative calcium entry, a refilling mechanism for depleted Ca^{2+} stores [23–25], and mutations in the PSEN2 gene enhance Ca^{2+} release from the endoplasmic reticulum (ER) through inositol trisphosphate receptors [26]. In turn, the increase in cytosolic calcium leads to calmodulin-mediated stimulation of the amyloidogenic protease BACE1 [27]. In addition, the treatment of neuronal and neuroblastoma cells with 1 μM soluble Aβ(1–42) increased BACE1 transcription, an effect that was reverted by an anti-Aβ(1–42) antibody [28]. Therefore, Aβ generates a positive feedback loop for Aβ production. Also, attenuated Ca^{2+} entry through store-operated calcium entry (SOCE) is consistently observed in sporadic AD and in skin fibroblasts from familial AD patients [29]. Recently, we showed that the Ca^{2+} entry through SOCE is highly sensitive to Aβ, because intracellular nanomolar concentrations of the Aβ oligomer can bind to stromal interaction molecule 1 (STIM1) and produce significant inhibition of Ca^{2+} entry [30]. On the other hand, the overexpression of plasma membrane calcium pumps (PMCAs) in striatal astrocytes has been shown to inhibit intracellular Ca^{2+} signals [31]. Interestingly, the modulation of PMCA activity has been suggested to be involved in the counterbalance of early cytosolic Ca^{2+} upregulation in primary cortical mouse astrocytes caused by Aβ [32]. These authors reported that the Aβ(25–35) fragment potentiated PMCA-mediated Ca^{2+}

extrusion in Aβ-conditioned primary cultures of astrocytes, leading to the diminution of cytosolic calcium concentration.

On these grounds, the aims of this work were to set up the experimental conditions of treatment with a cocktail of the cytokines IL-1α, TNFα and C1q to induce A1-like astrocytes in U251 cells in culture, in order to evaluate their capability to express APP and Aβ peptides, and to study the putative alterations of SOCE, resting cytosolic calcium concentration and PMCA expression levels in A1-like human astrocytic U251 cells compared to Control (untreated) cells.

2. Results

2.1. Selection of A1-like Astrocytes Using C3 Expression as Biomarker

After the treatment of U251 astrocytes with an inflammatory-mediator cocktail of cytokines, the larger cells with thick and large extensions display an expression of C3 several times higher than untreated Control U251 astrocytes, which are thinner and more elongated, and of much smaller size (see representative images in Figure 1). The analysis of the intensity of fluorescence in the images of cells stained with the anti-C3 antibody labeled with a secondary fluorescent antibody, acquired with the same exposure time (Figure 1), point out an increase in approximately 2.4 times (SEM ± 0.3) the expression level of C3 in the soma of A1-like astrocytes with respect to the non-transformed Control U251 astrocytes.

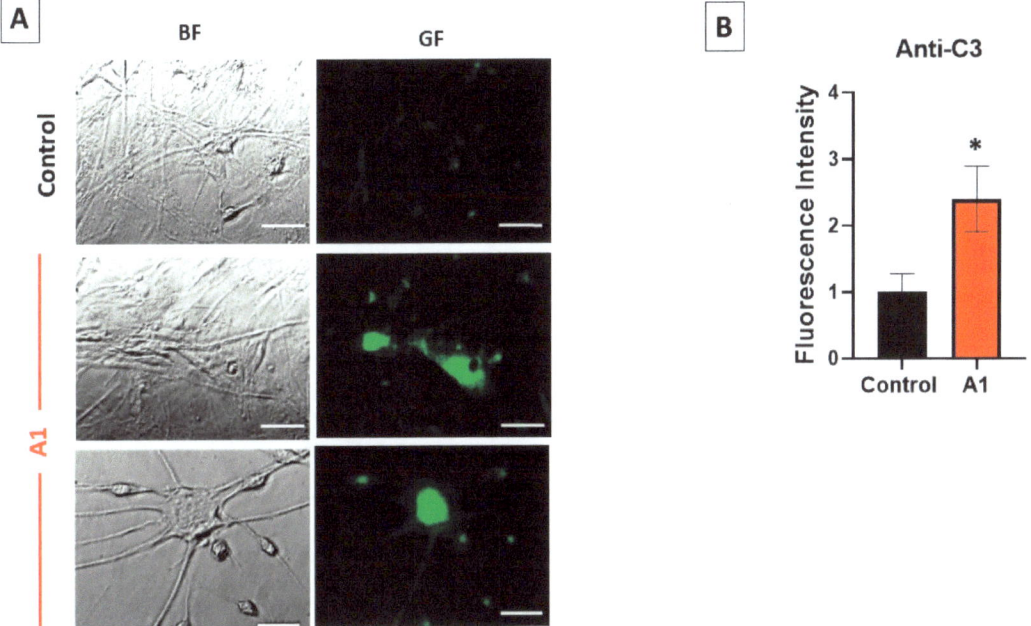

Figure 1. Enhanced expression of C3 in U251 astrocytes after treatment with the cytokines TNF-α (30 ng/mL), IL-1α (3 ng/mL) and C1q (400 ng/mL) for 24 h. (**A**) Representative fluorescence microscopy images of untreated U251 astrocytes (Control) and A1-like astrocytes induced by the treatment with a cocktail of cytokines stained with the anti-C3 antibody, as indicated in the Materials and Methods. All images were acquired with the same exposure time (0.3 s) using the Hamamatsu HCImage software of the fluorescence microscope. BF and GF stand for bright field and green fluorescence, respectively. The size of scale bars included in the microscopy images is 25 μm. (**B**) Mean ± SEM (standard error of the means) values of the fluorescence intensity of the soma of the Control (n = 21 cells) and A1-like astrocytes (n = 46 cells) stained with the anti-C3 antibody. Statistical analysis was carried out using the Student's t-test. (*) $p < 0.05$ with respect to the Control.

The enhanced expression of C3 in A1-like astrocytes was also experimentally assessed in the whole cell culture using Western blot. Figure 2A shows an increase in band intensities corresponding to C3b or C3 (~175–185 kDa) and to the C3α subunit (~116 kDa) in U251 astrocytes treated with cytokines (A1-like astrocytes), with respect to the untreated Control U251 astrocytes. The polyvinylidene difluoride (PVDF) membrane was cut below 70 kDa, and the lower part was used to quantify glyceraldehyde-3-phosphate dehydrogenase (GAPDH), which was selected as a marker to evaluate the protein load per lane. The quantitative analysis of band signal intensities relative to those of GAPDH shows a consistent increase in the expression of C3b or C3 and of the C3α subunit after the treatment of U251 astrocytes with cytokines (Figure 2B). Of note, the increase in C3/C3b expression is much higher than the increase in the C3α protein. Overall, the increase in the C3/C3b protein band is consistent with the large increase in immunoreactivity against the anti-C3 antibody observed via fluorescence microscopy in the giant cells with thick and large extensions after the treatment of U251 astrocytes with cytokines.

2.2. A1-like Astrocytes Express Higher Levels of Aβ Peptides Than Control U251 Astrocytes

Recently, we reported that an increase in A1 astrocytes during 3-nitropropionic acid-induced brain neurodegeneration was correlated with an increase in neurotoxic Aβ peptide production in the damaged brain areas [9]. Furthermore, several studies have shown that reactive astrocytes in culture can produce neurotoxic Aβ peptides [14,33,34]. On these grounds, we tested the possibility that U251-derived A1-like astrocytes also produce neurotoxic Aβ peptides.

Figure 3 shows that the treatment of U251 astrocytes with cytokines elicits enhanced immunostaining, with the anti-Aβ antibody labeled with a secondary fluorescent antibody. In addition, immunostaining with the anti-Aβ antibody reveals a non-homogeneous intracellular distribution of Aβ toxic peptides and APP (Figure 3A), suggesting its association with intracellular organelles, as we previously reported in the HT-22 neuronal cell line [30]. The intensity of fluorescence images of large cells of A1-like astrocytes with thick extensions, which are those strongly stained with the anti-C3 antibody, is approximately 5 times (SEM ± 0.5) higher in A1-like astrocytes with respect to the non-transformed Control U251 astrocytes acquired with the same exposure time (Figure 3B). An analysis of Aβ expression was also carried out via dot blot (Figure 3C), using the same anti-Aβ antibody. As shown, the treatment of U251 astrocytes with cytokines significantly increased the expression of Aβ peptides with respect to the non-treated cells.

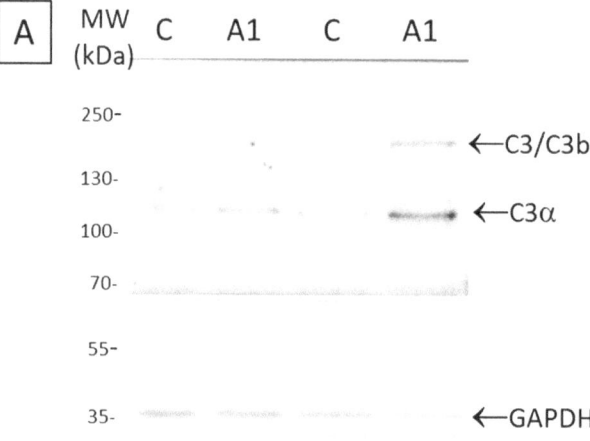

Figure 2. Cont.

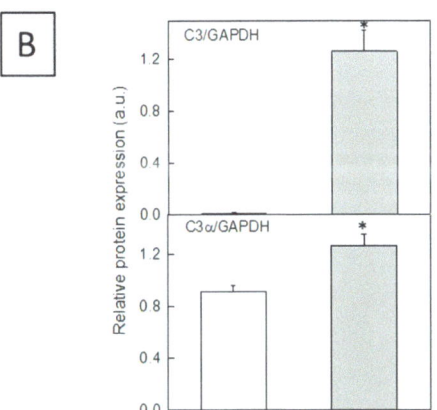

Figure 2. Expression of C3 in homogenates from astrocyte (U251 cell line) cultures. (**A**) Twenty-microgram homogenates from U251 cells untreated (C) or treated (A1-like) with TNF-α (30 ng/mL), IL-1α (3 ng/mL) and C1q (400 ng/mL) were loaded onto a 7.5–20% SDS-polyacrylamide gel, electro-transferred to a PVDF membrane, and immunostained with the anti-C3 antibody JF10-30. Representative blots from two different cultures are shown. The anti-GAPDH antibody was used as a protein loading Control. (**B**) The expression of C3 was quantified using Western blots from homogenates of four different Control and A1-like astrocytes cultures. Data were normalized to GAPDH and are represented as mean ± SEM values in arbitrary units. Statistical analysis was carried out using the Student's t-test. (*) $p < 0.05$ with respect to each Control.

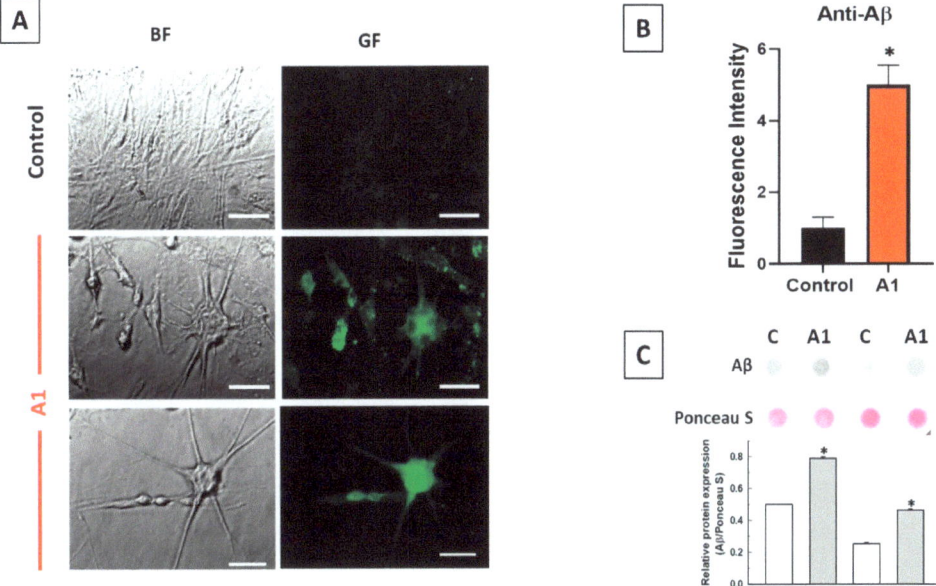

Figure 3. Enhanced expression of Aβ peptides in U251 astrocytes after treatment with the cytokines TNF-α (30 ng/mL), IL-1α (3 ng/mL) and C1q (400 ng/mL) for 24 h. (**A**) Representative fluorescence microscopy images of untreated U251 astrocytes (Control) and A1-like astrocytes induced by treatment with cytokines stained with the anti-Aβ antibody 6E10, as indicated in the Materials and

Methods. All images were acquired with the same exposure time (0.3 s) using the Hamamatsu HCImage software of the fluorescence microscope. BF and GF stand for bright field and green fluorescence, respectively. The size of scale bars included in the microscopy images is 25 µm. (**B**) Mean ± SEM values of the fluorescence intensity of the soma of the Control ($n = 19$ cells) and A1-like astrocytes ($n = 37$ cells) stained with the anti-Aβ antibody. Statistical analysis was carried out using the Student's *t*-test. (*) $p < 0.05$ with respect to the Control. (**C**) The expression of Aβ in homogenates from untreated (C) or treated (A1-like) U251 astrocytes was also quantified via dot blot, using 12 µg of homogenates and the anti-Aβ antibody, as described in the Materials and Methods. Representative dot blots from two different Control and A1-like astrocyte cultures are shown. Data were normalized to total protein stain using Ponceau S and are represented as mean ± SEM values in arbitrary units. (*) $p < 0.05$ with respect to each Control.

2.3. Store-Operated Calcium Entry (SOCE) Is Largely Decreased during the Transformation of U251 Astrocytes in A1-like Astrocytes

Neurotoxic Aβ peptides have been shown to impair intracellular calcium homeostasis in brain cells [21,35,36]. Moreover, several ER proteins have been shown to be involved in Aβ(1–42) production, and also in the Aβ(1–42) dysregulation of intracellular calcium, reviewed in [21]. In a recent work, we reported that nanomolar concentrations of the Aβ(1–42) peptide can inhibit SOCE [30]. Therefore, we experimentally measured the SOCE response in U251 astrocytes treated with cytokines and in untreated Control U251 astrocytes (Figure 4).

We selected as A1-like astrocytes the cells displaying a higher expression of C3, monitored with the anti-C3 antibody, after the treatment with cytokines. Among them, we selected for intracellular Ca^{2+} measurements only larger cells with thick extensions that also had higher levels of Aβ, detected with the anti-Aβ(1–42) antibody, because they are the most reliable for the analysis of fluorescence intensity changes using the region of interest (ROI) tool of the HCImage software of our fluorescence microscope. Figure 4B shows that the peaks of the thapsigargin (Tg)-induced release of Ca^{2+} from the ER and the Ca^{2+} entry after depletion of the ER with Tg are largely decreased in these A1-like astrocytes with respect to the Control U251 astrocytes not treated with cytokines. The analysis of the results show a $(75 \pm 10)\%$ decrease in Tg-induced Ca^{2+} release from the ER and $(85 \pm 10)\%$ inhibition of Ca^{2+} entry after depletion of the ER with Tg (Figure 4C).

2.4. The Cytosolic Ca^{2+} Concentration Does Not Increase during the Transformation of U251 Astrocytes in A1-like Astrocytes, Which Express Higher Levels of PMCA Than the Control U251 Astrocytes

The above results show a decrease in Ca^{2+} stored in the ER in A1-like astrocytes. In addition, large A1-like astrocytes with thick extensions loaded with Fluo3 display higher-intensity fluorescence than the Control U251 astrocytes untreated with cytokines. Therefore, we measured cytosolic Ca^{2+} concentration to experimentally assess the possibility that the enhanced release of Ca^{2+} from the ER can lead to a sustained increase in cytosolic calcium concentration in A1-like astrocytes. The cytosolic Ca^{2+} concentration was measured as described in the Materials and Methods. Although Fluo3-loaded A1-like astrocytes display a higher intensity of fluorescence, our results point out that the A1-like astrocytes uptake Fluo3 more efficiently than the Control astrocytes not treated with cytokines, because the analysis of these results show cytosolic Ca^{2+} concentrations of 66 ± 19 nM and 82 ± 24 nM for the A1-like astrocytes ($n = 8$ cells) and for the Control astrocytes ($n = 28$ cells), respectively. These results were further confirmed using Fura2-loaded astrocytes.

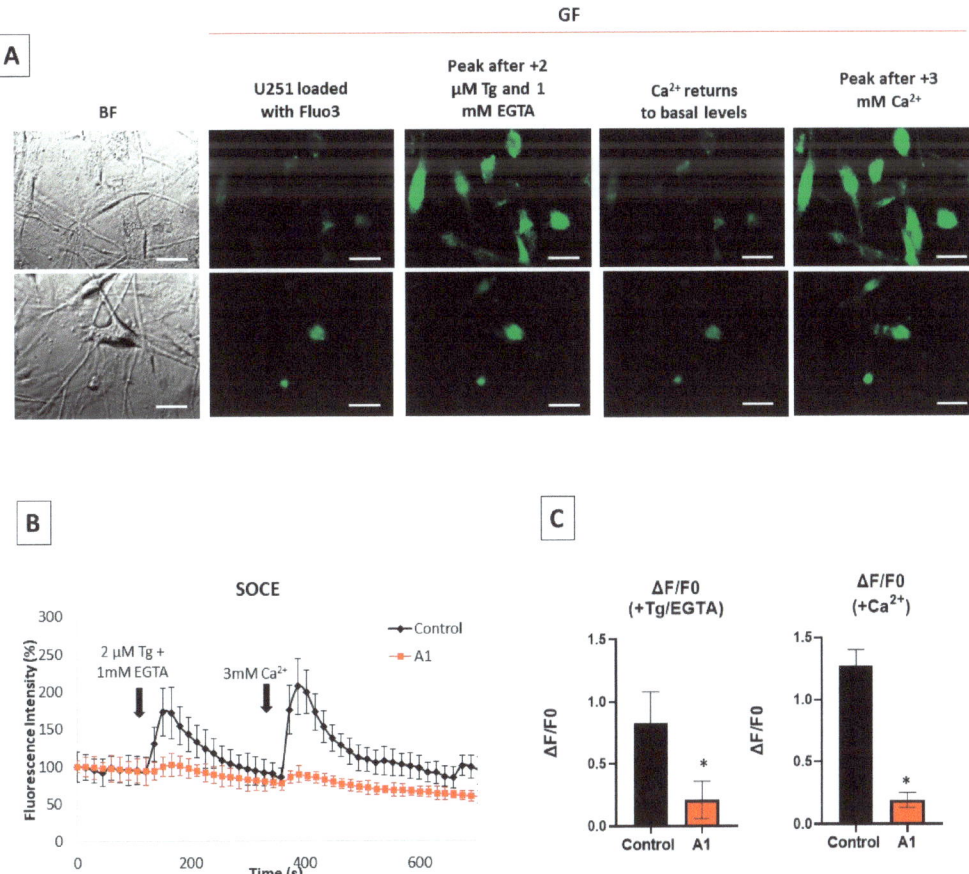

Figure 4. SOCE inhibition in U251 astrocytes after treatment with the cytokines TNF-α (30 ng/mL), IL-1α (3 ng/mL) and C1q (400 ng/mL) for 24 h. Untreated (Control) and treated U251 cells were loaded with 5 μM Fluo-3-pentaacetoxymethyl ester (Fluo3 AM) and 0.025% Pluronic® F-127 for 1 h to experimentally evaluate Ca^{2+} imaging of SOCE. (**A**) Representative microscopy images of Fluo3-loaded untreated U251 astrocytes (Control) and cells treated with the cytokines (reactive A1-like astrocytes), acquired during SOCE experiments. The size of the scale bars included in the microscopy images is 25 μm. (**B**) Representative kinetic traces of untreated U251 astrocytes (black trace) and reactive A1-like astrocytes (red trace) after the addition of 2 μM Tg plus 1 mM ethyleneglycoltetraacetic acid (EGTA), indicated by the first arrow, for Ca^{2+} release from stores and after the addition of 3 mM Ca^{2+} to monitor Ca^{2+} entry through the plasma membrane (indicated by the second arrow). (**C**) Means of the average fluorescence intensity (ΔF/F0) relative to the Control, after the addition of Tg + EGTA (Ca^{2+} release from stores) or after the addition of Ca^{2+} (Ca^{2+} entry). Data are presented as the mean ± SEM values of the experiments, performed in triplicate with $n = 30$ Control U251 cells, and $n = 9$ reactive A1-like astrocytes. Statistical analysis was carried out using the Student's *t*-test. (*) $p < 0.05$ with respect to each Control.

Since PMCAs play a key role in Ca^{2+} extrusion and an increase in PMCA expression during development has been showed in astrocytes cultured in vitro [37], next, we measured the putative changes in the expression level of PMCAs induced by the treatment of U251 astrocytes with cytokines (Figure 5). The results show that PMCA is upregulated in

A1-like astrocytes, which express around a three-fold (SEM ± 0.6) higher level of PMCAs relative to the Control U251 astrocytes not treated with cytokines.

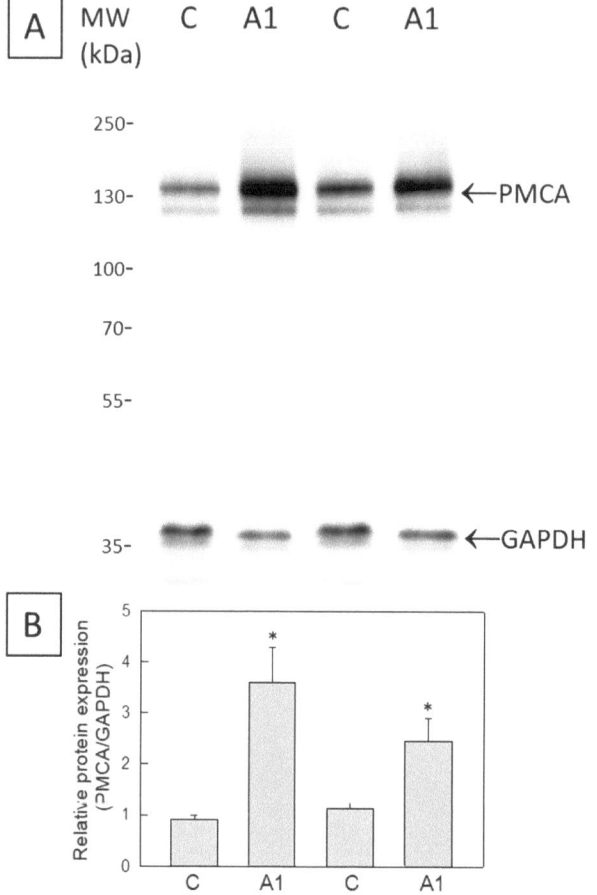

Figure 5. Expression of PMCA in homogenates from astrocyte (U251 cell line) cultures. (**A**) Twenty-microgram homogenates from U251 cells untreated (C) or treated (A1-like astrocytes) with TNF-α (30 ng/mL), IL-1α (3 ng/mL) and C1q (400 ng/mL), were loaded onto a 10% SDS-polyacrylamide gel, electrotransferred to a PVDF membrane, and immunostained with the PMCA antibody 5F10. The anti-GAPDH antibody was used as a protein loading control. (**B**) Quantification of PMCA protein levels in Control and A1-like astrocytes relative to GAPDH is shown as mean ± SEM values, in arbitrary units. Statistical analysis was carried out using the Student's t-test. (*) $p < 0.05$ with respect to each Control.

3. Discussion

The results of this work point out that treatment with the cytokines TNF-α (30 ng/mL), IL-1α (3 ng/mL) and C1q (400 ng/mL) for 24 h produces a large increase in C3 or C3b expression in U251 cells, and also around a two-fold increase in C3α expression, which are biomarkers of reactive A1 astrocytes [3]. Thus, this treatment with cytokines is sufficient to elicit the significant generation of A1-like astrocytes. Fluorescence microscopy images of cells stained with the anti-C3 antibody show that the increase in C3/C3b/C3α expression is stronger in the soma of large cells displaying thick and long extensions. Therefore, we selected this cell phenotype to study the effect of the transformation of U251 cells in A1-like astrocytes on Aβ production and on resting cytosolic Ca^{2+} homeostasis.

Many pro-inflammatory cytokines have been shown to upregulate APP in human neuroblastoma cells and non-neuronal cells such as human astrocyte cultures, as well as in the mouse brain [34]. For example, interleukin-1β has been shown to upregulate APP in human astrocytes and the U373MG human astrocytoma cell line [11,12]. Zhao et al. [14] have demonstrated that treatment for ≥48 h with cytokines including TNF-α and interferon-γ increase levels of endogenous BACE1 and APP, and stimulate amyloidogenic APP processing, in primary mouse astrocytes, leading to an increase in Aβ secretion. While there is little Aβ secretion from resting normal adult human astrocytes [38], a combination of interferon-γ and TNF-α has also been shown to induce Aβ secretion from primary human astrocytes and the U373 cell line [13]. In this work, we show that the treatment of U251 cells with the cytokines TNF-α (30 ng/mL), IL-1α (3 ng/mL) and C1q (400 ng/mL) for 24 h also produces a large increase in Aβ peptides immunoreactive with the anti-Aβ antibody in cells displaying an enhanced expression of C3/C3b/C3α, i.e., with the A1-like astrocyte phenotype. Of note, the anti-Aβ antibody 6E10 used in this work reacts to the toxic human Aβ peptides, such as Aβ(1–42) and Aβ(1–40), and also to their precursor forms, like APP, which contains the immunoreactive epitope against this antibody [39–41]. To the best of our knowledge, the production of toxic Aβ peptides by A1 astrocytes has not been reported elsewhere, and this is of particular relevance since A1 astrocytes are abundant in *post-mortem* brain samples of major human neurodegenerative diseases, including Alzheimer's, Huntington's and Parkinson's diseases, as well as amyotrophic lateral sclerosis and multiple sclerosis [3]. Although under normal conditions, astrocytes are less likely to be significant generators of Aβ because neurons express higher levels of BACE1 than astrocytes [42,43], it should be noted that astrocytes outnumber neurons over five-fold in the brain [44,45]. Indeed, several studies have shown that reactive astrocytes can contribute to Aβ production in AD [13,34,46]. Moreover, Aβ produced by astrocytes may be more pathogenic than that produced by neurons. A large fraction of the Aβ species present in Aβ plaques are N-truncated [47–49], and it has been reported that the percentage of N-truncated Aβ secreted by astrocytes is much higher than that of Aβ secreted by neurons, with values of 60% and 20%, respectively [50]. As Aβ can stimulate astrocytes to secrete pro-inflammatory molecules and cytokines in vitro and in vivo [51–53], these results suggest that a feed-forward loop may operate during neurodegeneration mediated by A1 astrocytes.

Aβ(1–42) and other neurotoxic β-amyloid peptides have been shown to alter intracellular Ca^{2+} homeostasis by acting on regulatory Ca^{2+}-dependent proteins and Ca^{2+} transport systems, reviewed in [21]. Much experimental evidence supports that ER Ca^{2+} dysregulation can lead to Aβ(1–42) generation [21]. In this work, we found that the treatment of U251 cells with the cytokines TNF-α (30 ng/mL), IL-1α (3 ng/mL) and C1q (400 ng/mL) for 24 h produced a large depletion of ER calcium content, and also a large attenuation of SOCE. The latter result can be seen as a direct effect of Aβ(1–42) generation in these A1-like astrocytes, because we previously demonstrated that only nanomolar concentrations of intracellular Aβ(1–42) are needed to inhibit SOCE activity [30]. In addition, the enhanced release of calcium from the ER can generate a feed-forward cycle, leading to potentiation of the production of neurotoxic Aβ peptides in A1-like reactive astrocytes, since it has been demonstrated that Aβ-induced BACE1 upregulation can be blocked by preventing calcium influx through treatment with 2-aminoethoxydiphenyl borate, an inhibitor of inositol trisphosphate-dependent calcium release from the ER, and U73122, an inhibitor of phospholipase C [54].

The activity of astrocytes, the major glial cell-type in the mammalian brain [55], is largely dependent on intracellular calcium signaling [15]. Lee et al. [16] have reported that picomolar amounts of Aβ peptides can enhance spontaneous intracellular calcium transient signaling. Also, it has been shown that pathological Aβ can cause abnormal calcium influx and intracellular signaling in astrocyte cultures [56,57], and aberrant Ca^{2+} signals have been noted as a hallmark of astrocyte functional remodeling in AD mouse models [19,20]. However, in this work, we found that the resting cytosolic Ca^{2+} concentration does not increase in A1-like astrocytes with respect to the Control (untreated) U251 cells, despite the fact that ER calcium content is markedly decreased. On the contrary, the mean values obtained for the cytosolic Ca^{2+} concentrations are 20% lower in A1-like astrocytes than in the Control U251 cells. This result points out that the extrusion of cytosolic calcium operates more efficiently in the A1-like astrocytes than in the Control U251 cells. Indeed, our results show around a three-fold higher PMCA expression level in the A1-like astrocytes than in the Control U251 cells. Due to the major role of PMCAs in the cytosolic calcium extrusion of brain cells [58,59], the upregulation of PMCA activity is likely to efficiently counterbalance, in a short time, the impact of ER calcium release on the resting cytosolic calcium concentration of A1-like astrocytes, unveiling a defense mechanism against Aβ-induced abnormal and harmful calcium signaling in these cells. Interestingly, Pham et al. [32] have recently reported that Aβ(25–35) lowered the cytosolic calcium concentration in Aβ-preconditioned primary cortical mouse astrocytes through potentiated Ca^{2+} extrusion via PMCAs triggered by a rise in cyclic AMP. The molecular mechanisms involved in the upregulation of PMCAs in A1-like astrocytes are unclear at present, and its elucidation will need extensive experimental work that is out of the scope of this article.

In summary, we found that treatment of U251 cells with the cytokines TNF-α, IL-1α and C1q for 24 h elicits significant generation of A1-like astrocytes, which display increased production of APP and Aβ peptides. Compared with the Control U251 cells, these A1-like astrocytes show more than 50% depletion of the Ca^{2+} stored in the ER without an increase in cytosolic Ca^{2+} concentration, since the attenuation of Ca^{2+} entry through SOCE and the upregulation of PMCA expression can efficiently counterbalance the enhanced Ca^{2+} release from the ER in A1-like astrocytes.

4. Materials and Methods

4.1. Materials

The human astroglioma U251 cell line was acquired from the American Type Culture Collection (Manassas, VA, USA). The primary antibody anti-C3 (JF10-30) and the fluorescent labeled secondary antibodies anti-rabbit IgG-Alexa488 (A11008) and anti-mouse IgG-Alexa488 (A11001) were from Invitrogen (Molecular Probes, Eugene, OR, USA). The primary antibody anti-Aβ (6E10) was purchased from Enzo Life Sciences (Farmingdale, NY, USA). The primary anti-PMCA antibody (clone 5F10) was purchased from Invitrogen. The primary anti-GAPDH antibody (GAPDH-0411) was obtained from Santa Cruz Biotechnology. IL-1α and TNF-α were supplied by Prepotech, and C1q was from BioRad. Fura-2 acetoxymethyl ester (Fura2 AM), Fluo3 AM, 4-Bromo-A23187 and Pluronic®F-127 were obtained from Biotium (Hayward, CA, USA). Thapsigargin (Tg) and ionomycin were purchased from Sigma-Aldrich.

4.2. Cell Culture and Preparation of Reactive Astrocytes

U251 cells were cultured in high-glucose Dulbecco's Modified Eagle's Medium (DMEM) supplemented with 2 mM L-glutamine, 100 units/mL penicillin, 0.1 mg/mL streptomycin and 10% fetal bovine serum (FBS). For all experiments, U251 cells were seeded in 35 mm dishes at a density of 2.2×10^4 cells/cm2 in the culture media described above and allowed to grow at 37 °C and 5% CO_2. After 48 h, reactive astrocytes (named A1-like) were prepared by replacing the culture medium with FBS-free DMEM supplemented with glutamine and antibiotics. The next day, cells were stimulated for 24 h with a cocktail of the pro-inflammatory cytokines IL-1α (3 ng/mL), TNF-α (30 ng/mL) and C1q (400 ng/mL), as detailed by Liddelow et al. [3]. Non-reactive astrocyte cells (Control group) were always maintained in DMEM supplemented with FBS.

4.3. U251 Cell Staining with C3 and Aβ Antibodies

A1-like astrocytes and Control (untreated U251) cells were seeded in 35 mm plates as described above. On the day of the experiment, cells were washed with MLocke's K5 buffer (4 mM $NaHCO_3$, 10 mM Tricine, 5 mM glucose, 2.3 mM $CaCl_2$, 1 mM $MgCl_2$, 154 mM NaCl and 5 mM KCl, pH 7.4 at 37 °C) to remove the phenol red remaining in the plates. Afterward, cells were fixed with 2.5% paraformaldehyde, 3 mM $MgCl_2$, 2 mM EGTA and 0.32 M sucrose in PBS (5 mM sodium phosphate, 137 mM NaCl and 27 mM KCl, pH 7). Fixed and permeabilized cells were blocked with 1% bovine serum albumin in PBS supplemented with 0.2% Triton X-100 (PBST) for 1 h at 37 °C and washed three times with PBS (washing step). Then, cells were incubated for 1 h at 37 °C with the respective target primary antibody in PBST: anti-C3 (dilution 1/200) or anti-Aβ (dilution 1/250 or 1/500). Thereafter, cells were washed and incubated for 1 h with the appropriate Alexa488-labeled secondary antibody in PBST (dilution 1/200) and rewashed. Green fluorescence (GF) images of Control and A1 cells were acquired with an excitation filter of 470 nm and a 510 nm dichroic mirror/520 nm emission filter, using the exposure times indicated for each case in the legends of the figures. Quantitative analysis of the average fluorescence intensity per pixel of selected neuronal soma was performed via HCImage software using the ROI tool, as in previous works [30,60–62].

4.4. Cell Homogenate Preparation, and Western Blot and Dot Blot Analyses

Cells were harvested, washed twice with PBS and centrifuged for 3 min at 1700 g to collect cell pellets. The Omni Tissue Master 125 with a 5 mm Probe was used to resuspend the pellet in 10 mM N-[2-hydroxyethyl] piperazine-N'-[2-ethanesulfonic acid] (HEPES)/KOH, at pH 7.4, with 0.32 M sucrose, 0.5 mM $MgSO_4$, 0.1 mM phenylmethanesulfonyl fluoride, 2 mM 2-mercaptoethanol and a protease inhibitor cocktail solution (Roche Diagnostics). The homogenate was then centrifuged for 1 min at 5000 g, and the supernatant was collected and stored at −80 °C in small aliquots. The protein concentration was determined using the Bradford method [63].

Proteins from 20 μg homogenates were separated using 10% or 7.5–20% gradient polyacrylamide sodium dodecyl sulfate (SDS) gels [64] and transferred onto PVDF membranes. Immunodetection of C3, PMCA and GAPDH was performed by incubating the PVDF membranes with the specific primary antibodies anti-C3 (dilution 1/1000), anti-PMCA (dilution 1/1000) and anti-GAPDH (dilution 1/3000) overnight at 4 °C, followed by 1 h of incubation at room temperature with the appropriate peroxidase-conjugated anti-mouse or anti-rabbit secondary antibodies, and developed using an Enhanced Chemiluminescence (ECL) substrate.

Immunodetection of total Aβ peptides was carried out via dot blot. Homogenates (12 μg) from U251 cells, untreated (C) or treated (A1-like astrocytes) with TNF-α (30 ng/mL), IL-1α (3 ng/mL) and C1q (400 ng/mL), were spotted onto a nitrocellulose membrane, sealed on a Bio-Dot® SF (Bio-Rad, Hercules, CA, USA). Total protein was visualized via Ponceau S protein staining. After blocking and washing, the membrane was incubated with the anti-Aβ antibody (6E10, dilution 1/1000) overnight at 4 °C. The membrane was incubated with peroxidase-conjugated anti-mouse secondary antibody and developed using the Enhanced Chemiluminescence (ECL) substrate.

4.5. Intracellular Cytosolic Ca^{2+} Measurements

Intracellular Ca^{2+} concentration ($[Ca^{2+}]i$) was measured in Control U251 cells and in A1-like astrocytes with the fluorescent probes Fluo3 AM and Fura2 AM, as previously described [30,60]. Briefly, cells were loaded with 5 μM of Fura2 AM or Fluo3 AM plus 0.025% Pluronic® F-127 with continuous and gentle mixing for 1 h at 37 °C and 5% CO_2. Afterward, cells were washed once with 1 mL of MLocke's K5 buffer, and the 35 mm culture dishes were placed on the thermostatic plate (Warner Instrument Co., Hamden, CT, USA) of a Nikon Diaphot 300 inverted epifluorescence microscope (Tokyo, Japan) at 37 °C with an NCF Plan ELWD 40× objective. Images of Fluo3-loaded cells were acquired using a Hamamatsu Orca-R2 CCD camera (binning mode 2 × 2) with an excitation filter of 470 nm, and a dichroic mirror of 510 nm with an emission filter of 520 nm [30]. Images of Fura2-loaded cells were recorded using 340 and 380 nm excitation filters and a 510 nm dichroic mirror/520 nm emission filter [60,62].

For the determination of $[Ca^{2+}]i$ using the Fluo3 probe, 5 mM $MnCl_2$ and 5 µg/mL of the nonfluorescent Ca^{2+} ionophore 4-Bromo-A23187 were added to Control U251 cells and to A1-like astrocytes, and the fluorescence microscopy images were recorded in kinetic mode to obtain the fluorescence intensity of Fluo3 saturated with Mn^{2+} [F(Mn-Fluo3)], which has been reported to be 20% of the value of fluorescence intensity upon saturating Ca^{2+} (Fmax) [65]. The fluorescence value of free Fluo3 (not bound to Ca^{2+}), Fmin, is about 0.01·Fmax [65]. $[Ca^{2+}]i$ was measured using the formula: $[Ca^{2+}]i = K_d$ [(F − Fmin)/(Fmax − F)], where F is the fluorescence intensity obtained with an excitation filter of 470 nm, and a 510 nm dichroic mirror/520 nm emission filter with a 0.1 s exposure time. The dissociation constant (K_d) for the Fluo3/Ca^{2+} complex used to obtain $[Ca^{2+}]i$ was 390 nM, reported in the *Molecular Probes Handbook: A Guide to Fluorescent Probes and Labeling Technologies*, Tenth Edition (2005).

For the determination of $[Ca^{2+}]i$ using the Fura2 probe, $[Ca^{2+}]i$ was calculated using the following equation: $[Ca^{2+}]i = K_d \times$ [(R − Rmin)/(Rmax − R)], where R is the measured fluorescence ratio (340/380), and Rmax and Rmin are the ratio values (340/380) for Ca^{2+}-bound and Ca^{2+}-free Fura2-loaded cells. Rmax and Rmin were experimentally determined from steady-state fluorescence ratio (340/380) measurements after sequential addition to the culture medium of Fura2-loaded cells of (i) nonfluorescent Ca^{2+} ionophore 4-Bromo-A23187 (5 µg/mL) or ionomycin (5 µg/mL), and (ii) 10 mM EGTA, respectively. To obtain the values of $[Ca^{2+}]I$, we used the reported dissociation constant (K_d) of Fura2/Ca^{2+} of 224 nM [66].

The response of SOCE was determined in Fluo3-loaded Control U251 cells and in A1-like astrocytes. The depletion of the Ca^{2+} stores was triggered by adding 2 µM of the sarcoendoplasmic calcium pump blocker Tg plus 1 mM EGTA in Ca^{2+}-free MLocke's K5 buffer [30]. Then, SOCE was measured after adding 3 mM of $CaCl_2$ to the Tg-containing medium. Data acquisition and analysis were carried out using HCImage software after the selection of the cells using the ROI tool of this software.

4.6. Statistics

Statistical analysis was carried out using the Student's *t* test, and the results are expressed as the mean ± standard error of the mean (SEM). A significant difference was defined as $p < 0.05$. All results were obtained at least in triplicate, with the number of cells (*n*) indicated for each experimental condition.

Author Contributions: Conceptualization: C.G.-M. and A.M.M.; methodology: J.P., M.B., L.S., C.G.-M. and A.M.M.; software: J.P. and C.G.-M.; validation: C.G.-M. and A.M.M.; formal analysis: J.P., M.B., C.G.-M. and A.M.M.; investigation: J.P., M.B., L.S., C.G.-M. and A.M.M.; resources: C.G.-M. and A.M.M.; data curation: J.P., M.B., C.G.-M. and A.M.M.; writing—original draft preparation: J.P., M.B., C.G.-M. and A.M.M.; writing—review and editing: J.P., M.B., C.G.-M. and A.M.M.; supervision: C.G.-M. and A.M.M.; project administration: A.M.M.; funding acquisition: C.G.-M. and A.M.M. All authors have read and agreed to the published version of the manuscript.

Funding: This work was funded by MCIN/AEI/ 10.13039/501100011033 (Grant PID2020-115512GB-100). And also, it was co-financed by Junta de Extremadura (GR21051) and by "ERDF A way of making Europe".

Institutional Review Board Statement: Not applicable.

Informed Consent Statement: Not applicable.

Data Availability Statement: Not applicable.

Acknowledgments: The gift of U251 cell samples from José Manuel Fuentes (Departamento de Bioquímica y Biología Molecular y Genética, Facultad de Veterinaria, Universidad de Extremadura, Cáceres, Spain) is gratefully acknowledged.

Conflicts of Interest: The authors declare no conflict of interest.

Sample Availability: Not available.

Abbreviations

Aβ	amyloid β peptide
AD	Alzheimer's disease
APP	amyloid β protein precursor
BACE1	β-site APP-cleaving enzyme 1
C1q	complement component 1q
DMEM	Dulbecco's modified Eagle's medium
EGTA	ethyleneglycoltetraacetic acid
ER	endoplasmic reticulum
Fluo3 AM	Fluo-3-pentaacetoxymethyl ester
Fura2 AM	Fura2 acetoxymethyl ester
GAPDH	glyceraldehyde-3-phosphate dehydrogenase
GF	green fluorescence
HEPES	N-[2-hydroxyethyl] piperazine-N'-[2-ethanesulfonic acid]
IL-1α	interleukin-1α
NPA	3-nitropropionic acid
PBS	phosphate-buffered saline
PBST	PBS supplemented with 0.2% 4-(1,1,3,3-tetramethyl butyl) phenyl-polyethylene glycol (Triton X-100®)
PMCA	plasma membrane calcium pump
PSEN	presenilin
PVDF	polyvinylidene difluoride
RF	red fluorescence
ROI	region of interest
SDS-PAGE	sodium dodecyl sulfate-polyacrylamide gel electrophoresis
SEM	standard error of the mean
SOCE	store-operated calcium entry
STIM1	stromal interaction molecule 1
Tg	thapsigargin
TNFα	tumor necrosis factor α

References

1. Zhang, Y.; Chen, K.; Sloan, S.A.; Bennett, M.L.; Scholze, A.R.; O'Keeffe, S.; Phatnani, H.P.; Guarnieri, P.; Caneda, C.; Ruderisch, N.; et al. An RNA-sequencing transcriptome and splicing database of glia, neurons, and vascular cells of the cerebral cortex. *J. Neurosci.* **2014**, *34*, 11929–11947. [CrossRef] [PubMed]
2. Bennett, M.L.; Bennett, F.C.; Liddelow, S.A.; Ajami, B.; Zamanian, J.L.; Fernhoff, N.B.; Mulinyawe, S.B.; Bohlen, C.J.; Adil, A.; Tucker, A.; et al. New tools for studying microglia in the mouse and human CNS. *Proc. Natl. Acad. Sci. USA* **2016**, *113*, E1738–E1746. [CrossRef] [PubMed]
3. Liddelow, S.A.; Guttenplan, K.A.; Clarke, L.E.; Bennett, F.C.; Bohlen, C.J.; Schirmer, L.; Bennett, M.L.; Münch, A.E.; Chung, W.S.; Peterson, T.C.; et al. Neurotoxic reactive astrocytes are induced by activated microglia. *Nature* **2017**, *541*, 481–487. [CrossRef] [PubMed]
4. Hawkins, B.T.; Davis, T.P. The blood-brain barrier/neurovascular unit in health and disease. *Pharmacol. Rev.* **2005**, *57*, 173–185. [CrossRef]
5. Escartin, C.; Galea, E.; Lakatos, A.; O'Callaghan, J.P.; Petzold, G.C.; Serrano-Pozo, A.; Steinhäuser, C.; Volterra, A.; Carmignoto, G.; Agarwal, A.; et al. Reactive astrocyte nomenclature, definitions, and future directions. *Nat. Neurosci.* **2021**, *24*, 312–325. [CrossRef]
6. Liddelow, S.A.; Barres, B.A. Reactive astrocytes: Production, function, and therapeutic potential. *Immunity* **2017**, *46*, 957–967. [CrossRef]
7. Lee, K.M.; MacLean, A.G. New advances on glial activation in health and disease. *World J. Virol.* **2015**, *4*, 42–55. [CrossRef]
8. Lopez-Sanchez, C.; Garcia-Martinez, V.; Poejo, J.; Garcia-Lopez, V.; Salazar, J.; Gutierrez-Merino, C. Early reactive A1 astrocytes induction by the neurotoxin 3-nitropropionic acid in rat brain. *Int. J. Mol. Sci.* **2020**, *21*, 3609. [CrossRef]
9. Lopez-Sanchez, C.; Poejo, J.; Garcia-Lopez, V.; Salazar, J.; Garcia-Martinez, V.; Gutierrez-Merino, C. Kaempferol prevents the activation of complement C3 protein and the generation of reactive A1 astrocytes that mediate rat brain degeneration induced by 3-nitropropionic acid. *Food Chem. Toxicol.* **2022**, *164*, 113017. [CrossRef] [PubMed]

10. Wang, T.; Sun, Q.; Yang, J.; Wang, G.; Zhao, F.; Chen, Y.; Jin, Y. Reactive astrocytes induced by 2-chloroethanol modulate microglia polarization through IL-1β, TNF-α, and iNOS upregulation. *Food Chem. Toxicol.* **2021**, *157*, 112550. [CrossRef] [PubMed]
11. Machein, U.; Lieb, K.; Hüll, M.; Fiebich, B.L. IL-1β and TNFα, but not IL-6, induce a1-antichymotrypsin expression in the human astrocytoma cell line U373 MG. *Neuroreport* **1995**, *6*, 2283–2286. [CrossRef] [PubMed]
12. Rogers, J.T.; Leiter, L.M.; McPhee, J.; Cahill, C.M.; Zhan, S.S.; Potter, H.; Nilsson, L.N. Translation of the Alzheimer amyloid precursor protein mRNA is upregulated by interleukin-1 through 50-untranslated region sequences. *J. Biol. Chem.* **1999**, *274*, 6421–6431. [CrossRef]
13. Blasko, I.; Veerhuis, R.; Stampfer-Kountchev, M.; Saurwein-Teissl, M.; Eikelenboom, P.; Grubeck-Loebenstein, B. Costimulatory effects of interferon-γ and interleukin-1β or tumor necrosis factor a on the synthesis of Aβ1–40 and Aβ1–42 by human astrocytes. *Neurobiol. Dis.* **2000**, *7*, 682–689. [CrossRef] [PubMed]
14. Zhao, J.; O'Connor, T.; Vassar, R. The contribution of activated astrocytes to Aβ production: Implications for Alzheimer's disease pathogenesis. *J. Neuroinflammation* **2011**, *8*, 150. [CrossRef]
15. Khakh, B.S.; McCarthy, K.D. Astrocyte calcium signaling: From observations to functions and the challenges therein. *Cold Spring Harb. Perspect. Biol.* **2015**, *7*, a020404. [CrossRef] [PubMed]
16. Lee, L.; Kosuri, P.; Arancio, O. Picomolar Amyloid-β Peptides Enhance Spontaneous Astrocyte Calcium Transients. *J. Alzheimers Dis.* **2014**, *38*, 49–62. [CrossRef]
17. Angulo, M.C.; Kozlov, A.S.; Charpak, S.; Audinat, E. Glutamate released from glial cells synchronizes neuronal activity in the hippocampus. *J. Neurosci.* **2004**, *24*, 6920–6927. [CrossRef]
18. Fellin, T.; Pascual, O.; Gobbo, S.; Pozzan, T.; Haydon, P.G.; Carmignoto, G. Neuronal synchrony mediated by astrocytic glutamate through activation of extrasynaptic NMDA receptors. *Neuron* **2004**, *43*, 729–743. [CrossRef]
19. Kuchibhotla, K.V.; Lattarulo, C.R.; Hyman, B.T.; Bacskai, B.J. Synchronous hyperactivity and intercellular calcium waves in astrocytes in Alzheimer mice. *Science* **2009**, *323*, 1211–1215. [CrossRef] [PubMed]
20. Delekate, A.; Fuchtemeier, M.; Schumacher, T.; Ulbrich, C.; Foddis, M.; Petzold, G.C. Metabotropic P2Y1 receptor signalling mediates astrocytic hyperactivity in vivo in an Alzheimer's disease mouse model. *Nat. Commun.* **2014**, *5*, 5422. [CrossRef]
21. Poejo, J.; Salazar, J.; Mata, A.M.; Gutierrez-Merino, C. The Relevance of Amyloid β-Calmodulin Complexation in Neurons and Brain Degeneration in Alzheimer's Disease. *Int. J. Mol. Sci.* **2021**, *22*, 4976. [CrossRef]
22. D'Andrea, M.R.; Nagele, R.G.; Wang, H.Y.; Peterson, P.A.; Lee, D.H. Evidence that neurons accumulating amyloid can undergo lysis to form amyloid plaques in Alzheimer's disease. *Histopathology* **2001**, *38*, 120–134. [CrossRef]
23. Leissring, M.A.; Akbari, Y.; Fanger, C.M.; Cahalan, M.D.; Mattson, M.P.; LaFerla, F.M. Capacitative Calcium Entry Deficits and Elevated Luminal Calcium Content in Mutant Presenilin-1 Knockin Mice. *J. Cell Biol.* **2000**, *149*, 793–798. [CrossRef]
24. Yoo, A.S.; Cheng, I.; Chung, S.; Grenfell, T.Z.; Lee, H.; Pack-Chung, E.; Handler, M.; Shen, J.; Xia, W.; Tesco, G.; et al. Presenilin-Mediated Modulation of Capacitative Calcium Entry. *Neuron* **2000**, *27*, 561–572. [CrossRef]
25. Popugaeva, E.; Pchitskaya, E.; Bezprozvanny, I. Dysregulation of neuronal calcium homeostasis in Alzheimer's disease—A therapeutic opportunity? *Biochem. Biophys. Res. Commun.* **2017**, *483*, 998–1004. [CrossRef]
26. Leissring, M.A.; Parker, I.; LaFerla, F.M. Presenilin-2 Mutations Modulate Amplitude and Kinetics of Inositol 1,4,5-Trisphosphate-mediated Calcium Signals. *J. Biol. Chem.* **1999**, *274*, 32535–32538. [CrossRef]
27. Chavez, S.E.; O'Day, D.H. Calmodulin binds to and regulates the activity of beta-secretase (BACE1). *Curr. Res. Alzheimers Dis.* **2007**, *1*, 37–47.
28. Giliberto, L.; Borghi, R.; Piccini, A.; Mangerini, R.; Sorbi, S.; Cirmena, G.; Garuti, A.; Ghetti, B.; Tagliavini, F.; Mughal, M.R.; et al. Mutant Presenilin 1 Increases the Expression and Activity of BACE1. *J. Biol. Chem.* **2009**, *284*, 9027–9038. [CrossRef] [PubMed]
29. Zeiger, W.; Vetrivel, K.S.; Buggia-Prévot, V.; Nguyen, P.D.; Wagner, S.L.; Villereal, M.L.; Thinakaran, G. Ca^{2+} Influx through Store-operated Ca^{2+} Channels Reduces Alzheimer Disease β-Amyloid Peptide Secretion. *J. Biol. Chem.* **2013**, *288*, 26955–26966. [CrossRef] [PubMed]
30. Poejo, J.; Orantos-Aguilera, Y.; Martin-Romero, F.J.; Mata, A.M.; Gutierrez-Merino, C. Internalized Amyloid-β (1-42) Peptide Inhibits the Store-Operated Calcium Entry in HT-22 Cells. *Int. J. Mol. Sci.* **2022**, *23*, 12678. [CrossRef] [PubMed]
31. Yu, X.; Taylor, A.M.W.; Nagai, J.; Golshani, P.; Evans, C.J.; Coppola, G.; Khakh, B.S. Reducing astrocyte calcium signaling in vivo alters striatal microcircuits and causes repetitive behavior. *Neuron* **2018**, *99*, 1170–1187.e9. [CrossRef] [PubMed]
32. Pham, C.; Hérault, K.; Oheim, M.; Maldera, S.; Vialou, V.; Cauli, B.; Li, D. Astrocytes respond to a neurotoxic Aβ fragment with state-dependent Ca2+ alteration and multiphasic transmitter release. *Acta Neuropathol. Commun.* **2021**, *9*, 44. [CrossRef] [PubMed]
33. Nadler, Y.; Alexandrovich, A.; Grigoriadis, N.; Hartmann, T.; Rao, K.S.J.; Shohami, E.; Stein, R. Increased expression of the gamma-secretase components presenilin-1 and nicastrin in activated astrocytes and microglia following traumatic brain injury. *Glia* **2008**, *56*, 552–567. [CrossRef] [PubMed]
34. Frost, G.R.; Li, Y.M. The role of astrocytes in amyloid production and Alzheimer's disease. *Open Biol.* **2017**, *7*, 170228. [CrossRef]
35. Kuchibhotla, K.V.; Goldman, S.T.; Lattarulo, C.R.; Wu, H.Y.; Hyman, B.T.; Bacskai, B.J. Aβ Plaques Lead to Aberrant Regulation of Calcium Homeostasis in Vivo Resulting in Structural and Functional Disruption of Neuronal Networks. *Neuron* **2008**, *59*, 214–225. [CrossRef]
36. Berridge, M.J. Calcium Signalling and Alzheimer's Disease. *Neurochem. Res.* **2011**, *36*, 1149–1156. [CrossRef]
37. Fresu, L.; Dehpour, A.; Genazzani, A.A.; Carafoli, E.; Guerini, D. Plasma membrane calcium ATPase isoforms in astrocytes. *Glia* **1999**, *28*, 150–155. [CrossRef]

38. Prà, I.D.; Whitfileld, J.F.; Pacchiana, R.; Bonafini, C.; Talacchi, A.; Chakravarthy, B.; Armato, U.; Chiarini, A. The amyloid-β42 proxy, amyloid-β25-35, induces normal human cerebral astrocytes to produce amyloid-β42. *J. Alzheimers Dis.* **2011**, *24*, 335–347. [CrossRef]
39. Kim, K.S.; Miller, D.L.; Sapienza, V.J.; Chen, C.M.J.; Bai, C.; Grundke-Iqbal, I.; Currie, C.J.; Wisniewski, H.M. Production and characterization of monoclonal antibodies reactive to synthetic cerebrovascular amyloid peptide. *Neurosci. Res. Commun.* **1988**, *2*, 121–130.
40. Hatami, A.; Albay, R., 3rd; Monjazeb, S.; Milton, S.; Glabe, C. Monoclonal antibodies against Abeta42 fibrils distinguish multiple aggregation state polymorphisms in vitro and in Alzheimer disease brain. *J. Biol. Chem.* **2014**, *289*, 32131–32143. [CrossRef]
41. Baghallab, I.; Reyes-Ruiz, J.M.; Abulnaja, K.; Huwait, E.; Glabe, C. Epitomic Characterization of the Specificity of the Anti-Amyloid Aβ Monoclonal Antibodies 6E10 and 4G8. *J. Alzheimers Dis.* **2018**, *66*, 1235–1244. [CrossRef] [PubMed]
42. Vassar, R.; Bennett, B.D.; Babu-Khan, S.; Kahn, S.; Mendiaz, E.A.; Denis, P.; Teplow, D.B.; Ross, S.; Amarante, P.; Loeloff, R.; et al. Beta-secretase cleavage of Alzheimer's amyloid precursor protein by the transmembrane aspartic protease BACE. *Science* **1999**, *286*, 735–741. [CrossRef]
43. Laird, F.M.; Cai, H.; Savonenko, A.V.; Farah, M.H.; He, K.; Melnikova, T.; Wen, H.; Chiang, H.C.; Xu, G.; Koliatsos, V.E.; et al. BACE1, a major determinant of selective vulnerability of the brain to amyloid-beta amyloidogenesis, is essential for cognitive, emotional, and synaptic functions. *J. Neurosci.* **2005**, *25*, 11693–11709. [CrossRef] [PubMed]
44. Kandel, E.R.; Schwartz, J.H.; Jessell, T.M. *Principles of Neural Science*, 4th ed.; McGraw-Hill Medical Press: New York, NY, USA, 2000.
45. Sofroniew, M.V.; Vinters, H.V. Astrocytes: Biology and pathology. *Acta Neuropathol.* **2010**, *119*, 7–35. [CrossRef] [PubMed]
46. Liang, Y.; Raven, F.; Ward, J.F.; Zhen, S.; Zhang, S.; Sun, H.; Miller, S.J.; Choi, S.H.; Tanzi, R.E.; Zhang, C. Upregulation of Alzheimer's Disease Amyloid-β Protein Precursor in Astrocytes Both in vitro and in vivo. *J. Alzheimers Dis.* **2020**, *76*, 1071–1082. [CrossRef]
47. Schieb, H.; Kratzin, H.; Jahn, O.; Mobius, W.; Rabe, S.; Staufenbiel, M.; Wiltfang, J.; Klafki, H.W. β-Amyloid peptide variants in brains and cerebrospinal fluid from amyloid precursor protein (APP) transgenic mice: Comparison with human Alzheimer amyloid. *J. Biol. Chem.* **2011**, *286*, 33747–33758. [CrossRef]
48. Moore, B.D.; Chakrabarty, P.; Levites, Y.; Kukar, T.L.; Baine, A.M.; Moroni, T.; Ladd, T.B.; Das, P.; Dickson, D.W.; Golde, T.E. Overlapping profiles of Aβ peptides in the Alzheimer's disease and pathological aging brains. *Alzheimers Res. Ther.* **2012**, *4*, 18. [CrossRef]
49. Bayer, T.A.; Wirths, O. Focusing the amyloid cascade hypothesis on N-truncated Aβ peptides as drug targets against Alzheimer's disease. *Acta Neuropathol.* **2014**, *127*, 787–801. [CrossRef]
50. Oberstein, T.J.; Spitzer, P.; Klafki, H.W.; Linning, P.; Neff, F.; Knölker, H.J.; Lewczuk, P.; Wiltfang, J.; Kornhuber, J.; Maler, J.M. Astrocytes and microglia but not neurons preferentially generate N-terminally truncated Aβ peptides. *Neurobiol. Dis.* **2015**, *73*, 24–35. [CrossRef]
51. Hu, J.; Akama, K.T.; Krafft, G.A.; Chromy, B.A.; Van Eldik, L.J. Amyloid-beta peptide activates cultured astrocytes: Morphological alterations, cytokine induction and nitric oxide release. *Brain Res.* **1998**, *785*, 195–206. [CrossRef]
52. Craft, J.M.; Watterson, D.M.; Frautschy, S.A.; Eldik, L.J.V. Aminopyridazines inhibit β-amyloid-induced glial activation and neuronal damage in vivo. *Neurobiol. Aging* **2004**, *25*, 1283–1292. [CrossRef]
53. White, J.A.; Manelli, A.M.; Holmberg, K.H.; Van Eldik, L.J.; LaDu, M.J. Differential effects of oligomeric and fibrillar amyloid-β1–42 on astrocyte-mediated inflammation. *Neurobiol. Dis.* **2005**, *18*, 459–465. [CrossRef]
54. Jin, S.M.; Cho, H.J.; Kim, Y.W.; Hwang, J.Y.; Mook-Jung, I. Aβ-induced Ca2+ influx regulates astrocytic BACE1 expression via calcineurin/NFAT4 signals. *Biochem. Biophys. Res. Commun.* **2012**, *425*, 649–655. [CrossRef]
55. Herculano-Houzel, S. The glia/neuron ratio: How it varies uniformly across brain structures and species and what that means for brain physiology and evolution. *Glia* **2014**, *62*, 1377–1391. [CrossRef] [PubMed]
56. Perez-Alvarez, A.; Navarrete, M.; Covelo, A.; Martin, E.D.; Araque, A. Structural and functional plasticity of astrocyte processes and dendritic spine interactions. *J. Neurosci.* **2014**, *34*, 12738–12744. [CrossRef] [PubMed]
57. Pham, C.; Moro, D.H.; Mouffle, C.; Didienne, S.; Hepp, R.; Pfrieger, F.W.; Mangin, J.M.; Legendre, P.; Martin, C.; Luquet, S.; et al. Mapping astrocyte activity domains by light sheet imaging and spatio-temporal correlation screening. *NeuroImage* **2020**, *220*, 117069. [CrossRef] [PubMed]
58. Stafford, N.; Wilson, C.; Oceandy, D.; Neyses, L.; Cartwright, E.J. The Plasma Membrane Calcium ATPases and Their Role as Major New Players in Human Disease. *Physiol. Rev.* **2017**, *97*, 1089–1125. [CrossRef]
59. Strehler, E.E.; Thayer, S.A. Evidence for a role of plasma membrane calcium pumps in neurodegenerative disease: Recent developments. *Neurosci Lett.* **2018**, *663*, 39–47. [CrossRef]
60. Fortalezas, S.; Marques-da-Silva, D.; Gutierrez-Merino, C. Creatine Protects Against Cytosolic Calcium Dysregulation, Mitochondrial Depolarization and Increase of Reactive Oxygen Species Production in Rotenone-Induced Cell Death of Cerebellar Granule Neurons. *Neurotox. Res.* **2018**, *34*, 717–732. [CrossRef]
61. Fortalezas, S.; Poejo, J.; Samhan-Arias, A.K.; Gutierrez-Merino, C. Cholesterol-Rich Plasma Membrane Submicrodomains Can Be a Major Extramitochondrial Source of Reactive Oxygen Species in Partially Depolarized Mature Cerebellar Granule Neurons in Culture. *J. Neurphysiol. Neurol. Dis.* **2019**, *5*, 1–22. [CrossRef]

62. Poejo, J.; Salazar, J.; Mata, A.M.; Gutierrez-Merino, C. Binding of Amyloid β(1–42)-calmodulin Complexes to Plasma Membrane Lipid Rafts in Cerebellar Granule Neurons Alters Resting Cytosolic Calcium Homeostasis. *Int. J. Mol. Sci.* **2021**, *22*, 1984. [CrossRef] [PubMed]
63. Bradford, M.M. A rapid and sensitive method for the quantitation of microgram quantities of protein utilizing the principle of protein-dye binding. *Anal. Biochem.* **1976**, *72*, 248–254. [CrossRef] [PubMed]
64. Laemmli, U.K. Cleavage of structural proteins during the assembly of the head of bacteriophage T4. *Nature* **1970**, *227*, 680–685. [CrossRef] [PubMed]
65. Kao, J.P.Y.; Li, G.; Auston, D.A. Chapter 5—Practical Aspects of Measuring Intracellular Calcium Signals with Fluorescent Indicators. In *Methods in Cell Biology*; Academic Press: Cambridge, MA, USA, 2010. [CrossRef]
66. McCormack, J.G.; Cobbold, P.H. *Cellular Calcium: A Practical Approach—The Practical Approach Series*; Oxford University Press: Oxford, UK, 1991.

Disclaimer/Publisher's Note: The statements, opinions and data contained in all publications are solely those of the individual author(s) and contributor(s) and not of MDPI and/or the editor(s). MDPI and/or the editor(s) disclaim responsibility for any injury to people or property resulting from any ideas, methods, instructions or products referred to in the content.

Communication

Mechanical Properties of 3-Hydroxybutyric Acid-Induced Vesicles

Seung Jun Jung [1], Kunn Hadinoto [2] and Jin-Won Park [1,*]

[1] Department of Chemical and Biomolecular Engineering, College of Energy and Biotechnology, Seoul National University of Science and Technology, Seoul 01811, Republic of Korea
[2] School of Chemical and Biomedical Engineering, Nanyang Technological University, Singapore 637551, Singapore
* Correspondence: jwpark@seoultech.ac.kr; Tel.: +82-2-970-6605

Abstract: The vesicle mechanical behaviors were studied upon its exposure to 3-hydroxybutyric acid using an atomic force microscope (AFM). Dipalmitoylphosphatidylcholine (DPPC) and 3-hydroxybutyric acid were used to manufacture the vesicles at their desired ratio. The deflection of an AFM probe with respect to its displacement was measured after characterizing the vesicle adsorption. The movement was analyzed with the Hertzian model to understand the physical behavior of the vesicles. However, in the deflection just prior to the first penetration, the model was a good fit, and the vesicle mechanical moduli were calculated. The moduli became lower with the higher ratio of 3-hydroxybutyric acid to DPPC, but the moduli were saturated at 0.5 of the ratio. These results appear to be the basis for the function of the metabolism associated with 3-hydroxybutyric acid, i.e., anesthetization and glycemic control, on the physical properties of cell membranes.

Keywords: 3-hydroxybutyric acid; mechanical properties; vesicles

1. Introduction

3-hydroxybutyric acid (synonym, β-hydroxybutyric acid) is associated with diabetes and cranial nerve symptoms [1,2]. This compound is used as an alternative when the level of glucose is scarce in a body, because 3-hydroxybutyric acid is synthesized from acetyl-CoA in the liver [3]. The compound plays a role in inhibiting histone deacetylase and, thus, increases brain-derived neurotrophic factor (BDNF) [2]. This knowledge may be clinically relevant to the treatment of psychological symptoms. Furthermore, 3-hydroxybutyric acid has been reported to be an anesthetic in animals and has been reported to modulate the glycine-receptor function [4]. The anesthetic action was caused by the compound to modify mechanical behaviors of cell membranes to modulate the membrane protein function [5].

Since the phospholipids distributed in the biological membranes are associated with the vesicle-derived process and the antimicrobial action through their physical behavior, the mechanical properties are critical to the biological phenomena [6–9]. An atomic force microscope (AFM) can provide the properties of a surface with the motion of an AFM probe at the sub-nano scale [10–12]. Especially for a surface against the probe, the probe approach has been considered to estimate steric and electrostatic properties of the sample surface. In addition, its retreat has been used to find the adhesiveness of the surface. Many investigations have been performed with AFM force data combined with theories such as Johnson-Kendall-Roberts theory, Poisson-Boltzmann theory, particle mesh Ewald method, Derjaguin-Muller-Toporov theory, and coarse-grained model [13–17]. In this study, it was aimed to investigate the mechanical properties of 3-hydroxybutyric acid-induced vesicles with respect to their ratio of 3-hydroxybutyric acid to lipids because little is known about the 3-hydroxybutyric acid metabolic mechanism in cell membranes. This research is relevant to fundamental biological functions of cellular processes such as anesthetic action and BNDF release.

2. Results

2.1. Surface Morphology

The image prior to the adsorption suggested that the height change was less than 1 nm (Figure 1A), while the averages of the height and the width after the adsorption were 10 and 190 nm, respectively (Figure 1B). The lipid bilayer was around 5 nm thick, and the squeezed vesicles are made of two bilayers [18]. Therefore, the thickness of the adsorbed vesicles was around 10 nm. The flatness difference between two images indicated that the vesicles adsorbed to the mica surface. Furthermore, according to the ratio of 3-hydroxybutyric acid to DPPC, the morphology was little changed. Little change was predicted because the multi-layers were converted into the large unilamellar vesicle at 65 °C higher than the lipid transition temperature. The morphological characterization was consistent with the results of DLS that the diameter was little affected by the ratio of 3-hydroxybutyric acid to DPPC. Since the radius of the vesicle was included in the Equation (1), the effect of the ratio on the change in the morphology was considered.

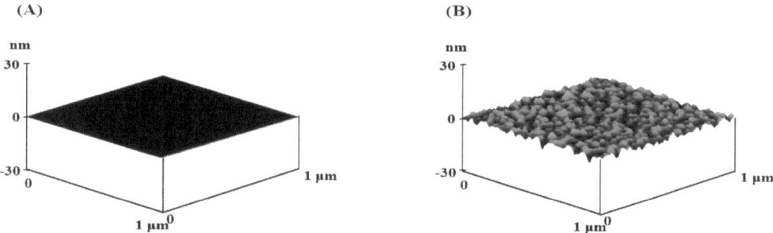

Figure 1. Surface morphology (**A**) before the lipid vesicle adsorption (**B**) after the adsorption.

2.2. Force Measurements

The deflection data represented the physical phenomena of the vesicle. Figure 2A showed the deflection with respect to the displacement of the AFM probe and was transformed into the force versus the distance between the probe and the surface (Figure 2B). The force was acquired from the multiplication of the deflection by the probe spring constant, and the distance was determined from the subtraction of the deflection from the displacement.

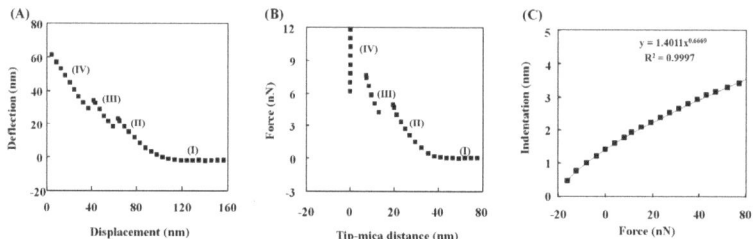

Figure 2. (**A**) Deflection with respect to displacement (z position) for the vesicle at 0% 3-hydroxybutyric acid; (**B**) force with respect to distance based on the data in (**A**); (**C**) indentation with respect to load force based on the region (II) data of (**A**,**B**).

These two graphs have identical distinct points which represent the sudden deflection of the probe and are divided into four different regions. In region (I), no contact of the probe occurred on the vesicle surface. Region (II) was from contact to the first vesicle penetration of the probe. Only region (II) was available to estimate the Young's modulus of the vesicle. Region (III) was from the first penetration to the second vesicle penetration, and region (IV) was from the second vesicle penetration to contact on the surface. The ratio of the deflection to the displacement with the probe on a hard surface is theoretically about

−1.0, and the ratio in the region (IV) was −0.99 [19]. Since the sterically repulsive distance was approximately 5 nm, no vesicle adsorption occurred on the probe. The ratio and the distance were mutually consistent with each other. In other words, the probe, after two penetrations, contacted the mica surface. This analysis was also identical to the results repeated in pure water.

2.3. Theoretical Analysis

The elasticity was explained with the slope of the force to the distance [16,20]. The slope corresponded to the resistance of each layer to the probe load. The slopes of region (II) and region (III) in Figure 2B are listed in Table 1 for the ratio of 3-hydroxybutyric acid to DPPC, and their variation ranges are less than 3%. The slope for the 0% 3-hydroxybutyric acid was 0.7 for region (II), while it was 3.6 N/m for region (III). The exponential value (b) was 0.667 for region (II) from the fitting $\delta = AF^b$ to the data, and it was 0.908 for region (III). In this formula, δ is the indentation [m] of the probe into the vesicle; F is the load force [N] of the probe; and A is the proportional constant from several parameters shown below. Therefore, the justification of the elasticity was performed using the values of b.

Table 1. Slopes of the force to the distance for the ratio of 3-hydroxybutyric acid to lipid.

Ratio of 3-Hydroxybutyric-Acid to Lipid	0	0.1	0.3	0.5	0.7	1.0
Slope of 1st steric force (N/m)	0.7 ± 0.01	0.69 ± 0.01	0.67 ± 0.01	0.65 ± 0.01	0.65 ± 0.01	0.65 ± 0.01
Slope of 2nd steric force (N/m)	3.6 ± 0.01	3.5 ± 0.01	3.4 ± 0.01	3.3 ± 0.01	3.3 ± 0.01	3.3 ± 0.01

3. Discussion

Since the exponential value of the load force for the indentation was 0.667, it was confirmed that the physical behavior of the vesicle prior to the first vesicle penetration was elastic. This confirmation led to further analysis to estimate Young's modulus, and the fits of the Hertzian model to data were the indentation (δ) for the load force (F) (Figure 2C). It was found for the physical behavior of the vesicle prior to the first vesicle penetration that the relation of the indentation to the force was in the range of exponential 0.656 to 0.676. Therefore, at least region (II) remained consistently elastic. From Young's modulus, the bending modulus was estimated. The Equations (1) and (2) provided the two vesicle moduli of the vesicle.

The increase in the ratio of 3-hydroxybutyric acid to lipid led to the decrease in Young's modulus until the ratio was 0.5. No further decrease was observed beyond 0.5. The vesicle without 3-hydroxybutyric acid showed 81×10^6 Pa as Young's modulus, which was consistent with the previous research [21]. Therefore, the dependence on the ratio was gradually decreased and saturated at 0.5. Interference of 3-hydroxybutyric acid in the lipid–headgroup arrangement may occur. The more 3-hydroxybutyric acid there is, the less moduli (Table 2). The value for each condition in Table 2 suggested an average along with a range of results.

Table 2. Mechanical moduli of the vesicle for the ratio of 3-hydroxybutyric acid/lipid, E_{ves}: Young's modulus and k_c: bending modulus.

	Ratio of 3-Hydroxybutyric Acid/Lipid					
	0	0.1	0.3	0.5	0.7	1.0
$E_{ves} \times 10^6$ (Pa)	81 ± 2	80 ± 2	78 ± 2	76 ± 2	76 ± 2	76 ± 2
$k_c \times 10^{-19}$ (J)	11.3 ± 0.3	11.1 ± 0.3	10.7 ± 0.3	10.5 ± 0.3	10.5 ± 0.3	10.5 ± 0.3

The previous study showed that a greater portion of 3-hydroxybutyric acid induced higher fluid [5]. In that research, the transition from solid to liquid happened in the solid phase. Those results are identical with those of this research because the vesicle state was in a solid phase. In addition, it has been also suggested that the association with 3-hydroxybutyric acid generated the distribution effect on the membrane to cause the change in the lipid layer.

4. Materials and Methods

Dipalmitoylphosphatidylcholine (DPPC) and 3-hydroxybutyric acid were from Sigma Aldrich (St. Louis, MO, USA). The molecules of DPPC formed the multi-layers on a glass vial bottom by evaporating chloroform with nitrogen, in which they were dissolved. The addition of the aqueous solution of Hepes 2 mM and 3-hydroxybutyric acid at pH 7 was performed in the vial to cover the layers completely overnight. The solution was vortexed 4 times every 20 min at 60° and sent through a 100-nanometer pore membrane to acquire the vesicle. The solution through the membrane was transferred for the measurement of the vesicle diameter, which was between 130 and 170 nm.

An AFM probe was located in a liquid cell and approached the mica peeled and transferred previously to the top of the AFM scanner (Nanoscope v5.12, Bruker, Billerica, MA, USA). Prior to the approach, a silicon O-ring was placed on the mica. After the approach, the vesicle solution was added to cover the mica surface completely at room temperature. After 2 hours for the adsorption, the non-adsorbed vesicles were washed out by injecting the buffer solution into the inside. After characterizing the adsorption, the deflection data were collected between the probe and the vesicle at room temperature [22]. The following theory was considered for the data with twice clear penetrations only.

The selection of data was for the analysis with the Hertzian model, which describes the elasticity of the sphere with the equation below [20,23].

$$\delta = 0.825 \left[\frac{(1-\nu_{ves}^2)^2 (R_{tip}+R_{ves})}{E_{ves}^2 R_{tip} R_{ves}} \right]^{\frac{1}{3}} F^{\frac{2}{3}} \quad (1)$$

$$\delta = |z - z_0| - (d - d_0), \quad F = k(d - d_0)$$

where ν_{ves} is Poisson's ratio of the vesicle; R_{tip} and R_{ves} are respectively the radius [m] of the probe and vesicle; E_{ves} is the Young's modulus [Pa] of the vesicle; and k is the spring constant [N/m] of the probe. The indentation was acquired from the difference between the probe displacement $|z - z_0|$ [m] and the probe deflection $(d - d_0)$ [m]. z_0 was the distance from the boundary between the regions, and d_0 was the deflection of the boundary. Therefore, the fitting of the experimental data was used through the least-square method to calculate E_{ves} using Equation (1), which was applied to the equation below to estimate the bending modulus k_c [J].

$$k_c = \frac{E_{ves} h^3}{12(1 - \nu_{ves}^2)} \quad (2)$$

where h is the thickness [m] of the vesicle bilayer.

5. Conclusions

The mechanical moduli of DPPC vesicles were investigated for the 3-hydroxybutyric acid ratio. The probe deflection was interpreted with the Hertzian model to investigate the physical behaviors of the DPPC vesicle neighboring 3-hydroxybutyric acid. The mechanical moduli were saturated at the 3-hydroxybutyric acid ratio of 0.5. This result may be caused by the degree of the lipids associated with 3-hydroxybutyric acid at the ratio. This study may be basis for biological mechanisms related to cellular processes such as anesthetization, glycemic regulation, and neuron responses.

Author Contributions: Conceptualization, J.-W.P.; methodology, S.J.J. and J.-W.P.; validation, K.H.; writing, S.J.J.; review and editing, K.H.; supervision, J.-W.P. All authors have read and agreed to the published version of the manuscript.

Funding: This research received no external funding.

Institutional Review Board Statement: Not applicable.

Data Availability Statement: Not applicable.

Acknowledgments: This study was supported by the Research Program funded by Seoul National University of Science and Technology.

Conflicts of Interest: The authors declare no conflict of interest.

References

1. Nowak, K.; Jurek, T.; Zawadzki, M. Postmortem Determination of Short-Term Markers of Hyperglycemia for the Purposes of Medicolegal Opinions. *Diagnostics* **2020**, *10*, 236. [CrossRef]
2. Sleiman, S.F.; Henry, J.; Alhaddad, R.; El Hayek, L.; Abou Haidar, E.; Stringer, T.; Ulja, D.; Karuppagounder, S.S.; Holson, E.B.; Ratan, R.R.; et al. Exercise promotes the expression of brain derived neurotrophic factor (BDNF) through the action of the ketone body beta-hydroxybutyrate. *Elife* **2016**, *5*, 5092. [CrossRef]
3. Chi, J.-T.; Lin, P.-H.; Tolstikov, V.; Oyekunle, T.; Chen, E.Y.; Bussberg, V.; Greenwood, B.; Sarangarajan, R.; Narain, N.R.; Kiebish, M.A.; et al. Metabolomic effects of androgen deprivation therapy treatment for prostate cancer. *Cancer Med.* **2019**, *9*, 3691–3702. [CrossRef]
4. Yang, L.; Zhao, J.; Milutinovic, P.S.; Brosnan, R.J.; Eger, E.I.; Sonner, J.M. Anesthetic properties of the ketone bodies beta-hydroxybutyric acid and acetone. *Anesth. Analg.* **2007**, *105*, 673–679. [CrossRef]
5. Hsu, T.T.; Leiske, D.L.; Rosenfeld, L.; Sonner, J.M.; Fuller, G.G. 3-Hydroxybutyric Acid Interacts with Lipid Mono layers at Concentrations That Impair Consciousness. *Langmuir* **2013**, *29*, 1948–1955. [CrossRef]
6. Lohner, K.; Latal, A.; Degovics, G.; Garidel, P. Packing characteristics of a model system mimicking cytoplasmic bacterial membranes. *Chem. Phys. Lipids* **2001**, *111*, 177–192. [CrossRef]
7. Zhu, Y.; Stevens, C.F. Probing synaptic vesicle fusion by altering mechanical properties of the neuronal surface membrane. *Proc. Natl. Acad. Sci. USA* **2008**, *105*, 18018–18022. [CrossRef]
8. Navarro-Hernandez, I.C.; López-Ortega, O.; Acevedo-Ochoa, E.; Cervantes-Díaz, R.; Romero-Ramírez, S.; Sosa-Hernández, V.A.; Meza-Sánchez, D.E.; Juárez-Vega, G.; Pérez-Martínez, C.A.; Chávez-Munguía, B.; et al. Tetraspanin 33 (TSPAN33) regulates endocytosis and migration of human B lymphocytes by affecting the tension of the plasma membrane. *FEBS J.* **2020**, *287*, 3449–3471. [CrossRef]
9. Khadka, N.K.; Teng, P.; Cai, J.; Pan, J. Modulation of lipid membrane structural and mechanical properties by a peptidomimetic derived from reduced amide scaffold. *Biochim. Biophys. Acta-Biomembr.* **2017**, *1859*, 734–744. [CrossRef]
10. Engler, A.J.; Richert, L.; Wong, J.Y.; Picart, C.; Discher, D.E. Surface probe measurements of the elasticity of sectioned tissue, thin gels and polyelectrolyte multilayer films: Correlations between substrate stiffness and cell adhesion. *Surf. Sci.* **2004**, *570*, 142–154. [CrossRef]
11. Wright, C.J.; Shah, M.K.; Powell, L.C.; Armstrong, I. Application of AFM from microbial cell to biofilm. *Scanning* **2010**, *32*, 134–149. [CrossRef]
12. Alam, F.; Kumar, S.; Varadarajan, K.M. Quantification of Adhesion Force of Bacteria on the Surface of Biomaterials: Techniques and Assays. *ACS Biomater Sci. Eng.* **2019**, *5*, 2093–2110. [CrossRef] [PubMed]
13. Park, J.-W. Probe chemistry effect on surface properties of asymmetric-phase lipid bilayers. *Colloids Surf. B* **2010**, *75*, 290–293. [CrossRef]
14. Ruiz-Cabello, F.J.M.; Trefalt, G.; Maroni, P.; Borkovec, M. Electric double-layer potentials and surface regulation properties measured by colloidal-probe atomic force microscopy. *Phys. Rev. E* **2014**, *90*, 012301. [CrossRef]
15. Black, J.M.; Zhu, M.; Zhang, P.; Unocic, R.R.; Guo, D.; Okatan, M.B.; Dai, S.; Cummings, P.T.; Kalinin, S.V.; Feng, G.; et al. Fundamental aspects of electric double layer force-distance measurements at liquid-solid interfaces using atomic force microscopy. *Sci. Rep.* **2016**, *6*, 32389. [CrossRef] [PubMed]
16. Iturri, J.; Toca-Herrera, J.L. Characterization of Cell Scaffolds by Atomic Force Microscopy. *Polymers* **2017**, *9*, 383. [CrossRef]
17. Kang, H.; Qian, X.; Guan, L.; Zhang, M.; Li, Q.; Wu, A.; Dong, M. Studying the Adhesion Force and Glass Transition of Thin Polystyrene Films by Atomic Force Microscopy. *Nanoscale Res. Lett.* **2018**, *13*, 5. [CrossRef] [PubMed]
18. Regan, D.; Williams, J.; Borri, P.; Langbein, W. Lipid Bilayer Thickness Measured by Quantitative DIC Reveals Phase Transitions and Effects of Substrate Hydrophilicity. *Langmuir* **2019**, *35*, 13805–13814. [CrossRef]
19. Weisenhorn, A.L.; Khorsandi, M.; Kasas, S.; Gotzos, V.; Butt, H.-J. Deformation and height anomaly of soft surfaces studied with an AFM. *Nanotechnology* **1993**, *4*, 106–113. [CrossRef]
20. Laney, D.E.; Garcia, R.A.; Parsons, S.M.; Hansma, H.G. Changes in the elastic properties of cholinergic synaptic vesicles as measured by atomic force microscopy. *Biophys. J.* **1997**, *72*, 806–813. [CrossRef]
21. Hur, J.; Park, J.-W. Trehalose-Induced Variation in Mechanical Properties of Vesicles in Aqueous Solution. *J. Membr. Biol.* **2015**, *248*, 1121–1125. [CrossRef]
22. Park, J.-W.; Lee, G.U. Properties of mixed lipid monolayers assembled on hydrophobic surfaces through vesicle adsorption. *Langmuir* **2006**, *22*, 5057–5063. [CrossRef]
23. Radmacher, M.; Fritz, M.; Kacher, C.M.; Walters, D.A.; Hansma, P.K. Imaging adhesion forces and elasticity of lysozyme adsorbed on mica with the atomic-force microscope. *Langmuir* **1994**, *10*, 3809–3814. [CrossRef]

Disclaimer/Publisher's Note: The statements, opinions and data contained in all publications are solely those of the individual author(s) and contributor(s) and not of MDPI and/or the editor(s). MDPI and/or the editor(s) disclaim responsibility for any injury to people or property resulting from any ideas, methods, instructions or products referred to in the content.

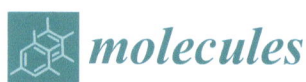 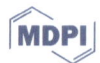

Article

New Functions of Intracellular LOXL2: Modulation of RNA-Binding Proteins

Pilar Eraso [1,†], María J. Mazón [1,†], Victoria Jiménez [1], Patricia Pizarro-García [1], Eva P. Cuevas [1,‡], Jara Majuelos-Melguizo [1], Jesús Morillo-Bernal [1], Amparo Cano [1,2,3] and Francisco Portillo [1,2,3,*]

[1] Departamento de Bioquímica UAM, Instituto de Investigaciones Biomédicas Alberto Sols, CSIC-UAM, 28029 Madrid, Spain; peraso@iib.uam.es (P.E.); mazonmaria@gmail.com (M.J.M.); victoria.jimenez@uam.es (V.J.); patripizgar@gmail.com (P.P.-G.); e.p.cuevas@csic.es (E.P.C.); jara_mm@hotmail.com (J.M.-M.); jmorillo@iib.uam.es (J.M.-B.); amparo.cano@inv.uam.es (A.C.)
[2] Instituto de Investigación Sanitaria del Hospital Universitario La Paz-IdiPAZ, 28029 Madrid, Spain
[3] Centro de Investigación Biomédica en Red, Área de Cáncer (CIBERONC), Instituto de Salud Carlos III, 28029 Madrid, Spain
* Correspondence: francisco.portillo@uam.es
† These authors contributed equally to this work.
‡ Current address: Centro de Investigaciones Biológicas Margarita Salas, 28040 Madrid, Spain.

Abstract: Lysyl oxidase-like 2 (LOXL2) was initially described as an extracellular enzyme involved in extracellular matrix remodeling. Nevertheless, numerous recent reports have implicated intracellular LOXL2 in a wide variety of processes that impact on gene transcription, development, differentiation, proliferation, migration, cell adhesion, and angiogenesis, suggesting multiple different functions for this protein. In addition, increasing knowledge about LOXL2 points to a role in several types of human cancer. Moreover, LOXL2 is able to induce the epithelial-to-mesenchymal transition (EMT) process—the first step in the metastatic cascade. To uncover the underlying mechanisms of the great variety of functions of intracellular LOXL2, we carried out an analysis of LOXL2's nuclear interactome. This study reveals the interaction of LOXL2 with numerous RNA-binding proteins (RBPs) involved in several aspects of RNA metabolism. Gene expression profile analysis of cells silenced for LOXL2, combined with in silico identification of RBPs' targets, points to six RBPs as candidates to be substrates of LOXL2's action, and that deserve a more mechanistic analysis in the future. The results presented here allow us to hypothesize novel LOXL2 functions that might help to comprehend its multifaceted role in the tumorigenic process.

Keywords: LOXL2; intracellular LOXL2; nuclear interactome; RNA-binding proteins; EMT

Citation: Eraso, P.; Mazón, M.J.; Jiménez, V.; Pizarro-García, P.; Cuevas, E.P.; Majuelos-Melguizo, J.; Morillo-Bernal, J.; Cano, A.; Portillo, F. New Functions of Intracellular LOXL2: Modulation of RNA-Binding Proteins. *Molecules* **2023**, *28*, 4433. https://doi.org/10.3390/molecules28114433

Academic Editors: Alejandro Samhan-Arias, Manuel Aureliano and Carmen Lopez-Sanchez

Received: 28 March 2023
Revised: 25 May 2023
Accepted: 26 May 2023
Published: 30 May 2023

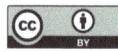

Copyright: © 2023 by the authors. Licensee MDPI, Basel, Switzerland. This article is an open access article distributed under the terms and conditions of the Creative Commons Attribution (CC BY) license (https://creativecommons.org/licenses/by/4.0/).

1. Introduction

LOXL2 belongs to the lysyl oxidase (LOX) protein family, which is constituted by five members: LOX, and four LOX-like enzymes (LOXL1–4). All members are characterized by a conserved carboxyl (C)-terminal amine oxidase catalytic domain that includes a histidine-rich copper-binding motif and a lysyl-tyrosyl-quinone cofactor, both of which are essential for the catalytic activity [1]. By contrast, the amino (N)-terminal region diverges among all members. In the case of LOXL2–4, they present four scavenger receptor cysteine-rich (SRCR) domains. Based on N-domain diversification and sequence comparison, the LOX protein family has been classssified into two subfamilies: one constituted by LOX and LOXL1, and the other including LOXL2, LOXL3, and LOXL4 [2,3]. The LOXL2–4 SRCR domains are identical to those that are widely distributed among members of the scavenger receptor superfamily [4]. The functional role of LOXL2's SRCR domains has not yet been well characterized. It is assumed that they could be involved in protein–protein interactions by analogy to the function of the SRCR domains present in other members of the scavenger receptor superfamily [5,6]. Nevertheless, it has been recently observed that specific LOXL2 and LOXL3 SRCR domains are able to deacetylate and deacetyliminate multiple acetyl-lysine residues of the STAT3 transcriptional factor by themselves [7]. Moreover, it has recently been described that the LOXL2 splice variant L2Δ13, which lacks the amino oxidase domain, is able to directly catalyze the deacetylation of aldolase A at Lys-13 [8]. These results may imply a new function of the SRCR domains that has not been described so far.

The canonical function of LOX enzymes is the maturation of the extracellular matrix (ECM). LOX enzymes catalyze the oxidative deamination of ε-amino groups of peptidyl-lysine and hydroxylysine residues to produce highly reactive aldehydes that undergo a spontaneous condensation, thereby establishing intra- or inter-crosslinkages in collagen and elastin [9,10]. Despite their well-established role in ECM maturation, lysyl oxidase proteins are also associated with diverse physiological and pathological processes, including fibrosis, cancer, and cardiovascular diseases (as reviewed in [9–13]).

Regarding LOXL2, increasing evidence has accumulated showing its role in several human cancers [14–16]. Interestingly, the role of LOXL2 in this pathological context has been associated with its intracellular location. Our previous studies in a large series of human tumor samples demonstrated that intracellular LOXL2 is associated with poor prognosis in laryngeal squamous-cell carcinomas and with distant metastasis in basal-like breast carcinomas [17,18]. Mechanistically, intracellular LOXL2 promotes tumorigenesis through transcriptional and posttranscriptional actions impinging on epithelial-to-mesenchymal transition (EMT)—a key process in the metastatic cascade. EMT is a genetic and reversible program that leads to the loss of epithelial status, apical–basal polarity, and cell–cell adhesions, as well as to the gain of mesenchymal traits, resulting in cells with a greater capacity for mobility, migration, and invasion [19]. Several transcription factors (TFs) have been described during the past decade as EMT inducers (EMT-TFs). A plethora of signaling pathways converge in the activation of one or more of the core EMT-TFs, including the zinc finger TFs of the SNAIL (SNAI1, SNAI2) and ZEB (ZEB1 and ZEB2) families, and the basic helix-loop-helix TFs TCF3 (also known as E47) and TWIST1 [20–23]. LOXL2 induces EMT through several mechanisms. It collaborates with SNAI1 to repress CDH1 (E-cadherin gene) expression by counteracting the SNAI1 GSK3β-dependent degradation, thereby increasing SNAI1's stability [24]. LOXL2 can also oxidize the trimethylated lysine 4 in histone 3 (H3K4me3) after SNAI1 binding to heterochromatin, thereby repressing CDH1 transcription [25,26]. Repression of E-cadherin expression is also mediated by the interaction between LOXL2 and TCF3/E47 and their direct binding to the CDH1 promoter region [27]. LOXL2 can also mediate the transcriptional downregulation of components of tight junctions and cell polarity complexes, including the *claudin-1* and *Lgl2* genes [18]. Moreover, in skin cancer cells, LOXL2 collaborates with KLF4 in the NOTCH1 promoter, where it oxidizes H3K4me3, thereby impairing RNA polymerase II recruitment and inhibiting NOTCH1 transcription, repressing epidermal differentiation [28]. More recently, we reported that LOXL2 overexpression promotes its accumulation in the endoplasmic reticulum, where it interacts with the HSPA5 chaperone, leading to the activation of the IRE1-XBP1s and PERK signaling pathways of the unfolded protein response, which, in turn, induces the expression of several EMT-TFs (SNAI1, SNAI2, ZEB2, and TCF3) [29]. Some of these actions are independent of LOXL2's amino oxidase catalytic activity [7,8,29–31].

As described above, many studies show that LOXL2 promotes the progression of many types of tumors. This implies that inhibitors decreasing LOXL2 expression or activity may be useful therapeutic agents for the treatment of many types of cancer. The development of LOX2 inhibitors started with simtuzumab—a humanized LOXL2-targeting antibody that failed to show clinical effectiveness in several phase 2 clinical trials in several types of cancer [32,33]. Recently, efforts have focused on the search for small-molecular-weight LOXL2 inhibitors. One example is PXS-S1A—a first-generation LOXL2 inhibitor derived from haloallylamine that has shown promising results in preclinical models. In MDA-MB-231 human model cells of breast cancer, PXS-S1A inhibited the growth of primary tumors and reduced primary tumor angiogenesis, although it was less efficient at blocking the overall metastatic burden in the lungs and liver [34]. In any case, we must be aware that lysyl oxidase family members may have overlapping functions, as recently shown for LOXL2 and LOXL3 [35]. Additionally, it should be considered that small-molecular-weight LOXL2 inhibitors are designed to block the catalytic activity of the enzyme, and we know that the classical oxidase activity is not required for many of the intracellular functions of LOXL2 in cancer, such as the induction of EMT.

Despite the accumulated evidence for LOXL2's intracellular functions, the mechanisms of LOXL2's actions promoting tumor progression are not yet fully understood. With the aim of further understanding the intracellular LOXL2 functions impinging on tumorigenesis, we explored the nuclear interactome of LOXL2. To this end, we performed immunoprecipitation experiments on a nuclear-enriched fraction of cells expressing a flag-tagged version of LOXL2, and we analyzed the proteins co-immunoprecipitating with LOXL2 by LC-MS/MS. The quality of the interactome was evaluated by co-immunoprecipitation analyses of endogenous LOXL2 and selected interacting proteins. LOXL2's nuclear interactome is composed of numerous RNA-binding proteins (RBPs) involved in all aspects of mRNA metabolism. The deletion of individual LOXL2-SRCR domains, combined with co-immunoprecipitation experiments, suggested that the SRCR-1 domain is required for LOXL2's interaction with nuclear proteins. To identify, among the possible RBPs targeted by LOXL2, those functionally relevant in tumorigenesis, a gene expression profile of cells silenced for LOXL2 was performed, followed by a selection of genes directly involved in EMT. This EMT signature was further scrutinized for genes containing binding sites for the RBPs identified in the LOXL2 interactome. After this study, six RBPs (ELAVL1, FMR1, IGF2BP1, TAF15, SRSF1, and U2AF2) emerged as solid candidates to be regulated by LOXL2, with potential implications in EMT regulation.

2. Results

2.1. Nuclear Interactome of LOXL2

To identify LOXL2's potential nuclear partners, we utilized HEK293T cells transfected with an empty flag vector or carrying a flag-tagged version of LOXL2. Nuclear-enriched extracts of duplicated cell cultures were immunoprecipitated with the corresponding anti-tag antibodies and subjected to LC-MS/MS identification. Prior to analysis, the hits identified in immunoprecipitates from flag-empty vector experiments were subtracted from the group of proteins immunoprecipitated with flag-LOXL2 (Dataset S1). Proteins identified with two or more peptides in the two experimental flag-LOXL2 immunoprecipitates were selected, resulting in a core set of 107 proteins (Figure 1A). While HSPA5 and IRS4 were identified as LOXL2 interactors in a previous study [36], most of the identified proteins in the present nuclear LOXL2 interactome represented novel interactions. To assess the robustness of the obtained interactome, we analyzed the interaction of endogenous LOXL2 with selected interactome proteins by co-immunoprecipitation assays in Hs578T cells (Figure 1B).

To gain insights into the biological functions associated with the nuclear LOXL2 interactome, Gene Ontology (GO) analyses were performed using the DAVID functional annotation tool [37,38]. Functional enrichment analysis of molecular functions using the GOTERM_MF_DIRECT category revealed several distinct groups of functionally related proteins involved in RNA metabolism (Figure 2A). The most significantly enriched term that originated from the analysis was related to the RNA-binding cluster. Comparison of the interactome with the RNA-binding protein (RBP) database [39] showed that 86% of the proteins (93 out 107) of the LOXL2 interactome were in fact RBPs (highlighted in red in Figure 1A). Indeed, the LOXL2 interactome functional enrichment analysis of biological processes using the GOTERM_BP_DIRECT category revealed that LOXL2-interacting RBPs cover all facets of RNA metabolism, including splicing, modification, intracellular trafficking, translation, and decay (Figure 2B) [40]. Additionally, most of the LOXL2-interacting RBPs identified in this study have been associated with different cancer traits [41–45] and are being used as potential targets for cancer therapeutics [46]. The finding of these RBPs as potential partners for LOXL2 allows us to hypothesize the modulation of RBPs' function as a new molecular mechanism of LOXL2's action in tumor progression.

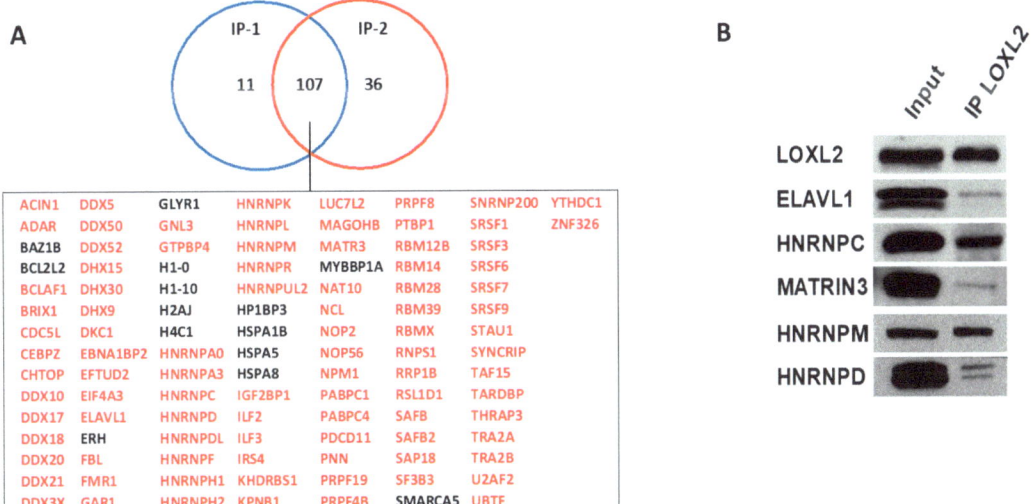

Figure 1. LOXL2's nuclear interaction partners: (**A**) Immunoprecipitation of flag-LOXL2 in two independent experiments (IP-1 and IP-2) in HEK293T cells identified 107 proteins, which are listed below the Venn diagram. RBPs are marked in red. (**B**) Co-immunoprecipitation of endogenous LOXL2 in Hs578T cells and selected RBPs.

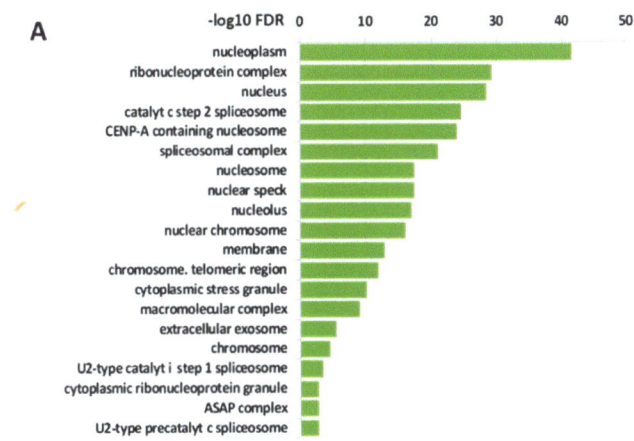

Figure 2. *Cont.*

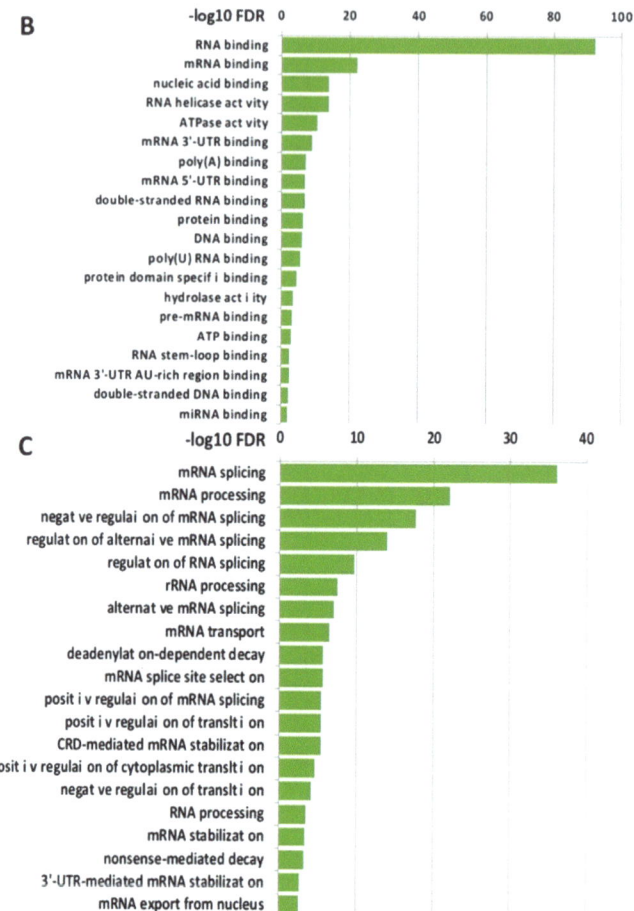

Figure 2. Molecular and biological functions of LOXL2's nuclear interaction partners: Enriched categories were obtained using the DAVID functional annotation tool and ranked by the FDR value (−Log10 FDR) shown on the x-axis. (**A**) Functional enrichment analysis of molecular function using the GOTERM_CC_DIRECT category. (**B**) Functional enrichment analysis of biological function using the GOTERM_MF_DIRECT category. (**C**) Functional enrichment analysis of biological function using the GOTERM_BP_DIRECT category.

2.2. LOXL2 Interacts with RBPs through the SRCR-1 Domain

SRCRs are evolutionarily conserved domains of about 110 amino acids that were first discovered in the type I macrophage scavenger receptor [5]. There are two types of SRCR domains: class A and B, which are characterized by the presence of six and eight cysteine residues, respectively. The spacing pattern between the cysteine residues is conserved within the domains, and they participate in the formation of intramolecular disulfide bridges [47,48]. The function of SRCRs is not fully understood, but they are believed to mediate the binding of the SRCR superfamily of proteins to their substrates, which can be lipids, polysaccharides, or other proteins [5]. LOXL2 contains four SRCR domains of class A, and cumulative evidence suggests that some of LOXL2's functions are independent of the amino oxidase catalytic domain but SRCR-domain-dependent [7,8,29–31,36,49,50].

To dissect the LOXL2 SRCR domain(s) involved in LOXL2's interaction with RBPs, HEK293T cells were transfected with four HA-tagged LOXL2 mutants carrying a deletion of each of the individual SRCR domains (Figure 3A). ELAVL1 (also known as HuR) was one of the RBPs identified as a member of LOXL2's nuclear interactome (Figure 1A); moreover, it constitutes one of the most intensively studied RBPs, and its association with tumorigenesis has been broadly reported [51]. Therefore, ELAVL1/HuR was selected to evaluate whether any of the LOXL2 mutants failed to bind this RBP. We performed co-immunoprecipitation assays using an antibody against HuR. The results (Figure 3B) showed that the mutant lacking the SRCR-1 domain (Δ-1) did not bind to ELAVL1/HuR. To expand this result to other proteins of the LOXL2 interactome, we performed LOXL2 and mutant Δ-1 co-immunoprecipitation assays with anti-HA antibody and analyzed the immunoprecipitates with antibodies against HSPA5, HNRNPC, MATRIN3, and HNRNPM. The results (Figure 3C) showed that the LOXL2 mutant devoid of SRCR-1 failed to bind to any of the evaluated proteins.

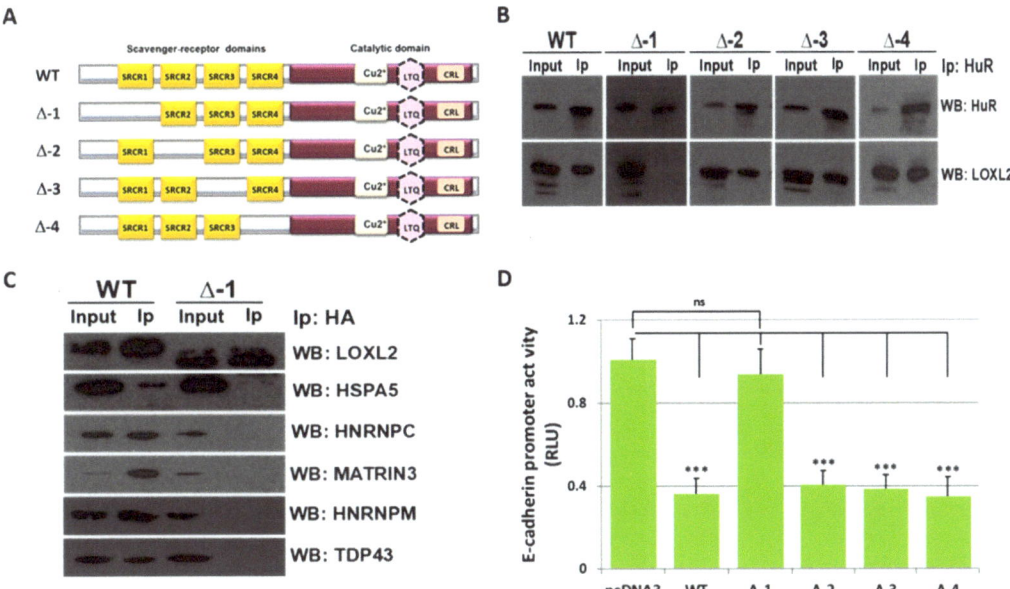

Figure 3. LOXL2's SRCR-1 domain is required for protein interaction: (**A**) Schematic representation of wild-type LOXL2 (WT) and mutants carrying a deletion of the following SRCR domains: SRCR-1 (Δ-1), SRCR-2 (Δ-2), SRCR-3 (Δ-3), or SRCR-4 (Δ-4). (**B**) Whole-cell lysates of HEK293T cells transfected with LOXL2 WT or indicated SRCR-deletion mutants were immunoprecipitated with anti-ELAVL1/HuR antibody and analyzed by WB, with anti-LOXL2 antibody and anti-HuR antibodies as controls. (**C**) HEK293T cells were transfected with LOXL2 (WT) or the mutant carrying the deletion of the SRCR-1 domain (Δ-1); LOXL2 was immunoprecipitated using anti-HA antibody and analyzed by WB with the indicated antibodies. (**D**) The activity of the *E-cadherin* promoter in HEK293T cells was measured in the presence of the indicated LOXL2 mutants. The activity was determined as relative luciferase units (RLU) and normalized to the activity detected in the presence of the control pcDNA3 vector. Results represent the mean ± SEM. of at least three independent experiments performed in triplicate (*** $p < 0.001$, ns, not significant).

We previously identified LOXL2 as a repressor of *E-cadherin* gene expression, and promoter assays indicated that the activity of the *E-cadherin* promoter was downregulated by LOXL2 through interaction with accessory proteins [29]. To analyze whether the transcriptional repression mediated by LOXL2 depends on its SRCR-1 domain, *E-cadherin* promoter assays were performed in the presence of wild-type LOXL2 or the LOXL2 mutants devoid of each individual SRCR domain. The results (Figure 3D) showed that repression of the

E-cadherin promoter is abolished in the presence of the mutant deleted of the SRCR-1 domain, suggesting that the interaction of LOXL2 with auxiliary proteins to repress *E-cadherin* gene expression is mediated by the SRCR-1 domain in vivo.

2.3. Identification of Putative RBP Candidates to Be Regulated by LOXL2

Due to the considerable number of RBPs identified in this study, we found it necessary to introduce selective criteria that could guide us to specific RBPs participating in transcriptionally related LOXL2 function. We reasoned that if LOXL2 was modulating the activity of any RBP, this should reflect on the gene expression profile of cells devoid of LOXL2. For the same reason, many of the mRNAs from LOXL2-regulated genes should be binding targets of the RBPs. As a first approach to identify those specific RBPs targeted by LOXL2, we analyzed the effects of LOXL2 silencing on gene expression profiles and, subsequently, examined whether the genes regulated by LOXL2 were potential targets of the RBPs. To this end, we performed an RNA sequence analysis of the gene expression profile of Hs578T-shLOXL2 compared to control cells after confirming the efficient LOXL2 silencing at the mRNA and protein levels (Figure S1). The RNA sequence analysis revealed a total of 4738 significantly expressed genes (p-value adjusted by FDR ≤ 0.05) (Dataset S2). Among them, we identified 621 differentially expressed genes with log2(fold change) ≥ 1 or ≤ -1, the majority being downregulated in shLOXL2 cells (488 genes out of 621) (Figure 4A).

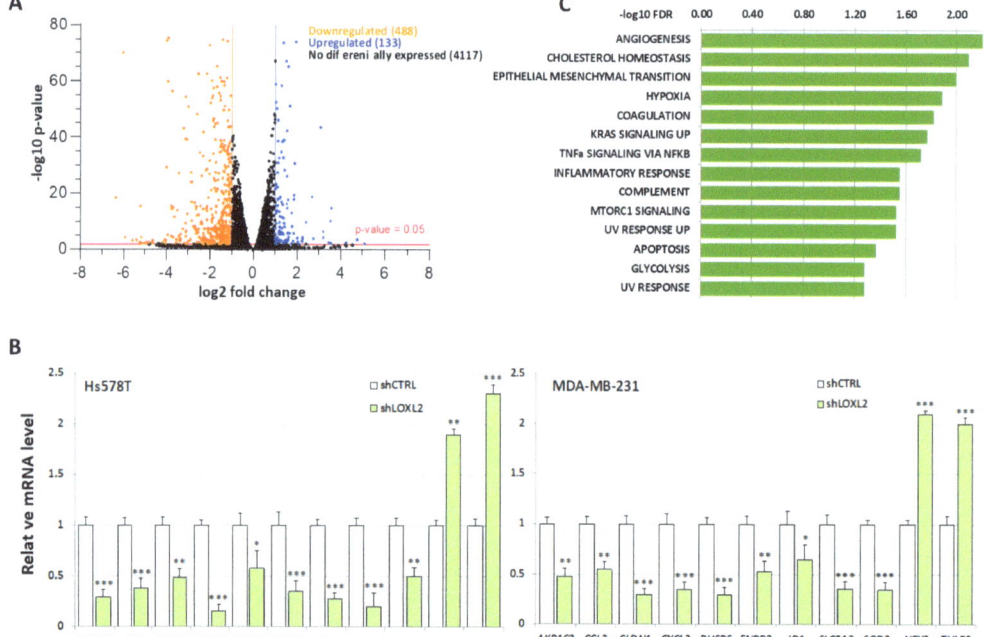

Figure 4. Gene expression profile of LOXL2-silenced cells: (**A**) Volcano plot showing transcriptome changes in LOXL2-depleted cells. The cutoffs were established at the log2 fold change > 1.0 or <−1.0 and the p-value < 0.05. Orange and blue dots represent significantly downregulated and upregulated genes, respectively. (**B**) Quantitative RT-qPCR confirming regulation of selected genes in LOXL2-ablated cells (dark green) compared to LOXL2 control cells (light green). Data are the mean ± SEM of three independent experiments assayed in triplicated samples in two independent breast cancer cell lines. The p-value was calculated by two-sided unpaired Student's t-test. (**C**) GSEA plot of differentially expressed genes (DEGs) showing enrichment of hallmark signatures. FDR values (−log10 FDR) of such enrichments are shown on the x-axis. (* p < 0.05, ** p < 0.01, *** p < 0.001).

None of the RBPs identified in the LOXL2 interactome exhibited altered levels in the RNA-Seq analysis. The data of the gene expression profile was confirmed by analyses of selected genes by RT-qPCR in Hs578T-shLOXL2 and MDA-MB-231-shLOXL2 cells compared to control cell lines. We observed that the pattern of gene expression was highly consistent between both cell lines (Figure 4B) and was comparable to the data obtained from the RNA-Seq analysis (Dataset S2).

To determine whether the DEGs belonged to a particular enriched pathway, we performed a gene set enrichment analysis (GSEA) using the "Hallmark" gene sets collection [52,53]. We observed several enriched pathways (p-value < 0.005) (Figure 4C), with EMT being one of the more significantly enriched signatures.

In fact, a search of the literature (Dataset S3) revealed that there is experimental evidence of involvement in EMT for 19.3% of the genes (120 out 621) (Figure 5A). Ninety-two of the EMT-related genes were downregulated, while the rest were upregulated (Figure 5B).

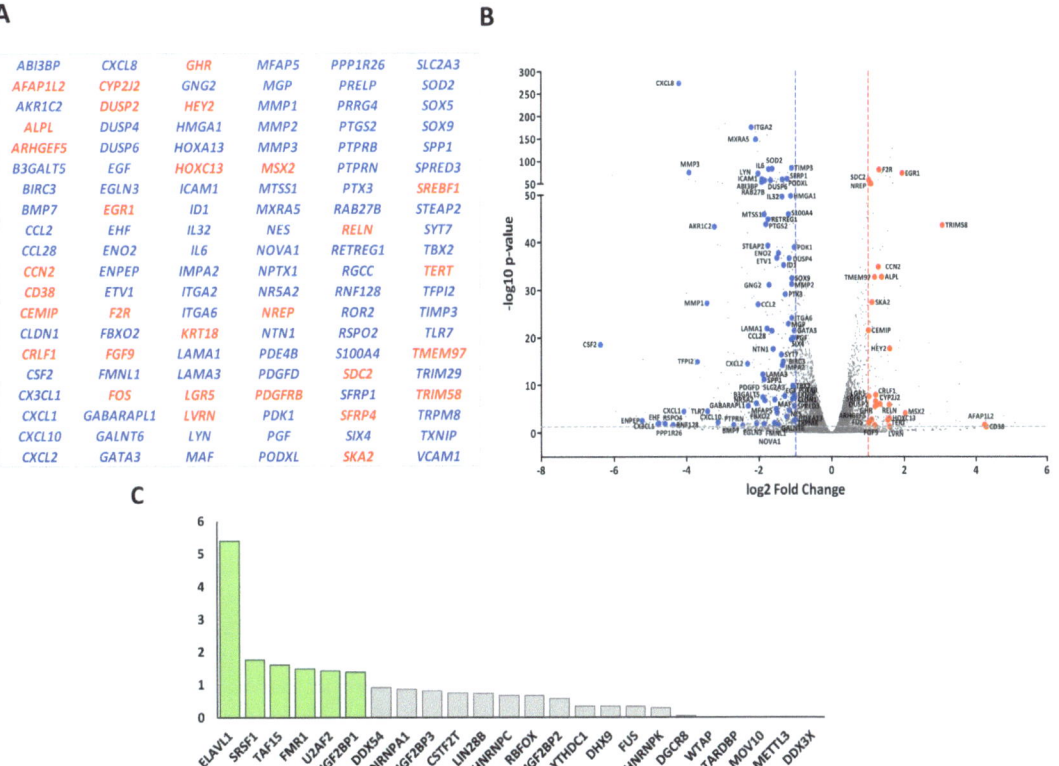

Figure 5. RBP candidates to be regulated by LOXL2: (**A**) List of differentially expressed genes in LOXL2-silenced cells with a described role in EMT. Up- and downregulated genes are marked in red and blue, respectively. (**B**) Volcano plot showing LOXL2-regulated EMT-related genes. The cutoffs were established at the log2 fold change > 1.0 (red line) or <−1.0 (blue line) and the p-value < 0.05 (grey line). Red and blue dots denote up- and downregulated EMT-related genes, respectively. (**C**) Enrichment plot of RBPs' targets in the EMT-related signature relative to the non-EMT-related signature. The p-values were obtained by using Fisher's exact test to compare the number of targets in both groups of genes. A p-value < 0.05 was considered statistically significant. Boxes marked in green represent significantly enriched RBPs.

Subsequently, we searched the ENCORI database [54] for the genes targeted by the RBPs identified in LOXL2's interactome. We extracted the gene target list for the 24 RBPs presenting high-stringency CLIP-Seq data (CLIP-Seq data from ≥ 5 different experiments) [54]. Next, we compared the list of genes targeted by each RBP with the gene set of the EMT-related signature and the remaining DEGs (not EMT-related). In three cases (DDX3X, METTL3, and WTAP), we could not find any target among the DEGs. The remaining RBPs targeted 107 and 402 genes of the EMT-related (Figure S2) and non-EMT-related signatures (Figure S3), respectively, with different frequencies. The numbers of RBP hits in both signatures are shown in Table S1. Fisher's exact test analysis of the RBPs targeting genes in the EMT-related versus non-EMT-related signatures showed that the binding sites of six RBPs (ELAVL1, FMR1, IGF2BP1, TAF15, SRSF1, and U2AF2) were significantly enriched in the EMT signature (p-value < 0.05) (Figure 5C) (Table S1), pointing to those RBPs as candidates to be regulated by LOXL2.

3. Discussion

The aim of this study was to identify new targets of LOXL2 that could be involved in the regulation of EMT. We performed LOXL2 co-immunoprecipitation experiments that revealed LOXL2's interactions with a large number of RBPs. Additionally, we also found that the LOXL2–RBP interactions were mediated by the SRCR-1 domain. The low-resolution structure of LOXL2 has recently been determined [55], revealing that the SRCR-1–3 domains project linearly away from the catalytic domain, with the SRCR-1 domain being the most external one—a situation that is compatible with our finding that SRCR-1 domain could participate in protein–protein interactions.

RBPs play essential roles in modulating gene expression by regulating splicing, RNA stability, and protein translation, and we reasoned that the impact of LOXL2 on the function of specific RBPs may leave an imprint on the gene expression profile of cells lacking LOXL2. A similar approach has been successfully used to uncover the contribution of hnRNPC to chemotherapy resistance in lung cancer [56]. The analysis of the gene expression profile of breast cancer cells silenced for LOXL2 revealed 120 DEGs involved in EMT. Subsequently, we identified the RBPs significantly targeting the EMT signature. Despite the limitations of this study, the results obtained point to six RBPs (ELAVL1, IGF2BP1, FMR1, TAF15, SRSF1, and U2AF2) as candidates to be regulated by LOXL2 in the context of EMT. The evidence in support of this proposal is based on the implication of these RBPs in EMT and the possible modulation of their function by LOXL2-mediated lysine oxidation.

ELAVL1 (ELAV-like RNA-binding protein 1), also known as HuR (human antigen R), is a member of the Hu family of RNA-binding proteins. This family comprises four members: the neuronal proteins HuB, HuC, and HuD, and the ubiquitously expressed HuR [57]. ELAVL1 binds to AU-rich elements located in the mRNA 3′-UTR region and contributes to stabilizing and controlling the translation of mRNAs containing those motifs [58]. Thousands of mRNAs are ELAVL1 targets, including factors fostering diverse cancer traits such as proliferation (cyclins A2, B1, D1, and E1), angiogenesis (HIF1a, PTGS2, and VEGFA), survival (BCL2 and MCL1), and invasion (MMP9 and SNAI1) [59,60]. In addition, ELAVL1 has also been described as an EMT modulator in breast and pancreatic cancers [61,62]. Furthermore, several modifications of lysine residues impact on ELAVL1's functions. For instance, ELAVL1's protein stability is controlled by bTrCP1-mediated Lys 182 ubiquitination and MDM2-mediated neddylation of Lys 283, 313, and 326 [63,64]. In addition, neddylation of Lys 313 and 326 also affects ELAVL1's RNA-binding activity [65]. Therefore, hypothetically, LOXL2 oxidization of those lysines could counteract ELAVL1's ubiquitination/neddylation, thereby altering the half-life and/or RNA-binding capacity of ELAVL1, which could impact on its EMT-regulatory function.

IGF2BP1 (insulin-like growth factor-2 mRNA-binding protein 1) belongs to a conserved family of RBPs that comprises three members: IGF2BP1, -2, and -3. IGFBPs control the stability, export, and translation of different mRNAs, including KRAS and MYC mRNAs [66]. IGF2BP1 has been reported to induce EMT by enhancing the expression of *LEF1* and *SNAI2* [67]. Mechanistically, IGF2BP1 is activated by FBXO45 ubiquitination of Lys 190 and 450 [68], suggesting that the oxidation of those lysines by LOXL2 could block IGF2BP1's ubiquitination and activation, thereby altering EMT.

FMR1 (fragile X messenger ribonucleoprotein 1) binds RNA, is associated with polysomes, and acts as regulator of translation [69]. When inactivated by a triplet nucleotide repeat expansion, it causes the neurodevelopmental disorder fragile X syndrome [70]. Despite its well-established role in the brain, in cancer cells FMR1 binds mRNAs involved in EMT and regulates their stability and translation [71]. FMR1's stability is controlled by the ubiquitin ligase Cdh1-APC through lysine ubiquitination [72]. Prevention of lysine ubiquitination by LOXL2-mediated oxidation would prevent FMR1's degradation and alter EMT status.

TAF15 (TATA-box-binding protein-associated factor 15) is a member of the TET family of proteins (which includes TLS, EWS, and TAF15). TAF15 (also known as TAFII68) was originally identified as a member of a subpopulation of the general transcription factor IID (TFIID) [73]. TFIID is the sequence-specific DNA-binding component of the RNA polymerase II transcriptional machinery. TFIID is composed of the TATA-binding protein (TBP) and at least 13 TBP-associated factors (TAF1-13). TAF15 is distinct from the other 13 best-known TAFs constituting the TFIID complex [74]. In this sense, TAF15 silencing does not affect general transcription but seems to impact a small subset of cell-cycle genes though miRNAs [74]. The TAF15/TBP complex is required for IL-6-activation-induced EMT and invasion [75]. Remarkably, LOXL2 is able to oxidize methylated lysines of TAF10—other components of the TFIID complexes—to represses TFIID-transcription-dependent genes [76]; therefore, it is conceivable that LOXL2 could exert a similar function on TAF15 to modify EMT status.

SRSF1 (RNA-binding protein serine/arginine splicing factor 1) is a splicing factor that, in addition to its function in alternative splicing, participates in nonsense-mediated mRNA decay, mRNA export, and translation [77]. Its involvement in EMT is well established as a regulator of alternative splicing of hundreds of genes, but recently it has been shown that it can induce EMT by stabilizing *RECQL4* mRNA [78]. SRSF1's stability is also restrained by lysine ubiquitination [79], which could eventually be altered by LOXL2-mediated lysine oxidation.

U2AF2 (U2 small nuclear RNA auxiliary factor 2) is a component of the spliceosome complex that appears mutated with low frequency in myelodysplastic syndromes [80], but to the best of our knowledge its role in EMT regulation has not been tested. U2AF2's stability is controlled by lysine ubiquitination [81]. In addition, JMJD6-mediated hydroxylation of Lys 15, 38, and 276 is required for the regulation of a large set of alternative splicing events [82]. Thus, lysine oxidation by LOXL2 could modify U2AF2's function.

Altogether, our results suggest that LOXL2's interaction with the candidate RBPs could alter cancer traits at different levels. LOXL2's interaction with ELAVL1 or IGF2BP1 may modulate the mRNA stability of proto-oncogenes, cytokines, and growth factors to promote cell survival, metastasis, and drug resistance [83,84]. By interaction with FMR1, LOXL2 may modify the mRNA translation of genes implicated in the hallmarks of cancer, such as *TP53*, *VEGF*, *hTERT*, *TGFB2*, and other essential oncogenes [85]. LOXL2 can collaborate with TAF15 in the regulation of genes such as *CDKN1A*, *CDK6*, *CCND1*, and other cell-cycle genes at the posttranscriptional level to control cell proliferation [74]. LOXL2 may also alter alternative splicing through interaction with SRSF1, which, in turn, may affect apoptosis and proliferation [86]. Finally, LOXL2–U2AF2 interaction may also alter pre-mRNA splicing. U2AF2 is an essential component required for the splicing of vertebrate pre-mRNAs, and it has been described to mediate the alternative splicing of CD44, which confers metastatic potential to tumors [81].

Our LOXL2 interactome analysis sheds light on new functions in EMT regulation for this multifaceted protein. Nevertheless, the large number of RBPs identified in this study suggests that LOXL2 could be implicated in many facets of mRNA metabolism that could impact on multiple cell functions beyond the EMT process, and that deserve future investigations. Concerning the LOXL2–RBPs–EMT link, further research to characterize the functional interplay between LOXL2 and selected RBPs, along with its impact on EMT, will help to uncover novel roles of intracellular LOXL2 in tumorigenesis.

4. Materials and Methods

4.1. Cell Culture and Plasmid Constructs

Human HEK293T, MDA-MB-231, and Hs578T cell lines were obtained from the American Type Culture Collection. Cells were grown in DMEM medium (Gibco, Grand Island, NY, USA) supplemented with 10% fetal bovine serum, 10 mmol/L glutamine (Life Technologies, Carlsbad, CA, USA), and 1% penicillin/streptomycin (Invitrogen, Waltham, MA, USA). All cell lines were grown at 37 °C in a humidified 5% CO_2 atmosphere. Cells were routinely tested for *Mycoplasma* contamination.

Human breast carcinoma Hs578T and MDA-MB-231 cells silenced for LOXL2 (shLOXL2) and control cells (shCTRL) were generated by stable transfection with pSuper-shLOXL2 and pSuper-shEGFP vectors, respectively, as described in [18]. Briefly, cells were transfected using Lipofectamine (Invitrogen) reagent with 5 µg of plasmids and selected in the presence of puromycin (1 µg/mL) for 2–3 weeks. LOXL2 silencing was confirmed by RT-qPCR and WB (Figure S1).

The human pcDNA3-Flag-LOXL2 vectors were as previously described in [87]. The human pReceiver-M06-HA-LOXL2 was purchased from GeneCopoeia (Ex-Y2020-M06). LOXL2 mutants carrying individual SRCR domain deletions (Δ1–Δ4) were generated from pReceiver-M06-HA-LOXL2 by site-directed mutagenesis and were performed by Mutagenex Inc. LOXL2 mutant Δ1 lacks amino acids 58 to 159, mutant Δ2 lacks amino acids 188–302, mutant Δ3 lacks amino acids 326–425, and mutant Δ4 lacks amino acids 435–544. The mouse *E-cadherin* promoter (-178 to $+92$) fused to the *luciferase* reporter gene was as previously described in [88].

4.2. Identification of Nuclear Proteins Associated with LOXL2

Nuclear protein extracts were obtained as described in [89]. Briefly, pcDNA3-Flag control and pcDNA3-Flag-LOXL2-transfected HEK293T cells were suspended in 10 mM HEPES pH 7.9, 10 mM KCl, 0.1 mM EDTA, 0.1 mM EGTA, 1 mM DTT, and a protease inhibitor cocktail (Roche). Cells were homogenized by adding 0.5% NP-40, and the tube was vigorously vortexed for 10 s. The homogenate was centrifuged for 5 min at $3000 \times g$, and the supernatant containing cytoplasmic proteins was discarded. The nuclear proteins were extracted in 20 mM HEPES pH 7.9, 400 mM NaCl, 1 mM EDTA, 1 mM EGTA, 1 mM DTT, and a protease inhibitor cocktail on ice for 30 min with occasional gentle shaking. The nuclear extracts were centrifuged for 10 min at $12,000 \times g$, and the supernatants were incubated overnight at 4 °C with 0.5 mg of Dynabeads Protein G (Thermo Fisher, Waltham, MA, USA) previously coated with 3 µg of anti-Flag antibody. The beads were washed three times with 20 mM HEPES pH 7.9, 1 mM EDTA, 1 mM EGTA, 1 mM DTT, and a protease inhibitor cocktail and then boiled in Laemmli sample buffer for 5 min. The supernatants were sent to the proteomic core facility of the Universidad Complutense de Madrid for protein identification by liquid chromatography–tandem mass spectrometry (LC-MS/MS).

4.3. Co-Immunoprecipitation

HEK293T cells were transiently transfected with pReceiver-LOXL2-HA and derivative mutants using Lipofectamine reagent (Invitrogen) with 2 µg of indicated plasmids. After 48 h, the cells were homogenized in 50 mM Tris-HCl pH 7.4, 150 mM NaCl, 5 mM EDTA, 1% Triton X-100 (IP buffer), and a protease inhibitor cocktail for 30 min at 4 °C with occasional gentle shaking. The homogenates were centrifuged for 15 min at $10,000 \times g$ and the pellet was discarded. Total lysates (0.5 mg) were incubated overnight at 4 °C with 3 µg of anti-ELAVL1 (Abcam, Cambridge, UK; ab136542) or anti-HA (Roche Life Science, Penzberg, Germany; 11-867-423-001) antibodies. Immune complexes were isolated by incubation with 1 mg of Dynabeads Protein G in IP buffer and a protease inhibitor cocktail for 3 h at 4 °C. After extensive washing (five times) with 1 mL of IP buffer, the immune complexes were eluted by incubation for 5 min at 95 °C in Laemmli sample buffer. Co-immunoprecipitation of endogenous LOXL2 in Hs578T cells and selected RBPs was performed as described above, except that the homogenate was incubated with anti-LOXL2 (Abcam; ab96233) or IgG antibody (Millipore, Burlington, MA, USA; cat. #PP64B). The proteins present in the eluted fractions were separated by SDS–polyacrylamide gel electrophoresis and analyzed by immunoblotting using an LOXL2 antibody from OriGene (TA807444); ELAVL1 (ab 200342), HSPA5 (ab21685), HNRNPC (ab133607), or MATRIN3 (ab151714) antibodies from Abcam; and HNRNPD (sc-166577) or HNRNPM (sc-20002) antibodies from Santa Cruz.

4.4. Promoter Assays

Luciferase reporter assays were performed as described in [90]. Briefly, transfections were carried out using Lipofectamine in the presence of 50 ng of empty pReceiver vector; pReceiver-LOXL2-HA, Δ1, Δ2, Δ3, or Δ4 expression vectors; 200 ng of mouse *E-cadherin* promoter; and 10 ng of pCMV-β-gal as a control for transfection efficiency. Luciferase and β-galactosidase activities were measured using the luciferase and β-Glo assay substrates (Promega) and normalized to the promoter activity detected in cells transfected with the empty pReceiver vector.

4.5. Gene Expression Profile Analysis

RNA from three independent clones of Hs578T-shCTRL control and Hs578T-shLOXL2 cells was used to perform RNA sequence analyses (Sistemas Genómicos, Valencia, Spain). Significant differentially expressed genes (DEGs) were selected by cutoff of *p*-values adjusted by false discovery rate (FDR) ≤ 0.05 and fold change greater than 2.

4.6. RNA Extraction, cDNA Synthesis, and Quantitative PCR (qPCR)

RNA was extracted and quality-tested in the Genomics Core Facility at the Instituto de Investigaciones Biomédicas Alberto Sols CSIC-UAM (Madrid, Spain). For cDNA synthesis, 1 μg of RNA was reverse-transcribed into cDNA using 200 units of M-MLV reverse transcriptase (Promega Corporation, Madison, WI, USA), 5 μL of M-MVL buffer (Promega), 0.5 μg of random primers (Promega), 10 mM dNTP mix (Bioron, Römerberg, Germany), and 25 units of RNaseOUT™ Recombinant Ribonuclease Inhibitor (Invitrogen) in a final reaction volume of 25 μL. Real-time qPCR was performed using Power SYBR Green Master Mix (Thermo Fisher) on the Applied Biosystems StepOne™ machine (Thermo Fisher). Each reaction was performed with 20 ng of cDNA and 9 pmol of specific forward and reverse primers (Supplementary Table S2). Values were normalized to the *GAPDH* housekeeping gene, and relative expression levels were analyzed by the $2^{-\Delta\Delta Ct}$ method. qPCRs were carried out in three independent samples assayed in triplicate.

4.7. Statistical Analysis

In the RT-qPCR assays, the *p*-values were generated using Student's *t*-test (unpaired, 2-tailed); *p*-values < 0.05 were considered statistically significant. Data are presented as the mean ± standard error of the mean (SEM).

The analyses of RBP targets' enrichment in the EMT signature with respect to the rest of the DEGs were performed by comparing the numbers of targets between both groups of genes using Fisher's exact test. A *p*-value < 0.05 was considered statistically significant.

5. Conclusions

This study intended to identify nuclear partners of LOXL2 involved in EMT regulation. We report that LOXL2's nuclear interactome is composed of numerous RBPs functioning in different aspects of mRNA metabolism. LOXL2 SRCR-1 was identified as the domain mediating interaction with RBPs. Analysis of mRNA changes associated with LOXL2 silencing, combined with the in silico identification of RBPs' targets, pointed to six RBPs as candidates to be modulated by LOXL2, with likely influence on EMT regulation. Our results link LOXL2 to RBPs' modulation in breast cancer; thus, using LOXL2 inhibitors in combination with RBP inhibitors may provide a more effective therapeutic strategy for treating breast cancer, as well as circumventing potential issues associated with targeting LOXL2 alone.

Supplementary Materials: The following supporting information can be downloaded at: https://www.mdpi.com/article/10.3390/molecules28114433/s1, Dataset S1: Data of LC-MS/MS of immunoprecipitations 1 and 2. Dataset S2: Data of RNAs-Seq analysis. Dataset S3: List of bibliographic references with experimental evidence of involvement of the EMT-related gene signature in EMT. Figure S1: Silencing of LOXL2 in Hs578T and MDA-MB-231 cell lines. Figure S2: Distribution of RBP targets among EMT-related DEGs. Figure S3: Distribution of RBP targets among non-EMT-related DEGs. Table S1: Number of genes targeted by the RBPs in EMT-related and non-EMT-related signatures. Table S2: List of primers used for qPCR analyses. Supplementary original figures: supplementary Western blot panels.

Author Contributions: A.C., M.J.M., P.E. and F.P. designed the experiments. P.E., M.J.M., V.J., P.P.-G., E.P.C., J.M.-M. and J.M.-B. performed the experiments. M.J.M., P.E. and F.P. analyzed the data. F.P. wrote the manuscript. A.C., P.E., M.J.M., V.J., P.P.-G., E.P.C., J.M.-M. and J.M.-B. revised the manuscript. F.P. and A.C. were responsible for project administration. A.C. and F.P. were responsible for funding acquisition. All authors have read and agreed to the published version of the manuscript.

Funding: This research was funded by grants from the Spanish Ministry of Science and Innovation MCIN (SAF2016-76504-R to A.C. and F.P., PID2019-111052RB-I00 to F.P.) and the Instituto de Salud Carlos III (CIBERONC-CB16/12/00295 to A.C.), all of which were partially supported by EU-FEDER funds.

Institutional Review Board Statement: Not applicable.

Informed Consent Statement: Not applicable.

Data Availability Statement: Not applicable.

Acknowledgments: We thank Vanesa Bermeo for her invaluable technical help with this study.

Conflicts of Interest: The authors declare no conflict of interest.

Sample Availability: Samples of the compounds are not available from the authors.

References

1. Finney, J.; Moon, H.-J.; Ronnebaum, T.; Lantz, M.; Mure, M. Human copper-dependent amine oxidases. *Arch. Biochem. Biophys.* **2014**, *546*, 19–32. [CrossRef] [PubMed]
2. Grau-Bové, X.; Ruiz-Trillo, I.; Rodriguez-Pascual, F. Origin and evolution of lysyl oxidases. *Sci. Rep.* **2015**, *5*, 10568. [CrossRef] [PubMed]
3. Lucero, H.A.; Kagan, H.M. Lysyl oxidase: An oxidative enzyme and effector of cell function. *Cell. Mol. Life Sci.* **2006**, *63*, 2304–2316. [CrossRef] [PubMed]
4. Canton, J.; Neculai, D.; Grinstein, S. Scavenger receptors in homeostasis and immunity. *Nat. Rev. Immunol.* **2013**, *13*, 621–634. [CrossRef] [PubMed]
5. Sarrias, M.R.; Gronlund, J.; Padilla, O.; Madsen, J.; Holmskov, U.; Lozano, F. The Scavenger Receptor Cysteine-Rich (SRCR) Domain: An Ancient and Highly Conserved Protein Module of the Innate Immune System. *Crit. Rev. Immunol.* **2004**, *24*, 38. [CrossRef] [PubMed]
6. Reichhardt, M.P.; Loimaranta, V.; Lea, S.M.; Johnson, S. Structures of SALSA/DMBT1 SRCR domains reveal the conserved ligand-binding mechanism of the ancient SRCR fold. *Life Sci. Alliance* **2020**, *3*, e201900502. [CrossRef]
7. Ma, L.; Huang, C.; Wang, X.-J.; Xin, D.E.; Wang, L.-S.; Zou, Q.C.; Zhang, Y.-N.S.; Tan, M.-D.; Wang, Y.-M.; Zhao, T.C.; et al. Lysyl Oxidase 3 Is a Dual-Specificity Enzyme Involved in STAT3 Deacetylation and Deacetylimination Modulation. *Mol. Cell* **2017**, *65*, 296–309. [CrossRef]
8. Jiao, J.-W.; Zhan, X.-H.; Wang, J.-J.; He, L.-X.; Guo, Z.-C.; Xu, X.-E.; Liao, L.-D.; Huang, X.; Wen, B.; Xu, Y.-W.; et al. LOXL2-dependent deacetylation of aldolase A induces metabolic reprogramming and tumor progression. *Redox Biol.* **2022**, *57*. [CrossRef]
9. Rodriguez-Pascual, F.; Rosell-Garcia, T. Lysyl Oxidases: Functions and Disorders. *Eur. J. Gastroenterol. Hepatol.* **2018**, *27*, S15–S19. [CrossRef]
10. Payne, S.L.; Hendrix, M.J.; Kirschmann, D.A. Paradoxical roles for lysyl oxidases in cancer—A prospect. *J. Cell. Biochem.* **2007**, *101*, 1338–1354. [CrossRef]
11. Barker, H.E.; Cox, T.R.; Erler, J.T. The rationale for targeting the LOX family in cancer. *Nat. Rev. Cancer* **2012**, *12*, 540–552. [CrossRef]

12. Trackman, P.C. Lysyl Oxidase Isoforms and Potential Therapeutic Opportunities for Fibrosis and Cancer. *Expert Opin. Ther. Targets* 2016, *20*, 935–945. [CrossRef] [PubMed]
13. Yang, N.; Cao, D.-F.; Yin, X.-X.; Zhou, H.-H.; Mao, X.-Y. Lysyl oxidases: Emerging biomarkers and therapeutic targets for various diseases. *Biomed. Pharmacother.* 2020, *131*, 110791. [CrossRef] [PubMed]
14. Cano, A.; Santamaría, P.G.; Moreno-Bueno, G. LOXL2 in epithelial cell plasticity and tumor progression. *Future Oncol.* 2012, *8*, 1095–1108. [CrossRef] [PubMed]
15. Wen, B.; Xu, L.-Y.; Li, E.-M. LOXL2 in cancer: Regulation, downstream effectors and novel roles. *Biochim. Biophys. Acta (BBA)-Rev. Cancer* 2020, *1874*, 188435. [CrossRef]
16. Wu, L.; Zhu, Y. The function and mechanisms of action of LOXL2 in cancer. *Int. J. Mol. Med.* 2015, *36*, 1200–1204. [CrossRef]
17. Peinado, H.; Moreno-Bueno, G.; Hardisson, D.; Perez-Gomez, E.; Santos, V.; Mendiola, M.; de Diego, J.I.; Nistal, M.; Quintanilla, M.; Portillo, F.; et al. Lysyl Oxidase–Like 2 as a New Poor Prognosis Marker of Squamous Cell Carcinomas. *Cancer Res.* 2008, *68*, 4541–4550. [CrossRef]
18. Moreno-Bueno, G.; Salvador, F.; Martín, A.; Floristán, A.; Cuevas, E.P.; Santos, V.; Montes, A.; Morales, S.; Castilla, M.A.; Rojo-Sebastián, A.; et al. Lysyl oxidase-like 2 (LOXL2), a new regulator of cell polarity required for metastatic dissemination of basal-like breast carcinomas. *EMBO Mol. Med.* 2011, *3*, 528–544. [CrossRef]
19. Yang, J.; Antin, P.; Berx, G.; Blanpain, C.; Brabletz, T.; Bronner, M.; Campbell, K.; Cano, A.; Casanova, J.; Christofori, G.; et al. Guidelines and definitions for research on epithelial–mesenchymal transition. *Nat. Rev. Mol. Cell Biol.* 2020, *21*, 341–352, Correction in *Nat. Rev. Mol. Cell Biol.* 2021, *22*, 834. [CrossRef]
20. Peinado, H.; Olmeda, D.; Cano, A. Snail, Zeb and bHLH factors in tumour progression: An alliance against the epithelial phenotype? *Nat. Rev. Cancer* 2007, *7*, 415–428. [CrossRef]
21. De Craene, B.; Berx, G. Regulatory networks defining EMT during cancer initiation and progression. *Nat. Rev. Cancer* 2013, *13*, 97–110. [CrossRef]
22. Goossens, S.; Vandamme, N.; Van Vlierberghe, P.; Berx, G. EMT transcription factors in cancer development re-evaluated: Beyond EMT and MET. *Biochim. Biophys. Acta (BBA)-Rev. Cancer* 2017, *1868*, 584–591. [CrossRef]
23. Brabletz, T.; Kalluri, R.; Nieto, M.A.; Weinberg, R.A. EMT in cancer. *Nat. Rev. Cancer* 2018, *18*, 128–134. [CrossRef] [PubMed]
24. Peinado, H.; Portillo, F.; Cano, A. Switching On-Off Snail: LOXL2 Versus GSK3? *Cell Cycle* 2005, *4*, 1749–1752. [CrossRef] [PubMed]
25. Millanes-Romero, A.; Herranz, N.; Perrera, V.; Iturbide, A.; Loubat-Casanovas, J.; Gil, J.; Jenuwein, T.; de Herreros, A.G.; Peiró, S. Regulation of Heterochromatin Transcription by Snail1/LOXL2 during Epithelial-to-Mesenchymal Transition. *Mol. Cell* 2013, *52*, 746–757. [CrossRef] [PubMed]
26. Herranz, N.; Dave, N.; Millanes-Romero, A.; Pascual-Reguant, L.; Morey, L.; Díaz, V.M.; Lórenz-Fonfría, V.; Gutierrez-Gallego, R.; Jerónimo, C.; Iturbide, A.; et al. Lysyl oxidase-like 2 (LOXL2) oxidizes trimethylated lysine 4 in histone H3. *FEBS J.* 2016, *283*, 4263–4273. [CrossRef] [PubMed]
27. Canesin, G.; Cuevas, E.P.; Santos, V.; López-Menéndez, C.; Moreno-Bueno, G.; Huang, Y.; Csiszar, K.; Portillo, F.; Peinado, H.; Lyden, D.; et al. Lysyl oxidase-like 2 (LOXL2) and E47 EMT factor: Novel partners in E-cadherin repression and early metastasis colonization. *Oncogene* 2014, *34*, 951–964. [CrossRef]
28. Martin, A.; Salvador, F.; Moreno-Bueno, G.; Floristán, A.; Ruiz-Herguido, C.; Cuevas, E.P.; Morales, S.; Santos, V.; Csiszar, K.; Dubus, P.; et al. Lysyl oxidase-like 2 represses Notch1 expression in the skin to promote squamous cell carcinoma progression. *EMBO J.* 2015, *34*, 1090–1109. [CrossRef]
29. Cuevas, E.P.; Moreno-Bueno, G.; Canesin, G.; Santos, V.; Portillo, F.; Cano, A. LOXL2 catalytically inactive mutants mediate epithelial-to-mesenchymal transition. *Biol. Open* 2014, *3*, 129–137. [CrossRef]
30. Lugassy, J.; Zaffryar-Eilot, S.; Soueid, S.; Mordoviz, A.; Smith, V.; Kessler, O.; Neufeld, G. The Enzymatic Activity of Lysyl Oxidas-like-2 (LOXL2) Is Not Required for LOXL2-induced Inhibition of Keratinocyte Differentiation. *J. Biol. Chem.* 2012, *287*, 3541–3549. [CrossRef]
31. Umana-Diaz, C.; Pichol-Thievend, C.; Marchand, M.F.; Atlas, Y.; Salza, R.; Malbouyres, M.; Barret, A.; Teillon, J.; Ardidie-Robouant, C.; Ruggiero, F.; et al. Scavenger Receptor Cysteine-Rich domains of Lysyl Oxidase-Like2 regulate endothelial ECM and angiogenesis through non-catalytic scaffolding mechanisms. *Matrix Biol.* 2019, *88*, 33–52. [CrossRef]
32. Hecht, J.R.; Benson, A.B.; Vyushkov, D.; Yang, Y.; Bendell, J.; Verma, U. A Phase II, Randomized, Double-Blind, Placebo-Controlled Study of Simtuzumab in Combination with FOLFIRI for the Second-Line Treatment of Metastatic *KRAS* Mutant Colorectal Adenocarcinoma. *Oncologist* 2017, *22*, 243-e23. [CrossRef]
33. Benson, A.B.; Wainberg, Z.A.; Hecht, J.R.; Vyushkov, D.; Dong, H.; Bendell, J.; Kudrik, F. A Phase II Randomized, Double-Blind, Placebo-Controlled Study of Simtuzumab or Placebo in Combination with Gemcitabine for the First-Line Treatment of Pancreatic Adenocarcinoma. *Oncologist* 2017, *22*, 241-e15. [CrossRef] [PubMed]
34. Chang, J.; Lucas, M.; Leonte, L.E.; Garcia-Montolio, M.; Singh, L.B.; Findlay, A.D.; Deodhar, M.; Foot, J.S.; Jarolimek, W.; Timpson, P.; et al. Pre-clinical evaluation of small molecule LOXL2 inhibitors in breast cancer. *Oncotarget* 2017, *8*, 26066–26078. [CrossRef]
35. Santamaría, P.G.; Dubus, P.; Bustos-Tauler, J.; Floristán, A.; Vázquez-Naharro, A.; Morales, S.; Cano, A.; Portillo, F. Loxl2 and Loxl3 Paralogues Play Redundant Roles during Mouse Development. *Int. J. Mol. Sci.* 2022, *23*, 5730. [CrossRef] [PubMed]
36. Cuevas, E.P.; Eraso, P.; Mazón, M.J.; Santos, V.; Moreno-Bueno, G.; Cano, A.; Portillo, F. LOXL2 drives epithelial-mesenchymal transition via activation of IRE1-XBP1 signalling pathway. *Sci. Rep.* 2017, *7*, srep44988. [CrossRef] [PubMed]

37. Sherman, B.T.; Hao, M.; Qiu, J.; Jiao, X.; Baseler, M.W.; Lane, H.C.; Imamichi, T.; Chang, W. DAVID: A web server for functional enrichment analysis and functional annotation of gene lists (2021 update). *Nucleic Acids Res.* **2022**, *50*, W216–W221. [CrossRef]
38. Huang, D.W.; Sherman, B.T.; Lempicki, R.A. Systematic and integrative analysis of large gene lists using DAVID bioinformatics resources. *Nat. Protoc.* **2009**, *4*, 44–57. [CrossRef]
39. Gerstberger, S.; Hafner, M.; Tuschl, T. A census of human RNA-binding proteins. *Nat. Rev. Genet.* **2014**, *15*, 829–845. [CrossRef]
40. Hentze, M.W.; Castello, A.; Schwarzl, T.; Preiss, T. A brave new world of RNA-binding proteins. *Nat. Rev. Mol. Cell Biol.* **2018**, *19*, 327–341. [CrossRef]
41. Pereira, B.; Billaud, M.; Almeida, R. RNA-Binding Proteins in Cancer: Old Players and New Actors. *Trends Cancer* **2017**, *3*, 506–528. [CrossRef]
42. Kang, D.; Lee, Y.; Lee, J.-S. RNA-Binding Proteins in Cancer: Functional and Therapeutic Perspectives. *Cancers* **2020**, *12*, 2699. [CrossRef] [PubMed]
43. Qin, H.; Ni, H.; Liu, Y.; Yuan, Y.; Xi, T.; Li, X.; Zheng, L. RNA-binding proteins in tumor progression. *J. Hematol. Oncol.* **2020**, *13*, 1–23. [CrossRef] [PubMed]
44. Li, W.; Deng, X.; Chen, J. RNA-binding proteins in regulating mRNA stability and translation: Roles and mechanisms in cancer. *Semin. Cancer Biol.* **2022**, *86*, 664–677. [CrossRef] [PubMed]
45. Wang, S.; Sun, Z.; Lei, Z.; Zhang, H.-T. RNA-binding proteins and cancer metastasis. *Semin. Cancer Biol.* **2022**, *86*, 748–768. [CrossRef]
46. Mohibi, S.; Chen, X.; Zhang, J. Cancer the 'RBP'eutics–RNA-binding proteins as therapeutic targets for cancer. *Pharmacol. Ther.* **2019**, *203*, 107390. [CrossRef] [PubMed]
47. Resnick, D.; Pearson, A.; Krieger, M. The SRCR superfamily: A family reminiscent of the Ig superfamily. *Trends Biochem. Sci.* **1994**, *19*, 5–8. [CrossRef]
48. Hohenester, E.; Sasaki, T.; Timpl, R. Crystal structure of a scavenger receptor cysteine-rich domain sheds light on an ancient superfamily. *Nat. Struct. Biol.* **1999**, *6*, 228–232. [CrossRef]
49. de Jong, O.G.; van der Waals, L.M.; Kools, F.R.W.; Verhaar, M.C.; van Balkom, B.W.M. Lysyl oxidase-like 2 is a regulator of angiogenesis through modulation of endothelial-to-mesenchymal transition. *J. Cell. Physiol.* **2018**, *234*, 10260–10269. [CrossRef]
50. Peng, T.; Deng, X.; Tian, F.; Li, Z.; Jiang, P.; Zhao, X.; Chen, G.; Chen, Y.; Zheng, P.; Li, D.; et al. The interaction of LOXL2 with GATA6 induces VEGFA expression and angiogenesis in cholangiocarcinoma. *Int. J. Oncol.* **2019**, *55*, 657–670. [CrossRef]
51. Srikantan, S. HuR function in disease. *Front. Biosci.* **2012**, *17*, 189–205. [CrossRef]
52. Subramanian, A.; Tamayo, P.; Mootha, V.K.; Mukherjee, S.; Ebert, B.L.; Gillette, M.A.; Paulovich, A.; Pomeroy, S.L.; Golub, T.R.; Lander, E.S.; et al. Gene set enrichment analysis: A knowledge-based approach for interpreting genome-wide expression profiles. *Proc. Natl. Acad. Sci. USA* **2005**, *102*, 15545–15550. [CrossRef] [PubMed]
53. Liberzon, A.; Birger, C.; Thorvaldsdóttir, H.; Ghandi, M.; Mesirov, J.P.; Tamayo, P. The Molecular Signatures Database Hallmark Gene Set Collection. *Cell Syst.* **2015**, *1*, 417–425. [CrossRef]
54. Li, J.-H.; Liu, S.; Zhou, H.; Qu, L.-H.; Yang, J.-H. starBase v2.0: Decoding miRNA-ceRNA, miRNA-ncRNA and protein–RNA interaction networks from large-scale CLIP-Seq data. *Nucleic Acids Res.* **2013**, *42*, D92–D97. [CrossRef] [PubMed]
55. Schmelzer, C.E.H.; Heinz, A.; Troilo, H.; Lockhart-Cairns, M.P.; Jowitt, T.A.; Marchand, M.F.; Bidault, L.; Bignon, M.; Hedtke, T.; Barret, A.; et al. Lysyl oxidase-like 2 (LOXL2)-mediated cross-linking of tropoelastin. *FASEB J.* **2019**, *33*, 5468–5481. [CrossRef] [PubMed]
56. Krismer, K.; Bird, M.A.; Varmeh, S.; Handly, E.D.; Gattinger, A.; Bernwinkler, T.; Anderson, D.A.; Heinzel, A.; Joughin, B.A.; Kong, Y.W.; et al. Transite: A Computational Motif-Based Analysis Platform That Identifies RNA-Binding Proteins Modulating Changes in Gene Expression. *Cell Rep.* **2020**, *32*, 108064. [CrossRef] [PubMed]
57. Antic, D.; Keene, J.D. Embryonic Lethal Abnormal Visual RNA-Binding Proteins Involved in Growth, Differentiation, and Posttranscriptional Gene Expression. *Am. J. Hum. Genet.* **1997**, *61*, 273–278. [CrossRef]
58. Khabar, K.S.A. Hallmarks of cancer and AU-rich elements. *Wiley Interdiscip. Rev. RNA* **2016**, *8*, e1368. [CrossRef]
59. Abdelmohsen, K.; Gorospe, M. Posttranscriptional regulation of cancer traits by HuR. *Wiley Interdiscip. Rev. RNA* **2010**, *1*, 214–229. [CrossRef]
60. Kotta-Loizou, I.; Vasilopoulos, S.N.; Coutts, R.H.; Theocharis, S. Current Evidence and Future Perspectives on HuR and Breast Cancer Development, Prognosis, and Treatment. *Neoplasia* **2016**, *18*, 674–688. [CrossRef]
61. Dong, R.; Chen, P.; Polireddy, K.; Wu, X.; Wang, T.; Ramesh, R.; Dixon, D.A.; Xu, L.; Aubé, J.; Chen, Q. An RNA-Binding Protein, Hu-antigen R, in Pancreatic Cancer Epithelial to Mesenchymal Transition, Metastasis, and Cancer Stem Cells. *Mol. Cancer Ther.* **2020**, *19*, 2267–2277. [CrossRef]
62. Latorre, E.; Carelli, S.; Raimondi, I.; D'Agostino, V.; Castiglioni, I.; Zucal, C.; Moro, G.; Luciani, A.; Ghilardi, G.; Monti, E.; et al. The Ribonucleic Complex HuR-MALAT1 Represses CD133 Expression and Suppresses Epithelial–Mesenchymal Transition in Breast Cancer. *Cancer Res.* **2016**, *76*, 2626–2636. [CrossRef] [PubMed]
63. Doller, A.; Pfeilschifter, J.; Eberhardt, W. Signalling pathways regulating nucleo-cytoplasmic shuttling of the mRNA-binding protein HuR. *Cell. Signal.* **2008**, *20*, 2165–2173. [CrossRef] [PubMed]
64. Abdelmohsen, K.; Srikantan, S.; Yang, X.; Lal, A.; Kim, H.H.; Kuwano, Y.; Galban, S.; Becker, K.G.; Kamara, D.; de Cabo, R.; et al. Ubiquitin-mediated proteolysis of HuR by heat shock. *EMBO J.* **2009**, *28*, 1271–1282. [CrossRef]
65. Grammatikakis, I.; Abdelmohsen, K.; Gorospe, M. Posttranslational control of HuR function. *Wiley Interdiscip. Rev. RNA* **2016**, *8*, e1372. [CrossRef] [PubMed]

66. Bell, J.L.; Wächter, K.; Mühleck, B.; Pazaitis, N.; Köhn, M.; Lederer, M.; Hüttelmaier, S. Insulin-like growth factor 2 mRNA-binding proteins (IGF2BPs): Post-transcriptional drivers of cancer progression? *Cell. Mol. Life Sci.* **2012**, *70*, 2657–2675. [CrossRef]
67. Zirkel, A.; Lederer, M.; Stöhr, N.; Pazaitis, N.; Hüttelmaier, S. IGF2BP1 promotes mesenchymal cell properties and migration of tumor-derived cells by enhancing the expression of LEF1 and SNAI2 (SLUG). *Nucleic Acids Res.* **2013**, *41*, 6618–6636. [CrossRef]
68. Lin, X.-T.; Yu, H.-Q.; Fang, L.; Tan, Y.; Liu, Z.-Y.; Wu, D.; Zhang, J.; Xiong, H.-J.; Xie, C.-M. Elevated FBXO45 promotes liver tumorigenesis through enhancing IGF2BP1 ubiquitination and subsequent PLK1 upregulation. *eLife* **2021**, *10*, e70715. [CrossRef]
69. Richter, J.D.; Zhao, X. The molecular biology of FMRP: New insights into fragile X syndrome. *Nat. Rev. Neurosci.* **2021**, *22*, 209–222. [CrossRef]
70. Hagerman, R.J.; Berry-Kravis, E.; Hazlett, H.C.; Bailey, D.B., Jr.; Moine, H.; Kooy, R.F.; Tassone, F.; Gantois, I.; Sonenberg, N.; Mandel, J.L.; et al. Fragile X syndrome. *Nat. Rev. Dis. Primers* **2017**, *3*, 17065. [CrossRef]
71. Lucá, R.; Averna, M.; Zalfa, F.; Vecchi, M.; Bianchi, F.; La Fata, G.; Del Nonno, F.; Nardacci, R.; Bianchi, M.; Nuciforo, P.; et al. The Fragile X Protein binds m RNA s involved in cancer progression and modulates metastasis formation. *EMBO Mol. Med.* **2013**, *5*, 1523–1536. [CrossRef] [PubMed]
72. Huang, J.; Ikeuchi, Y.; Malumbres, M.; Bonni, A. A Cdh1-APC/FMRP Ubiquitin Signaling Link Drives mGluR-Dependent Synaptic Plasticity in the Mammalian Brain. *Neuron* **2015**, *86*, 726–739. [CrossRef] [PubMed]
73. Bertolotti, A.; Lutz, Y.; Heard, D.J.; Chambon, P.; Tora, L. hTAF(II)68, a novel RNA/ssDNA-binding protein with homology to the pro-oncoproteins TLS/FUS and EWS is associated with both TFIID and RNA polymerase II. *EMBO J.* **1996**, *15*, 5022–5031. [CrossRef]
74. Ballarino, M.; Jobert, L.; Dembélé, D.; de la Grange, P.; Auboeuf, D.; Tora, L. TAF15 is important for cellular proliferation and regulates the expression of a subset of cell cycle genes through miRNAs. *Oncogene* **2012**, *32*, 4646–4655. [CrossRef]
75. Su, Z.; Sun, Z.; Wang, Z.; Wang, S.; Wang, Y.; Jin, E.; Li, C.; Zhao, J.; Liu, Z.; Zhou, Z.; et al. TIF1γ inhibits lung adenocarcinoma EMT and metastasis by interacting with the TAF15/TBP complex. *Cell Rep.* **2022**, *41*, 111513. [CrossRef]
76. Iturbide, A.; Pascual-Reguant, L.; Fargas, L.; Cebrià, J.P.; Alsina, B.; de Herreros, A.G.; Peiró, S. LOXL2 Oxidizes Methylated TAF10 and Controls TFIID-Dependent Genes during Neural Progenitor Differentiation. *Mol. Cell* **2015**, *58*, 755–766. [CrossRef]
77. Das, S.; Krainer, A.R. Emerging Functions of SRSF1, Splicing Factor and Oncoprotein, in RNA Metabolism and Cancer. *Mol. Cancer Res.* **2014**, *12*, 1195–1204. [CrossRef] [PubMed]
78. Ye, Y.; Yu, F.; Li, Z.; Xie, Y.; Yu, X. RNA binding protein serine/arginine splicing factor 1 promotes the proliferation, migration and invasion of hepatocellular carcinoma by interacting with RecQ protein-like 4 mRNA. *Bioengineered* **2021**, *12*, 6144–6154. [CrossRef]
79. Moulton, V.R.; Gillooly, A.R.; Tsokos, G.C. Ubiquitination Regulates Expression of the Serine/Arginine-rich Splicing Factor 1 (SRSF1) in Normal and Systemic Lupus Erythematosus (SLE) T Cells. *J. Biol. Chem.* **2014**, *289*, 4126–4134. [CrossRef]
80. Douet-Guilbert, N.; Soubise, B.; Bernard, D.G.; Troadec, M.-B. Cytogenetic and Genetic Abnormalities with Diagnostic Value in Myelodysplastic Syndromes (MDS): Focus on the Pre-Messenger RNA Splicing Process. *Diagnostics* **2022**, *12*, 1658. [CrossRef]
81. Zhang, P.; Feng, S.; Liu, G.; Wang, H.; Fu, A.; Zhu, H.; Ren, Q.; Wang, B.; Xu, X.; Bai, H.; et al. CD82 suppresses CD44 alternative splicing-dependent melanoma metastasis by mediating U2AF2 ubiquitination and degradation. *Oncogene* **2016**, *35*, 5056–5069. [CrossRef]
82. Yi, J.; Shen, H.-F.; Qiu, J.-S.; Huang, M.-F.; Zhang, W.; Ding, J.-C.; Zhu, X.-Y.; Zhou, Y.; Fu, X.-D.; Liu, W. JMJD6 and U2AF65 co-regulate alternative splicing in both JMJD6 enzymatic activity dependent and independent manner. *Nucleic Acids Res.* **2016**, *45*, 3503–3518. [CrossRef]
83. Wu, X.; Xu, L. The RNA-binding protein HuR in human cancer: A friend or foe? *Adv. Drug Deliv. Rev.* **2022**, *184*, 114179. [CrossRef]
84. Glaß, M.; Misiak, D.; Bley, N.; Müller, S.; Hagemann, S.; Busch, B.; Rausch, A.; Hüttelmaier, S. IGF2BP1, a Conserved Regulator of RNA Turnover in Cancer. *Front. Mol. Biosci.* **2021**, *8*, 632219. [CrossRef]
85. Majumder, M.; Johnson, R.H.; Palanisamy, V. Fragile X-related protein family: A double-edged sword in neurodevelopmental disorders and cancer. *Crit. Rev. Biochem. Mol. Biol.* **2020**, *55*, 1–16. [CrossRef] [PubMed]
86. Anczuków, O.; Rosenberg, A.Z.; Akerman, M.; Das, S.; Zhan, L.; Karni, R.; Muthuswamy, S.K.; Krainer, A.R. The splicing factor SRSF1 regulates apoptosis and proliferation to promote mammary epithelial cell transformation. *Nat. Struct. Mol. Biol.* **2012**, *19*, 220–228. [CrossRef]
87. Peinado, H.; del Carmen Iglesias-de la Cruz, M.; Olmeda, D.; Csiszar, K.; Fong, K.S.K.; Vega, S.; Nieto, M.A.; Cano, A.; Portillo, F. A molecular role for lysyl oxidase-like 2 enzyme in Snail regulation and tumor progression. *EMBO J.* **2005**, *24*, 3446–3458. [PubMed]
88. Bolós, V.; Peinado, H.; Perez-Moreno, M.A.; Fraga, M.F.; Esteller, M.; Cano, A. The transcription factor Slug represses E-cadherin expression and induces epithelial to mesenchymal transitions: A comparison with Snail and E47 repressors. *J. Cell Sci.* **2003**, *116*, 499–511. [CrossRef] [PubMed]
89. Schreiber, E.; Matthias, P.; Müller, M.M.; Schaffner, W. Rapid detection of octamer binding proteins with 'mini extracts', prepared from a small number of cells. *Nucleic Acids Res.* **1989**, *17*, 6419. [CrossRef]
90. Moreno-Bueno, G.; Peinado, H.; Molina, P.; Olmeda, D.; Cubillo, E.; Santos, V.; Palacios, J.; Portillo, F.; Cano, A. The morphological and molecular features of the epithelial-to-mesenchymal transition. *Nat. Protoc.* **2009**, *4*, 1591–1613. [CrossRef]

Disclaimer/Publisher's Note: The statements, opinions and data contained in all publications are solely those of the individual author(s) and contributor(s) and not of MDPI and/or the editor(s). MDPI and/or the editor(s) disclaim responsibility for any injury to people or property resulting from any ideas, methods, instructions or products referred to in the content.

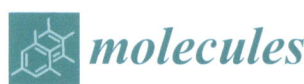

Article

Resazurin Reduction-Based Assays Revisited: Guidelines for Accurate Reporting of Relative Differences on Metabolic Status

Beatriz Vieira-da-Silva and Miguel A. R. B. Castanho *

Instituto de Medicina Molecular, Faculdade de Medicina, Universidade de Lisboa, 1649-028 Lisboa, Portugal
* Correspondence: macastanho@medicina.ulisboa.pt; Tel.: +351-217985136

Abstract: Cell viability and metabolic activity are ubiquitous parameters used in biochemistry, molecular biology, and biotechnological studies. Virtually all toxicology and pharmacological projects include at some point the evaluation of cell viability and/or metabolic activity. Among the methods used to address cell metabolic activity, resazurin reduction is probably the most common. At variance with resazurin, resorufin is intrinsically fluorescent, which simplifies its detection. Resazurin conversion to resorufin in the presence of cells is used as a reporter of metabolic activity of cells and can be detected by a simple fluorometric assay. UV–Vis absorbance is an alternative technique but is not as sensitive. In contrast to its wide empirical "black box" use, the chemical and cell biology fundamentals of the resazurin assay are underexplored. Resorufin is further converted to other species, which jeopardizes the linearity of the assays, and the interference of extracellular processes has to be accounted for when quantitative bioassays are aimed at. In this work, we revisit the fundamentals of metabolic activity assays based on the reduction of resazurin. Deviation to linearity both in calibration and kinetics, as well as the existence of competing reactions for resazurin and resorufin and their impact on the outcome of the assay, are addressed. In brief, fluorometric ratio assays using low resazurin concentrations obtained from data collected at short time intervals are proposed to ensure reliable conclusions.

Keywords: resazurin; cell viability; metabolic activity; fluorometric assay; UV–Vis assay; cytotoxicity

Citation: Vieira-da-Silva, B.;
Castanho, M.A.R.B. Resazurin
Reduction-Based Assays Revisited:
Guidelines for Accurate Reporting of
Relative Differences on Metabolic
Status. *Molecules* **2023**, *28*, 2283.
https://doi.org/10.3390/
molecules28052283

Academic Editors: Alejandro
Samhan-Arias, Manuel Aureliano,
Carmen Lopez-Sanchez and
Yun-Bae Kim

Received: 28 December 2022
Revised: 21 February 2023
Accepted: 24 February 2023
Published: 1 March 2023

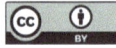

Copyright: © 2023 by the authors.
Licensee MDPI, Basel, Switzerland.
This article is an open access article
distributed under the terms and
conditions of the Creative Commons
Attribution (CC BY) license (https://
creativecommons.org/licenses/by/
4.0/).

1. Introduction

The use of molecules able to report the intracellular reducing environment through simple assays is extremely ubiquitous in biochemistry, molecular biology, and pharmacy laboratories. Molecules such as MTT, (3-(4,5-dimethylthiazol-2-yl)-2,5-diphenyltetrazolium bromide) tetrazolium, or resazurin (7-Hydroxy-3H-phenoxazin-3-one 10-oxide) are able to penetrate cells, undergo reduction in the intracellular space, and report the change in their oxidation state by colorimetric or fluorometric techniques. This process is used as a tool to draw conclusions regarding the metabolic activity of cells as the reducing environment can only be maintained through an operative intermediary metabolism.

When addressing methods to evaluate cytotoxicity, one should bear in mind that resazurin, like MTT, does not report the viability of cells as it does not report cell death, only metabolic activity. It may be used to compare the intrinsic reducing power of two different cell types, or the impact of a solute on a specific cell type in terms of metabolic dysfunction or impairment, but it cannot be used to unequivocally evaluate cell death. Direct cell death count by microscopic morphological alterations in cytoplasmic or nuclear structures, for instance, are methods appropriate to study cell death. Here, the focus is on resazurin reduction to study quantitative fold variations in metabolic activity.

The advantages and disadvantages of using resazurin over MTT have been reviewed before [1,2] and will be left out of the scope of this paper. Likewise, a broader comparison of different methods to address metabolic activity and viability is not within the realm of this study. Here, we will focus on the conditions that validate the resazurin assay as a reliable method to report on variations of cell activity. These conditions are frequently overlooked. Moreover, oversimplistic and erroneous assumptions are frequently adopted, explicitly or implicitly. For instance, the conversion of resazurin to resorufin is not a simple, irreversible reaction of two species, the reactant and the product. In addition, resorufin is frequently detected by fluorometry. At variance with electronic spectrophotometry/UV–Vis absorption, calibration in fluorometry is not straightforward [3].

2. Results

2.1. The Consecutive Reactions of Resazurin and Their Kinetics

The details of resazurin redox and acid-base reaction were addressed thoroughly by voltammetry with a mercury electrode [4], which is a suitable model for biological redox reactions. The basics of resazurin redox reaction at different pHs is represented in reaction Scheme 1:

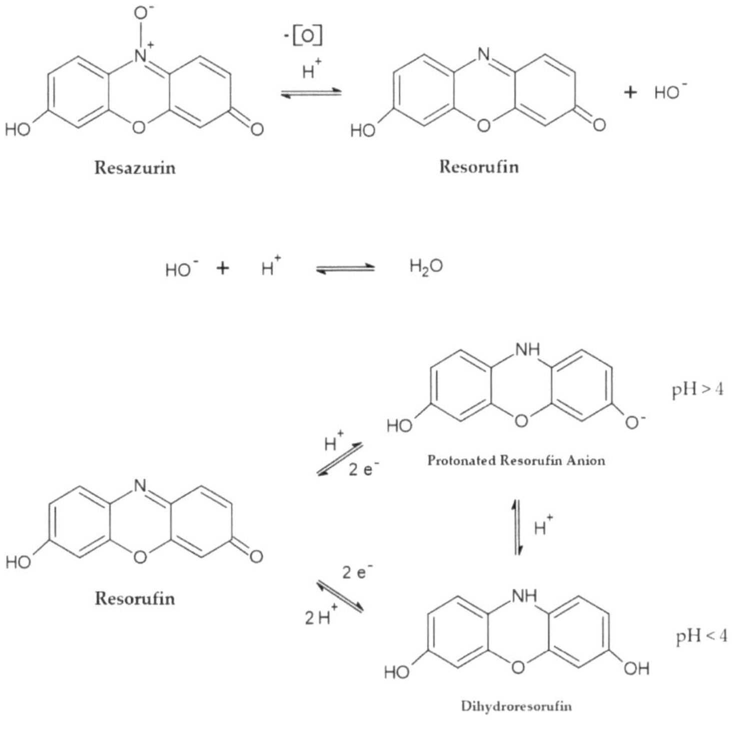

Scheme 1. Reaction scheme of resazurin redox and acid-base reaction into resorufin. At different pHs further products are formed; protonated resorufin anion for pH > 4 and dihydroresorufin when pH < 4.

For the sake of simplicity, we will represent this reaction scheme by:

$$A \xrightarrow{k_1} B \xrightarrow{k_2} C \qquad (1)$$

in which A is resazurin, B is resorufin, and C are the end products of degradation (mainly protonated resorufin anion when pH > 4); the reaction rate constant k_1 is dependent on the intrinsic rate of the reaction and the quantity of reducing species in the environment (NAD(P)H) or cytochrome c oxidase in the case of cells [1]. By approximation, k_1 can then be decomposed in:

$$k_1 = k_1' \cdot [C_v] \qquad (2)$$

k_1' is the intrinsic rate constant and $[C_v]$ is the number of viable cells per unit volume.

The fluorescence quantum yield of B at or close to λ_{exc} = 570 nm is much higher than the one of A or C, so the kinetics of the reaction can be followed by the time evolution of the intensity of fluorescence emission of B, $I_{f,B}(t)$. $I_{f,B}(t)$ is proportional to [B] in circumstances in which the inner filter effect [5] is not significant and interfering processes such as aggregation are not operative.

The time dependence of [B], [B](t), can be quantitatively established using the iterative method at short fixed-time intervals, Δt [6]:

$$[B](t+\Delta t) = [k_1[A](t) - k_2[B](t)] \cdot \Delta t + [B](t) \quad (3)$$

The following condition applies:

$$[B](t=0) = 0 \quad (4)$$

Using $I_{f,B}(t)$ instead of [B](t):

$$I_{f,B}(t) = k \cdot [B](t) \quad (5)$$

$$I_{f,B}(t+\Delta t) = \left[k \cdot k_1 \cdot [A](t) - k_2 I_{f,B}(t)\right] \cdot \Delta t + I_{f,B}(t) \quad (6)$$

k is a proportionality constant dependent on the fluorescence quantum yield of B. The slope of $I_{f,B}(t)$ at t = 0 is:

$$\lim_{t \to 0}\left[\frac{I_{f,B}(t+\Delta t)}{\Delta t}\right] = k \cdot k_1 \cdot [A](t=0) \quad (7)$$

Comparing two distinct experimental conditions, hereafter named (a) and (b), such as absence and presence of a toxic solute, for instance, the slope ratio is:

$$\frac{slope_{(a)}}{slope_{(b)}} = \frac{k_{1\,(a)}}{k_{1\,(b)}} = \frac{k'_{1\,(a)}[C_v]_{(a)}}{k'_{1\,(b)}[C_v]_{(b)}} \quad (8)$$

assuming k and [A](t = 0) are equal in the two conditions, (a) and (b). Additionally, assuming that k'_1 is invariant between conditions (a) and (b):

$$\frac{slope_{(a)}}{slope_{(b)}} = \frac{[C_v]_{(a)}}{[C_v]_{(b)}} \quad (9)$$

I.e., variations in the number of viable cells can be directly measured from the slope of the fluorometric kinetics monitoring of resorufin formation. In another type of experimental design, when comparing cells from different tissues at the same density, the slopes ratio corresponds to the ratio of the intrinsic reducing power of the two cell types $k'_{1\,(a)}/k'_{1\,(b)}$.

Slopes can be replaced by $I_{f,B}(t)$ measurements at a fixed time point, t_x, as long as t_x is short:

$$\frac{I_{f,B}(t_x)_{(a)}}{I_{f,B}(t_x)_{(b)}} \approx \frac{[C_v]_{(a)}}{[C_v]_{(b)}} \quad (10)$$

This equation and its deduction constitute a quantitative validation to the assumptions qualitatively performed in some critical appraisals of the resazurin assay by others [7,8].

2.2. Assumptions and Limitations

Equation (10) is important as it establishes the theoretical framework for a truly quantitative deployment of the resazurin reduction assay to draw conclusions on variations of cell metabolic activity. Nonetheless, several assumptions were made while deriving it. These assumptions are practical limitations that cannot be overlooked as they need to be experimentally checked when applying the method.

2.2.1. All Living Cells Have Equal Reducing Power and Non-Cellular Conversion of A to B Is Non-Significant

In practice, assuming Equation (2) is valid implies that viable cells are homogenous in their reducing power, and conversion of A to B caused by agents other than cells is non-significant. A can be converted to B by cells through electron transfer from NAD(P)H or by substituting molecular oxygen as an electron acceptor [1]. Either way, it reflects the activity of live cells.

In contrast, reduction may also occur through non-cellular electron donors, which may compromise the validity of Equation (4), therefore making Equation (10) not applicable. Although the resazurin assay is not as susceptible as similar assays, such as MTT, to small molecule interference, this is a possibility [2,9]. Nevertheless, a specific study using *E. faecalis* found that, under anaerobic conditions, resazurin conversion to resorufin can only happen intracellularly, while resorufin reduction can happen both intracellularly and extracellularly [10].

2.2.2. Instrumental Factors in Fluorimetry

Equation (5) is only valid in specific conditions, which are critically dependent on instrumental ("geometric") factors. The linear dependence of the fluorescence emission intensity on the concentration of a given solute requires the absence of significant inner filter effects [3,5], i.e., solute concentration sufficiently high to attenuate the intensity of the excitation bean at the focus point from where fluorescence emission is collected. Moreover, high concentrations of B may lead to binding to interfering agents with alteration of the fluorescence quantum yield. B concentrations should be kept as low as possible so that the sensitivity at the specific experimental conditions used is not jeopardized. Furthermore, A is associated with cytotoxic effects [1,9], which constitutes further reason to use as low a resazurin concentration as possible in an experiment.

It should also be stressed that fluorescence signals are not registered by fluorometers relative to a blank sample signal, at variance with UV–Vis absorption. Therefore, the fluorescence intensity recorded is specific to each apparatus at any given experimental session. This means that k, in Equation (5), is specific to a certain batch of samples, assayed in a specific spectrofluorometer, for a specific experimental session. While UV–Vis absorption could be used in alternative to fluorimetry because absorbance is also proportional to solute concentration, without having this limitation the sensitivity of the technique is much lower, therefore demanding higher concentrations of resazurin.

2.2.3. Only $[C_v]$ Varies While Other Factors Are Constant When Comparing Conditions (a) and (b)

While comparing the two different experimental conditions (a) and (b), such as the absence and the presence of a given toxic solute, Equation (10) only applies if $[C_v]$ is the only variable. Changes in the reduction power of the cells or differential interference from other solutes renders k different in conditions (a) and (b). The consequences are Equations (8)–(10) are no longer valid and, therefore, the resazurin assay will lead to biased results.

2.2.4. Viability vs. Metabolic Activity

Overall, one should bear in mind that although sometimes abusively referred to evaluate cell viability, the resazurin reduction assay, in fact, assesses metabolic activity. Under certain conditions (e.g., some bacteria-forming biofilms), cells having very low metabolic activity may be mistakenly taken for non-viable cells. Proper controls are needed to assure that there is sufficient metabolic activity to unequivocally distinguish viable from non-viable cells.

2.3. Practical Examples from Literature

The experimental conditions used to implement the resazurin assay and subsequent data analysis are frequently based on empirics and chemical intuition. Although thorough studies are scarce but well-interpreted [7,8], they miss detailed quantitative analyses. Application of the data analysis methodology developed in Section 2.1 enables more robust conclusions and further proof of the validity of the procedure.

2.3.1. Comparing the Reducing Power of Different Types of Cells

The data presented by Uzarski et al. [7] on the reducing power of three different cell lines, immortalized human renal fibrotic fibroblasts (TK 188), distal Madin–Darby canine kidney cells (MDCK), and proximal primary renal tubule epithelial cells (RPTE), can be fit by Equation (6) (Figure 1A). The ratio obtained with any two of the three cell lines, assuming there is an equal number of cells, is the estimated ratio of k_1', the intrinsic reducing power of the cells.

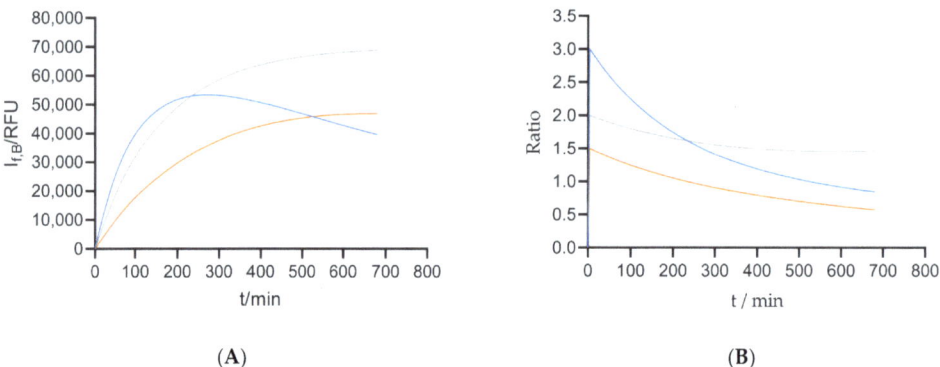

(A) (B)

Figure 1. Fitting curves of the data presented by Uzarski et al. [7] on the reducing power of three different cell lines (panel **A**-TK188 fibroblasts, grey; Distal MDCK cells, blue; Proximal RPTE cells, orange) and ratio of the fitted curves obtained with any two out of the three cell lines (panel **B**-MDCK/RPTE, blue; MDCK/TK188, orange; TK188/RPTE, grey). For the fitted curves in panel A, k_2/k_1 was 0.11, 0.20 and 0.00 for MDCK, RPTE and TK188, respectively. [A](t = 0) was set equal for the three cell lines. Aditional data can be found in reference [7].

The intrinsic power of reducing resazurin is different in the three cell lines (Figure 1B) and the fate of resorufin is quite different as reflected by k_2 and denoted by the curves on Figure 1A after there is a decrease of the fluorescence intensity in MDCK cells and the formation of a plateau regarding the other two cell lines.

The ratio of $I_{f,B}(t)$ (Figure 1B) is clearly dependent on t for each pair of the three cell lines. The ratio at very short times ($t \approx 0$) shows that MCCK cells are three-fold more reducing than RPTE cells but only 1.5-fold more than TK188, which is twice more reducing than RPTE. The relative scale of reducing power is thus MDCK > (1.5-fold) TK188 > (2-fold) RPTE.

It should be stressed that at longer times ($t \gg 0$), $I_{f,B}(t)$ ratios vary greatly and may even fall below one. Therefore, when fluorescence intensities are not measured at sufficiently short intervals, the relative reducing power may be completely biased. This happens mainly in cases in which $I_{f,B}(t)$ curves have a significant descendent curve at long t, as seen in Figure 1A for the MDCK cells.

2.3.2. Cytotoxicity: The Effect of Solutes on Cell Metabolic Activity

Lavogina et al. [8] determined the kinetics of the formation of resorufin by HeLa cells in the absence and presence of 10μM doxorubicin, among other experimental data. Equation (7) was fit to the data (Figure 2A). The drop in the number of viable cells caused by doxorubicin was 7.4-fold, as shown by Figure 2B at $t \approx 0$.

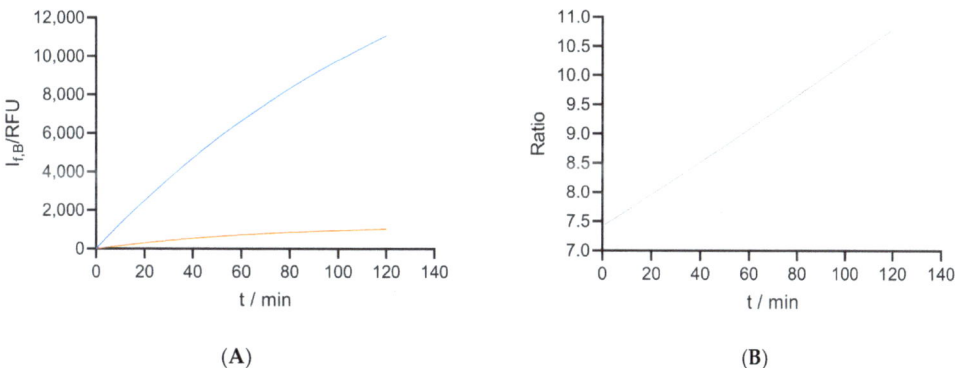

Figure 2. Fitting curves of the data presented by Lavogina et al. [8] on the metabolic activity of HeLa cells in the absence (blue) and presence of 10 μM doxorubicin (orange) (panel **A**) and ratio of the two fitted curves (panel **B**). For the fitted curves in (panel **A**), k_2/k_1 was 14.4 and 0.00 for the sample with and without doxorubicin, respectively. $[A](t = 0)$ was set equal in both conditions.

The examples of Figures 1 and 2 demonstrate how a quantitative analysis over the resazurin assay can be performed to draw conclusions on the intrinsic reducing power of different cell lines or changes on cell cytotoxicity, depending on the experimental setup.

3. Conclusions

The resazurin reduction assay is ubiquitously used for its simplicity, low cost, and sensitivity. Nonetheless, its use up to now has relied on empirics and chemical intuition rather than on solid biochemical knowledge. We have derived the equations describing the kinetics of resorufin production and consumption and related the kinetic parameters to experimental conditions. The approach was validated by application of published data by independent laboratories. Such a quantitative approach opens new avenues to bridge chemistry, biology, toxicology, and pharmaceutical science into consensual and comparable applications of the resazurin assay.

It should be stressed that the nature of cells in culture and the variability of the levels of markers of cell viability among the individual cells in a population was not taken into account but may be relevant for more detailed expert approaches when viability is considered. In this case, specific approaches to cell viability, such as directly counting cells, could be considered. The use of multiplexed orthogonal methods to estimate the number of viable cells can be considered for more robust approaches [9].

Good Practice in MTT and Resazurin Assay

The practical implications of our work for the end user can be condensed in a set of good practice rules. From a user's perspective, the relevance of our work is the identification of the experimental conditions that make resazurin assay reliable to evaluate the toxicity of a certain compound on a given cell type or to evaluate the intrinsic reducing power of any two cell types. The latter challenge is similar to the evaluation of two different growth conditions on a given cell type.

Practical tips for a meaningful application of resazurin, or any other reducing power-based viability assay, are as follows:

(1) Use as low a resazurin concentration as possible because toxicity issues and technical spectroscopic biases may arise. The minimal concentration you can use depends on the signal-to-noise ratio of your detection system.
(2) Test for the reducing power of the medium in the absence of cells. Make sure it is non-significant when compared to cell reducing power in the absence of any toxic agents.

(3) Use data obtained at the shortest time interval possible, i.e., resazurin reduction data (formation of resorufin) should be registered as soon as possible after resazurin addition to cells, provided that the read-out is above the detection limit of the experimental setup you are using.

(4) Observance of the three previous rules allows quantitative ratiometric analysis, i.e., the fold variation of the measured response (fluorescence intensity or UV-Vis. absorption) is the fold variation of metabolic activity or intrinsic reducing power of cells.

Author Contributions: Conceptualization, M.A.R.B.C.; methodology, M.A.R.B.C.; formal analysis, M.A.R.B.C. and B.V.-d.-S.; investigation, M.A.R.B.C. and B.V.-d.-S.; resources, M.A.R.B.C. and B.V.-d.-S.; writing—original draft preparation, M.A.R.B.C.; writing—review and editing, B.V.-d.-S.; supervision, M.A.R.B.C.; project administration, M.A.R.B.C.; funding acquisition, M.A.R.B.C. All authors have read and agreed to the published version of the manuscript.

Funding: The project leading to these results has received funding from "la Caixa" Foundation and FCT, I.P. under the project code [LCF/PR/HR21/00605], BREAST-BRAIN-N-BBB.

Institutional Review Board Statement: Not applicable.

Informed Consent Statement: Not applicable.

Data Availability Statement: Not applicable.

Conflicts of Interest: The authors declare no conflict of interest.

Sample Availability: Not applicable.

References

1. Aslantürk, Ö.S. In Vitro Cytotoxicity and Cell Viability Assays: Principles, Advantages, and Disadvantages. In *Genotoxicity—A Predictable Risk to Our Actual World*; InTechOpen: London, UK, 2018; Chapter 1. ISBN 978-1-78923-419-0.
2. Neufeld, B.H.; Tapia, J.B.; Lutzke, A.; Reynolds, M.M. Small Molecule Interferences in Resazurin and MTT-Based Metabolic Assays in the Absence of Cells. *Anal. Chem.* **2018**, *90*, 6867–6876. [CrossRef] [PubMed]
3. Lakowicz, J.R. *Principles of Fluorescence Spectroscopy*; Springer: Berlin/Heidelberg, Germany, 2006. ISBN 0387312781.
4. Çakir, S.; Arslan, E. Voltammetry of Resazurin at a Mercury Electrode. *Chem. Pap.* **2010**, *64*, 386–394. [CrossRef]
5. Coutinho, A.; Prieto, M. Ribonuclease T1 and Alcohol Dehydrogenase Fluorescence Quenching by Acrylamide: A Laboratory Experiment for Undergraduate Students. *J. Chem. Educ.* **1993**, *70*, 425–428. [CrossRef]
6. da Poian, A.T.; Castanho, M.A.R.B. *Integrative Human Biochemistry*, 2nd ed.; Springer International Publishing: Cham, Switzerland, 2021; Chapter 4. ISBN 978-3-030-48739-3.
7. Uzarski, J.S.; DiVito, M.D.; Wertheim, J.A.; Miller, W.M. Essential Design Considerations for the Resazurin Reduction Assay to Noninvasively Quantify Cell Expansion within Perfused Extracellular Matrix Scaffolds. *Biomaterials* **2017**, *129*, 163–175. [CrossRef]
8. Lavogina, D.; Lust, H.; Tahk, M.-J.; Laasfeld, T.; Vellama, H.; Nasirova, N.; Vardja, M.; Eskla, K.-L.; Salumets, A.; Rinken, A.; et al. Revisiting the Resazurin-Based Sensing of Cellular Viability: Widening the Application Horizon. *Biosensors* **2022**, *12*, 196. [CrossRef]
9. Riss, T.L.; Moravec, R.A.; Niles, A.L.; Duellman, S.; Benink, H.A.; Worzella, T.J.; Minor, L. *Cell Viability Assays*; Markossian, S., Grossman, A., Brimacombe, K., Arkin, M., Auld, D., Austin, C., Baell, J., Chung, T.D.Y., Coussens, N.P., Dahlin, J.L., et al., Eds.; Eli Lilly & Company and the National Center for Advancing Translational Sciences: Bethesda, MD, USA, 2004. Available online: https://pubmed.ncbi.nlm.nih.gov/23805433/ (accessed on 15 December 2022).
10. Chen, J.L.; Steele, T.W.J.; Stuckey, D.C. Metabolic Reduction of Resazurin; Location within the Cell for Cytotoxicity Assays. *Biotechnol. Bioeng.* **2018**, *115*, 351–358. [CrossRef]

Disclaimer/Publisher's Note: The statements, opinions and data contained in all publications are solely those of the individual author(s) and contributor(s) and not of MDPI and/or the editor(s). MDPI and/or the editor(s) disclaim responsibility for any injury to people or property resulting from any ideas, methods, instructions or products referred to in the content.

MDPI AG
Grosspeteranlage 5
4052 Basel
Switzerland
Tel.: +41 61 683 77 34

Molecules Editorial Office
E-mail: molecules@mdpi.com
www.mdpi.com/journal/molecules

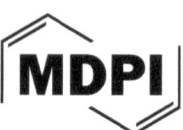

Disclaimer/Publisher's Note: The title and front matter of this reprint are at the discretion of the Guest Editors. The publisher is not responsible for their content or any associated concerns. The statements, opinions and data contained in all individual articles are solely those of the individual Editors and contributors and not of MDPI. MDPI disclaims responsibility for any injury to people or property resulting from any ideas, methods, instructions or products referred to in the content.

www.ingramcontent.com/pod-product-compliance
Lightning Source LLC
LaVergne TN
LVHW072322090526
838202LV00019B/2334